Man, Food, and Nutrition

Strategies and Technological Measures for Alleviating the World Food Problem

Editor:

Miloslav Rechcigl, Jr., Ph. D.

Nutrition Advisor and Chief
Research and Institutional Grants Division
Agency for International Development
U.S. Department of State
Washington, D.C.

published by:

CRC PRESS

A division of The Chemical Rubber Co. 18901 Cranwood Parkway, Cleveland, Ohio 44128

International Standard Book Number 0-87819-040-6

Library of Congress Card Number 73-78163

THE EDITOR

Miloslav Rechcigl, Jr. is Nutrition Advisor and Chief of Research and Institutional Grants Division in the Agency for International Development, U.S. Department of State.

He has a B.S. in biochemistry (1954), a Master of Nutritional Science degree (1955), and a Ph.D. in nutrition, biochemistry and physiology (1958), all from Cornell University. He was formerly a Research Biochemist in the National Cancer Institute, National Institutes of Health and subsequently served as Special Assistant for Nutrition and Health in the Health Services and Mental Health Administration, U.S. Department of Health, Education, and Welfare.

Dr. Rechcigl is a member of some 30 scientific and professional societies, including being a Fellow of the American Association for the Advancement of Science, Fellow of the Washington Academy of Sciences, Fellow of the American Institute of Chemists, and Fellow of the International College of Applied Nutrition. He holds memberships in the Cosmos Club, the Honorary Society of Phi Kappa Phi, and the Society of Sigma Xi, and is recipient of numerous honors, including an honorary membership certificate from the International Social Science Honor Society Delta Tau Kappa. In 1969 he was a delegate to the White House Conference on Food, Nutrition, and Health and currently serves as President of the District of Columbia Institute of Chemists.

His bibliography extends over 100 publications, including contributions to books, articles in periodicals, and monographs in the fields of nutrition, biochemistry, physiology, pathology, enzymology, and molecular biology. Most recently he authored and edited *Food, Nutrition and Health. A Multidisciplinary Treatise Addressed to the Major Nutrition Problems from a World Wide Perspective* (Karger, 1973), following his earlier pioneering treatise on *Enzyme Synthesis and Degradation in Mammalian Systems* (Karger, 1971) and that on *Microbodies and Related Particles. Morphology, Biochemistry, and Physiology* (Academic Press, 1969).

CONTRIBUTORS

Dr. James R. Anderson
Chief Geographer
Office of the Director
Geological Survey
U.S. Department of the Interior
Washington, D.C. 20242

Dr. John C. Ayres
Head, Department of Food Science
University of Georgia
College of Agriculture
Athens, Ga. 30601

J. M. Bengoa, M.D.
Chief, Nutrition Unit
World Health Organization
1211 Geneva 27
Switzerland

Dr. K. L. Blaxter
Director, The Rowett Research Institute
Bucksburn
Aberdeen AB2 9SB
Scotland, Great Britain

Dr. Ricardo Bressani
Head, Division of Agricultural and Food Sciences
Instituto de Nutricion de Centro America y Panama
Carretera Roosevelt Zona 11
Guatemala, C.A.

Dr. Luigi Chiarappa
Plant Pathologist
Plant Protection Service
Plant Production and Protection Division
Food and Agriculture Organization of the United Nations
Via delle Terme di Caracalla
00100 – Rome, Italy

Dr. Colin Clark
Institute of Economic Progress
Mannix College
Monash University
Clayton, Victoria, 3168
Australia

Dr. C. Anthonie de Vries
Agricultural Scientist
Royal Tropical Institute
63 Mauritskade
Amsterdam-Oost
The Netherlands

Dr. L. G. Elías
Scientist
Division of Agricultural and Food Sciences
Instituto de Nutricion de Centro America y Panama
Guatemala, C.A.

Patrick François
Food Policy and Nutrition Division
Food and Agriculture Organization of the United Nations
Via delle Terme di Caracalla
00100 – Rome, Italy

Mr. Marcel Ganzin
Director, Food Policy and Nutrition Division
Food and Agriculture Organization of the United Nations
Via delle Terme di Caracalla
00100 – Rome, Italy

Dr. Homer T. Hopkins
Hittman Associates, Inc.
Environmental and Geosciences Department
Columbia, Md. 21045

Dr. M. L. Kakade
Senior Biochemist
Research and Product Development
Land O'Lakes, Inc.
614 McKinley Place
Minneapolis, Minn. 55413

Dr. Charles E. Kellogg
4100 Nicholson Street
Hyattsville, Md. 20782

Dr. Irvin E. Liener
Professor, Department of Biochemistry
University of Minnesota
St. Paul, Minn. 55101

Dr. G. A. Lodge
Chief, Monogastric Nutrition
Nutrition Laboratory
Animal Research Institute
Canada Department of Agriculture
Ottawa, Ontario, KIA OC6
Canada

Dr. Maija Pekkarinen
Department of Nutritional Chemistry
University of Helsinki
00710 Helsinki 71
Suomi, Finland

Julien Périssé
Food Policy and Nutrition Division
Food and Agriculture Organization of the United Nations
Via delle Terme di Caracalla
00100 – Rome, Italy

Dr. Ralph W. Phillips
Director, International Organizations Staff
Office of Assistant Secretary
U.S. Department of Agriculture
Washington, D.C. 20250

Dr. N. W. Pirie
Head, Biochemistry Department
Rothamsted Experimental Station
Harpenden, Herts.
England

Dr. Miloslav Rechcigl, Jr.
Nutrition Advisor and Chief,
Research and Institutional Grants Division
Agency for International Development
U.S. Department of State
Washington, D.C. 20523

Dr. George F. Sprague
Professor of Plant Breeding and Genetics
Department of Agronomy
University of Illinois
Urbana, Ill. 61801

Dr. John Boyd Turner
Institute of Economic Progress
Mannix College
Monash University
Clayton, Victoria, 3168
Australia

Dr. Les J. Teply
Senior Nutritionist
United Nations Children's Emergency Fund
United Nations
New York, N.Y. 10017

PREFACE

This treatise offers a comprehensive integrated critical review of the nature and the scope of the world food problem, and presents strategies and discusses various technological approaches to overcoming world hunger and malnutrition.

Although accurate data are lacking, it is estimated that some half of today's world population is afflicted to some degree by hunger or malnutrition. As a consequence of the introduction of public health measures, there has been a marked reduction in the death rates, without significant alteration in the birth rates. This has resulted in an unprecedented rise in the rate of population growth, particularly among the developing nations. Inasmuch as the existing population control measures have been, so far, largely ineffective in checking the population explosion, there has been a reemergence of neo-Malthusian thought. The newly self-appointed apostles of this philosophy are again promulgating the notion that food production will not be able to keep pace with population growth and are forecasting the inevitable famine and self-wrought doom for mankind.

A team of 24 leading authorities from the United States and eight other countries, including scientists from government, university and industrial sectors, as well as specialists from UNESCO, WHO, and FAO, who have contributed to this volume, are challenging this view. The authors reason that the earth resources and the technological advances, if properly used, could not only avert such catastrophe but would actually lead to the improvement of the nutritional status and the well-being of the many now malnourished peoples throughout the world.

The book is comprised of six sections. The first section is devoted to the description of the world food problem, including such topics as the state of world nutrition, and world food consumption patterns, the state of world food production, and world population growth and future food needs. The four sections which follow concern themselves with strategies and technological measures for alleviating the world food problem. Specific measures discussed have been organized under four major headings, namely: (a) expanding food production; (b) reducing wastes and spoilage of foodstuffs; (c) using unconventional sources of food; and (d) improving nutritional quality of food. The last section deals with the aspects of food and nutrition policy.

From its inception the treatise has been conceived as an interdisciplinary effort, encompassing a multitude of areas, i.e., agricultural economics, economic geography, demography, population, dietetics, clinical nutrition, agronomy, crop science, plant breeding, plant nutrition, plant pathology, pest control, animal husbandry, animal breeding, animal nutrition, animal pathology, pest control, food microbiology, food toxicology, biochemistry, food preservation, food processing, food composition, food fortification, new food technology, and food and nutrition policy.

The emphasis throughout has been on integration and synthesis rather than on detail. As such, the book should, therefore, appeal to a large audience of readers, be they technicians, researchers, teachers, students, policy makers, or humanitarians and concerned laymen with interest in the problems of international development. Apart from its value as a guide or reference source, we feel that the volume is particularly well suited for teaching purposes.

My editorial responsibilities were greatly facilitated by esprit de corps and competence of individual contributors and I am greatly indebted to each and every one for this. I wish to also express my appreciation to Mrs. Phyllis S. Jarvis of CRC Press for her invaluable assistance in undertaking the many chores incident to publication. Mrs. Eva Rechcigl, Karen Marie and Jack Rechcigl rendered indispensable help during the compilation of the subject index. Last but not least, the encouraging and gracious guidance of Mr. B. J. Starkoff, President of The Chemical Rubber Co. and Mr. Gerald A. Becker, Director of CRC Editorial Operations, is recognized with many thanks.

Miloslav Rechcigl, Jr.
Washington, D.C.

TABLE OF CONTENTS

Preface

The World Food Problem

The State of World Nutrition 1
J. M. Bengoa

World Food Consumption Patterns 15
M. Pekkarinen

The State of World Food Production 35
J. R. Anderson

World Population Growth and Future Food Trends 55
C. Clark and J. Turner

Expanding Food Production

Expanding Farm Production: Extending the Area of Soils Used 79
Charles E. Kellogg

Increasing Crop Yields: Technical Measures for Increasing Productivity 91
G. F. Sprague

Increasing Crop Yields: Relative Potential of Specific Crops by Region and/or Country 109
C. A. de Vries

Increasing Output of Animal Production: Technical Measures for Increasing Productivity 127
K. L. Blaxter

Increasing Output of Animal Production: Relative Potential of Specific Meat-producing Animals by Region and/or Country 147
R. W. Phillips

Reducing Wastes and Spoilage of Foodstuffs

Reducing Crop Losses 163
L. Chiarappa

Reducing Food Spoilage and Deterioration 177
J. C. Ayres

Use of Unconventional Sources of Food

Production and Use of Unconventional Sources of Food 189
N. W. Pirie

Improving Nutritional Quality of Food

Improving Nutrient Composition of Plants 203
H. T. Hopkins

Improving Nutrient Composition of Meat-producing Animals 215
G. A. Lodge

The Increased Availability of Nutrients from Plant Foodstuffs through Processing 231
I. E. Liener and M. L. Kakade

Food Fortification 243
L. J. Teply

Development of Highly Nutritious Products 251
R. Bressani and L. G. Elías

Food and Nutrition Policy

Need for Food and Nutrition Policies 278
M. Ganzin, J. Périssé, and P. François

Abbreviations and Symbols 287
Tables and Figures 289

Indexes 293

THE STATE OF WORLD NUTRITION

J. M. Bengoa

TABLE OF CONTENTS

Introduction 1

Trends in Age-specific Death Rates 2

Death Rates due to Malnutrition 2

Protein-calorie Malnutrition (PCM) 3
- Definition 3
- Prevalence 4
- The Pattern of PCM in Community Surveys 7

Nutritional Anemias 7

Xerophthalmia 8

Endemic Goiter and Cretinism 10

Pellagra 10

Scurvy 10

Rickets and Osteomalacia 10

Beriberi 11

Final Remarks 11
- Acknowledgment 11

References 12

INTRODUCTION

Any attempt to appraise the nutrition situation in the world today meets with difficulty and a quantitative evaluation is particularly hard to make. Some trends in the magnitude of different forms of malnutrition and their present significance have recently been summarized by Aykroyd[1] in his excellent historical review of the world's deficiency diseases. Since the period when acute specific deficiency diseases, particularly vitamin deficiency diseases, were easily identifiable there has been a clear trend toward forms of malnutrition that are less defined, more moderate, and therefore more difficult to quantify. The difficulties and limitations encountered may be summarized as follows:

a. Mortality statistics based on information provided by physicians were a more reliable indication of the magnitude of deficiency diseases in the past than at present because the cause of death was more clearly identifiable (pellagra, beriberi, scurvy, rickets, etc.).

b. Many deaths in children are recorded as due to infectious diseases when, in fact, malnutrition is the underlying or associated cause.

c. In morbidity studies of all except extremely severe forms of malnutrition, such as kwashiorkor and nutritional marasmus, there is no universal agreement on clinical features and classification.

d. In prevalence studies of malnutrition, little attention has been paid to the moderate forms which are the most important from the public health point of view.

e. Prevalence studies at a given period of time do not reflect seasonal changes which are usually considerable.

f. In such prevalence studies, the samples of the population used are not always representative of the community or the country concerned.

Despite these limitations, more reliable information on the worldwide magnitude of malnutrition than was available some years ago can now be obtained through the interchange of views among persons interested in this field, frequent meetings held at the international level, and reference to published work.[2–4]

TRENDS IN AGE-SPECIFIC DEATH RATES

The present decline in mortality in children under five years of age is impressive in some countries but does not necessarily mean that the nutritional status has been improved. It is probably due more to specific public health activities, better medical care, and more ready availability of antibiotics and other new drugs than to any improvement in the standard of living, including nutritional conditions. This argument has already been developed elsewhere.[5,6]

During recent years the mortality rate in the age group one to four years has been widely used as an indirect indication of the nutritional situation in a given country.[7] Some few years ago the mortality rate in this age group was 30 times and even more than 40 times higher in developing countries than in developed countries. This is, moreover, the age group where the greatest reduction of mortality has been observed. Yet, as indicated by Gordon et al.,[8] the second year death rate is a still better indicator of the nutritional situation. One important fact is that the present decline in mortality among young children in developing countries has been much more rapid than was the corresponding decline in the advanced countries 50 to 100 years ago. At that time, child mortality in the advanced countries stood as high as it does today in some developing countries, but the fall, when it occurred, was relatively slow and probably due more to higher standards of living than to public health action. This point has been well documented by Brown and McKeown[9] and McKeown and Record[10] in their analyses of the trends in mortality in England and Wales.

DEATH RATES DUE TO MALNUTRITION

In principle, specific death rates due to malnutrition should be extremely useful in assessing the nutritional situation in a given country. As previously mentioned, they were valuable in assessing trends in the past when the diagnosis of vitamin deficiency diseases did not present much difficulty. At present, in practice, the classification of deaths associated with malnutrition is so unreliable "as to be almost worthless," as was stated at the last meeting of the Joint FAO/WHO Expert Committee on Nutrition.[11] An analysis of this problem in Latin America was recently published by Bengoa.[5]

For these reasons, the preliminary results of the Inter-American Investigation of Mortality in Childhood are of paramount importance. This study, developed in 18 widely separated areas of the Americas, is a continental collaborative effort sponsored by the Pan American Health Organization, with the objective of developing valid and comparable statistics related to causes of death in children under five years of age.[12] Although the prevailing conditions vary widely in different parts of the world, some of the findings and conclusions of this study might be applicable to other regions or countries. The methodology of the study has been published elsewhere.[12] Tables 1, 2, and 3 give the preliminary results.

Table 1 shows that malnutrition is an *underlying cause* of death in children under five years in 7% of the total deaths and an *associated cause* in 46.2%. As a whole, malnutrition is directly or indirectly responsible for deaths of

TABLE 1

Mortality due to Nutritional Deficiency (as an Underlying and Associate Cause) in Children under Five Years of Age*

Place	Total number of deaths under 5	Nutrition, underlying cause No.	%	Nutrition, associated cause No.	%	Total number of deaths in which nutrition was involved No.	%
Cali	667	106	16.0	266	39.9	372	55.8
Cartagena	403	74	18.4	176	43.7	250	62.1
Kingston	413	26	6.3	131	31.7	157	38.2
La Paz	1,366	50	3.7	556	40.7	606	44.4
Medellin	501	54	10.8	254	50.7	308	61.5
Monterrey	1,465	64	4.4	721	49.2	785	53.6
Recife	1,471	84	5.7	880	59.8	964	65.5
Resistencia	298	20	6.7	170	57.0	190	63.8
Ribeirao Preto	143	3	2.1	96	67.1	99	69.2
San Juan	65	2	3.1	24	36.9	26	40.0
San Salvador	973	58	6.0	414	42.5	472	48.5
Santiago	606	36	5.9	235	38.8	271	44.7
Sao Paulo	1,235	72	5.8	558	45.2	630	51.0
Chaco, rural	318	9	2.8	153	48.1	162	50.9
Franca	141	12	8.5	69	48.9	81	57.4
San Juan (suburban)	207	19	9.2	80	38.6	99	47.8
San Juan (rural)	357	29	8.1	140	39.2	169	47.3
San Salvador (rural)	392	56	14.3	173	44.1	229	58.4
Total	11,021	774	7.0	5,096	46.2	5,870	53.2

*Does not include neonatal deaths.

From Pan American Health Organization, 1971, Provisional Report on the Inter-American Investigation of Mortality in Childhood, First Year of Investigation.

children under five years of age in 53.2% of cases. These figures are quite different from the data recorded in the vital statistics publications and are of much greater public health significance.

Table 2 shows the pattern of malnutrition in deaths of children under one year of age. Of the 3,873 infant deaths due to malnutrition analyzed in the study, 108 (4.6%) were due to kwashiorkor, 995 (25.7%) to nutritional marasmus, and 2,698 (69.7%) to other (intermediate) forms. The pattern is quite different in deaths due to malnutrition among children of one to four years of age. Table 3 shows that of the 2,189 deaths due directly or indirectly to malnutrition, 685 (31.3%) were due to kwashiorkor, 391 (17.9%) to nutritional marasmus, and 1,113 (50.8%) to other forms. However, the variations in different geographical areas are very great, and the range is 0 to 61.7% for kwashiorkor cases and 7.0 to 28.9% for nutritional marasmus cases. This is probably due to differences in the pattern of weaning.

PROTEIN-CALORIE MALNUTRITION (PCM)

Definition

The term "protein-calorie malnutrition" is most commonly used to describe a complex syndrome of malnutrition mainly affecting young children and comprising not only protein and calorie deficiencies but also other nutrient deficiencies and certain infections. PCM is always accompanied by retardation of growth and development, but its clinical manifestations vary widely according to

TABLE 2

Pattern of Nutritional Deficiency in Mortality of Infants under One Year of Age

Place	Number of deaths due to malnutrition	Kwashiorkor		Marasmus		Other	
		No.	%	No.	%	No.	%
Cali	185	18	9.7	65	35.0	102	55.1
Cartagena	137	35	25.5	31	22.6	71	51.8
Kingston	104	4	3.8	29	27.9	71	68.3
La Paz	335	15	4.5	43	12.8	277	82.7
Medellin	153	2	1.3	64	41.8	87	56.9
Monterrey	571	17	3.0	111	19.4	443	77.6
Recife	608	50	8.2	190	31.3	368	60.5
Resistencia	146	3	2.1	35	24.0	108	74.0
Ribeirao Preto	71	1	1.4	18	25.4	52	73.2
San Juan	25	–	–	7	28.0	18	72.0
San Salvador	270	11	4.1	62	23.0	197	73.0
Santiago	228	2	0.9	69	30.3	157	68.9
Sao Paulo	559	8	1.4	152	27.2	399	71.4
Chaco, rural	103	3	2.9	7	6.8	93	90.3
Franca	61	1	1.6	17	27.9	43	70.5
San Juan (suburban)	90	–	–	34	37.8	56	62.2
San Juan (rural)	139	1	0.7	50	36.0	88	63.3
San Salvador (rural)	88	9	10.2	11	12.5	68	77.3
Total	3,873	108	4.6	995	25.7	2,698	69.7

From Pan American Health Organization, 1971, Provisional Report on the Inter-American Investigation of Mortality in Childhood, First Year of Investigation.

the nature of the causative factors and the age of the child. Two severe forms are recognized: nutritional marasmus and kwashiorkor. Nutritional marasmus is a condition characterized by muscle wasting, loss of subcutaneous fat, and very low body weight, and, in many places, occurs mainly in infants under one year of age. Kwashiorkor is characterized by retarded growth, edema, dermatosis, hair changes, mental apathy, and misery. It is most frequently seen in children of one to three years of age, during or after weaning, and is usually precipitated by one or more infections.

Between these severe forms a wide range of variation and gradation exists. There is general agreement that five forms constitute the PCM syndrome, namely, nutritional marasmus, kwashiorkor, intermediate forms (marasmic kwashiorkor), moderate forms, and nutritional dwarfing.

There has been a tendency to overemphasize the importance of either protein or calorie deficiency alone, whereas in fact the two almost always occur together, as stated by the Joint FAO/WHO Expert Committee on Nutrition.[11] The following section provides information on the prevalence and pattern of PCM in different regions of the world.

Prevalence

Mention has been made of the difficulties and limitations encountered in community studies on the prevalence of malnutrition. Such studies are, however, the best available method of assessing the magnitude of the problem. In two previous publications[13,14] summaries were made of the data available up to 1965 and up to 1968, respectively. In the present section we shall try to present a general review of the results obtained

TABLE 3

Pattern of Nutritional Deficiency in Mortality of Children 1–4 Years of Age

Place	Number of deaths due to malnutrition	Kwashiorkor		Marasmus		Other	
		No.	%	No.	%	No.	%
Cali	188	73	38.8	28	14.9	87	46.3
Cartagena	115	71	61.7	8	7.0	36	31.3
Kingston	55	13	23.6	13	23.6	29	52.7
La Paz	304	42	13.8	37	12.2	225	74.0
Medellin	155	53	34.2	12	7.7	90	58.1
Monterrey	245	65	26.5	44	18.0	136	55.5
Recife	376	152	40.4	94	25.0	130	34.6
Resistencia	45	8	17.8	13	28.9	24	53.3
Ribeirao Preto	28	11	39.3	5	17.9	12	42.9
San Juan	4	–	–	1	25.0	3	75.0
San Salvador	208	70	33.8	51	24.5	87	41.8
Santiago	46	6	13.0	9	19.6	31	67.4
Sao Paulo	135	30	22.2	28	20.7	77	57.0
Chaco, rural	61	7	11.5	7	11.5	47	77.0
Franca	23	3	13.0	2	8.7	18	78.3
San Juan (suburban)	15	–	–	4	26.7	11	73.3
San Juan (rural)	41	3	7.3	7	17.1	31	75.6
San Salvador (rural)	145	78	53.8	28	19.3	39	26.9
Total	2,189	685	31.3	391	17.9	1,113	50.8

From Pan American Health Organization, 1971, Provisional Report on the Inter-American Investigation of Mortality in Childhood, First Year of Investigation.

during the last ten years (1963–1972) in 77 nutritional surveys carried out at the community level in 46 developing countries. The surveys have involved the clinical examination of about 200,000 children, mostly under 5 years of age.

Since the diagnostic criteria sometimes differ and the samples are not always really representative of the total population, some caution is needed in interpreting the data.

In most of the surveys the Gomez classification* has been used with or without a slight modification.[16] In other surveys clinical criteria have been adopted. In surveys using the Gomez classification the prevalence rates are, in general, higher than in those where clinical criteria have been adopted. The reason is that the Gomez classification not only measures the present nutritional status of the children, but also reflects the influence of past malnourishment. If it were possible to have information on the weight-height ratio instead of the weight-age ratio, a more reliable indication of the present nutritional status

*Gomez et al.[15] classify malnutrition in three degrees as follows:

Degree of malnutrition	Deviation from reference weight for age
1st	10–25%
2nd	25–40%
3rd	over 40%

could be obtained.[17–19] At present, the weight-height ratio is difficult to use because of the absence of reference values to estimate degrees of malnutrition.

Table 4 gives a summary of the range of prevalence in three continents. The extreme values show great variation which makes it difficult to reach any valid conclusions. The variations are due not only to differences in nutrition levels in different areas, but also to differences in the criteria used in collecting data and, particularly, differences in the sampling methods; in many cases the number of children examined is too small to give valid results. It should also be mentioned that, for obvious reasons, the data given in Table 4 and succeeding tables do not include cases of malnutrition occurring during natural or social disasters.

Table 5 includes only those surveys where the number of children examined is higher than 1,000 in any given area. This does not necessarily mean that such a sample is considered fully representative of the area or country concerned, but simply that it was the best available. This table summarizes the results of 25 surveys in 17 countries, the total number of children examined being approximately 175,000.

Severe forms of PCM are found in a percentage ranging between 0.5 and 20.0, the median being 2.6%. Moderate forms are found in a percentage between 3.5 and 46.4, the median being 18.9%.

There are regional differences which probably reflect the different patterns of malnutrition in the three continents. In Latin America the proportion of children with either severe or moderate malnutrition is of the order of 19%, in Africa, of 26%, and in Asia of 31%. It is evident that within each of these continents there are also great differences in the ranges of prevalence occurring in individual countries.

The risks involved in trying to reach definitive conclusions from fragmentary data are especially great when the latter are obtained from a limited number of surveys and are not always truly representative of the area or country concerned. But in view of the pressure of public opinion to know the real magnitude of undernutrition in the

TABLE 4

Range of % Prevalence of PCM in Community Surveys (1963–1972)

Area	No. of communities surveyed	No. of surveys	No. of children examined	% Prevalence of PCM		
				Severe forms	Moderate forms	Total
Latin America	20	29	116,179	0–12.0	3.5–32.0	4.6–37.0
Africa	16	32	34,184	0– 9.8	5.6–66.0	7.3–73.0
Asia	10	16	43,326	0–20.0	13.0–73.8	14.8–80.3
Total	46	77	193,689	0–20.0	3.5–73.8	4.6–80.3

TABLE 5

Range and Median of % Prevalence of PCM in Community Surveys (Selected surveys with more than 1,000 children examined)

Area	No. of countries	No. of surveys	No. of children examined	Severe forms		Moderate forms	
				Range %	Median %	Range %	Median %
Latin America	8	11	108,715	0.5– 6.3	1.6	3.5–32.0	18.9
Africa	5	7	24,739	1.7– 9.8	4.4	5.4–44.9	26.5
Asia	4	7	39,494	1.1–20.0	3.2	16.0–46.4	31.2
Total	17	25	172,948	0.5–20.0	2.6	3.5–46.4	18.9

world, it is preferable to use the best, if still unsatisfactory, information available in the hope of counteracting the distorted information given in some circles and of checking the tendency either to underestimate or to overestimate the problem.

Although the extrapolation is undertaken with some reluctance, an attempt will be made to estimate roughly the number of malnourished children in the world on the basis of the data available at present. If the median values shown in Table 5 for the percentage prevalence of severe and moderate forms of PCM, respectively, are applied to the population aged 0 to 4 years of Latin America, Africa, and Asia (excluding China and Japan) it appears that about 10 million children suffer from severe malnutrition (700,000 in Latin America, 2,700,000 in Africa, and 6,600,000 in Asia) and about 89 million from moderate malnutrition (9 million in Latin America, 16 million in Africa, and 64 million in Asia). The total number of malnourished children in the age group 0 to 4 years in the world would thus be around 100 million. But this represents only the point prevalence and the number of cases in a given year may be several times higher, particularly regarding acute kwashiorkor.

As we have seen, the data available up to now on the prevalence of malnutrition in the world are very scanty and of limited value. There is a need for better information and a more uniform methodology in collecting it. The WHO Monograph, "The Assessment of the Nutritional Status of the Community," by D. B. Jelliffe may help in this respect.[16]

The Pattern of PCM in Community Surveys

The pattern of PCM at hospital level as summarized by a Joint FAO/WHO Expert Committee[11] may be seen in Table 6. It is clear that the age of the onset of PCM is an important factor; nutritional marasmus is more frequent when PCM affects children under one year of age, and kwashiorkor when older children are affected.

The results obtained in surveys carried out at community level are presented in Table 7. In 39 of the 77 nutrition surveys made in the 10 years 1963–72 the type of PCM, either marasmus or kwashiorkor, was recorded. In 10 of these 39 surveys no cases of either kwashiorkor or marasmus were found, and in 7 the results were given as a total of both types without specification. These 17 surveys have not been included in Table 7 which therefore gives the results of only 22 of the 77 surveys mentioned above.

In 17 surveys, mainly in the African Region, more cases of nutritional marasmus than of kwashiorkor were found. In four surveys the reverse was noted and in one, in Nigeria, an equal number of the two conditions was recorded.

However, these findings require careful analysis and interpretation. Kwashiorkor is an acute and severe condition and the child sufferer who does not receive medical attention usually dies within a few days or weeks. A child with nutritional marasmus, however, may survive and "adapt" to the condition for several months. The turnover rate of cases in a community is usually much higher in kwashiorkor than in nutritional marasmus, even where the two conditions have the same point prevalence; therefore, more children are affected with kwashiorkor than with nutritional marasmus in any one year. This subject has already been discussed by Bengoa[38] and by the Joint FAO/WHO Expert Committee on Nutrition.[11] It is difficult, therefore, to compare point prevalence rates of the two conditions, one being acute and the other chronic.

NUTRITIONAL ANEMIAS

Of the various criteria for defining iron-deficiency anemia, hemoglobin concentration in the blood is the one most frequently used in prevalence studies. A WHO Scientific Group[39] proposed that anemia should be considered to exist when hemoglobin was below certain specific levels established according to age.

The nutritional anemia problem in the world is much more serious and of greater social significance than is generally realized. In a WHO publication[40] we read that "a great deal of ill-health, sapping energy and productiveness in many countries and causing tragedies in childbirth, is due to anaemia." Prevalence studies show the following results in different parts of the world.[41]

In South America, iron deficiency anemia has been found in the range of 5 to 15% for men and 10 to 35% for women. The proportion of children with anemia varies between 15% and 50%, the highest being found in hookworm-infected areas.

In the U.S. iron deficiency anemia is common and the prevalence has been estimated at 20% of the population. In a very careful study made in

TABLE 6

Regional Differences in the Pattern of PCM (Hospital Cases)*

Country	Percentage of cases classified as			Percentage of cases less than 1 year of age
	Kwashiorkor	Marasmus	Unspecified	
Chile (Santiago)	3	97	–	83
Iran	33	67	–	45
Jamaica	32	34	34	52
Jordan	24	15	61	
Senegal (Dakar)	45	55	–	
South Africa (Johannesburg)	96	4	–	48
Sudan	92	8	–	50
Thailand	44	46	10	18

*Joint FAO/WHO Expert Committee on Nutrition, Eighth Report, *W.H.O. Tech. Rep. Ser.*, No. 477, 1971.

Tennessee[42] 18% of 74,027 apparently healthy children under the age of 6 were anemic.

In Africa, 6 to 17% of men and 15 to 50% of women (Bantus of South Africa excepted) have been found to suffer from iron deficiency. In children up to the age of 15, the incidence of anemia varies between 30% and 60% and still higher figures have been reported in children below 7 years of age.

In Asia, about 10% of men suffer from iron deficiency anemia and in women the prevalence is higher than 20%, rising even to 40% in pregnancy. Several surveys have indicated a prevalence above 50% in children and the extremely high figure of 92% has been reported in children below two years of age.

In Europe, it is estimated that the prevalence in women is between 10% and 25%.

In the Middle East, 25 to 70% of children and about 20 to 25% of pregnant women have been found to be anemic.

Mortality due to anemias (most of them probably nutritional anemias) has been recorded for Latin America, the U.S., and Canada.[5] While in the U.S. and Canada the mortality rate per 100,000 population for deaths due to anemia is of the order of 1.8, in Latin America several countries show figures of the order of 10, 20, and even 40.

Information on the prevalence of megaloblastic anemia, usually due to a deficiency of folic acid, vitamin B_{12}, or both, is more scanty but in general its public health significance has been underestimated. Folate deficiency is a far more common cause of nutritional megaloblastic anemia than deficiency of vitamin B_{12}.[41] It occurs commonly in pregnancy, when the folate requirement increases, but may also be precipitated by relatively minor degrees of malabsorption, a condition very common in India, the Caribbean Islands, etc.

In developed countries the prevalence of clinically recognizable megaloblastic anemia among pregnant women attending hospital clinics is between 2.5% and 5.0%, and in developing countries it is present clinically in approximately 20% of such women.

In conclusion, nutritional anemias are of great public health significance because of their repercussions on productivity and because they aggravate many other diseases and thus contribute to an increase in mortality.

XEROPHTHALMIA

Xerophthalmia is an eye disease due to vitamin A deficiency; its most severe form is called keratomalacia. Xerophthalmia is the cause of half the cases of total blindness in young children in some areas of the Far East. According to Wilson,[43] more than 14,000 infants in India went

TABLE 7

% Prevalence of Kwashiorkor and Nutritional Marasmus in Young Children: Community Surveys

Country	Year of survey	No. of children	Age	Kwashiorkor	Marasmus	Total	Ref.
Africa							
Central African Republic	1971–72	10,503	0–5	2.6	0.4	3.0	20
Malawi							
South	1969	619	0–5	0.5	2.7	3.2	21
Nkhotakota District	1970	445	0–4	0.2	2.7	2.9	22
Lower Shire	1970	547	0–4	0.2	0.7	0.9	23
Nigeria	1965	432	0–5	1.6	1.6	3.2	24
Rwanda	1971	7,021	0–5	6.6	3.2	9.8	25
Tanzania							
Hombolo	1965	401	0–4	0	3.2	3.2	26
Kisarawe	1968	630	0–5	0.8	6.8	7.6	27
Tabora	1969	551	0–5	0.2	0.3	0.5	28
West	1969	393	0–5	0.3	1.2	1.5	28
Uganda							
Ankole	1965	286	0–7	0.3	1.2	1.5	29
Buganda	–	133	0–3	0.8	0	0.8	30
Karamoja	–	298	0–3	0	1.3	1.3	30
Latin America							
Barbados	1969	248	0–5	0	1.2	1.2	31
Guyana	1971	964	0–5	0	1.3	1.3	31
Honduras	1967	633	0–4	0	0.2	0.2	32
Jamaica	1970	489	0–4	0	1.5	1.5	31
Nicaragua	1967	708	0–4	0	0.1	0.1	33
Panama	1967	624	0–4	0	0.3	0.3	34
Asia							
India	1969	15,000	–	0.4–0.9	1.0–2.0	1.4–2.9	35
India	–	3,115	0–5	0.6	1.0	1.6	36
Pakistan	1962–64	1,020	0–4	1.5	1.2	2.7	37

blind in 1970 from keratomalacia. Xerophthalmia is usually associated with protein-calorie malnutrition and it is most common in children of one to three years of age.

In 1964, a "global survey of xerophthalmia" was undertaken by three WHO consultants.[44] Data on xerophthalmia were sought by questionnaires, discussions with doctors, the study of health statistics, and personal observations. The condition occurs in most of the developing countries, but is specially common in large urban areas in South and East Asia. The prevalence is very high in Indonesia, South India, and Bangladesh. In the Eastern Mediterranean countries, Africa, and Latin America it is not very severe, although a few places have a relatively high prevalence. In West Africa, it is rare because the red palm oil generally used for cooking is rich in carotene.

Long-term efforts to prevent xerophthalmia are mainly concentrated on increasing production of foods which are rich sources of vitamin A and education of the public, but more immediate measures such as food fortification and the administration of large doses of vitamin A to preschool children are being introduced. It is expected that such measures will succeed in reducing the present prevalence of xerophthalmia, which constitutes a serious public health problem.

ENDEMIC GOITER AND CRETINISM

Since 1958, when Kelly and Snedden[45] made a comprehensive world review of endemic goiter, no other analysis of such a magnitude has been undertaken. However, some more recent information has emerged from international conferences and seminars.[46–48]

Kelly and Snedden estimated that in 1958 there were as many as 200 million goitrous people in the world. In Europe goiter has been almost completely controlled. Great progress has been achieved elsewhere and particularly in Colombia, Guatemala, and the Himalayan region of India.

Most of the highly endemic goiter areas are located in a few isolated regions, where endemic cretinism is also found. During recent years greater attention has been given to the cretinism problem which has obvious repercussions on intellectual development.[49,50] In some areas in Nepal, Zaire, Bolivia, and other countries, the prevalence of endemic cretinism may be as high as 1 to 5% of the total population.

New methods for goiter control include the injection or the oral administration of iodized oil; research on the use of the latter route is still under way. These, together with the older method of iodization of salt, may be expected to reduce the prevalence of the condition.

PELLAGRA

Pellagra occurs sporadically in many parts of the world, and is still prevalent in Egypt, India, Lesotho, Malawi, parts of the Republic of South Africa, and elsewhere. Epidemiologically, however, the disease appears to present a variety of features. While in Lower Egypt the main causative factor is probably maize, in Upper Egypt, where the staple food is sorghum millet, maize is not consumed to any great extent. In India also, pellagra cases have been found on sorghum diets and Gopalan and Srikantia[51] have advanced the hypothesis of amino acid imbalance. In Lesotho, in addition to maize, alcoholism (fermented maize) may be an important precipitating factor.[52]

Patwardhan and Darby[53] recently made an extensive review of pellagra in Egypt in the years 1964–66 and concluded that in Upper Egypt the pellagra prevalence per 100,000 population was of the order of 10.3 and in the Lower Egypt area of 83.2. In India, about 1% of all cases admitted to hospitals in Hyderabad are cases of pellagra, and 8 to 10% of admissions to mental hospitals are due to this cause.[1] According to Pretorius,[54] it is not rare to see pellagrous skin lesions in half or more of the patients attending medical clinics in Bantu areas of South Africa.

An important feature is the great seasonal variations in the incidence of pellagra. Whether this is due to changes in solar radiation or to differences in staple foods at different times of the year is a matter of controversy. Because of the mental symptoms in pellagra, the psychiatrists are becoming interested in the epidemiological factors involved, but perhaps pellagra will soon disappear from the world, leaving such obscure and controversial questions without an answer.

SCURVY

Today, scurvy is uncommon and occurs chiefly in old people and in infants weaned on diets poor in ascorbic acid. In adults, scurvy may be linked with poverty, alcoholism, or neglect. In some developed countries, where the population relies largely on potatoes, vitamin C deficiency may be a cause of concern.

An evaluation of 33 surveys conducted by the United States Interdepartmental Committee on Nutrition and National Defense (ICNND) in 29 countries between 1956 and 1967 confirms that frank scurvy is rare in most parts of the world.[41]

RICKETS AND OSTEOMALACIA

Contrary to what was thought some years ago, rickets and osteomalacia are still prevalent in varying degrees in infants and young children in certain developing countries in the tropics and particularly in the subtropics.

Nutrition surveys in Vietnam, India, Israel, Egypt, Nigeria, and South Africa, among other countries, indicate a prevalence ranging from 0.1% to 20% of clinically diagnosed cases of rickets. In a recent WHO survey in North Africa, 45 to 60% of the children examined were found to show signs of rickets. Children with severe rickets ranged between 3% and 18% of the 1,160 children examined.[55]

It is expected that through the traditional preventive measures and particularly through the periodic administration of massive doses of vitamin D, a measure that is already being employed in many countries, the prevalence of rickets will be reduced to levels of less public health significance.

BERIBERI

It would be an overstatement to say that beriberi has already been eradicated all over the world. Infantile beriberi, in particular, is still a controversial problem. Some countries, such as the Philippines, still report several thousand deaths from infantile beriberi annually although, as indicated by Aykroyd,[1] the accuracy of the diagnosis has been questioned. Cases have been reported recently in some Asian countries with rice-eating populations, but an accurate estimate of the prevalence is very hard to make. One difficulty lies in the fact that infants affected by beriberi usually die suddenly. A peak in infant mortality between the second and sixth month of life is highly suggestive of infantile beriberi. No data are available on this interesting indicator suggested by Aykroyd.[1]

FINAL REMARKS

The real significance of malnutrition in its diversified forms as described in this paper cannot be conveyed simply by quoting mortality rates and the results of prevalence studies. The problem is too complex for that. To begin with, two, three, or more of the conditions described above may occur simultaneously; this happens relatively frequently in many developing countries. Children suffering from PCM and at the same time from anemia and some vitamin deficiency are a common feature in many areas. What is more, the children affected by several nutritional deficiency conditions are often affected simultaneously by some infectious diseases; indeed, it has been estimated that many two-year-old children suffer from some infection or other during 25 to 30% of their lives.[56]

Another important fact is that besides the host of severely or moderately malnourished children, there are an even greater number with a poor diet, some degree of growth retardation, lowered learning capacity, and a permanent feeling of dissatisfaction and hunger. They always seem tired and generally live under very poor hygienic conditions. They are, in a word, both witnesses to and participants in the social deprivation syndrome, so well described by Ramos Galvan et al.[57] The behavior of these children in the future of society is unpredictable. In the nutritional surveys in developing countries, these children are classified as "apparently healthy children" because they are compared with children who show frank clinical evidence of being malnourished. These "deprived" children are in the majority in many developing countries; they are living under a permanent risk of falling into a more or less frank form of malnutrition. These children are subject to a continuum of stress of which incidents of severe malnutrition are only one of the more dramatic side effects. They belong to a generation which may never achieve, either physically or intellectually, what Brock terms "their genetically installed potential," as quoted by Moodie et al.[58]

Finally, and in contrast to what has been described above, there is a group in many societies which is indulging in an excessive intake of foods and is affected by quite different forms of malnutrition – they stand, so to speak, as a symbol of the great differences among people all over the world.

Acknowledgment

I wish to acknowledge with thanks the assistance provided by Mr. Gérard Plouidy, Scientist, Nutrition Unit, World Health Organization, Geneva, in the collection of the data which appear in this paper.

REFERENCES

1. **Aykroyd, W. R.,** *Conquest of Deficiency Diseases,* Freedom from Hunger Campaign Basic Study No. 24, World Health Organization, Geneva, 1970.
2. *Proceedings of the Seventh International Congress of Nutrition,* Hamburg, 1966, F. Vieweg & Sohn, Braunschweig, 1967.
3. *Proceedings of the Eighth International Congress of Nutrition,* Prague, 1969, Excerpta Medica, Amsterdam, 1970.
4. *Proceedings of the Ninth International Congress of Nutrition,* Mexico, 1972, S. Karger, Basel, in press.
5. **Bengoa, J. M.,** Nutritional significance of mortality statistics, in *Proceedings of the Third Western Hemisphere Nutrition Congress,* Miami Beach, 1971, Futura Publishing Co., New York, 1972, 270.
6. **Arriaga, E. E. and Davis, K.,** The pattern of mortality change in Latin America, *Demography,* 6, 223, 1969.
7. **Bengoa, J. M., Jelliffe, D. B., and Perez, C.,** Some indicators for a broad assessment of the magnitude of protein-calorie malnutrition in young children in population groups, *Am. J. Clin. Nutr.,* 7, 714, 1959.
8. **Gordon, J. E., Wyon, J. B., and Ascoli, W.,** The second year death rate in less developed countries, *Am. J. Med. Sci.,* 254, 357, 1967.
9. **Brown, R. G. and McKeown, T.,** Medical evidence related to English population changes in the eighteenth century, *Popul. Stud.,* 9, 119, 1955.
10. **McKeown, T. and Record, R. G.,** Reasons for the decline of mortality in England and Wales during the nineteenth century, *Popul. Stud.,* 16, 94, 1962.
11. Joint FAO/WHO Expert Committee on Nutrition, Eighth Report, Food fortification, protein-calorie malnutrition, *WHO Tech. Rep. Ser.,* No. 477, World Health Organization, Geneva, 1971.
12. Inter-American investigation of mortality in childhood, first year of investigation, provisional report, Pan American Health Organization, Washington, 1971.
13. **Bengoa, J. M.,** Priorities in public health nutrition problems, in *Proceedings of the Seventh International Congress of Nutrition,* Vol. 4, Hamburg, 1966, F. Vieweg & Sohn, Braunschweig, 1967, 811.
14. **Bengoa, J. M.,** Recent trends in public health nutrition: protein-calorie malnutrition, in Nutrition, *Proceedings of the Eighth International Congress,* Prague, 1969, Excerpta Medica, Amsterdam, 1970, 14.
15. **Gomez, F., Ramos Galvan, R., Cravioto, J., and Frenk, S.,** Malnutrition in infancy and childhood with special reference to kwashiorkor, in *Advances in Pediatrics,* Vol. 7, Levine, S., Ed., Year Book Publishers, New York, 1955.
16. **Jelliffe, D. B.,** *The Assessment of the Nutritional Status of the Community,* WHO Monogr. Ser., No. 53, World Health Organization, Geneva, 1966.
17. **Seoane, N. and Latham, M. C.,** Nutritional anthropometry in the identification of malnutrition in childhood, *J. Trop. Pediat.,* 17, 98, 1971.
18. **McLaren, D. S. and Read, W. W. C.,** Classification of nutritional status in early childhood, *Lancet,* 2, 146, 1972.
19. **Waterlow, J. C.,** Classification and definition of protein-energy malnutrition, to be published.
20. **Martineaud, M. L. L.,** *Rapport de Mission en Nutrition dans la République Centre Africaine,* WHO Regional Office for Africa, Brazzaville, 1972.
21. **Burgess, H. J. L. and Cole-King, S. M.,** Report on a survey of nutritional status of preschool children in Namitambo, Local Court area, Chiradzulu sub-district, *Malawi Med. Bull.,* 3, 99, 1969.
22. **Burgess, H. J. L. and Driessen, F.,** *A Report on a Nutritional Status Survey Carried out in Chief Malenga Chanzi Area, Nkhotakota District,* Ministry of Health, Nkhotakota, 1970.
23. **Burgess, H. J. L. and Wheeler, E.,** *A Report of a Nutritional Status and Dietary Survey Carried out in Ngabu Area,* Ministry of Health, Blantyre, 1970.
24. United States Office of International Research, Nutrition Section, *Republic of Nigeria: Nutrition Survey, February-April, 1965,* National Institutes of Health, Bethesda, Md., 1967.
25. **Martineaud, M. L. L.,** *Enquête Clinique Nutritionnelle au Rwanda, Rapport de Mission,* WHO Regional Office for Africa, Brazzaville, AFR/NUT/49, 1971.
26. **Burgess, H. J. L., Maletnlema, T. N., and Burgess, A. P.,** The nutritional status of young children in Hombolo, Tanzania, *East Afr. Med. J.,* 45, 605, 1968.
27. **Burgess, H. J. L., Maletnlema, T. N., and Burgess, A. P.,** The health of children in Kisarawe district, Tanzania, *Trop. Geogr. Med.,* 21, 39, 1969.
28. **Burgess, H. J. L.,** personal communication.
29. **Cook, R.,** Critères d'évaluation de la santé de l'enfant dans le région rurale d'Ankole (Ouganda), in *Living Conditions of the Child in Rural Environment in Africa,* Proceedings of a Colloquium, Dakar (Senegal), February 20-25, 1967, Centre International de l'Enfance, Paris, 1967.
30. **Rutishauser, I. H. E. and Whitehead, R. G.,** Field evaluation of two biochemical tests which may reflect nutritional status in three areas of Uganda, *Br. J. Nutr.,* 23, 1, 1969.
31. **Jelliffe, D. B.,** personal communication.
32. *Evaluacion nutricional de la poblacion de Centro America y Panama, Honduras,* Instituto de Nutricion de Centro America y Panama, Guatemala City, 1969.
33. *Evaluacion nutricional de la poblacion de Centro America y Panama, Nicaragua,* Instituto de Nutricion de Centro America y Panama, Guatemala City, 1969.

34. *Evaluacion nutricional de la poblacion de Centro America y Panama, Panama,* Instituto de Nutricion de Centro America y Panama, Guatemala City, 1969.
35. **Gopalan, C.,** personal communication.
36. **Rao, N. P., Singh, D., and Swaminathan, M. C.,** Nutritional status of pre-school children of rural communities near Hyderabad City, *Indian J. Med. Res.,* 57, 2132, 1969.
37. Pakistan, Directorate of Nutrition and Research, *Pakistan :Nutrition Survey of East Pakistan, March 1962–January 1964,* A report in collaboration with the University of Dacca and the Nutrition Section, Office of International Research, National Institutes of Health, U.S. Public Health Service, Washington, D.C., 1966.
38. **Bengoa, J. M.,** Clinical and socio-economic aspects of PCM, in *Protein-calorie Malnutrition,* von Muralt, A., Ed., Springer-Verlag, Berlin, 1969, 126.
39. Nutritional anaemias, Report of a WHO scientific group, *WHO Tech. Rep. Ser.,* No. 405, World Health Organization, Geneva, 1968.
40. *Malnutrition and Disease,* Freedom from Hunger Campaign Basic Study No. 12, World Health Organization, Geneva, 1963.
41. *Requirements of Ascorbic Acid, Vitamin D, Vitamin B.12, Folate and Iron,* Report of a Joint FAO/WHO Expert Group, *WHO Tech. Rep. Ser.,* No. 452, World Health Organization, Geneva, 1970.
42. **Hutcheson, R. H. and Hutcheson, J. K.,** Iron and vitamins C and D deficiencies in a large population of children, *Health Serv. Rep.,* 87, 232, 1972.
43. **Wilson, J.,** Fighting blindness with vitamin A, *UNICEF News,* No. 71, 1972.
44. **Oomen, H. A. P. C., McLaren, D. S., and Escapini, H.,** A global survey on xerophthalmia, *Trop. Geogr. Med.,* 16, 271, 1964.
45. **Kelly, F. C. and Snedden, W. W.,** Prevalence and geographical distribution of endemic goitre, in *Endemic Goitre, WHO Monogr. Ser.,* No. 44, World Health Organization, Geneva, 1960.
46. *Endemic Goitre,* Stanbury, J. B., Ed., Pan American Health Organization, Washington, 1969.
47. Seminario sobre yodization de la sal para prevencion del bocio endemico, Salta, Argentina, Junio de 1965, informe final, Organizacion Panamericana de la Salud, Washington, 1965.
48. Report of a seminar on goitre control, New Delhi, October-November 1967, World Health Organization Regional Office for South-East Asia, New Delhi, 1967.
49. *Endemic Cretinism,* Hetzel, B. S. and Pharoah, P. O. D., Eds., Institute of Human Biology, Papua-New Guinea, 1971.
50. Proceedings of a Symposium on endemic cretinism, Kroc Foundation, Santa Ynez Valley, California, January 1972, Stanbury, J. B., Ed., to be published.
51. **Gopalan, C. and Srikantia, S. G.,** Leucine and pellagra, *Lancet,* 1, 954, 1960.
52. **Munoz, A.,** personal communication.
53. **Patwardhan, V. N. and Darby, W. J.,** *The State of Nutrition in the Arab Middle East,* Vanderbilt University Press, Nashville, 1972, Chap. 3.
54. **Pretorius, P. J.,** The clinical nature and extent of protein malnutrition in South Africa, *South Afr. Med. J.,* 42, 956, 1968.
55. Joint FAO/WHO Expert Committee on Nutrition, Seventh Report, *WHO Tech. Rep. Ser.,* No. 377, World Health Organization, Geneva, 1967.
56. **Bengoa, J. M.,** Malnutrition and infectious diseases – the "surviving child," *Biotech. Bioeng. Symp.,* 1, 253, 1969.
57. **Ramos Galvan, R., Mariscal, C., Viniegra, A., and Perez Ortiz, B.,** *Desnutricion en el Nino,* Hospital Infantil de Mexico, Mexico, 1969.
58. **Moodie, A. D., Keet, M. P., Evans, D. E., Wittmann, W., and Hansen, J. D. L.,** Environmental stress and the underprivileged child – kwashiorkor in perspective, *Ecol. Food Nutr.,* 1, 95, 1972.

WORLD FOOD CONSUMPTION PATTERNS

M. Pekkarinen

TABLE OF CONTENTS

Introduction 16

Material 16

Cereals 16
  Varieties of Grain 18
    Rice 18
    Wheat 18
    Maize 19
    Other grain 19

Starchy Foods 20
  Variety 20
    Potatoes 20
    Sweet Potatoes and Yams 21
    Cassava 22
    Plantains 22

Pulses, Nuts, and Seeds 22

Vegetables 24

Fruits 25

Meat 26

Milk and Milk Products 28
  Cheese 29

Eggs and Fish 30

Fats and Oils 30

Sugar 31

Beverages 32

Summary 32

References 33

INTRODUCTION

Food consumption patterns denote both the selection and quantity of the foodstuffs used by a population. The patterns vary greatly in the different regions of the world. While the selection of foods is rich and the consumption of many foods is even too abundant from the nutrition point of view in the developed areas, simultaneously a large part of the population in the developing regions suffers from lack of food. In addition, their food is often imbalanced to the extent that the requirements of nutrients, those of proteins in particular, are not met.

The most important factor affecting the food consumption patterns is the available food supply, which is distributed very unevenly in the world. The food supply is influenced by the food production, the quantity and quality of which varies from one region to another, depending on the natural conditions and economic possibilities. The quantity and selection of foods may be increased in the developed areas through import, but this is not possible in most of the developing countries due to unsufficient economic resources. The regional distribution of foods is uneven also in the developing countries because of a lack of transportation. Although there would be enough food in some developing region or food could be produced, religious customs sometimes prevent the appropriate use of foods, e.g., among Hindus, Muslims, and Jews. Many food taboos also affect the use of food, particularly in Africa. There is also much ignorance in the world. If it could be removed, this would improve the food consumption patterns even within the limits of the food supplies available, especially in the developing regions, but faulty food habits and problems resulting from overnutrition in the developed parts of the world could also be corrected. The improvement of the economic situation of the developing countries is, however, the best way of changing the food consumption patterns into more favorable ones so that at least the minimum food requirements would be met.

MATERIAL

The data introduced in the present article are taken from the Production Yearbook 1971,[1] the Food Balance Sheets 1964–66 by FAO,[2] and the Food Consumption Statistics 1960–1968 by OECD.[3] In these statistics the food consumption figures for individual countries are based on the food supplies available for the use of people. Although these quantities are not very exact, particularly regarding the developing countries, they give a general picture of the food consumption patterns for comparison between the various regions and different parts of a region. In addition, there are considerable differences in individual countries between different areas and population groups.

The comparison between the regions has been done using the region division of the FAO, in which the U.S.S.R. is a part of Europe; Egypt, Libya, and Sudan in Africa are included in the Near East; and Australia and New Zealand belong to Oceania. The food consumption comparisons are made by dividing the countries into groups based on the per capita per day consumption of different foods.[1] Statistical data are available from 7 regions and 133 countries in all, which cover practically the whole world. The comparisons are made by food groups.

CEREALS

The consumption of cereals varies greatly in different parts of the world both quantitatively and qualitatively, reflecting very clearly the differences between the standards of living of the people in various regions. The total consumption of cereals is the lowest in highly developed countries. According to statistics,[1] the consumption of cereals has decreased considerably during the last 20 years, and the decreasing trend will probably continue in several countries. The areas of a high standard of living and low cereal consumption are North America in particular and a large part of Europe (Table 1). But also in some countries of the developing areas, in Latin America and Africa in particular, the consumption of cereals is very small. In these, cereals are replaced by starchy roots to a considerable degree. However, cereals are the main food in the Far East, the largest part of Africa, and in many countries in the Near East and Latin America as well as in some European countries. Contrary to the developed countries, the consumption of cereals has increased in the developing countries during the last 10 to 20 years, with the exception of Japan, where the standard of living has risen very fast and already attained the level of developed countries.

TABLE 1

Different Levels of Cereal Consumption per capita in Countries in Different Regions of the World[1]

Per capita consumption	Europe 27	North America 2	Latin America 26	Near East 15	Far East 23	Africa 38	Oceania 2
Cereals, total range, g per day	157–534	176–180	156–379	270–565	323–572	54–544	212–216
less than 200	6	2	4			10	
200–300	9		15	2		6	2
300–400	7		7	7	10	11	
400–500	3			4	11	9	
500 and more	2			2	2	2	
Rice, kg per year							
less than 10	26	2	11	8	1	21	2
10–30	1		4	6		3	
30–50			6			2	
50–100			4		8	4	
100 and more			–		14	3	
Wheat, kg per year							
less than 10	–		1	1	7	25	
10–30	–		12	1	14	5	
30–50	5		6	–	1	3	
50–100	14	2	5	5		1	2
100 and more	8		1	8	1	2	
Maize, kg per year							
less than 10	14	2	3	11	14	11	
10–30	3		4		4	12	
30–50			6	1		7	
50–100	2		1	1	2	2	
100 and more			5			5	
Millet and sorghum, kg per year							
less than 10	2	2		5	6	10	2
10–30				2	3	8	
30–50						4	
50–100				2		8	
100 and more				1		4	
Rye, kg per year							
less than 10	9	2	5	1	2		1
10–30	9			1			
30–50	1						
50–100	1						
Barley, kg per year							
less than 10	20	2	4	6	6	2	
10–30				2	1	3	
30 and more				2	1	1	
Oats, kg per year							
less than 10	16	2	11		2	1	2

The consumption of cereals varies greatly even in the same area, as can be seen from Table 1. The lowest cereal consumption figures in Europe are in Iceland and Sweden and generally in Scandinavia and Central Europe, whereas the highest figures are in east Europe, particularly in Bulgaria, Romania, and Yugoslavia. The cereal consumption is also quite high in the U.S.S.R.

Little cereal is used in the North American countries, Canada and the U.S. In Latin America the differences in the consumption of cereals are rather small between the countries, as compared to many other areas. The least amount of cereal is consumed in the Dominican Republic, Colombia, Ecuador, and Paraguay; the highest figures are found in the Central American countries.

In the Near East, the highest cereal consumption countries are Egypt, Afghanistan, Turkey, and the Arab countries. Cereals are very important food in all the countries in the Far East, the daily consumption being over or about 500 g in South Korea, Laos, Pakistan, South Vietnam, and Nepal.

Among the African countries the cereal consumption varies greatly from the very low 50 to 60 g/day in countries such as Gabon and Congo to over 500 g/day in Malawi and Rhodesia.

In Oceania, the cereal consumptions in Australia and New Zealand are at the level of the developed countries in Europe.

Varieties of Grain

The different areas of the world vary from each other also in respect to the consumption of different kinds of cereals. Climate conditions determine which cereals can be grown in each area and thus also the consumption.

The three most important cereals of the world are rice, wheat, and maize. Rice and wheat are staple food to about four fifths of the population of the world.[4]

Rice

Rice is the staple food to almost a half of the human population. The main consumption area of rice is the Far East, where about 88% of the total rice produced is consumed. Only 5% is consumed in Latin America, 5% in Africa and the Near East, and as little as 2% of the total production in North America and Europe.[5] The highest rice consumption area in the Far East is that formed by Laos, Cambodia, Thailand, Vietnam, Malaysia, and Burma, where the annual consumption varies between 175 and 140 kg per capita per year.[2] The consumption varies greatly even within a country, e.g., in India from 230 kg in the rice-eating eastern areas to a negligible quantity in the wheat-eating northwestern area.[5] With the exception of Mongolia, where the annual consumption of rice amounts to only 3.5 kg per capita,[2] rice is the main cereal in the Far East.

Outside the Far East rice is the main cereal only in a restricted area in Africa, i.e., the island of Madagaskar (144 kg) and in the coastal area of western Africa (Liberia 122 kg, Sierra Leone 106 kg, Gambia, Guinea, and Senegal). In most of the African countries the yearly consumption is less than 10 kg per capita. The consumption is nearly as small in the Near East, where the highest figures are found in Saudi Arabia and Iran.

In Latin America rice is a more important cereal than in the areas mentioned. In some countries it is even the main cereal, such as Brazil, Surinam, Guyana, and Panama, whereas in the southern states of South America and in most of the states of Central America the consumption is fairly low.

The lowest rice consumption areas are in North America, Oceania, and Europe. It is more than 10 kg per capita in only one European country, Portugal.

In the developing countries rice is nearly always eaten in boiled form, but cooking methods vary and consumer preferences are very marked.

Wheat

There are four areas in the world where the consumption of wheat is about equal, i.e., Europe, Near East, North America, and Oceania, where wheat is the main cereal. The Mediterranean countries lead in wheat consumption: Bulgaria (167 kg), Yugoslavia, Italy, and Greece; of the Near East countries, Turkey (140 kg), Syria, and Jordan. This group also includes the African countries Tunisia (125 kg), Algeria, and Morocco. The wheat consumption in the U.S.S.R. is also considerable (122 kg). In the more developed countries of Europe and in North America the consumption of wheat is smaller than in the Mediterranean countries, which is a sign of a higher standard of living. Considerable amounts of wheat are also consumed in Latin America, especially in Chile (119 kg) and in Argentina, where it is the most important cereal as in many other South American countries. The lowest consumption figures are found in Central America and Colombia.

The consumption of wheat is rather small in the Far East, with the exception of Mongolia (133 kg). However, the consumption of wheat increases with a higher standard of living. The wheat consumption is the highest in Pakistan (41 kg), Japan, India, and China, where the natural conditions for growing wheat are more favorable than in many other parts of the Far East or where there are economic resources to import wheat, as in Japan.

In Africa the wheat consumption is relatively modest, with the exception of the Mediterranean countries, South Africa, and Ethiopia. It is less than 10 kg per person per year in most of the countries.

In the developed countries wheat is used mainly in the form of bread. In the Far East, northern India, and Pakistan, the main wheat foods are porridge, small cakes, and unleavened products; Japan and Korea use their domestic wheat for noodles. In the developing regions of North Africa hard durum wheat is consumed mainly in the form of couscous, in Near Eastern regions in the form of pancake bread called bulgur. Pastes are common wheat food in Latin America.[4]

Maize

Maize is the third main cereal of the world, and the main cereal in Central America, where it comprises 74% of the total cereal consumption.[6] Leading maize consumption countries are Guatemala (197 kg), Honduras, Nicaragua, El Salvador, and Mexico.[2] In South America, where wheat is the main cereal, the proportion of maize of the total cereal is about 30%.[6] As a foodstuff, maize outweighs wheat only in Bolivia, Colombia, and Paraguay. In South America the consumption of cereals is more varied and distributed more evenly between the various kinds than in Central America.

The other important maize region of the world is southeast Africa, where maize is the staple food of the population of Malawi (215 kg), Zambia, Rhodesia, South Africa, and Kenya. Maize is also the most important cereal in many countries in the coastal area of northeast and west Africa, although its consumption in this region is considerably lower than in the maize countries mentioned.

Maize does not play a major role in the food of the countries in the Far East, as in Africa, although some of them, such as North Korea and Nepal (both 55 kg), use more maize than other Far East regions. When the standard of living rises, there is a tendency to move away from the cheap cereals, such as maize and millet, and to replace them by rice.

A digression from the typical maize consumption pattern is seen in Afghanistan in the Near East, as well as in Albania, Romania, Portugal, and Yugoslavia in Europe. Very little maize is used in the other Near East and European countries or in North America.

Maize is eaten in Central America and Mexico in the form of baked cakes or bread called tortillas and as porridge. In Africa various dishes are made from it, such as doughy balls called kenke, or it is eaten as gruel or paste.[4]

Other Grain

Important items in the total cereal consumption of the whole world are also *millet* and *sorghum*, which are staple foods in Africa, especially among the population in the savanna regions in Niger, Chad, Upper Volta, and Mali (168 to 127 kg). Closely connected with this area are Sudan and Yemen in the Near East, where the consumption of millet and sorghum is very high. The importance of these cereals is also reflected in the fact that they outweigh all other cereals in 15 African countries. In the Far East only a few countries use them, the leading ones being India (about 30 kg), North Korea, and China. In other parts of the world their consumption is minimal.

Rye, barley, and oats are cereals which are insignificant in the food consumption patterns of the whole world. Rye is grown in North and Central Europe and in the U.S.S.R. and it is eaten chiefly as bread. The quantitative significance of rye is smaller than that of wheat. Outside of Europe rye is consumed only in North America and in some countries in Latin America, the Far and Near East; the amounts used are very small except in Turkey. More barley is consumed outside of Europe than in it; the highest consumption figures in the Far East are found in North Korea; in the Near East, in Irak, Syria, and Libya; in Africa in the Mediterranean countries and Ethiopia; and in Latin America in Peru. The use of oats as human food is very rare throughout the world, except in some places in Europe.

To summarize, the consumption of cereals is the highest in the developing countries of the Far East and Africa, as well as in the developing regions of Europe, and the lowest European and North American countries with a high standard of living. Low consumption figures are also found in Latin America and some African countries, where the main part of the cereals is replaced by starchy roots. The Far East is typically a rice region. The Near East, the Mediterranean countries of Africa and Europe, as well as North America and Oceania are wheat regions, whereas Central America and the coastal areas of Africa are maize consumers, and the savanna areas in Africa and the Near East use millet and sorghum.

STARCHY FOODS

The starchy food group consists of starchy roots and tubers, including potatoes, sweet potatoes, yams, and cassava. This group also contains plantains and bananas and other starchy foods, such as dates and figs, if they are staple food in the diet of a people.[2]

The development of the consumption of starchy food in the world has proceeded along the same lines as that of cereals. In the developed countries their use is decreasing with a rising standard of living, whereas in many developing countries their consumption has continued to increase. In addition to cereals, they constitute the staple food of a large part of the population of the world since they are inexpensive and rich in carbohydrates. This, too, indicates that the standard of living has not risen in the developing countries or that the rise has been very slow.

When the total consumption of starchy foods is considered, it is observed that it has decreased everywhere else in Europe except in Portugal and Yugoslavia, where it has remained on the same level, whereas it has risen somewhat in Greece and Italy. In North America the consumption of starchy foods has decreased, while in Latin America it has either decreased or remained the same, except in Brazil, Colombia, Panama, and Paraguay, where it has increased. Of the Near East countries, the consumption has decreased in Israel and Libya and remained the same in all other countries where it has been possible to follow this development. In those Far East countries where consumption statistics have been available for the last 10 to 20 years, the use of starchy food has somewhat decreased, with the exception of those countries where the consumption was originally very small. Only a few African countries have had consumption statistics for longer periods of time. In those places where the consumption has been low, it has usually remained on the same level, whereas in the countries with high consumption figures, they seem to increase continuously. Only a few countries, e.g., Kenya, show a decrease in the consumption of starchy food.

The total consumption of starchy food varies greatly in different parts of the world and even within one region, as in the wide areas of Latin America and Africa (Table 2). The lowest total consumption is found in southern Europe, North America, the Near and Far East, and in Oceania. The low consumption of starchy food in the Far and Near East should be considered together with the consumption of cereals since these foodstuffs replace each other. In countries where only small quantities of starchy food are used, the consumption of cereals is high and vice versa. Starchy food is the staple food of the population in the states on both sides of the equator; this is a relatively consistent area (Ivory Coast, Ghana, Togo, C.A. Rep., Congo, Gabon, Zaire, Rwanda, Uganda, and Burundi). In all these countries the consumption is very high, on the average 1,000 to 1,800 g per person per day. Correspondingly, the consumption of cereals is very low in most of these countries. In Latin America, starchy food predominates the diet of the peoples of Paraguay, Brazil, and Peru.

Variety

There are many varieties of starchy food used in the different parts of the world.

Potatoes

Potatoes are both produced and consumed to the largest extent in Europe, where they constitute the only starchy food. Typical areas of potato consumption also include North America, Oceania, and the Near East. Potatoes are also a common food in the Far East, but the consumption is small; the leading country there is North Korea (59 kg per year), where it is the chief starchy food. Some other potato countries are China, Mongolia, and Nepal. Pototoes are also familiar in Africa, but excluding the Mediterranean countries and South Africa, they have no significance in the diet. On the contrary, in Latin America potatoes are used abundantly in Bolivia, Peru, Argentina, and Chile, where they are an important food. The use of potatoes in Central America is minimal, although they are commonly known there.

TABLE 2

Different Levels of Starchy Food Consumption per capita in Countries in Different Regions of the World[1]

Per capita consumption grams per day	Europe 27	North America 2	Latin America 26	Near East 15	Far East 23	Africa 38	Oceania 2
Starchy food, total range, g	53–383	151–215	35–836	2–421	6–247	6–1,832	154–183
less than 200	10	1	11	14	20	17	2
200–300	10	1	5		3	2	
300–400	7		4				
400–500			3	1		2	
500–1,000			3			7	
1,000 and more						10	
Potatoes							
less than 100	5		19	14	19	29	
100–200	5	1	4	1	1		2
200–300	10	1	2				
300–400	7						
Sweet potatoes and yams							
less than 100		2	16	3	18	18	2
100–200			1		2	5	
200–300					1	2	
300–400						5	
Cassava							
less than 100			19		14	12	
100–200						3	
200–300					1	7	
300 and more			1	1		7	
Plantains							
less than 100			10			5	
100–200			6			5	
200–300			2			4	
300–400			1				
600 and more						2	
Others							
less than 100			19	3	6	12	
100–200			1	1			
200–300						2	

Potatoes are used in numerous ways in various regions and countries. They are used mainly, however, as natural products. Potato flour is the most important industrial product in Europe. In countries with a high standard of living and a highly developed food industry, such as the U.S., various potato products have an increasing role in the diet.

Sweet Potatoes and Yams

These starchy foods are important in tropical and subtropical regions, especially in the west coast of Africa (Ivory Coast, Ghana, Dahomey, Nigeria, Gabon) and in east Africa in Burundi. Very few of the Near East countries use small amounts of sweet potatoes. They are also eaten in the Far East, where they are staple food in North Korea, China, and Taiwan. The quantities consumed are lower than in Africa, however. In Latin America sweet potatoes and yams are used mainly in South America, but their consumption is not very high. The leading country is Paraguay (38 kg per year), followed by Uruguay and Cuba; in the latter they are the most important starchy food. The consumption of sweet potatoes is very small in North America and Oceania, where both sweet potatoes and yams are eaten in the same manner as potatoes.

Cassava

Cassava is common in Latin America, the Far East, and Africa; however, its consumption is fairly small in most of the countries in Latin America and the Far East. In Paraguay, however, it is the main starchy food of the population (181 kg per year), as well as in Brazil, where its consumption is much lower (56 kg). In the Far East, Indonesia in particular is a cassava country. Quantitatively it is the predominant starchy food in both Vietnams, Ceylon, and some parts of Malaysia, although the consumption is modest. In the Near East, only Sudan uses cassava (126 kg). Geographically, Sudan belongs to Africa, where the use of cassava as human food is the highest in the world, besides Latin America. Consumption patterns are, however, diverse in various parts of Africa. The highest consumption area is in the equator region, where the use of starchy foods in general is abundant. The highest consumption figures for cassava (354 to 102 kg) are found in Central Africa Republic, Mozambique, Congo, Liberia, Angola, Gabon, Dahomey, Cameroon, Nigeria, and Togo. Of these, Gabon, Dahomey, and Nigeria are also countries where considerable quantities of yams are consumed.

Sweet cassava is used in the same manner as potatoes and prepared in various ways.[6] The main cassava root product is a coarse meal or a flour. Some countries manufacture tapioca flour, which is used as food or bakery products. In some areas of the Far East, cassava is eaten as a substitute for rice or maize, while in Latin America cassava bread is made from flour or meal.[4]

Plantains

Plantains are a fruit of the banana family and used as staple food in most of the tropic regions. Because of their high starch content, they are included in the starchy food group. In many tropical countries bananas are also staple food and included in the consumption figures of plantains.

Regionally, plantains and bananas are considered starchy food only in Latin America and Africa, in the countries situated by the equator. The consumption of plantains is fairly high in both areas, higher in Latin America than in Africa. Only in the southern states of South America and Mexico are no plantains used according to consumption statistics; here bananas are included in the fruit group. The highest quantities of plantains and bananas are consumed in the Dominican Republic (143 kg per person per year), Venezuela, and in the small countries of Central America; the latter are also users of guineous.

Of the African countries, Rwanda (297 kg) and Uganda (237 kg) are the greatest consumers of plantains and bananas. In the other equator countries the consumption varies between 12 and 100 kg per person per year.

In addition to the above-mentioned starchy foods, many others are also used in the world, but they have more local than regional significance, and the quantities consumed are often small. The largest selection is found in Latin America. Breadfruit is common in Jamaica (66 kg). The Far East, the Philippines and Taiwan use small amounts of taro. In Africa, taro is used especially in Ghana (86 kg), Cameroon (80 kg), and Ivory Coast; small amounts are also consumed in their neighbor countries.

When comparing the different regions, it is observed that the highest starchy food consumption is in Africa and Latin America, and the lowest in the Near and Far East. The greatest differences within a region occur in Africa. Europe, including the U.S.S.R., North America, Oceania, and the Near East belong to the potato consumption area. Almost equal amounts of cassava, sweet potatoes (and yams), and potatoes are used in the Far East, mainly cassava and sweet potatoes in the eastern and southeastern parts of the region, and potatoes in the north. The consumption of all starchy foods is very small in the southern parts of the region. In Latin America, both cassava and plantains are used abundantly, cassava particularly in Paraguay, in Central America, and the northern parts of South America. The use of potatoes is also common, although not to the same extent as cassava and plantains in South America, with the exception of the countries on the southern and western coasts. Sweet potatoes and yams are consumed less than potatoes, chiefly in the eastern coast of South America and in the West Indies. African staple starchy foods are cassava, sweet potatoes, yams, and plantains, bananas included. The role of potatoes is small considering the whole area.

PULSES, NUTS, AND SEEDS

This group of foods comprises a large variety of edible leguminous seeds, called pulses in most English-speaking countries, as well as nuts and seeds. These foods are very important as sources of proteins to a large part of the population of the world with no economic resources to obtain enough animal protein.

In developed areas the consumption of pulses has remained practically the same, although some increase seems to have occurred in some central and south European countries. Their consumption has generally risen in Central America, too, especially in Mexico. In the Near East the consumption has increased in Israel and Libya. In the Far East the use of pulses has more than doubled during the past 20 years in Japan and Taiwan; it has also increased in the Philippines (70%), Korea, and Ceylon, whereas in Indonesia and Pakistan, among others, the consumption has decreased somewhat. Of the African countries, more pulses than before are consumed in Burundi and Ethiopia, but less in South Africa and some others.

When the present consumption of pulses is studied in different parts of the world (Table 3), it is seen that it is the lowest in North America and Oceania and in most European and Near East countries. The consumption of pulses, nuts, and seeds is the highest in Africa, the Far East, and Latin America. Large variations in the amounts consumed are seen within the regions.

In Europe pulses are used mainly in the Mediterranean countries, especially in Malta, whereas the consumption is the smallest in Scandinavia and the countries around the Baltic Sea. The most common pulses are dry beans, dry peas (very common in the U.S.S.R.), dry broad beans, and in some southern countries, chickpeas and small amounts of lentils. Small quantities of nuts are eaten in all European countries, as well as cacao and even soya flour in some countries. Seeds are used only in very few countries.

In North America and Oceania both dry beans and peas, nuts, and cacao are consumed in about equal amounts, contrary to Europe, where the consumption of pulses is the highest.

In Latin America, pulses play a more predominant role in the food in Central America than in South America. Of individual countries the consumption is, however, the highest in Brazil. The most commonly used varieties of pulses are kidney beans and broad beans,[7] whereas much smaller amounts of dry peas, lentils, and lupines are consumed. Part of the leguminous plants are eaten as such, particularly in South America. Nuts are of minor significance in the diet and no seeds are used.

In the Near East the use of pulses is fairly equal in different countries. Many varieties of pulses and small amounts of nuts and seeds are used.

TABLE 3

Different Levels of Pulses, Vegetables, and Fruit Consumption per capita in Countries in Different Regions of the World[1]

Per capita consumption grams per day	Europe 27	North America 2	Latin America 26	Near East 15	Far East 23	Africa 38	Oceania 2
Pulses, nuts and seeds, range, g	4–90	12–22	6–81	13–36	11–100	8–140	10–13
less than 20	17	1	4	5	8	7	2
20–40	7	1	14	10	8	16	
40–60	2		4		4	6	
60 and more	1		4		2	9	
Vegetables, range, g	27–466	213–318	35–265	30–381	10–362	5–146	192–234
less than 100	4		21	5	9	34	
100–200	11		3	4	11	4	1
200–300	7	1	2	4	2		1
300–400	4	1		2	1		
400 and more	1						
Fruits, range, g	58–397	230–276	69–356	49–410	6–186	11–180	211–275
less than 100	6		5	4	14	31	
100–200	9		14	2	9	5	
200–300	9	2	5	3			2
300–400	2		2	4			
400 and more	1			2			

In almost all Far East countries pulses are an important protein source for the population, especially in India and other countries in south Asia. The greatest consumption figures are in Ceylon, North Korea, India (53 kg), Thailand, Japan, and Indonesia. Many varieties of pulses are produced and consumed in the Far East, but quantitatively the most important ones are chickpeas, dry beans, and pigeon peas, which are both produced and consumed abundantly, particularly in India, but also in China. As the source of high-quality protein, soybean is an important leguminous plant in many countries, particularly in Japan, where the diet includes many soybean products such as flours, soybean paste miso, and soybean sauce called shoyu. Soybean is also common in China, South Korea, Singapore, and Malaysia. In Taiwan it is used abundantly as curd.

In spite of the large variety of nuts, they have small significance in the food of any people, with the exception of the countries using coconut: Thailand, Malaysia, Singapore, and the Philippines. Seeds are used only in very small amounts, mostly in North Korea, sesame seeds being the most common variety.

Pulses are common food in Africa, but their consumption varies greatly in different countries. East Africa is the foremost area in this respect; the consumption is high, especially in Rwanda, Burundi, and Uganda, where pulses sometimes replace cereals and root crops as the staple food,[7] and in the countries by the Guinean Gulf. The number of varieties is not, however, quite as large as in the Far East. It is the greatest in the Mediterranean countries, where the most common variety is dry broad bean. The available detailed information on their consumption indicates that dry beans are the most abundant leguminous plant in Africa. In the coastal states of Niger and Nigeria, the largest part of the world's cow pea crop is harvested;[1] probably the consumption also centers mainly in this area.

In Africa, more nuts are used as food than anywhere else in the world; their consumption is even higher than that of leguminous plants in many countries along the Gulf of Guinea and in the Central Africa Republic. Groundnuts are the most common species; coconuts are also prominent, and even more important than groundnuts in some countries. The use of seeds seems to be very rare, and only sesame seeds and melon seeds are eaten as food.

VEGETABLES

The consumption statistics are incomplete concerning vegetables, in developing countries in particular, and it seems likely that the true consumption figures are higher than the officially estimated ones in many countries because they do not include vegetables produced in private gardens and eaten mainly within one household.

The use of vegetables has become increasingly common in all parts of Europe, which is evidently a result of the rising living standard, particularly in central and north Europe. In North and Latin America the consumption has been fairly constant, with the exception of Argentina, where it has doubled. The consumption has also increased in the Near East, but in the Far East it has remained the same or risen only slightly. In Japan, where the economic development has been very rapid, the use of vegetables has more than doubled in 20 years. In those African countries from which consumption trends are available, the consumption has remained on an equal level.[1]

The regions of high vegetable consumption are Europe, North America, Australia, New Zealand, and the Near East, whereas low consumption regions are Africa, Latin America, and the Far East (Table 3). Excluding North America and Oceania, the differences in the consumed quantities are very great within the regions, depending on conditions favorable for production, economic factors, and food habits.

According to the statistics of OECD,[3] the leading vegetable consumers in Europe are Portugal (197 kg per capita per year), Italy (144 kg), Greece (139 kg), France (127 kg), and Spain (120 kg), i.e., southern Europe as a whole, where the conditions are favorable for growing vegetables. The smallest consumers are the Scandinavian countries (Iceland 10 kg, Finland 16 kg, Norway and Sweden 35 kg, Denmark 41 kg), where the climate restricts the production of vegetables; especially in the winter most of the vegetables consumed are imported. The choice of vegetables is very abundant everywhere. The most common are tomatoes, in the Mediterranean countries in particular, onions, cucumbers, carrots, cauliflowers, cabbages, green beans and peas, and green leafy vegetables, although the mutual shares vary greatly from one country to another.

Most of the vegetables are eaten as fresh products either raw or cooked in various ways.

Tomatoes are usually eaten cooked in the Mediterranean countries, in contrast to other parts of Europe.[8] Part of the vegetable crop is processed; the most common products are tomato paste, ketchup, and juice, which are both produced and consumed mainly in the Mediterranean countries. Since freezing vegetables has become common, the seasonal variations in their use have been leveled out, particularly in north Europe.

The consumption patterns of vegetables concerning both the quantities and varieties are very similar in North America, Oceania, the Near East, and south and west Europe. In the Near East all the Mediterranean countries are large vegetable consumers, particularly Jordania (137 kg) and Israel (119 kg);[2] the number of varieties is also very high in them. But relatively few vegetables are used in Yemen, Sudan, and Iran. The most common vegetable in all these countries is the tomato, which, as well as other vegetables, is almost exclusively eaten fresh. Contrary to Europe and the other regions mentioned above, in North America the majority of the tomatoes consumed are in the processed form, especially as ketchup, sauce, juice, and as canned whole tomatoes.[8] Processed vegetables play an important role, especially in the U.S. According to statistics of OECD,[3] 63.5 kg per capita per year of vegetables were consumed as fresh, 4.3 kg as frozen, 23.8 kg as canned, and 7.6 kg as canned vegetable soups. During the last ten years the amounts of fresh vegetables have decreased and those of frozen and canned increased.

In the Far East, Japan uses the highest quantity of vegetables per person per year, 125 kg, followed by North Korea and Taiwan, whereas the consumption in India is minimal. Due to the lack of detailed consumption statistics, no data are available on the kinds of vegetables used nor of the quantities. From production statistics[1] it may be concluded that onions, tomatoes, cabbages, cauliflowers, green beans and peas, cucumbers, gherkins, and melons are known in the Far East. The largest quantities of these are produced in Japan, where their consumption is also the highest. Small quantities of processed vegetables, tomato products in particular, are also eaten in Japan.

In Latin America the consumption of vegetables is the largest in Argentina and Chile. However, the consumption is very low in many of the Latin American countries; the abundant consumption of starchy foods replaces the use of vegetables in Paraguay, Brazil, and Venezuela. The most abundant vegetables are the tomato and onion, but other common vegetables are included in the diet of the population. Many unspecified vegetables are also used.

Throughout Africa the use of vegetables is very modest. Only Tunisia, Sierra Leone, Gabon, and Tanzania approach the European level. The available detailed consumption data indicate that tomatoes, onions, and leafy vegetables are the most common vegetables. North Africa produces and consumes the same kinds of vegetables as the Mediterranean countries.

FRUITS

Fruits are an important food all over the world; their consumption is continually increasing everywhere except in the Far East and Africa. The increase has been the largest in Europe and in Japan, where the consumption of fruits has increased to 4 times the amount consumed 20 years ago.[1]

With the exception of the Far East and Africa, the consumption of fruits is relatively great throughout the world, although the differences within regions are equally great regarding the consumption of vegetables (Table 3). The leading fruit producer and consumer countries are the Mediterranean countries in Europe and the Near East. The highest consumption figures are, however, found in Switzerland, where fruit juices add to the figures (18 kg per person per year).[3] The leading consumers of fresh fruit in Europe are Greece and Italy and in the Near East, Israel and Lebanon. Plenty of fruit is also used in many central European countries and in Sweden, where the consumption is based mostly on imported fruits. The smallest consumption figures are found in some east European countries (U.S.S.R., Poland, Albania) and in Iceland, as well as in Sudan, Yemen, and Afghanistan in the Near East.

In both Europe and the Near East the consumption of fruits is very diversified both in import and export countries, varying somewhat with the season of the year. The percentage of citrus fruits is 20 to 30% of the fresh fruits in Europe, except in Greece and Yugoslavia, where it is under 10%.[3] From the beginning of the 1960's the portion of citrus fruits has increased in many countries by 1 to 13%, mostly in Italy; in some it has remained unchanged or even decreased, as in Greece from 26 to 9%. Citrus fruits are also important in the Near East, particularly in Israel. Apples, pears, peaches, plums, and apricots are common fruits. Grapes are abundant, especially in the Mediterranean countries, where melons are also common. Dates are grown and consumed in large quantities in some Near East countries (Egypt, Yemen); in Libya and Saudi Arabia they are staple food to the extent that they are included in the starchy food group in statistics.[2]

A typical feature of the fruit consumption in Europe is the fairly abundant use of cultivated berries, strawberries in particular. Many delicious wild berries are consumed in Scandinavia.

Dried fruits, mainly raisins and plums, are used both in Europe and the Near East. Canned fruits are consumed mostly in Spain, Sweden, and Norway, and juice especially in Switzerland, Sweden, and Austria.[3]

The use of fruits is abundant and varies in North America and Oceania. The most common varieties in the U.S. are citrus fruits, apples, bananas, and melons,[9] but many other fresh fruits and berries are also common. The use of canned fruits is very widespread in North America and Australia, and more citrus juice is used in North America and Canada than anywhere in the world.[3,8] In the consumption of citrus products, the U.S. is the leading country in the world. The consumption of citrus products both in North America and Europe has risen faster than that of fresh citrus fruits.

Dried fruits are used scantily in North America, but in Australia their consumption is very high (12 kg per capita per year).[2]

In Latin America fruits are used frequently, the leading countries being the Dominican Republic and Paraguay, while the smallest consumers are Guatemala and Bolivia. The number of varieties is very great. In most countries citrus fruits are the most common fruits, and in many countries bananas, when they are not included in the group of starchy food. Avocado, mango, and pineapple are also abundant in many countries, as well as many locally grown fruits not encountered anywhere else in the world.

In most of the Far East countries the daily per capita consumption of fruit is less than 100 g, in Mongolia only 6 g per day and in China 14 g. The highest figures are in Cambodia, West Malaysia, Singapore, and Japan. According to production statistics, the main fruit in the Far East is banana, followed by orange, pineapple, and apple.[1] Other fruits seem to have less significance. Japan is the only country where strawberries are grown. Small amounts of dried and preserved fruits are used in the Far East.

The use of fruits is very limited in all African countries. It should be noted, however, that bananas are considered a staple starchy food in Africa and are not, therefore, included in the fruit consumption figures. The largest fruit consumers are Tanzania, the Mediterranean countries, and Central African Republic. The assortment of fruit is not very great, with the exception of the Mediterranean countries; the most common are citrus fruits, bananas, pineapples, and apples. Grapes are grown mainly in Algeria and South Africa, but almost the whole production is used for wine-making.

MEAT

Nutritionally, meat is a very important food as a source of high-quality proteins. But the gap regarding the consumption of meat continues to widen between the developing and developed regions. In regions where the consumption of meat is high, it tends to rise further along with a rising standard of living, even quicker than the consumption of other foods.[10] For example, in Europe its consumption has risen by 20 to 40% during the last 15 to 20 years and in some countries it has more than doubled (Greece, Italy, the Netherlands, Spain), and in Canada and the U.S. the increase has been over 30%. In most of the developing countries, where the use of meat is very scarce, it has either risen only very slowly or not at all. Exceptions are the Near East countries Israel and Libya, where the consumption has increased threefold during the corresponding period of time. Of the Far East countries the consumption has doubled in South Korea and Taiwan, and in Japan it is 9 times higher than 20 years ago. When the increases in the meat consumption are judged, it should be taken into account that the starting point has been quite different in the developed countries as compared to the developing ones. Improvements in the economic situation of the developing countries might create conditions for increasing the meat consumption, unless the rapidly growing population would baffle it.

Europe, North America, Oceania, and part of South America are regions of high meat consumption (Table 4). The average meat consumption is the highest in Argentina, the U.S., New Zealand, and Australia. In the developing regions of Africa, the Far East, and the Near East the use of meat is very moderate.

In the European countries the daily meat consumption per person varies considerably. The lowest figures are encountered in Albania, Yugoslavia, and Portugal, the highest again in France, Ireland, and Germany. Pig meat is the most common meat in Europe, especially in the east and north European countries. Beef surpasses pork only in Malta and Italy, Belgium, France, Spain, Portugal, and Finland. Mutton and lamb, including goat, are the chief meats in Greece, Albania, and particularly Iceland. The use of poultry meat is common all over Europe, but the amounts consumed are considerably smaller than those of pork or beef. Poultry meat consumers are mainly the countries of south Europe, Hungary, the U.K., and Ireland. Edible offals are used everywhere; their amounts vary depending on the total meat consumption.

Other kinds of meat besides those mentioned above are of no importance in Europe. The ratio between processed and unprocessed meat varies in different countries; in most of them unprocessed meat is more common. An exception is at least West Germany, where the proportion of processed meat is higher.[10] The assortment of processed meats also varies from one country to another.

In North America and other developed regions, the relative consumption of various meats is greatly affected by consumer preference, as well as the price. Beef and poultry are preferred in North America. Beef is a main meat, but even poultry is prominent since it accounts for one fifth of the total meat consumption,[1,10] i.e., it is higher than anywhere else in the world over such a large region. The consumption of pork is only slightly higher than that of poultry in North America. There is a tendency to replace fat meat by less fat meat; the same tendency is also seen in west and north Europe. Mutton and lamb as well as other meats are not prominent in North America.

A typical feature of North America is the high consumption of processed meat, accounting for about one half of the total meat consumption.[10]

In Australia and New Zealand, which are cattle breeding countries, the consumption of meat is very abundant, mainly because the prices of meat are low. The percentage of beef, including veal, is over 40% in both countries, that of mutton and lamb a little less, and that of pork 10 to 13%. Poultry is the most important other kind of meat.

TABLE 4

Different Levels of Meat, Egg, and Fish Consumption per capita in Countries in Different Regions of the World[1]

Per capita consumption grams per day	Europe 27	North America 2	Latin America 26	Near East 15	Far East 23	Africa 38	Oceania 2
Meat, range, g	84–229	257–310	22–335	29–155	4–302	13–113	294–301
less than 50			6	10	19	29	
50–100	3		12	3	2	7	
100–150	11		5	1	1	2	
150–200	7		1	1			
200 and more	6	2	2		1		2
Eggs, range, g	4–44	41–50	4–20	2–62	1–45	1–8	34–48
less than 10	2		8	12	14	37	
10–30	12		18	2	7		
30–60	13	2			1		2
60 and more				1			
Fish, range, g	2–107	15–18	1–37	1–30	1–88	1–35	36–42
less than 10	7		14	12	4	15	
10–30	13	2	10	1	9	19	2
30–60	5		2	1	7	2	
60 and more	2				2		

The southern states of South America specialize in meat production, due to the mild climate; they are also considerable meat consumers. Argentina is the leading meat consumption country in the world, but plenty of meat is also used in Uruguay. With the exception of these southern countries, meat is consumed much less in other parts of Latin America because there are no possibilities of producing it sufficiently and not enough economic resources to import it. Of the various kinds of meat, beef is the most important; for example, in Argentina about 80% of the meat consumed is beef.[2,10] Besides beef, only pig meat and poultry play some role in the total consumption. Small amounts of mutton are eaten in South American countries.

In the Near East the consumption of meat is smaller than in Latin America. It is the highest in Israel, where the standard of living is higher than in the other Near East countries, and in Cyprus. Mutton and lamb are the most important kinds of meat in many countries in the Near East, although beef is also very common. Poultry is common in Israel and its neighbor Lebanon, goat meat in Yemen, and buffalo meat in Egypt; camel meat is the main kind of meat eaten in Libya, and it is not rare in Sudan and Saudi Arabia either. Due to religious reasons, the use of pork is very rare in the Near East.

In the Far East, where the general standard of living of the population is very low indeed, minimal amounts of meat are consumed, the smallest meat consumption countries being India, Ceylon, and Indonesia. Pig meat is the main meat in most of the countries, although beef is common in spite of the low consumption figures. Goats are also grown in the Far East, and goat meat provides a small addition to the meager meat consumption. In India with its almost 500 million people, the minimal amount of meat consumed consists of goat, sheep, buffalo, and poultry. Cattle meat cannot be used for religious reasons, although cattle breeding is common in the country.

Similar to the Far East, Africa, too, is a region of a low standard of living and low consumption of meat. Only in South Africa and Gabon is the consumption of meat at a satisfactory level. Beef plays the most prominent part in the consumption. A great variety of meats are consumed in these countries, such as sheep, goat, pig, poultry, buffalo, camel, game, and even snails.

In summary, it is seen that plenty of meat is consumed in developed areas and in the countries having a high standard of living in Europe and in North America. Its consumption is also high in such areas where it can be produced inexpensively, as in Oceania and the southern parts of South America. But the consumption of meat is very low in the developing areas in Latin America, the Near East, the Far East, and in Africa. Beef is the main meat in North America, Latin America, and Africa; pig meat in most European countries and the Far East; mutton and lamb in the Near East; and beef, mutton, and lamb in Oceania. Poultry meat and processed meat are used mainly in North America.

MILK AND MILK PRODUCTS

In addition to meat, milk is an important source of proteins of good quality. However, too little or no milk is available where it is needed most, and too much milk is produced in areas where its consumption is high already. The three regions of high milk consumption in the world are Europe, North America, and Oceania (Table 5). In the countries with high milk consumption, Scandinavia and Canada, the trend has been slightly decreasing during the last 20 years, whereas in the U.S. and Australia it has been increasing slightly. The increase in the milk consumption has been the highest in southern Europe, particularly in France, where it has previously been lower than in the other European countries. In the developing countries, where the consumption of milk is very low as a rule, it has remained practically the same.

According to statistics,[1] the ten leading milk consumer countries are Finland, Ireland, Iceland, Denmark, Sweden, Norway, the U.S., the Netherlands, New Zealand, and Australia. Of these, seven are in Europe, two in Oceania, and one in North America. Milk is mainly used as whole milk; its fat percentage varies in different countries. Denmark, Sweden, and the Netherlands have started to replace whole milk by low-fat liquid milk products to a large extent. The same phenomenon is also observed in the U.S., while the use of low-fat milk products is minimal in Canada, Australia, and New Zealand.[2] Condensed milk and dried milk are used mainly in central Europe, North America, and Oceania. Only cow milk is used, both as such and in milk products.

Of the Latin American countries, only Uruguay

TABLE 5

Different Levels of Milk and Cheese Consumption per capita in Countries in Different Regions of the World[1]

Per capita consumption	Europe 27	North America 2	Latin America 26	Near East 15	Far East 23	Africa 38	Oceania 2
Milk, range, g per day	183–861	619–689	25–557	89–403	1–237	7–494	646–661
less than 100			2	3	17	28	
100–200	1		11	7	4	7	
200–300	5		8	4	2	1	
300–500	7		4	1		2	
500–700	8	2	1				2
700 and more	6						
Cheese,[1,3] range, kg per year	2.1–14.3	4.7–6.8	0.3–6.7	0.3–8.1	0.1–0.8	0.1–3.0	3.3–3.5
less than 1			8	3	2	10	
1–3	5		13	4		2	
3–6	11	1	2	1			2
6–9	6	1	1	5			
9 and more	5						

is a prominent milk consumer. There seem to be no definite differences in the milk consumption of the other countries. Latin America nearly exclusively uses cow milk, but a few countries also consume goat and sheep milk.

In the Far East the consumption of milk is almost on the same level as in Latin America. The leading country is Israel, and the last in the list are Afghanistan, Saudi Arabia, and Yemen. Of the milk produced in this area, 55% is cow milk, 20% sheep milk, 13% goat milk, and 11% buffalo milk,[1] a considerable part of which is, however, used for cheese production.[2,11] In Jordania, Libya, and Yemen, sheep milk is quantitatively the most important milk, in Saudi Arabia and Yemen, goat milk. Buffalo milk is important in Egypt.

The consumption of milk is minimal in both the Far East and Africa. Although cattle are often bred, milk production is very low. Mongolia and Pakistan are the leading milk users in the Far East, and Mauretania, Somali, and South Africa in Africa. Quite negligible amounts of milk are used in both Koreas and China and in many west African countries. Of the milk produced in the Far East, 50% is buffalo milk, a little less cow milk, and the rest goat and sheep milk.[1] It may be mentioned that in India the consumption of cow milk and buffalo milk is almost equal, although beef is not accepted as food. Of the milk produced in Africa over 80% is cow milk and only 10% goat and sheep milk. Camel milk is also used in some countries in east and west Africa.[2]

Cheese

The quantity of milk used for preparing cheese varies greatly in different parts of the world. Cheese is used mostly in developed areas, where the total consumption of milk is high (Table 5). With a rising standard of living the use of cheese also increases. France is the leading cheese consumer in the world; prominent consumers are also Bulgaria, Greece, Switzerland, and the Scandinavian countries, excluding Finland. Other milks (goat, sheep) besides cow milk are unimportant in this connection.

North America is also a relatively large cheese consumer. But surprisingly Australia and New Zealand, where the milk consumption is high, use only moderate amounts of cheese. The emigrants from Europe have increased the cheese consumption in these parts of the world.[12]

In addition to the regions mentioned here, many countries in the Far East (Cyprus, Jordania, Egypt, Israel, Syria) use large quantities of cow, goat, sheep, and buffalo milk cheese. Cheese is also a common food in Latin America, although the amounts consumed are considerably lower than in the regions mentioned above. Argentina, Uruguay, and El Salvador, which are cattle breeding countries, use the largest quantities of cheese. Mostly cow milk cheese is eaten in this area.

The consumption of cheese is only casual and very low in the Far East. In Africa cheese plays some role in the food of the populations of Niger, Tunisia, and Morocco.

EGGS AND FISH

As seen in Table 4, the consumption of eggs is common but quantitatively small all over the world. The consumption has risen in most of the European countries, as well as in some countries in Latin America, the Near East, and the Far East, chiefly in Japan. No changes worth mentioning have occurred in other parts of the world in the consumption of eggs.

The leading egg consumer countries are Israel, the U.S., New Zealand, Japan, the United Kingdom, Canada, and Central Europe. The very low egg consumption in the vast developing regions is no solution to the lack of proteins in the food of the population.

What was said about the consumption of eggs also applies to a great extent to fish. Their consumption has gone up only in a few countries in Europe, mainly in south Europe, and in some countries in the Far East, Japan and Taiwan in particular. Everywhere else the consumption of fish has remained the same as previously, as far as the reliable data on the development of the consumption and the amounts consumed show.

The highest fish consumption figures are found in countries where fishing is of great importance as a means of living for at least part of the population. Such countries are Iceland, Portugal, and Norway in Europe, and Japan and some other island countries in the Far East. It is surprising to note that very little fish are used in several countries all over the world which have a long coastal region. In many areas and many individual countries where fish play some role in the diet, their consumption is restricted to the coast and around rivers and lakes because of difficulties in transporting far off and the rapid spoilage.

Many varieties of fresh-water and pelagic fish are used in different parts of the world. Also crustaceans and mollusks are eaten. A considerable part of the fish is consumed fresh, frozen fish included, but the use of canned products is rather common, too, both in developed and developing countries. Fish are also consumed salted, smoked, and dried, particularly in Japan but also in Europe, e.g., in Portugal, Norway, and Greece.[3]

FATS AND OILS

The fat consumption patterns of the world may be studied from the point of view of total consumption and the quality of the fats consumed. The highest consumption figures are found in Europe and North America, the lowest in Africa, the Far East and in several countries in the Near East and Latin America (Table 6). The fat consumption has continued to increase in most countries of Europe, the U.S., the Near East, and in Japan, and remained the same or even decreased somewhat in Norway, Australia, and New Zealand. The countries in central and north Europe, mainly the Netherlands, Belgium, and Luxembourg, Denmark, and France use great quantities of fats. According to the quality of the fats consumed, the countries may be divided into three groups: (1) the users of large quantities of butter fat, (2) large quantities of margarine, and (3) almost exclusively oil. The first group includes Finland, West Germany, and Ireland. Norway, the Netherlands, Denmark, and Sweden use large quantities of margarine.[3] Both butter and margarine are used in many countries. The countries almost exclusively using oil, chiefly olive oil, are mainly in south Europe, especially Greece, Italy, Spain, and Bulgaria.[2,3] Slaughter fats are used to a small degree in most countries.

In North America, the U.S. is the largest user of shortenings and other vegetable oils, in addition to margarine, butter, and lard. The main food fat in Canada is butter, beside shortenings and margarine.

The leading butter fat consumption country in the world is New Zealand followed by Finland. Butter is also the most important food fat in Australia. Both countries also use margarine and some vegetable oils and animal fats.

In Latin America the fat consumption is the highest in Argentina. In this region oil is quantitatively the most important fat, however. The varieties of oil used are very many, and several kinds of oils are used in every country. Butter and animal fats are also common, but the amounts consumed are small.

In the Near East, the consumption of fat is rather small, with the exception of Israel and Libya. The use of oils is common, and the

TABLE 6

Different Levels of Fat, Sugar, and Beverage Consumption per capita in Countries in Different Regions of the World[1]

Per capita consumption	Europe 27	North America 2	Latin America 26	Near East 15	Far East 23	Africa 38	Oceania 2
Fats and oils, range, g	14–90	51–66	4–51	3–52	1–32	1–37	36–42
less than 20	1		10	6	18	32	
20–40	4		15	7	5	6	1
40–60	11	1	1	2			4
60 and more	11	1					
Sugar and sweets, range, g	48–150	136–140	50–135	10–107	3–104	2–104	123–141
less than 50	2			7	14	33	
50–100	12		16	7	8	2	
100–150	13	2	10	1	1	2	2
Beverages, kg per year							
Beer, range, kg	1.5–156.5		3.0–47.4	0.5–82.9	0.1–16.1	0.3–253.8	
less than 20	8		16	7	10	20	
20–50	6		5	1		4	
50–100	4			1		5	
100 and more	3					2	
Wine, range, kg	0.5–115.7		0.1–63.6	0.9–24.9		0.1–45.5	
less than 20	6		8	4		18	
20–50	14		1	1		3	
50–100	1		1				
100 and more	3						
Other, range, kg	0.2–13.8		1.2–7.4	0.4–6.6	0.1–38.8		
	11		13	4	9		

proportional consumption of oils varies in different countries. In most countries olive oil is the predominant oil, as in the Mediterranean countries in general. Little butter and animal fats are used. Israel also uses margarine.

Oils are the main food fat in the Far East and their choice is large. Some animal fats and small amounts of butter are also consumed.

In Africa the almost exclusive food fat is oil, palm oil being the most important. Groundnut oil and cottonseed oil are common in many places, and olive oil in the Mediterranean countries. Butter is rather rare. The use of oils and fats is altogether lower than in the rest of the world.

SUGAR

Sugar has become increasingly common in all parts of the world. In some developing countries its consumption has risen even more than in the developed countries, where the consumption seems to be slightly decreasing in some cases (Sweden, Canada, Australia, New Zealand). But the use of sugar is very high in North America, Oceania, most European and Latin American countries, and in the more developed countries in the Near and Far East and Africa (Table 6). The ten leading sugar consumption countries of the world are Iceland, Australia, Ireland, the U.S., Colombia, Denmark, the Netherlands, Canada, the United Kingdom, and Cuba. Five of these are in Europe, two in North America, two in Latin America, and one in Oceania. The smallest sugar consumption figures are found in Africa and the Far East.

There are regional differences in the sugar consumption in Europe. It is the highest in Central and North Europe and the lowest in South Europe. In Latin America the differences between the various countries are not as marked, although the consumption in South America is often higher than in other parts of the region. The poor population particularly in the northern parts of South America, in Central America, and in the Garibian region use remarkably high amounts of sugar.[13]

The consumption of sugar is smaller in the Near and Far East than in the areas mentioned. Israel and the other Mediterranean countries lead, while Singapore and Japan are quite large sugar consumers, too. Particularly in Japan the consumption has increased very strongly along with the increasing consumption of many other foodstuffs. With the exception of South Africa and Mauritius, very little sugar is used in Africa so far, which is an advantage considering the general nutritional status of the population.

Small amounts of honey, besides sugar, are also used in various parts of the world, mainly in Europe and North America, according to statistics.

BEVERAGES

When considering the food consumption patterns of the world, beverages cannot be excluded, since they belong to the daily diet of the population in many countries and, in addition, they are an important source of energy. Beer and wine are common beverages, but their main consumption areas are in Europe (Table 6). Marked amounts of beer are consumed in Germany and Czechoslovakia, but the other central European countries, Scandinavia, and the U.S.S.R. consume much beer, too. Beer consumption in the U.S. is on the same level as in most of the European countries.[9] Although the use of beer is quite common in all parts of the world, in Africa in particular, the quantities consumed are small compared to those consumed in Europe. Exceptions are, however, Uganda and Burundi in east Africa; in these the consumption surpasses even that in Europe. The neighboring countries also use large quantities of beer. Everywhere beer is brewed from national cereals. In Europe, Near and Far East, malt is used for this purpose; malt, maize, millet, sorghum, and plantains in Africa; and malt, millet, maize, and rice in Latin America.

Wine countries in Europe are the Mediterranean countries, Italy and France, as well as Portugal, where wine belongs to the normal diet. Little wine is used in other parts of the world, in Latin America mostly in Chile, in Africa in Cameroon, and in the Near East in Cyprus. Wine is mainly made from grapes everywhere, and in Africa almost the whole grape crop is used for preparing wine.

In all parts of the world, other alcoholic beverages are used besides beer and wine, mainly spirit. Europe is the leading area here, too. In Japan the use of liqueur is common and fairly abundant. Spirit is made in various countries from different materials such as cereals, molasses, sugar, cane, sweet potatoes, paddy, dried dates, grapes, plums, etc. Most countries have their own special products. Although spirit and other alcoholic beverages do not belong to the daily diet in the same manner as beer and wine, they still reflect the usage patterns of beverages in various parts of the world.

SUMMARY

The food consumption patterns vary greatly in different parts of the world, depending on the level of development and conditions for production. Typically, developed areas consume plenty of animal foods, vegetables, fruit, sugar, fats, and beverages and small quantities of cereals and starchy foods, whereas developing countries consume large quantities of cereals and starchy foods, which partly replace each other. The use of vegetables and fruit is lower than in the developed regions, and that of animal foods is minimal, the main protein source being pulses. Europe, the Near East, North America, and Oceania are wheat regions, whereas rice is the main cereal in the Far East, maize in Latin America and Africa, and millet and sorghum in Africa. Staple starchy food are potatoes in Europe, North America, Oceania, and the Near East; cassava and sweet potatoes in the Far East; cassava and plantains in Latin America; and cassava, sweet potatoes and yams, and plantains in Africa. Pig meat is the most common meat in Europe and the Far East, mutton and lamb in the Near East and partly in Oceania, and beef in all other regions of the world. Milk and cheese are consumed chiefly in Europe, North America, and Oceania, cheese also in the Near East. Butter and/or margarine are the predominant fats in Europe, excluding south Europe, as well as in North America and Oceania; and oils predominate in the Mediterranean countries, the Far East, Africa, and Latin America. Beer is the most common beverage in central and north Europe, wine in south Europe.

REFERENCES

1. Food and Agriculture Organization of the United Nations, *Production Yearbook Vol. 25, 1971,* Rome, 1972.
2. Food and Agriculture Organization of the United Nations, *Food Balance Sheets 1964–68 Average,* Rome, 1971.
3. Organization for Economic Co-operation and Development, *Food Consumption Statistics 1960–1968,* Paris, 1970.
4. Food and Agriculture Organization of the United Nations, *The Economic Relationships between Grains and Rice,* Commodity Bulletin Series 39, Italy, 1965.
5. Food and Agriculture Organization of the United Nations, *The World Rice Economy,* Trends and Forces, Volume 2, Commodity Bulletin Series 36, Rome, 1963.
6. Lehmann, G., Lebensmittel- und Ernährungsprobleme in Entwicklungsländern. 1. Mitteilung – Über die Brotversorgung, *Ernährungs-Umschau,* 18, 505, 1971.
7. Food and Agriculture Organization of the United Nations, *Legumes in Human Nutrition,* FAO Nutritional Studies No. 19, Rome, 1964.
8. Food and Agriculture Organization of the United Nations, *Processed Fruit and Vegetables,* Trends in world production and trade of citrus products, canned peaches and apricots, and tomato products, Commodity Bulletin Series 47, Rome, 1970.
9. U.S. Department of Agriculture, Agricultural Research Service, *Food Consumption of Households in the United States,* Seasons and Year 1965–66, Household Food Consumption Survey 1965–66, Report No. 12, Washington, 1972.
10. Food and Agriculture Organization of the United Nations, *The World Meat Economy,* Commodity Bulletin Series 40, Rome, 1965.
11. Food and Agriculture Organization of the United Nations, *Report of the Nutrition Committee for the Middle East,* FAO Nutrition Meetings Report Series No. 24, 1959.
12. Food and Agriculture Organization of the United Nations, *A Review of Cheese Production, Consumption and Trade in Some Developed Countries,* Commodity Bulletin Series 41, Rome, 1966.
13. Food and Agriculture Organization of the United Nations, *Report of the Fourth Conference on Nutrition Problems in Latin America,* FAO Nutrition Meetings Report Series No. 18, Rome, 1959.

THE STATE OF WORLD FOOD PRODUCTION

J. R. Anderson

TABLE OF CONTENTS

Introduction 35
Principal Sources of Food 35
Trends and Patterns in Food Production 37
Use of Land Resources 42
Agricultural Systems 45
Increasing World Food Production 52
References 54

INTRODUCTION

One of the most basic questions of today's world relates to food production. How can enough food be produced to give the world's people an adequate diet? Is it possible to increase food production fast enough to match the current rate of population growth? Or will a general slowdown in population growth be necessary in order to attain a better way of life for more people? The following examination of the present state of world food production should offer some insights into this fundamental problem in spite of the likely continuing disagreement on how the problem should be resolved in different parts of the world.

PRINCIPAL SOURCES OF FOOD

The main components of world food production are crops, livestock, and fish. Of these, crops account for approximately 75% of the world's food production by weight with only about 23% contributed by livestock and a mere but vital 2% derived from fish and other products of the world's fisheries (Table 1). Most of the world's people use crops directly for food, since animals are extravagant converters of feed grains and other crops into human food. Although much used as a source of food in some parts of the world, fish and other products of oceans, lakes, and streams are not readily and cheaply accessible to many people.

A great variety of crops are grown for food;

TABLE 1

Major Components of World Food Production, 1969

	Million metric tons	Percent
Food crops	1,612[1]	75
Livestock and livestock products	487[2]	23
Fishery products	63	2
Total	2,162	100

[1] Includes pulses and starchy root crops in addition to the food products listed in Annex Table 1A of *The State of Food and Agriculture, 1970.*
[2] A considerable part of the weight contributed by livestock is of course derived from crops.

(Source: FAO, *The State of Food and Agriculture, 1970,* 196 and *Production Yearbook,* 1970.)

however, relatively few crops account for most of the world's food supply derived from that source. In its annual *Production Yearbook,* the Food and Agriculture Organization of the United Nations (FAO) reports production data for 9 cereal crops, 2 sugar crops, 3 starchy root crops, 9 pulses, 14 oil crops, 14 fruit crops with some reported in combination, and 6 vegetable crops. Except for fruits and vegetables, the area and production of most of these crops are shown in Table 2. Of course, statistical information gathered on a worldwide basis has serious limitations, including a wide variation in the reliability of the data and a probable serious underreporting of some kinds of crops compared with others. However, such information, if used judiciously, can contribute to a better understanding of the state of world food production.

From the study of Table 2 it is quite obvious that cereal and starchy root crops dominate world food production by weight, accounting for about 88% of the average total production for 1966–70, as derived from the crops included in Table 2; cereals alone account for 60% of the total. Of course, weight alone does not give an adequate indication of the world's food situation, since

TABLE 2

World Area and Production of Major Crops and Groups of Crops, 1948–52 and 1966–70

	Area (million hectares)		Production (million metric tons)	
	1948–52	1966–70	1948–52	1966–70
Cereals				
Wheat	176.6	217.7	176.0	313.2
Rye	38.9	21.6	37.9	31.0
Barley	52.1	74.0	59.4	123.5
Oats	53.2	31.6	62.0	52.0
Maize	88.2	105.9	139.9	253.6
Millets and sorghums	94.5	111.3	47.8	85.8
Rice (paddy)	102.8	129.7	167.3	283.0
Total	606.3	691.8	692.5	1,142.1
Starchy roots				
Potatoes	22.6	22.3	247.6	297.1
Sweet potatoes and yams	10.2	16.5	69.5	133.8
Cassava	6.9	9.6	50.6	86.9
Total	39.7	48.4	367.7	517.8
Sugar				
Sugar cane	6.6	10.4	25.7	51.0
Sugar beets	4.2	7.9	12.7	29.2
Total	10.8	18.3	38.4	80.2
Pulses[1]	50.9	59.3	29.6	41.6
Oil crops[2]	83.9	114.4	57.2	110.4
Grand total	791.6	932.2	1,185.4	1,892.1

[1] Includes dry beans, dry peas, broad beans, chickpeas, lentils, pigeon peas, cow peas, vetch, lupins, and miscellaneous pulses.

[2] Includes soybeans, groundnuts in shell (peanuts), cottonseed, linseed, rapeseed, sesame seed, sunflower seed, olives for oil, palm oil, and palm kernels.

(Source: FAO *Production Yearbooks, 1966–70.*)

composition of the production from a nutritional standpoint is vitally important. Particularly the problem of proteins is not adequately reflected by such data. Fruits and vegetables which occupy a rather small part of the arable land used for food production are especially significant components of an adequate diet. Similarly, the calorie contribution of sugar crops to the world's food supply is markedly understated with tonnage data.

About half of the world's arable land (cropland) is now being used to produce cereal crops. Oil crops account for 8% of the total arable land and starchy roots, sugar, and pulses make up another 9%. Fruits and vegetables occupy about 2 to 3% of total arable land. Thus, approximately 70% of the world's arable land, totaling 1,424 million hectares, is devoted to the production of crops that can be used directly as food crops for human consumption. However, in some parts of the world, particularly in some of the developed countries, a substantial part of the grain production, especially maize, sorghum, barley, rye, and oats, is fed to livestock. The remaining 30% of the arable land base is mainly used for the production of hay and forage crops. However, about 3 to 4% is used for fiber and beverage crop production.

TRENDS AND PATTERNS IN FOOD PRODUCTION

Between the 1948–52 and the 1966–70 periods, the area in major food crops excluding fruits and vegetables increased by 141 million hectares, which amounted to an 18% increase in the area being used for food crop production (see Table 3). Some of this increase resulted from a shift from hay and forage crops to food areas in some parts of the world. However, much of this substantial increase in the area devoted to food crops resulted from new arable land being developed from forest land, grazing land, and other uses. Significant gains in all of the major crop categories occurred; however, the most outstanding percentage gain was in sugar crops, which had a 70% increase from a relatively small base of 10.8 million hectares. Other percentage increases ranged from 14% for cereals from a big base area of 606 million hectares to 24% for oil crops.

Among the several major crops, significant increases in the area of all the cereal crops occurred except for oats and rye, which underwent a major decline in area. For the most part, wheat and barley gained at the expense of these crops. Potatoes remained practically stationary in area, while sweet potatoes, yams, and cassava, grown mainly in the subtropics and tropics, had substantial increases. Both sugar cane and sugar beets had increases. Among the pulses, dry beans showed the most significant gain. Among the oil crops, groundnuts and particularly soybeans had major area gains.

A brief analysis of regional variations in food crop trends reveals marked contrasts among the several world regions shown in Tables 3 and 4. Europe, Canada, and especially the U.S. experienced a decline in the area in cereals; however, very substantial increases in production were associated with outstanding increases in yields. All other world regions had increases in area in cereal crops, with the Far East, Latin America, and the U.S.S.R. having the largest absolute gains in area and Oceania having the highest percentage gain. Similarly, Europe, U.S.S.R., and the U.S. and Canada had declines in root crop area with all other world regions except Oceania showing increases. The area in sugar crops was expanded in all world regions. The area in pulses likewise increased in most world regions, with the exception of Europe and the U.S. and Canada. Oil crops underwent areal increases in all regions. In the U.S. a major increase in the area in soybeans was counterbalanced to some extent by decreases in cottonseed, flaxseed, and groundnuts (peanuts).

Increases in the production of food crops have occurred in every world region (Table 4). Total world production of food crops increased by 707 million metric tons between the 1948–52 and 1966–70 periods. This amounts to a 59% increase for the 18-year period, which represents an increase of about 3.3% a year, compared with the annual percentage increase in area of about 18% for the same period for an annual percentage increase of only about 1%. Thus, production gains per hectare have significantly outstripped the areal expansion of food production, which quite clearly indicates that increases in capital and labor, particularly capital, have been considerably more important contributors to increased food crop production than has land.

About half of the present tonnage of food crops of the world is being produced on 38% of the total area used for food crops that is found in Europe, U.S.S.R., U.S. and Canada, and Oceania. Since these world regions only have 26% of the

TABLE 3

Summary of Major Food Crops by Region and Area, 1948–52 and 1966–70

	World (million hectares)		Europe (million hectares)		U.S.S.R. (million hectares)		U.S. and Canada (million hectares)		Latin America (million hectares)	
	1948–52	1966–70	1948–52	1966–70	1948–52	1966–70	1948–52	1966–70	1948–52	1966–70
Cereals										
Wheat	176.6	217.7	28.0	28.1	42.6	67.3	38.3	31.0	7.5	8.6
Rye	38.9	21.6	12.2	7.8	24.0	11.7	1.3	0.8	0.8	0.6
Barley	52.1	74.0	8.9	15.6	8.6	20.5	6.9	7.5	1.2	1.3
Oats	53.2	31.6	12.5	7.6	16.2	8.6	19.8	10.2	0.9	0.7
Maize	88.2	105.9	10.4	11.3	4.4	3.9	30.0	23.5	14.1	26.0
Millets and sorghums	94.5	111.3	0.1	0.2	3.9	3.3	3.1	5.6	0.7	2.9
Rice (paddy)	102.8	129.7	0.3	0.4	0.1	0.3	0.8	0.9	2.7	6.0
Total	606.3	691.8	72.4	71.0	99.8	115.6	100.2	79.5	27.9	46.1
Starchy roots										
Potatoes	22.6	22.3	9.5	7.5	8.6	8.2	0.8	0.7	0.8	1.1
Sweet potatoes and yams	10.2	16.5	–	–	–	–	0.2	0.1	0.4	0.5
Cassava	6.9	9.6	–	–	–	–	–	–	1.4	2.4
Total	39.7	48.4	9.5	7.5	8.6	8.2	1.0	0.8	2.6	4.0
Sugar										
Sugar cane	6.6	10.4	–	–	–	–	0.2	0.2	3.5	4.8
Sugar beets	4.2	7.9	2.4	3.0	1.4	3.7	0.3	0.6	–	–
Total	10.8	18.3	2.4	3.0	1.4	3.7	0.5	0.8	3.5	4.8
Pulses[1]	50.9	59.3	6.6	5.9	2.7	5.3	1.0	0.8	4.0	4.8
Oil crops[2]	83.9	114.4	2.6	2.8	8.1	10.1	18.0	23.8	6.8	9.5
Grand total	791.6	932.2	93.5	90.2	120.6	142.9	120.7	105.7	44.8	69.2

TABLE 3 (continued)

Summary of Major Food Crops by Region and Area, 1948–52 and 1966–70

	Near East (million hectares)		Far East (million hectares)		China[3] (million hectares)		Africa (million hectares)		Oceania (million hectares)	
	1948–52	1966–70	1948–52	1966–70	1948–52	1966–70	1948–52	1966–70	1948–52	1966–70
Cereals										
Wheat	12.0	19.7	14.7	21.8	23.0	25.2*	5.8	7.0	4.7	9.0
Rye	0.5	0.7	0.1	–	–	–	–	–	–	–
Barley	5.0	6.6	5.1	4.6	11.1	12.0	4.8	4.5	0.5	1.4
Oats	0.3	0.4	0.2	0.1	2.0	2.1	0.4	0.3	0.9	1.6
Maize	1.7	1.9	8.1	14.1	9.6	9.2	9.8	15.9	0.1	0.1
Millets and sorghums	2.1	2.8	35.1	40.5	27.7	28.0	21.7	27.8	0.1	0.2
Rice (paddy)	0.9	1.3	68.7	87.4	26.8	30.2	2.5	3.2	–	–
Total	22.5	33.4	132.0	168.5	100.2	106.7	45.0	58.7	6.3	12.3
Starchy roots										
Potatoes	0.1	0.2	0.6	1.0	1.9	3.2	0.2	0.3	0.1	0.1
Sweet potatoes and yams	–	–	1.4	1.7	5.7	11.0	2.5	3.2	–	–
Cassava	–	–	1.4	2.3	–	–	4.1	4.9	–	–
Total	0.1	0.2	3.4	5.0	7.6	14.2	6.8	8.4	0.1	0.1
Sugar										
Sugar cane	–	0.1	2.4	4.0	0.2	0.4	0.2	0.6	0.1	0.3
Sugar beets	0.1	0.3	–	0.1	–	0.2	–	–	–	–
Total	0.1	0.4	2.4	4.1	0.2	0.6	0.2	0.6	0.1	0.3
Pulses[1]	1.2	1.3	22.1	25.7	7.9	8.5	5.4	7.0	–	–
Oil crops[2]	2.3	4.0	21.4	29.5	17.8	24.9	6.9	9.7	–	0.1
Grand total	26.2	39.3	181.3	232.8	133.7	154.9	64.3	84.4	6.5	12.8

*1965 figure only.

[1] Includes dry beans, dry peas, broad beans, chickpeas, lentils, pigeon peas, cow peas, vetch, lupins, and miscellaneous pulses.

[2] Includes soybeans, groundnuts in shell (peanuts), cottonseed, linseed, rapeseed, sesame seed, sunflower seed, olives for oil, palm oil, and palm kernels. Area used for olives for oil, palm oil, and palm kernels is not available.

[3] Data for China (mainland) are not available for all years included in averages.

TABLE 4

Summary of Major Food Crops by Region – Production, 1948–52 and 1966–70.

	World (million metric tons)		Europe (million metric tons)		U.S.S.R. (million metric tons)		U.S. and Canada (million metric tons)		Latin America (million metric tons)	
	1948–52	1966–70	1948–52	1966–70	1948–52	1966–70	1948–52	1966–70	1948–52	1966–70
Cereals										
Wheat	176.0	313.2	41.2	69.3	35.8	89.0	44.5	56.3	8.0	11.2
Rye	37.9	31.0	17.8	15.5	18.0	13.2	1.0	1.1	0.6	0.4
Barley	59.4	123.5	15.0	44.9	6.4	28.4	10.1	16.1	1.3	1.4
Oats	62.0	52.0	20.0	17.6	13.0	11.3	25.2	18.2	0.9	0.8
Maize	139.9	253.6	12.9	34.7	5.8	10.3	74.7	113.6	15.2	35.3
Millets and sorghums	47.7	85.8	0.1	0.4	1.7	3.1	3.9	18.6	0.6	5.1
Rice (paddy)	169.6	283.0	1.3	1.7	0.2	1.0	1.9	4.1	4.6	10.4
Total	692.5	1,142.1	108.3	184.1	80.9	156.3	161.3	228.0	31.2	64.6
Starchy roots										
Potatoes	247.6	297.1	130.2	134.0	80.2	94.9	12.5	16.4	4.7	8.7
Sweet potatoes and yams	69.5	133.8	0.2	0.1	–	–	1.0	0.6	2.6	4.1
Cassava	50.6	86.9	–	–	–	–	–	–	15.6	33.0
Total	367.7	517.8	130.4	134.1	80.2	94.9	13.5	17.0	22.9	45.8
Sugar										
Sugar cane	25.7	51.0	–	–	–	–	1.3	2.2	13.7	21.2
Sugar beets	12.7	29.2	7.8	14.4	2.7	9.5	1.6	3.0	–	–
Total	38.4	80.2	7.8	14.4	2.7	9.5	2.9	5.2	13.7	21.2
Pulses[1]	29.6	41.6	3.4	3.4	1.9	7.1	1.1	1.1	2.3	4.6
Oil crops[2]	57.2	110.4	5.6	9.4	4.4	11.1	14.8	36.1	4.0	8.5
Grand total	1,185.4	1,892.1	255.5	345.4	170.1	278.9	193.6	287.4	74.1	144.7

TABLE 4 (continued)

Summary of Major Food Crops by Region – Production, 1948–52 and 1966–70.

	Near East (million metric tons)		Far East (million metric tons)		China[3] (million metric tons)		Africa (million metric tons)		Oceania (million metric tons)	
	1948–52	1966–70	1948–52	1966–70	1948–52	1966–70	1948–52	1966–70	1948–52	1966–70
Cereals										
Wheat	11.0	20.3	11.5	23.1	15.9	27.8	3.4	5.1	4.7	11.1
Rye	0.5	0.8	–	–	–	–	–	–	–	–
Barley	4.7	6.7	5.6	6.0	12.4	14.7*	3.3	3.6	0.6	1.7
Oats	0.3	0.5	0.2	0.2	1.5	1.7*	0.3	0.2	0.6	1.5
Maize	2.6	4.2	6.6	15.7	14.1	22.7*	7.9	16.9	0.1	0.2
Millets and sorghums	2.3	3.2	13.3	19.2	13.9	17.1*	11.8	18.7	0.1	0.4
Rice (paddy)	2.1	4.3	98.7	163.6	58.2	93.2	2.5	4.5	0.1	0.2
Total	23.5	40.0	135.9	227.8	116.0	177.2	29.2	49.0	6.2	15.1
Starchy roots										
Potatoes	1.1	2.8	5.1	10.4	12.1	27.0*	1.1	1.9	0.6	1.0
Sweet potatoes and yams	–	0.1	13.0	16.0	36.4	90.0*	16.2	22.7	0.1	0.2
Cassava	0.1	0.1	9.7	19.7	–	–	25.1	34.0	0.1	0.1
Total	1.2	3.0	27.8	46.1	48.5	117.0*	42.4	58.6	0.8	1.3
Sugar										
Sugar cane	0.2	0.6	7.2	17.5	0.6	2.8	1.7	3.9	1.0	2.8
Sugar beets	0.2	1.2	–	0.3	0.4	0.7	–	0.1	–	–
Total	0.4	1.8	7.2	17.8	1.0	3.5	1.7	4.0	1.0	2.8
Pulses[1]	1.1	1.4	10.3	12.8	6.9	7.5	2.5	3.6	0.1	0.1
Oil crops[2]	2.0	4.3	9.1	14.7	11.9	18.1	5.4	8.1	–	0.1
Grand total	28.2	50.5	190.3	319.2	184.3	323.3	81.2	123.3	8.1	19.4

*1965 figures only

[1] Includes dry beans, dry peas, broad beans, chickpeas, lentils, pigeon peas, cow peas, vetch, lupins, and miscellaneous pulses.
[2] Includes soybeans, groundnuts in shell (peanuts), cottonseed, linseed, rapeseed, sesame seed, sunflower seed, olives for oil, palm oil and palm kernels. Area used for olives for oil, palm oil, and palm kernels is not available.
[3] Data for China (mainland) are not available for all years included in averages.

(Source: FAO *Production Yearbooks, 1966–70.*)

world's people, there is a striking imbalance in world food production that requires correction. The question of how this can be accomplished has of course become one of the major problems of the present-day world. The fact that livestock production in the more developed nations of the four world regions included above absorbs a very substantial part of the crop production of these regions further accentuates the dietary contrasts between the developing and developed nations.

Altogether, two fifths of the total *value* of world agricultural production is accounted for by livestock products. Meat comprises nearly three fifths of this value, whole milk about one fourth, eggs about one tenth, and wool about one twentieth. The production of livestock products used for food (excluding wool) is particularly concentrated in the U.S. and Western Europe. These two regions alone now account for about two fifths of the total value of all livestock products being produced in the world.

The extravagant use of land resources in livestock production is particularly evident in the U.S., where livestock and livestock products now account for well over half of the total value of all farm products sold. The feed that is needed to produce livestock in the U.S. is derived from three main sources: 923 million acres (374 million hectares) of pasture and grazing land; 100 or more million acres (40 million hectares) which is suitable for use as arable land (cropland); 65 million acres (26 million hectares) of hay crops; and about 113 million acres (46 million hectares) of feed grains. Thus, of the 297 million acres (170 million hectares) of land used for harvested crops in 1964, about 178 million acres (72 million hectares) were used to produce feed for livestock. Altogether about a third of the livestock feed was made up of corn, sorghum, oats, barley, and other grains which can be consumed directly as human food.

USE OF LAND RESOURCES

About a third of the world's land area is used to some extent for agriculture and the grazing of livestock (Table 5). However, as emphasized earlier, most of the food production comes from the arable land (cropland), which constitutes only about a tenth of the world's land area. About 45% of this arable land is in Europe, U.S.S.R., U.S. and Canada, and Oceania, which are the economically more advanced world regions; yet these regions have only 26% of the world's population. Among the world regions, Europe and the Far East have the highest proportion of the total land area in arable land with 30 and 24%, respectively. None of the other regions have more than 12% and Latin America and Oceania only have 6% of the total land area used as arable land or cropland (Table 6).

Not only is the arable land of the world unevenly distributed among the major regions, but there is marked unevenness of distribution within regions. Particularly noticeable are the vast cold and dry parts of the world that have practically no cropland at all except where some water is available for irrigation within or on the periphery of the world's deserts. About one fifth of the world is too cold for wheat, which is one of the most widely grown crops and another two fifths of land area of the world is too dry. Extensive areas of the wet tropics are also currently little used for crop production. Areas of steep slopes and poor soils, although climatically suitable for growing crops, are unlikely to be of much value for that purpose.

The quality of the arable land area also varies greatly. Thus, one must be quite careful about making comparisons on the basis of area alone. Generally, land that is irrigated is more productive than land which is not irrigated.

This is particularly true of arable land in subhumid and semiarid climatic situations. In 1970, FAO reported 192 million hectares irrigated in specified countries which include most of the countries where irrigation is a significant practice.[1]

In marked contrast to the high yielding irrigated lands of subhumid and semiarid areas, much arable land in those regions of the world has relatively low yields because of inadequate precipitation. In some countries, such as the U.S., Soviet Union, Canada, and Australia, the practice of dry farming is widely used. Under this practice cropland lies idle or fallow in a cultivated condition every other year so that enough moisture can be accumulated to produce a grain crop, mainly wheat, every other year. Thus, the U.S. has had an average of about 15 million hectares of cultivated summer fallow during the past few years, while producing wheat on about 20 million hectares. The likelihood of crop failure is also high in areas where dry farming is practiced. Although higher yields result from the practice of dry farming, it is obvious that a much more extensive area is used

TABLE 5

Major Uses of Land by World Regions[1]

Region	Total area	Arable land[2]	Permanent meadows and pastures	Forest land	Other area
	Million hectares	Million hectares	Million hectares	Million hectares	Million hectares
Europe[3]	493	148	93	139	113
U.S.S.R.	2,240	233	375	910	722
U.S. and Canada	1,968	220	280	739	729
Latin America	2,057	123	502	1,003	429
Near East[4]	1,207	81[7]	183[7]	138	805
Far East[5]	1,117	270[7]	114[7]	448	285
China (mainland)	956	110	177	77	592
Africa[6]	2,503	192	817	555	939
Oceania	851	47	460	82	262
Total	13,392	1,424	3,001	4,091	4,876

[1] As reported in the *FAO Production Yearbook 1970.*
[2] Includes land under permanent crops such as fruit and nut orchards and groves.
[3] Excludes U.S.S.R.
[4] Includes Libya, Sudan, and the United Arab Republic and Asian countries west of Pakistan.
[5] Includes Pakistan and all countries to east except China mainland and U.S.S.R.; Indonesia and the Philippines are included.
[6] Excludes Libya, Sudan, and United Arab Republic.
[7] Adjustment made for underreporting in Iran.

TABLE 6

Arable Land and Population by World Regions as of 1970.[1]

	1970		1970	1969
	Arable land (million hectares)	Total world land area (Percent)	As a percent of world's arable land (Percent)	Population (millions)
Europe[2]	148	30	10	458
U.S.S.R.	233	10	16	240
U.S. and Canada	220	11	16	224
Latin America	123	6	9	276
Near East[3]	81[4]	7	6	165
Far East[5]	270	24	19	1,136
China (mainland)	110	12	8	832
Africa[6]	192	8	13	297
Oceania	47	6	3	19
Total	1,424	11	100	3,647

[1] Source: FAO *Production Yearbook, 1970*
[2] Excludes U.S.S.R.
[3] Includes Libya, Sudan, and the United Arab Republic and Asian countries west of Pakistan.
[4] Adjustment made for under-reporting in Iran.
[5] Includes Pakistan and all countries to the east except China (mainland) and U.S.S.R. Indonesia and the Philippines are included.
[6] Excludes Libya, Sudan, and United Arab Republic.

for wheat culture in semiarid and subhumid areas than the area from which wheat is actually harvested.

Another significant variation in the quality of arable land relates to the length of the frost-free season or the period during which crops may be grown. In the high latitudes, the period that is free of frost hazard is very short and thus a relatively limited variety of crops can be grown and often losses occur due to frost in spring after crops have been planted or in autumn before being harvested. By contrast, in many tropical and subtropical areas of the world more than one crop can be raised on the same tract of land without a freeze hazard. This practice is known as double cropping. In some areas where double cropping is a common practice, the hazard of drought exists, thus sometimes curtailing the usefulness of the practice as a means of increasing food production.

In evaluating the present state of world food production, the changes in amount of arable land being used to produce food in different parts of the world are of considerable significance. Although data on arable land reported by the Food and Agriculture Organization are difficult to compare between 1950 and 1970, a general estimate of the changes in the arable land area of some of the different regions of the world is possible. In spite of precautions that must be taken in using the data on land use available for 1950 and 1970, it is possible to make some significant generalizations. In the first place, there has been very little overall change in the total arable area of Europe and the U.S. and Canada during this 20-year period. Although some new lands have been brought into the cropland base in irrigated areas of the western U.S. and in the lower Mississippi alluvial valley, much cropland has been reverting to forest land and to pasture in the southeastern and northeastern parts of the country. In Europe a very stable arable land base has been established and very little change is now occurring. Since these two world regions have relatively reliable land use information, these conditions of land use stability have been analyzed in considerable detail by experts.

In the Soviet Union and in Oceania, particularly in Australia, some expansion of the arable land area has occurred over this 20-year period. Although the new lands program of the Soviet Union experienced considerable difficulty, expansion of areal land to the east of the well-established agricultural areas has occurred. In the Esperance Region of Western Australia and in Queensland "on land covered with Brigalow (a leguminous tree that leaves nitrogen-rich soil)"[2] several million hectares of new land are being developed for crop and livestock production. Also, the Commonwealth War Service Land Development Scheme for ex-servicemen has been responsible for the development of land in Queensland, New South Wales, Western Australia, South Australia, and Victoria.[3] Thus, among the economically more highly developed world regions, Europe and the U.S. and Canada have reached a level of considerable stability, while a moderate expansion continues to take place in the U.S.S.R. and Oceania.

In the other five world regions the available land use information is generally much less reliable than for the four regions just discussed. However, in spite of the difficulties in making accurate comparisons, it is fairly obvious that some substantial increases in arable land have taken place since 1950. In the Near East significant expansion of arable land has occurred in Turkey and Israel and to a lesser extent in Iran. In the latter country there is some modest possibility for some further expansion of arable land; however, such expansion will be expensive and does not appear likely in the near future.[4] In Northern Africa, where relatively little expansion of the arable land area has occurred over the past 20 years, there appears to be a considerable area of land in Sudan and in Ethiopia which is potentially productive land. However, no thorough land surveys have been made; therefore, it is difficult to determine the feasibility of increasing the arable land of these countries at this time.

In sub-Saharan Africa potentially useable land for growing crops is available; however, the political, economic, and other conditions, such as the presence of the tsetse fly, seem to preclude much widespread development of potentially arable land in the near future. Nigeria, Liberia, Ghana, Tanzania, and South Africa are among the countries with sufficiently reliable land use information to indicate quite clearly that substantial increases in arable land have occurred between 1950 and 1970. Generally, throughout Africa increases in the arable land area are evidenced from available information.

Among the Far East countries, India, Pakistan, and China (mainland) have registered increases in the arable land base between 1950 and 1970.

Smaller countries such as those of Southeast Asia and the Philippines have also had some additions to the arable land base. Very little change in the arable land area of Japan has taken place. Future substantial additions to the arable land bases of countries in this part of the world are not likely, since the dense populations have already exerted great pressure on the land resources of the region. There are, however, some remaining opportunities for expansion of the arable land such as in the Mekong Delta and the "outer" islands of Indonesia.

In Latin America the most substantial increases in the arable land base have occurred in Brazil, Mexico, and Venezuela between 1950 and 1970. Although 1950 data are probably not highly reliable in all of these countries, it does seem probable that about 25 to 30 million hectares have been added to the arable land base in those countries. Argentina has probably added about 3 million hectares during this same span of time. Other smaller countries have also made some marked percentage increases in arable land. Several of the countries of Middle America are among those countries which have had significant proportional increases. Among the major world regions that have just been reviewed, probably Latin America has the greatest opportunities for further expansion of the arable land base in the near future. With a rapidly growing population and with a considerable undeveloped area, Brazil will very likely continue to expand its arable land base substantially. There are also opportunities elsewhere for further expansion, particularly in the wet tropical areas of Latin America.

The expansion of the arable land base of the world from an approximate 1.27 billion hectares in 1950 to 1.42 billion hectares in 1970 represents a very modest increase of about 12% or 0.6% a year. While this expansion of the arable land base has contributed to an increase in world food production, this increase has not been nearly so significant as increases resulting from a substantial improvement of productivity on the arable land already being used for crop production prior to 1950.

The potential for further expansion of arable land was recently carefully studied by Kellogg in terms of the major soil groups of the world and the capability of these soils to be used for crop production. Table 7 summarizes Kellogg's analysis. From this analysis of the potentially arable land, the following areas of the world seem to have the greatest potential for expanding the arable land area: (1) some of the forested humid tropics and subtropics, particularly of Africa and South America; (2) some of the extensive forested areas in the mid-latitudes, particularly the U.S., and (3) some of the areas presently used for grazing in the U.S., U.S.S.R., Australia, New Zealand, and parts of Latin America.

When the present area of arable land totaling 1,424 million hectares is compared with the Kellogg estimate of potentially arable land area of 2,668 million hectares, an approximate doubling of the present arable land area is conceivable. However, it is quite improbable that any significant acceleration in the rate at which additions have been made to the arable land base over the past 20 years is likely to occur unless a number of important political, economic, and demographic circumstances are appreciably altered. Even if a doubling of the expansion rate for arable land is assumed as reasonable for the future, it will take many years to utilize the potential arable land completely. In the foreseeable future capital investments in additional technological inputs for food production seem likely to yield a more substantial return than the investment of available capital in land clearing, drainage, flood control, irrigation, and the numerous other improvements needed to use new land for food production. However, in some areas with a good supply of land potentially useable for crops, the expansion of the area in crops may be economically feasible if a sufficient rising demand for food continues.

AGRICULTURAL SYSTEMS

A very significant influence on the production of food is the system or type of agriculture that has evolved over time in a particular part of the world. One of the most basic questions that surely needs to be raised in evaluating the potentials for increased food production relates to the gains and losses that may result from making major changes in the system or systems of farming being used to produce food; when the U.S. made its dramatic shift to the mechanized agriculture, a significant gain in the cropland base for the production of human food was made since the farmers no longer had to raise the feed on their farms for their horses and mules. Yet from a long-run standpoint, the substitution of oil for soil may not be such a

TABLE 7

Estimated Potentially Arable Land in the World

Soil group on acccompanying soil map	Percent of soil group potentially arable	Hectares potentially arable (millions)
Prairie soils, degraded chernozems	80.0	97
Chernozems and reddish chestnut	70.0	267
Dark gray and black soils of subtropics and tropics	50.0	250
Chestnut, brown, reddish brown	30.0	361
Sierozems, desert	.5	14
Podsols and weakly podsolized	10.0	130
Gray-brown podsolic	65.0	394
Latosols, red-yellow podsolics	35.0	1,126
Red-yellow mediterranean	15.0	17
Soils of mountains	.5	12
Tundra	.0	0
Total		2,668

These criteria were used to define arable land:

1. That reasonably good management would be used including appropriate combinations of adapted crop varieties, water control methods, pest control, and method of plant nutrient maintenance, including some chemical fertilizers.
2. Crops include the ordinary food, fiber, and industrial crops that are normally cultivated as well as fruits, nut crops, rubber, sisal, coffee, tea, cocoa, palms, vines, and meadow crops that may not be cultivated.
3. All regular fallow land is counted, including the natural fallow under shifting cultivation.
4. Irrigation of arid soils is limited by water from streams and wells. Sea water is excluded as a potential source.

(Source: *Farmer's World: The Yearbook of Agriculture,* U.S. Department of Agriculture, Washington, D.C., 1964, 62.)

sweeping step forward for a nation that is rapidly running out of petroleum resources. Certainly the modernization of the production process and the abandonment of systems of agriculture that have evolved over time may not necessarily be the best solution to the resolution of food shortages. When a more specialized monoculture is substituted for a more highly diversified system of agriculture, serious problems may arise in a country not fully prepared for the vagaries of international trade and insect and disease problems.

A great variety of systems or types of agricultural production exist in the world today. These systems have been influenced by environmental conditions and by such cultural circumstances as tradition, technology, and population density. Thus, the paddy rice culture of southeastern Asia exists in a subtropical setting as does rice production in the American Southeast, with both locations reflecting the influence of climate. However, in Southeast Asia the labor intensive approach to rice culture, which has evolved under conditions of dense population, little use of modern technology, and a certain combination of traditions, is strikingly different from the capital intensive system of rice culture of southeastern U.S., which has developed under conditions of low population density, application of much modern technology, and a set of European traditions.

On a worldwide basis, agriculture can be classified into the following four major systems and subtypes:

Ecological or near-ecological primitive migrating systems

Gathering (often combined with hunting and fishing)
Nomadic grazing
Shifting cultivation (sometimes classed as primitive migratory subsistence)

Subsistence systems
Primitive sedentary subsistence
Intensive sedentary subsistence
Near-subsistence Mediterranean

Commercial systems
Tropical and subtropical plantation
Mid-latitude grain farming
Vegetable and fruit culture
Mixed crop and livestock farming
Dairy farming
Livestock ranching

Collective systems
Several of the commercial systems are similar to the collective systems in terms of products produced but the organization and decision-making in the production process differs markedly from that of the commercial systems.

An examination of these several systems of agricultural production clearly indicates that some have been far more significant than others in contributing to the world's supply of food. Looking to the future, it is obvious that very little increase in the production of food is likely to occur under some of the existing systems although a change to other systems of production may lead to significant increases in production in areas where agricultural systems now exist that are not conducive to major increases in food production. A brief review of some of these possibilities is pertinent to an understanding of the status of world food production.

Particularly significant possibilities exist for more food production in some of the areas where the ecological or near-ecological primitive migrating systems now prevail. The gathering subtype occurs mainly in the (1) tropical Amazon and Orinoco River Basins of South America, (2) Congo Basin, Guinea Coast, Kalahari Desert, interior Mozambique, and adjacent areas of Rhodesia and Malawi in Africa, (3) interior areas of Indonesia and New Guinea, (4) interior parts of southwestern Asia, (5) interior western Australia and the Arnhem Land area of northern Australia, and (6) high northern latitudes. Nomadic grazing is found principally in Saharan Africa, the interior steppes of southern Africa, eastern Africa, southwestern Asia, and interior Asia including some of the central Asia area of the U.S.S.R. Shifting cultivation occurs in many parts of the wet tropics of Middle and South America, southeastern Asia, and Africa.

When information on soil quality obtained under the World Soil Geography Project of the U.S. Department of Agriculture is analyzed, it is obvious that much potential cropland not currently being used for that purpose is available in some parts of the world. As previously discussed, the most significant area of potential cropland is in the humid tropics and subtropics of Africa and South America. Thus, such areas as the Amazon and Orinoco River Basins, Indonesia, New Guinea, the Congo Basin, and the areas of shifting cultivation in the wet tropics now have systems of agricultural production which are not compatible with the potential for additional food production in those areas.

In contrast, the high northern latitudes and the desert and steppe areas of primitive migrating systems of agriculture have considerably less promise of increased food production. Lack of water in the interior desert and steppe areas is not likely to be effectively resolved over extensive areas. For some dry coastal areas, desalinization of sea water may permit a change from an extensive to an intensive system of agriculture. The cold northern areas of the U.S.S.R., Canada, Scandinavia, and Alaska have little or no promise of contributing effectively to world food production in spite of considerable experimentation, particularly in the Soviet Union.

The amount of food produced in the areas of subsistence agriculture differs greatly. Nearly all the food produced is consumed by the farm operator and his family. Large inputs of manual labor rather than the use of capital for labor-saving machinery are characteristic of this system of agriculture. Primitive sedentary agriculture is most commonly seen in the highland areas of the tropics. However, in some parts of the wet tropical lowlands, farmers have acquired a sufficient understanding of soil management to remain on the same land without shifting from place to place as does the shifting cultivator. Since much of the primitive sedentary agriculture of the tropical highlands is carried on under adverse conditions of topography and soils, it does not appear that such areas are likely to improve food production substantially in the near future.

Intensive sedentary subsistence agriculture is the way of life for nearly half of the world's people; about two thirds of the world's farmers are operating subsistence farms on an intensive basis. The major concentrations of these farms are in eastern and southern Asia. Only in the Tigris and Euphrates Valleys of Iraq and in the Nile Valley of Egypt are subsistence farms of widespread importance outside eastern and southern Asia. A very high man-land ratio characterizes the areas of intensive sedentary agriculture. Much labor furnished by the farmer and his family is used. Irrigation is a widespread though not a universal practice. Crops dominate the agriculture of such areas since the amount of food that could be obtained from milk, eggs, meat, and other livestock products is much less than through the direct human consumption of the crops grown. However, a hog or two, some chickens, or goats may be kept as scavengers to use crop and other vegetative wastes. In India, millions of cattle are retained without making a really significant contribution to the food supply.

Although great quantities of food are produced under this system of agriculture, it is in these areas of intensive sedentary farming that a great need exists for further improvements. Great ingenuity and much hard work have brought high returns per unit area farmed, but opportunities exist for further increases in yields through the use of higher yielding varieties, fertilizers, pesticides, and other improved practices, which have not been available to these farmers because of a lack of capital or other reasons.

Perhaps in no other system of agriculture is tradition so strong in determining the farming operation. The continuity from one generation to the next has been very strong, since lack of mobility generally prevails among the people of these areas. Japan, however, is an interesting and informative example of a marked change from the traditional subsistence pattern of agriculture to a semisubsistence or semicommercial type. The rapid introduction of small tractors to Japanese farms has brought substantial change, although many of the characteristics of subsistence agriculture still remain on the relatively small farms which produce mainly crops. However, many Japanese farmers now sell a substantial amount of produce.

In the Mediterranean world of western Asia, southern Europe, and northern Africa, a distinctive type of agriculture has evolved under the dry summer subtropical climate. Wheat and barley are grown under winter rainfall with some supplemental irrigation sometimes used. Pulses are also raised in winter for both human food and livestock feed. A great variety of crops are produced during the summer under irrigation. Olives, grapes, and several other fruits are an integral part of the agriculture of this part of the world. Great contrast exists between some of the Mediterranean areas of near-subsistence agriculture and the highly commercialized approach to agricultural production found in the similar climatic regime of southern California. In recent years, some remarkable agricultural gains have occurred in Israel where near-subsistence conditions formerly prevailed in several places. Perhaps the Israeli experience may be duplicated elsewhere; however, it does not appear probable the present Mediterranean areas of near-subsistence agriculture will soon match the much higher levels of production found in California where massive amounts of capital have been invested.

Although large quantities of food are produced under the intensive sedentary subsistence system of agriculture, the main areas of surplus food production are associated with the commercial and collective systems of production. In the U.S., one farmworker is now capable of producing enough food for himself and 50 others.[5] Thus, only about 6% of the economically active population of the U.S. is engaged in agriculture. This capability to produce and sell surplus food is the main characteristic of commercial agriculture. This does not necessarily mean that a country having commercial systems of agriculture is necessarily a net exporter of agricultural commodities, but it does mean that the farmers in an area of commercial agriculture are supplying urban and other nonfarm segments of the population with food. Much use of capital also characterizes commercial agriculture, and purchases of tractors and machinery, fertilizers, pesticides, herbicides, improved plants, better breeds of animals, and other technological innovations are common. Therefore, the commercial farmer becomes quite dependent upon the world around him not only because he needs markets for his products but also because he must buy many things for the farm operation and for the use of his family.

Among the several commercial agricultural systems, the tropical and sub-tropical plantations have played a significant role in some parts of the world. However, with the main exceptions of sugar and bananas, most of the plantations have specialized more in nonfood crops such as natural rubber, cotton, and tea than in the production of food crops. Historically, relatively large numbers of unskilled workers have comprised the labor force for plantation agriculture. Ownership of plantations and the supply of capital for their operation have generally not been indigenous to the areas where plantations are found. Products have been exported to mid-latitude countries.

An interesting transformation of plantation agriculture in the southeastern U.S. is taking place which may have considerable significance for other plantation areas. In recent years a greater emphasis on food crops such as soybeans and rice and the raising of beef cattle has gradually been replacing the historical dominance of cotton and tobacco as the main plantation crops. Many of these neoplantations of the lower alluvial valley of the Mississippi are, for example, among the most efficient units of agricultural production in the U.S. today. A significant question related to the development of a viable commercial agriculture in parts of the wet tropics such as the Amazon Basin may well be: Is the modern neoplantation of the American South likely to be a useful unit of production for such areas?

Mid-latitude grain farming has been renowned for the large quantities of grain produced for consumption elsewhere. The farms are highly mechanized and are situated mainly in areas having a relatively sparse population. Major areas have been the semiarid and subhumid parts of the U.S., Canada, Australia, Argentina, and the U.S.S.R. Although a collective approach to production characterizes the agriculture of the U.S.S.R., the main crops of that part of the world are wheat, barley, rye, and oats which are also grown in the other areas. Grain sorghums have also become a major crop of the southern Great Plains of the U.S. Although the grain farming areas of the mid-latitudes have been major contributors to the world's food supply, it is questionable as to whether or not grain farming should be expanded much further into drier areas in order to increase world supplies of grain. Experience in the U.S.S.R. and in the U.S. and Canada indicates that crop production becomes quite hazardous on these drier margins. In the past, economic incentives associated with World Wars I and II led to excessive expansion of wheat farming in Canada and the U.S. Successive years of severe drought in the 1930's and the 1950's have convinced many farmers that a more extensive system of agriculture such as cattle ranching may be a better long-run adjustment to the climatic conditions of the western part of the American Great Plains. In Siberia, the Soviet Union had a similar unfortunate experience with the plowing up of extensive areas of native grasslands for wheat culture. From these experiences, a cautious concern about the possibility of a substantial increase in food supplies from these areas seems warranted.

In the eastern U.S.; western, central, and eastern Europe; South Africa; and in southern Brazil, northeastern Argentina, and in Chile, south of about the 38° parallel, the mixing of crop and livestock production on the same farm unit on a commercial basis has resulted in a highly productive agricultural system supplying great quantities of food. For the most part the farms are not as large in the areas of mixed crop and livestock farming as in the areas of commercial grain farming. However, one of the most pervasive trends in the American Midwest has been an increase in the size of the farm since the 1920's. The degree to which the mixing of crop and livestock production occurs varies greatly. In the American Midwest, corn, soybeans, alfalfa, and some oats and wheat constitute the main crops grown. Hogs and beef and dairy cattle are the main livestock raised. However, it is not likely that all of these crops and livestock would be raised on any one farm.

In Europe mixed crop and livestock farming generally require smaller farms and less mechanization than American farms. There is also less emphasis on beef cattle and hogs. However, the use of animal manures is still an integral part of European farming to a much greater degree than in the U.S., where a much greater reliance is being placed on inorganic fertilizers. Sugar beets, potatoes, and rye are much more important crops in parts of Europe than in the American Midwest. Much less corn is grown except in the Danube Basin and practically no soybeans are raised.

In the areas of mixed crop and livestock farming, most of the land resources capable of being used for agriculture are now being used for that purpose. Consequently, there is little opportunity to expand the agricultural base in these parts of the world. However, in spite of the fact that areas such as the American Midwest have made great use of a wide array of technological innovations, there is still a significant potential for further increases in agricultural output through the investment of still more capital in such things as fertilizers, improvements in plant and animal breeding, better conservation practices, pesticides, herbicides, and improvement in storage facilities to reduce losses. However, a favorable price structure for agricultural commodities will be needed to encourage more use of capital in agricultural production in these parts of the world, for lucrative alternative investment opportunities are available in these same geographical areas.

Commercial production of vegetables and fruits is found in association with urban concentrations of population, although not necessarily in close proximity to urban centers. A great variation in the size of vegetable and fruit producing farms exists in different parts of the world and even within the same geographical areas. Large corporate- or family-owned units such as the pineapple plantations of Hawaii or the citrus groves of Florida contrast markedly with small family-operated market gardens found close to many European cities. Many different fruits and vegetables are produced and marketed in a great variety of ways and under different circumstances of location. Fruits are sold canned, dried, frozen, and fresh. Vegetables are shipped fresh from Florida, Texas, California, and Arizona during fall, winter, and spring months to northern markets; the quick-freezing and canning of vegetables is of much significance in the U.S. but of much less importance elsewhere. Some of the production of these crops takes place under highly artificial circumstances such as in greenhouses and with the use of plastic coverings. On the other hand, fruit production in particular, as well as many vegetable-producing areas, is located in those areas having the most favorable natural conditions for efficient production.

In the U.S. and to some extent in Europe, the production of fruits and vegetables is being greatly affected by the rising cost of labor and a relative inability to mechanize the harvesting of these crops. Unionization of farm labor in California and Florida is making a significant impact on the cost of production, processing, and marketing in areas where migratory and other relatively large pools of inexpensive labor previously could be found. While an improvement in the wages for such workers has long been overdue, the American housewife is now being faced with substantial price increases for such products, which may cause a significant shift in the patterns of food consumption. Synthetic orange drinks, for example, are giving Florida citrus growers severe competition at the present time.

Similarly, but under different circumstances, commercial dairying has a labor problem that is more subtle in its impact upon milk production. The three major areas of commercial dairying are found in (1) northwestern Europe, southern Scandinavia, the Baltic-Moscow area of the Soviet Union, and the Baltic area of East Germany and Poland; (2) the northeastern states and the southern parts of the Great Lakes States (Wisconsin, Michigan, and Minnesota) in the U.S.; (3) New Zealand, Tasmania, and adjacent coastal areas of Australia. Secondary and smaller areas of considerable importance in the U.S. are found in the Puget Sound-Willamette Valley areas of Washington and Oregon and in California. Milk and other dairy products have long been an integral part of the diet of millions of people, particularly in western, central, and eastern Europe, U.S., Canada, Australia, New Zealand, and South Africa. In many areas having dense populations and a high man-land ratio with little opportunity to trade, milk has been a much less important food.

Particularly in the major milk-producing areas of the U.S., a considerable change in the type of dairy farm is taking place. Dairying needs much labor and capital. Cows must be milked seven days a week and all year long. As the present generation of dairy farmers is retiring, many dairy farms are shifting to the production of other agricultural commodities since the younger generation is generally not willing to operate farms requiring such large amounts of responsible labor when other jobs are available in the nearby urban centers at much higher wages. Thus, a significant change in the system of dairying is occurring in some places. Farms are being greatly increased in size and corporate ownership and salaried managers are becoming more common in many parts of the U.S.

An assessment of livestock ranching results in a general conclusion that the major areas of the world where livestock ranching is the dominant or a significant system for the production of food are not likely to experience any major shift to a more intensive type of agriculture in the near future. Livestock ranching is now found mainly in those areas of the world which are not well suited to crop production; therefore, a serious physical limitation exists which will be generally quite expensive or even economically impossible to correct in the near future. The major regions of livestock ranching are (1) western U.S. and Canada and northern Mexico; (2) much of Australia except eastern, southern, and northern coastal areas and the dry interior desert; (3) much of the South Island of New Zealand; (4) southern interior Africa south of approximately 12° S latitude; (5) llanos of Venezuela and eastern Colombia; (6) eastern Brazil and Bolivia, Paraguay, Uruguay, central Chile, and Argentina except the pampas; (7) U.S.S.R. immediately east and southeast of the Caspian Sea and the Kirghiz steppe area.[6]

Although livestock ranching makes a significant contribution to the world's supply of beef and mutton, the amount of food produced per unit of area is generally quite low. The carrying capacity of arid and semiarid grazing land is low and several hectares are needed to support one animal unit. In the U.S. cattle are generally shipped from the range lands to areas of surplus feed such as the Midwest and California. Some irrigated areas within the western states have also developed the capability of producing sufficient feed to establish important feedlot operations.

In some parts of the world collective systems of agriculture have now been operating for several years. Particularly in the U.S.S.R. and in Eastern Europe much change in the systems of agriculture has resulted from the reorganization of production under a system of collective and state farms. However, the kinds of crops and livestock being grown have not changed as much as have the production processes used in raising them. The completeness of the changes made in producing agricultural commodities on collective and state farms of the Soviet Union, in contrast to the former peasant agriculture, raises an interesting question relevant to resolving the growing demand for food. Has a significant increase in food output resulted from the changes instituted in Soviet agriculture? A reliable answer to such a sweeping question is of course extremely difficult to obtain, since there is little opportunity to make valid historical comparisons with peasant agriculture operating under similar environmental conditions. However, some of the experiences under foreign aid programs of the U.S. indicate rather clearly that decision-making divorced from the cultural milieu of a particular system of agriculture may not necessarily lead to significant progress in raising levels of food production. Generally it is very difficult to change an agricultural system without first winning the confidence of the prospective participants, which seems a necessary first step to make an effective break with tradition. Experience with new federal agricultural programs in the U.S. during the 1930's offers substantial documentation of considerable difficulty in making changes. Yet change will be a necessary ingredient of any major expansion in agricultural output.

Undoubtedly many changes in systems of agricultural production are needed and in many instances such changes may have to be induced. However, the careful study of the existing system and a careful evaluation of the gains and losses that may be expected from induced changes both in the short run and the long run should precede any large-scale efforts to effectuate changes in systems of agriculture in order to expand food production.

Significant but often subtle changes in agriculture have occurred as direct or indirect results of events or outside interference. Three major new crops have been introduced into American agricultural systems within the past 50 years because of a combination of circumstances including the institution of crop allotments on such crops as wheat and cotton. In 1920 there were fewer than 8 million hectares (18 million acres) of alfalfa, grain sorghums, and soybeans on American farms. In 1970 the harvested area of these three crops amounted to 32 million hectares (88 million acres). Increased emphasis on poultry, particularly broilers, and the use of a large-scale mass production process have been other major changes in American agriculture. Concurrently a de-emphasis of such crops as cotton, oats, and wheat has occurred. Thus, the product mix may change significantly without concurrent major changes in the process taking place.

The substitution of soybeans for oats and cotton and sorghums for wheat is an example of a change in the product mix that has not been accompanied by any significant reorganization of the production process. In contrast, broiler production is now organized quite differently in the U.S. from the 1920's when most chickens were produced in small flocks on nearly every American farm. Product changes such as these are of course most likely to occur in those parts of the world where the physical environment permits a greater variety of crops to be grown. Yet the introduction of grain sorghums into the agriculture of the southern Great Plains is an example of a major shift occurring in a more restrictive natural environment.

INCREASING WORLD FOOD PRODUCTION

A review of the prospects of increasing food production in different parts of the world reveals a great variety or combinations of possible approaches and conditions. The resource base, capital and labor availability, access to a wide array of technology, degree of economic incentive, and the framework of social, political, and other institutional conditions are all worthy of careful attention in assessing the prospects for increasing the food production of any country. It is also quite important to understand the complementarity of circumstances that contribute to successful breakthroughs in food production. Furthermore, it is important to recognize that the increases in food production are not so likely to be immediate and striking, but rather such changes may be gradual and uneven in occurrence. There is a rather inevitable lag in the farmer's response to a changing set of conditions. For example, it took fully a quarter of a century to make the change from animate to inanimate power on American farms. Similarly, hybrid corn took a considerable period of time for adoption throughout the U.S., even though agricultural research and extension personnel throughout the country were quite aware of its potential for increasing yields.

An examination of the world's land resources has clearly established the fact that much land not currently being used to produce food could be so used from the standpoint of physical capability. However, the development of new lands for agricultural production will face many obstacles in the future just as in the past. An historical examination of the agricultural development of the North American continent is replete with economic, political, and social impediments that hindered progress. In the colonial period the emphasis on the production of export crops often prevented a well-rounded agricultural economy from developing. Later the great clash between the industrial North and the agricultural South had a major impact. More recently several regional problems have delayed the harmonious culmination of an efficient and balanced pattern of agriculture in the U.S. and Canada.

Remoteness of undeveloped areas historically has been, and still is today for extensive areas of the wet tropics, a major handicap to balanced agricultural development. Lack of an effective transportation system which offers contact with those areas needing agricultural commodities has generally been one of the first major difficulties to be surmounted in bringing new lands into production. In the U.S. major subsidies were given by the several states for canal building and soon thereafter both state and the federal governments began a massive subsidization of railroad building. There were many false starts and failures, but in the end an efficient system of transportation evolved, which has contributed greatly to the success of American agriculture. And so today Brazil and other countries of Latin America as well as the countries of tropical Africa need to develop a network of transportation facilities that permit the efficient movement of commodities. Such a transportation system costs much money and takes time to develop – at least a half a century in the U.S. For today's world a crucial question to be asked is: Can the developmental period be reduced?

In order to bring about agricultural development on new lands, a considerable economic incentive will be needed. Not only must this incentive include large initial outlays of capital but also a continued willingness to provide subsidies from capital resources that may be woefully small in relation to the many demands for such capital. The need for manufacturing industries and the prestige of industrial development have often led to a general neglect of the agricultural sector. Certainly documentary evidence of such neglect could be found in American history. Ideally, progress in increasing agricultural output should go hand in hand with the creation of new opportunities for employment and investment of capital in the nonagricultural sectors of a developing economy. However, this has generally been extremely difficult to achieve.

Yet another internal condition which generally plays a major role in agricultural development is the pattern of land ownership and tenancy which exists. All too frequently it has been extremely difficult to bring about necessary land reforms to accommodate the rapidly changing conditions of an expanding agricultural economy. In the U.S. the ownership of land by the federal government necessitated the establishment of governmental policy for the disposal of the public domain. The Homestead Act of 1862, which had been preceded by numerous other acts dealing with the sale of public lands, was not adequate at the time it was passed. The frontier of agriculture of the 1860's had reached lands where physical conditions dictated the need for much more land than 160 acres for the creation of successful new farms. Tradition, tribal ownership, problems of federation, existence of large landholdings, need for long-term credit, and many other problems confront those nations needing to expand their agricultural production onto new lands as well as to increase output per unit area.

If these problems, which, except for the availability of capital, are mainly internal in nature, are not enough, there are other conditions which hamper the development of new land for agriculture in some parts of the world. Paramount in the realm of international deterrents are the many restrictions on the movement of people and commodities among countries. Since 1923, the U.S. has had a strict quota on the number of persons who can enter the country from abroad. While one may effectively agree that the transfer of people from one part of the world to another may not necessarily lead to any marked improvement in the level of living for the world as a whole, there is the probability that freer movement of people among the nations of the world might eventually eliminate some striking inequities that now exist.

Restrictions on the flow of commodities of various kinds have long been a factor influencing agricultural development. Not only has the reality of trade restrictions been present for a long time, but also there has been endless change and vacillation which often leads to the commitment of scarce capital and other resources for development to produce commodities which may become disadvantaged in world trade because of the action taken by another nation or a group of countries. In the past two decades the growing importance of economic communities of countries such as the European Economic Community has not led to any major diminution in the level of restrictions on the movement of goods in international trade. Rather some agonizing readjustments have been taking place and several countries that are organizing into regional blocs have replaced some of the more heterogeneous and haphazard arrangements for international trade. It certainly remains to be seen whether or not such arrangements will contribute to any general improvement in world living conditions.

During the next decade or two if not longer, improvements in the present status of world food production will probably come from continuing application of new technology rather than from bringing new lands into agricultural production. Yet, it must be emphasized that in some parts of the world, advances on both of these fronts offer considerable promise if certain impediments can be overcome. Changes in the systems of agriculture now prevailing must be made with great care. The present patterns of food production have for the most part developed over a span of many years, even hundreds of years. Peasant farmers in many different parts of the world have generally continued to use the same farming practices as used by their ancestors, the same crops, and the same varieties of seed. These approaches to food production have proved to be the most reliable and have sustained life from generation to generation for those who do not have the educational background to understand how other practices and other varieties might yield better results. In those parts of the world where a bare level of existence prevails, experimentation with new ideas may be disastrous. Acceptance of technological innovation may come slowly and only after new techniques have clearly been proved reliable.

Much technological innovation in agriculture has become available in recent years. For example, new varieties of rice, wheat, and corn have been developed; because each of these crops is an important source of food in different parts of the developing world, the introduction of these high-yielding varieties could play a significant role in bringing about increased food production. Since many of the peasant farmers of the world are keenly aware of their plight, clear demonstration of opportunities for improved yields may lead these farmers to break with tradition and to adopt the new seeds, fertilizers, and pesticides if the necessary credit or money can be obtained. Certainly this is not an easy accomplishment to achieve over extensive areas, but the remarkable initial impact of new rice and wheat varieties developed in the Philippines and in Mexico, respectively, gives good reason for the hope that substantial improvement can be achieved. Yet it obviously will not be easy to sustain the momentum of the striking initial impact of the introduction of new technology in the face of highly diverse and long-established traditional systems of agriculture. For example, expansion of irrigation will be needed to make the introduction of new crop varieties possible in some areas. This will cost money and the competition for scarce capital may lead to delays in providing for the total package of improvement that will yield the greatest return. It is often very difficult to impress persons in positions of responsibility of the great importance of an integrated and comprehensive approach to the adoption of new techniques rather than a piecemeal selection of innovation over an extended period of time. Pressures are often too great to permit the "package" approach to acceptance of innovation. It is much easier to accept one or two new ideas at a time rather than a whole complex of interrelated technology.

As in the analysis of expanding agricultural activity onto lands not previously used for the purpose, it is quite evident that technological expansion will be confronted by many of the same difficult problems. Among these are lack of capital and credit, need for general and technical education, resolution of the difficult and longstanding need for land reform in some areas, and the obvious need for strong stable economic incentives that will assure that the initial momentum of acceptance of improved technology can be maintained and even deployed to meet other needs.

The relation of agriculture to other sectors of the economy is in many countries an unfavorable circumstance in terms of economic incentive. Maintenance of a balance among the several sectors of the economy has been extremely difficult in the more industrialized countries of the world and has often led to a de-emphasis of the agricultural sector. Even in developing countries, agriculture is often in the less favored position. Employment opportunities and wage scales offer considerable incentives for labor to leave the rural areas for the city. Sometimes this movement of labor off the farm occurs in advance of the creation of new employment opportunities in other sectors of the economy, thus leading to unemployment and social and political unrest. Ideally the introduction of technological improvements in the agricultural sectors should go hand in hand with the development of other sectors of the economy in developing nations. The enhanced productivity of agriculture possible with a reduced labor force would support the need for food and some of the raw materials for the other sectors of the economy, thus reducing to some extent the dependence on international markets for both the agricultural and nonagricultural products of a developing country.

Most difficult and complex of all of the conditions that are barriers to changing the status of world food production are the political, social, and other institutional arrangements and traditions that exist today. Change comes slowly, and sometimes such change is regressive rather than progressive. Attempts to interfere in the internal affairs of nations in order to facilitate economic improvements are often unsuccessful. Yet there is an obvious need for international assistance and cooperation if improvements are to be made. Certainly improvements in diets and increased food production are among the world's most pressing needs now and in the foreseeable future.

REFERENCES

1. U.N., Food and Agriculture Organization, *Production Yearbook, 1970,* Rome, 1971, 9.
2. **Abbott, G. W.,** *Agriculture in Australia: With Emphasis on Trade with Far East Countries,* Economic Research Service, U.S. Department of Agriculture, Washington, D. C., 1969, 3.
3. **Abbott, G. W.,** *Agriculture in Australia: With Emphasis on Trade with Far East Countries,* Economic Research Service, U.S. Department of Agriculture, Washington, D. C., 1969, 2.
4. **Tegeler, H. H.,** *Agriculture of West Asia,* Economic Research Service, U.S. Department of Agriculture, Washington, D.C., 1966, 4.
5. U.S. Department of Agriculture, *Farm Index,* Washington, D.C., July, 1972, 4.
6. **Anderson, J. R.,** *A Geography of Agriculture,* Wm. C. Brown Co., Dubuque, Iowa, 1970, 99.

WORLD POPULATION GROWTH AND FUTURE FOOD TRENDS

C. Clark
J. Boyd Turner

TABLE OF CONTENTS

Introduction 55

Population 56

Calorie Requirements 64

Protein Requirements 67

Calorie Protein Interaction 67

Requirement and Availability 70

Spending Income 70

Policy Implications 75
- Food Supply Fertility Linkage 75
- Quantity Before Quality - The Peasant Is No Fool 75
- Income to Buy Food 75
- Food at Low Prices 75
- Employment to Get Income 76
- Transport to Distribute Food 76

Conclusion 76

References 76

INTRODUCTION

Barring major famine, epidemic, or war, the world population is likely to increase from about 3,600 million in 1970 to about 6,500 million in the year 2000 AD. At that time world population will still be growing rapidly. As an almost entirely abstract estimate, using the United Nations medium variant of population projection, world population may stop growing at a size of 13,500 million in 2100 AD. However, it is during the next 15 years, to 1985, that population will be growing at the rate of 2% annually. Thereafter, the rate is likely to be lower, though for several decades large absolute increases in population will continue.

Following population growth, food needs will at least double between 1970 and 2000. Current undernutrition, desire for greater variety of diet, and the fact that, where possible, food consumption is greater than strict physiological needs combine to make the demand for food increase more rapidly than population increase.

POPULATION[1]

During the 19th century, the total world population increased at 0.5% annually, and at 0.8% annually during the first half of this century. Since 1950, despite the marked fertility declines in the more developed regions, the unprecedented declines in world mortality rates, without a corresponding decrease in fertility rates of the less developed regions, has brought about a rapid increase in world population, at a rate of 1.8% annually in the 1950's and at 2.0% annually in the 1960's. How long will this rate of increase continue?

The United Nations variant of rate of population increase "considered the most plausible" is the medium variant. It postulates a continuing 2.0% annual increase until 1985, with a gradual slowdown thereafter. Population is not evenly distributed around the earth and there is considerable variation about this aggregate growth rate. Table 1 shows the total population for 1960 to 2000, crude birth rate and crude death rate for 1965 to 2000, and expectation of life at birth and gross reproduction rates for the years 1965 to 1985, in major areas and regions of the world.

The largest increase in population is expected in South Asia, which contains about one third of the world's population – predominantly India, Indonesia, and Pakistan (now Pakistan and Bangla Desh). The next region of importance is East Asia. Although its population is increasing only at an estimated moderate rate, the sheer size of China leads to large absolute increases. A considerable increase in population is also expected in Latin America and Africa. Table 2 shows the current and conjectured population of selected countries.

The decade of the 1970's may show a rate of world population increase reaching a maximum, to plateau for a period, and then decline. Medium variant projections show little change in the total world rate of 2.0 to 2.1% annually for the period 1970 to 1985. More developed regions (Europe, the U.S.S.R., Northern America, Japan, Temperate South America, Australia, and New Zealand) will grow at 1.0 to 1.1% annually, and the less developed regions (the remainder of the world) at 2.4 to 2.5% annually. Currently, rates of growth are highest in Latin America and South Asia. Because of its already low mortality rates compared with other less developed regions, the Latin American rate of population increase is likely to continue at 2.8 to 2.9% annually for the period. In South Asia, a decline in the natural increase rate is expected, from 2.8% annually in 1965 to 1970 to 2.6% annually in 1980 to 1985. With low fertility levels in Japan and an estimated moderate fertility rate in China, East Asian growth rates of population in 1965 to 1970, 1.8% annually, currently the lowest among the less developed regions, are expected to decline to 1.5% annually during the forecast period. On the other hand, in Africa, the rate of increase in 1965 to 1970, 2.6% annually, may rise to 3.0% annually in 1980 to 1985, as African mortality rates, currently the highest in the world, fall and approach those of other less developed regions. The very low death rates of some countries, such as Japan at 7.5 per thousand, are due to youthful populations. Such death rates are projected to pass through a minimum and then approach the death rates of the more developed regions.

Crude birth rates and crude death rates in the more developed regions are projected to remain virtually constant at 19 and 9 per 1,000, respectively. Slight variations in crude birth rates are due mainly to favorable changes in population age structure. Increase in death rates is entirely due to continued aging of the population. The Soviet Union is expected to have a slight increase in fertility and Eastern Europe a decline.

The less developed regions present a different picture. Large increases in life expectancy and declines in crude death rates are expected for all countries of this group. Life expectancy at birth will increase on the average by 8 years, from 50 to 58. In South Asia, life expectancy at birth may rise from 49 to 58 years during the two decades 1965 to 1985, in East Asia from 52 to 61 years, in Africa from 43 to 51 years, and in Latin America, the smallest increase, from 60 to 66½ years. Projected African gross reproduction rates are stable throughout the forecast period; the decline in crude birth rate from 47 per 1,000 to 45 per 1,000 is the result of change in age structure with decline in mortality. In Latin America, the fertility decline is likely to be moderate, with a large drop in Tropical South America and a small decline in Temperate South America. Substantial declines in fertility are expected in South Asia and East Asia. Fertility declines in Korea, Taiwan, Singapore, and Hong Kong have already been large.[2] In these less developed regions, a virtually constant rate of population growth of 2.4 to 2.5% annually results as birth rates and death rates decline equally.

TABLE 1

Part 1: Total Population and Expectation of Life (U.N. Medium Variant)

Areas and regions	Total population 1960	1970	1980	1990	2000	Expectation of life at birth 1965-1970	1970-1975	1975-1980	1980-1985
			(In millions)				(Years)		
World total[a,b]	2986	3632	4457	5438	6494	53	56	58	60
More developed regions[a]	976	1090	1210	1336	1454	70	71	72	72
Less developed regions[a]	2010	2542	3247	4102	5040	50	52	55	58
East Asia	785	930	1095	1265	1424	52	55	58	61
Mainland region	645	765	901	1043	1176	50	53	56	59
Japan	93	103	116	125	133	71	73	74	74
Other East Asia	47	61	78	97	115	60	63	65	68
South Asia	865	1126	1486	1912	2354	49	52	55	58
Middle South Asia	588	762	1001	1280	1565	48	51	54	57
Southeast Asia	219	287	380	492	608	50	53	56	59
Southwest Asia	58	77	104	140	181	51	54	57	60
Europe	425	462	497	533	568	71	72	72	73
Western Europe	135	149	158	169	179	72	72	73	73
Southern Europe	118	128	140	152	163	70	71	72	72
Eastern Europe	97	104	112	120	127	71	72	73	73
Northern Europe	76	81	86	93	99	72	73	73	74
Soviet Union	214	243	271	302	330	70	71	71	72
Africa	270	344	457	616	818	43	46	49	51
Western Africa	80	101	133	180	240	39	42	44	47
Eastern Africa	77	98	129	174	233	42	45	47	50
Middle Africa	29	36	46	60	80	39	42	44	47
Northern Africa	65	87	119	163	214	50	53	56	59
Southern Africa	18	23	29	38	50	48	50	53	55
Northern America	199	228	261	299	333	70	71	71	71
Latin America	213	283	377	500	652	60	62	65	67
Tropical South America	112	151	204	272	358	60	62	64	67
Middle American Mainland	48	67	95	132	180	60	63	65	67
Temperate South America	33	39	47	55	63	65	66	68	69
Caribbean	21	26	32	40	50	58	60	62	64
Oceania	15.8	19.4	24.0	29.6	35.2	65	66	68	64
Australia and New Zealand	12.7	15.4	18.8	22.7	26.2	72	72	72	73
Melanesia	2.2	2.8	3.6	4.7	6.1	47	50	53	56
Polynesia and Micronesia	0.9	1.2	1.7	2.2	2.9	61	64	66	68

[a]Totals for the world, more developed, and less developed regions have been adjusted for discrepancies between regional assumptions of immigration and emigration.
[b]1965-1985 projections based on country-by-country basis and are provided by 5-year-age groupings for each sex and by single years for 5 to 24 years.

(Source: *U.N. Population Study, No. 49,* September, 1971).

TABLE 1 (Continued)

Part 2: Crude Birth Rates, Crude Death Rate, and Gross Reproduction Rate (U.N. Medium Variant)

Areas and regions	Crude birth rate						Crude death rate						Gross reproduction rate			
	1965–1970	1970–1975	1975–1980	1980–1985	1985–1990	1990–2000	1965–1970	1970–1975	1975–1980	1980–1985	1985–1990	1990–2000	1965–1970	1970–1975	1975–1980	1980–1985
	Per thousand						Per thousand									
World total[a,b]	33.8	33.2	32.1	30.9			14.0	12.8	11.6	10.5			2.3	2.2	2.1	2.0
More developed regions[a]	18.6	18.9	19.5	19.5			9.1	9.2	9.3	9.4			1.3	1.3	1.3	1.3
Less developed regions[a]	40.6	39.0	37.0	34.9			16.1	14.3	12.5	10.9			2.7	2.6	2.5	2.3
East Asia	31.5	29.1	27.0	25.1	22.9	20.2	14.0	12.3	11.0	10.0	9.2	8.3	2.0	1.8	1.7	1.5
Mainland region	33.1	30.2	27.8	25.9			15.3	13.4	11.9	10.6			2.1	1.9	1.7	1.6
Japan	18.0	18.6	18.1	15.9			7.0	6.6	6.8	7.5			1.0	1.0	1.1	1.1
Other East Asia	34.7	32.5	31.4	30.1			9.7	8.4	7.4	6.6			2.5	2.3	2.1	1.9
South Asia	44.3	43.9	40.0	36.9	33.7	28.3	16.8	14.8	12.7	10.9	9.3	7.6	3.0	3.0	2.8	2.5
Middle South Asia	44.4	42.9	39.8	36.6			17.2	15.3	13.1	11.2			3.0	3.0	2.7	2.5
Southeast Asia	44.2	42.6	39.9	36.9			16.1	14.1	12.1	10.4			3.0	3.0	2.8	2.6
Southwest Asia	43.6	43.0	41.7	39.9			15.6	13.8	12.0	10.4			3.1	3.1	3.0	2.8
Europe	18.0	17.9	17.9	17.9	17.7	17.0	10.2	10.3	10.4	10.6	10.6	10.4	1.3	1.3	1.2	1.2
Western Europe	17.5	17.1	17.1	17.4			11.0	11.1	11.2	11.3			1.3	1.3	1.3	1.3
Southern Europe	19.4	19.1	18.9	18.9			9.3	9.3	9.4	9.8			1.3	1.3	1.3	1.3
Eastern Europe	17.3	17.4	17.4	16.8			9.5	9.6	9.8	10.2			1.2	1.1	1.1	1.1
Northern Europe	17.6	18.0	18.3	18.6			11.1	11.1	11.2	11.0			1.3	1.3	1.3	1.3
Soviet Union	17.9	18.5	19.8	20.4	19.4	17.8	7.7	8.0	8.3	8.7	9.1	9.1	1.2	1.2	1.3	1.3
Africa	46.8	46.6	46.1	45.2	43.4	39.5	21.3	19.2	17.2	15.4	13.6	11.2	3.1	3.1	3.1	3.1
Western Africa	48.8	48.7	48.4	47.9			24.3	22.1	20.2	18.3			3.2	3.2	3.2	3.2
Eastern Africa	46.6	46.4	46.0	45.5			21.8	19.8	17.9	16.1			3.1	3.1	3.1	3.1
Middle Africa	45.3	45.8	45.3	45.7			24.3	22.2	20.2	18.4			2.9	2.9	2.9	3.0
Northern Africa	46.9	46.5	45.4	42.9			16.9	14.8	12.9	10.9			3.2	3.2	3.2	3.0
Southern Africa	40.7	40.4	40.1	39.7			17.4	15.8	14.3	13.0			2.7	2.7	2.8	2.8

TABLE 1 (Continued)

Part 2: Crude Birth Rates, Crude Death Rate, and Gross Reproduction Rate (U.N. Medium Variant)

Areas and regions	Crude birth rate						Crude death rate						Gross reproduction rate			
	1965–1970	1970–1975	1975–1980	1980–1985	1985–1990	1990–2000	1965–1970	1970–1975	1975–1980	1980–1985	1985–1990	1990–2000	1965–1970	1970–1975	1975–1980	1980–1985
Northern America	19.3	20.3	21.7	22.1	21.3	18.7	9.4	9.5	9.4	9.2	9.0	8.8	1.4	1.3	1.3	1.3
Latin America	38.4	37.6	36.6	35.5	34.1	32.0	10.0	8.9	7.9	7.0	6.4	5.6	2.7	2.6	2.5	2.4
Tropical South America	39.8	38.9	37.8	36.3			10.0	8.8	7.7	6.8			2.8	2.7	2.6	2.4
Middle American Mainland	43.7	42.7	41.4	40.2			10.1	8.7	7.6	6.6			3.1	3.1	2.9	2.8
Temperate South America	26.3	25.5	24.8	24.1			9.1	8.8	8.5	8.3			1.8	1.7	1.6	1.6
Caribbean	35.0	33.8	33.0	32.3			10.9	9.9	9.1	8.5			2.4	2.3	2.2	2.1
Oceania	24.5	25.6	25.9	26.3	25.6	22.6	10.0	9.3	8.9	8.5	8.1	7.7	1.7	1.7	1.7	1.7
Australia and New Zealand	29.2	21.7	22.5	22.6			8.7	8.3	8.2	8.1			1.4	1.4	1.4	1.4
Melanesia	41.7	41.4	39.6	40.1			17.6	15.7	13.8	12.2			2.9	2.9	2.8	2.8
Polynesia and Micronesia	39.7	38.0	35.4	36.4			8.8	7.5	6.4	5.8			2.9	2.6	2.4	2.4

[a]Totals for the world, more developed, and less developed regions have been adjusted for discrepancies between regional assumptions of immigration and emigration.
[b]1965-1985 projections based on country-by-country basis and are provided by 5-year-age groupings for each sex and by single years for 5 to 24 years.

(Source: *U.N. Population Study No. 49*, September, 1971.)

TABLE 2

Estimated Population of Selected Countries

(millions)

	1965	1970	1975	1980	1985
India	487	555	633	717	808
Indonesia	105	121	140	161	184
Pakistan*	116	137	162	191	224
China	695	760	826	894	965

*Includes Bangla Desh

(Source: *U.N. Population Study No. 49,* September, 1971.)

Regarding population age structure, Table 3 shows the percentage age distribution of the world and major regions for 1965 and 1985, distribution by number for 1970 and 1980, and average annual rates of increase for each group. In the more developed regions, children under 15 years of age compose 28% of the total population, 42% in less developed regions. Working age group (15 to 64 years of age) is 63% and 55%, respectively. Thus, the more developed regions have a lower dependency ratio as well as a higher labor productivity. Persons 65 years of age and over compose 9% and 3% of the population, respectively. In all regions except Africa, the proportion of children is likely to decline. In Africa during 1965 to 1985, the proportion of children is likely to increase, from about 43.5% to 45%, and the proportion of economically active persons is expected to fall by 2% to 52%.

In the more developed regions, between 1965 and 1985, the proportion of economically active population is stable at about 63%, the percentage of children declining by 2% to 26%. In less developed regions the rate of growth of working age population is steady at 2.5% annually; the rate of increase of young children (0 to 4 years) shows a steady decline and that of school children (5 to 14 years) is projected to reach a maximum in 1975 to 1980, and decline thereafter. Both regions show high initial rates of aging of population. While that of the more developed regions is projected to decline rapidly, in less developed regions the rate of increase of persons aged 65 and over rises to a high 3.3% annually. As life expectancy at birth in less developed regions rises markedly and fertility begins to decline faster than mortality, this rapid aging of population is likely to continue. From 1970 to 1980, the absolute increase in aged in the more developed regions is 21% of regional total population increase, against 5% of population increase in less developed regions.

Of major importance is internal migration, notably from rural to urban areas. Table 4 shows that in 1970 to 1980, the highest rates of urban growth are found in Africa, 5% per annum, then in South Asia 4.5% per annum, Latin America 4.2% per annum and East Asia 3.8% per annum. While absolute numbers in urban groups are projected to increase rapidly, rural populations will also continue to increase at a moderately high rate. For the decade 1970 to 1980, regarding rural populations in the less developed regions, South Asia has the highest rate of increase, 2.3% annually, then Africa 2.2%, Latin America 1.0%, and East Asia 0.8% annually. Considerable variation is found within these broad divisions, especially in Latin America.

Major war has been found to retard population growth in the region of conflict by about ten years.

As life expectancy at birth rises, and a healthy life is the common lot, a situation of demographic immortality, to use Borrie's[3] phrase, is emerging. World potential fertility approaches its biological maximum, i.e., its fecundability, when nearly all women live healthily from menarche to menopause. A steady-state population has, by definition, constant age-specific fertility rates, a birth rate equal to the death rate, at 13 per 1,000, and, assuming only biological mortality, that is, with no exogenous causes of death, the age structure is constant at 24% of population 65 years of age and above.[4] The net reproduction rate of such a population is 1.0.

Much current discussion, reasonable and un-

TABLE 3

Age Distribution Population Size
Annual Growth Rate of Age Groups:
Percentage Distribution of Age Groups
(U.N. Medium Variant)

	(In millions)		(In percent)			
	1970	1980	1965–1970	1970–1975	1975–1980	1980–1985
World total						
All ages	3632	4457	2.0	2.0	2.1	2.0
0–4	508	612	2.1	2.0	1.8	1.6
5–14	836	1021	1.6	1.8	2.2	2.0
15–64	2098	2577	2.0	2.1	2.0	2.2
65 and over	189	246	2.6	2.7	2.5	1.8
More developed regions						
All ages	1090	1210	1.0	1.0	1.1	1.1
0–4	96	113	–0.5	1.5	1.7	1.1
5–14	196	199	0.4	–0.2	0.5	1.6
15–64	693	768	1.2	1.1	1.0	1.0
65 and over	105	130	2.5	2.4	1.9	0.4
Less developed regions						
All ages	2542	3247	2.4	2.5	2.4	2.4
0–4	412	500	2.8	2.1	1.8	1.7
5–14	640	822	2.0	2.4	2.6	2.1
15–64	1405	1809	2.5	2.6	2.5	2.7
65 and over	84	117	2.8	3.2	3.3	3.3

(In percent)

	1965				1985			
Major Area	0–4	5–14	15–64	65 and over	0–4	5–14	15–64	65 and over
World total	37.4		57.6	5.0	36.3		58.2	5.5
More developed regions	28.1		63.0	8.9	26.2		63.4	10.4
Less developed regions	41.6		55.1	3.3	39.8		56.4	3.8
East Asia	12.9	24.0	59.0	4.1	11.1	20.6	63.0	5.3
South Asia	16.9	26.1	54.0	3.0	15.5	26.5	54.6	3.4
Europe	8.7	16.7	64.1	10.5	8.6	16.2	63.3	11.8
U.S.S.R.	10.2	20.4	62.1	7.4	9.7	16.5	64.3	9.4
Africa	17.7	25.8	53.7	2.8	18.1	26.9	52.0	3.0
Northern America	10.6	20.4	59.8	9.2	10.5	18.2	61.6	9.8
Latin America	16.5	26.0	53.9	3.6	15.8	25.6	54.5	4.1
Oceania	11.8	21.0	59.9	7.3	12.0	20.4	60.1	7.5

(**Source:** *U.N. Population Study No. 49,* September, 1971.)

TABLE 4

Urban and Rural Population: Number and Rate of Growth 1960–2000

	Urban population (millions)					Rural population (millions)					Urban growth rates (percent)				Rural growth rates (percent)			
	1960	1970	1980	1990	2000	1960	1970	1980	1990	2000	1960–1970	1970–1980	1980–1990	1990–2000	1960–1970	1970–1980	1980–1990	1990–2000
World total	985	1352	1854	2517	3329	1997	2283	2614	2939	3186	3.2	3.2	3.1	2.8	1.4	1.4	1.2	0.8
More developed regions	582	717	864	1021	1174	394	374	347	316	280	2.1	1.9	1.7	1.4	–0.5	–0.8	–0.9	–1.2
Less developed regions	403	635	990	1496	2155	1603	1910	2267	2623	2906	4.6	4.5	4.2	3.7	1.8	1.7	1.5	1.0
East Asia	179	266	387	541	722	610	664	708	725	703	4.1	3.8	3.4	2.9	1.0	0.7	0.2	0.3
Mainland region	103	164	252	371	518	537	601	649	672	658	4.8	4.4	4.0	3.4	1.1	0.8	0.3	–0.2
Japan	59	75	93	108	120	34	29	23	18	13	2.4	2.2	1.5	1.1	–1.8	–2.1	–2.8	–3.2
Other East Asia	17	27	43	62	83	30	34	35	35	32	5.1	4.4	3.9	3.0	1.2	0.5	0.0	–0.9
South Asia	154	238	370	556	793	711	888	1116	1355	1561	4.4	4.5	4.2	3.6	2.2	2.3	2.0	1.4
Middle South Asia	99	150	229	339	476	490	612	772	941	1089	4.3	4.4	4.0	3.5	2.3	2.3	2.0	1.5
Southeast Asia	39	60	94	140	203	180	227	286	350	405	4.5	4.5	4.2	3.6	2.3	2.4	2.0	1.5
Southwest Asia	17	28	47	76	114	42	49	57	65	67	5.3	5.3	4.9	4.1	1.6	1.6	1.2	0.5
Europe	246	292	339	388	438	179	170	158	145	131	1.7	1.5	1.4	1.2	–0.5	–0.7	–0.9	–1.0
Western Europe	91	108	122	137	151	44	41	36	32	28	1.7	1.2	1.2	1.0	–0.7	–1.2	–1.3	–1.4
Southern Europe	53	65	80	95	111	65	63	60	57	52	2.2	2.0	1.8	1.6	–0.2	–0.4	–0.6	–0.9
Eastern Europe	47	57	69	80	92	50	47	44	39	35	2.0	1.8	1.5	1.4	–0.6	–0.7	–1.0	–1.1
Northern Europe	55	62	68	76	84	20	19	18	17	15	1.1	1.0	1.0	1.0	–0.6	–0.7	–0.7	–0.8
Soviet Union	106	139	174	214	252	108	104	97	89	77	2.7	2.3	2.1	1.7	–0.4	–0.7	–0.9	–1.3
Africa	48	77	125	203	320	221	268	332	413	498	4.7	5.0	5.0	4.7	1.9	2.2	2.2	1.9
Western Africa	12	20	34	58	96	67	81	99	122	144	5.2	5.4	5.4	5.1	1.9	2.0	2.1	1.7
Eastern Africa	6	9	16	29	50	71	88	112	145	184	5.4	5.6	5.8	5.6	2.2	2.4	2.6	2.4
Middle Africa	3	6	11	19	33	26	30	35	42	48	5.7	5.9	6.0	5.6	1.4	1.6	1.7	1.4
Northern Africa	20	30	49	76	113	46	56	71	87	101	4.5	4.8	4.6	4.0	2.0	2.3	2.1	1.5
Southern Africa	8	10	15	21	29	11	12	15	18	21	3.3	3.4	3.5	3.4	1.6	1.8	1.9	1.7
Northern America	138	169	204	145	284	60	59	56	54	50	2.0	1.9	1.8	1.5	–0.3	–0.4	–0.5	–0.8
Latin America	103	158	238	350	495	110	125	139	150	157	4.4	4.2	3.9	3.5	1.3	1.0	0.8	0.5

TABLE 4 (Continued)

Urban and Rural Population: Number and Rate of Growth 1960–2000

	Urban population (millions)					Rural population (millions)					Urban growth rates (percent)				Rural growth rates (percent)			
	1960	1970	1980	1990	2000	1960	1970	1980	1990	2000	1960–1970	1970–1980	1980–1990	1990–2000	1960–1970	1970–1980	1980–1990	1990–2000
Tropical South America	51	84	131	198	286	60	67	72	74	73	5.0	4.6	4.2	3.7	1.1	0.7	0.3	-0.2
Middle America Mainland	22	35	55	84	125	27	33	40	48	55	4.8	4.7	4.5	4.0	2.1	2.0	1.8	1.4
Temperate South America	23	30	38	46	56	10	10	9	8	7	2.7	2.4	2.1	1.9	-0.4	-0.6	-0.9	-1.2
Caribbean	7	11	15	21	28	13	15	17	20	22	3.6	3.4	3.3	3.2	1.5	1.3	1.2	1.1
Oceania	10	13	17	21	25	5	6	7	9	10	2.5	2.5	2.3	1.8	1.3	1.5	1.7	1.5
Australia and New Zealand	10	13	16	20	24	2	3	3	2	2	2.4	2.4	2.2	1.7	-0.1	-0.1	-0.3	-0.8
Melanesia	0	0	0	0	0	2	2	3	4	6	5.5	5.6	5.8	5.5	2.4	2.5	2.7	2.4
Polynesia and Micronesia	0	0	1	1	1	1	1	1	2	2	5.0	4.8	4.7	4.0	2.9	2.6	2.6	1.9

(**Source:** *U.N. Population Study N. 49*, September, 1971.)

reasonable, on the dimensions of present and future food needs and the capacity of the world to support the likely population, is founded on the population data presented here. How reliable are these data? The *United Nations Demographic Yearbook 1970* poses the question of whether or not there has been an increase in reliability of data during the decade 1959 to 1969, for in 1959 knowledge of population size and rate of growth was rather inadequate. "Very tentatively one might conclude that there has been a slight improvement in knowledge of the size of the world's population but none or very little in knowledge about its rate of growth. A considerable improvement is to be expected however within the next two years when the results of numerous new censuses become available for analysis. Pending substantial progress in the registration of vital statistics, however, the estimated rates of increase for current years will remain considerably in doubt."[5] As most countries hold censuses at decade intervals, estimates of population reach a nadir in the year before a new census is taken. Preliminary results from the 1971 Indian census show a smaller population than had been projected for 1971 on the basis of the growth rates derived from the 1961 census. Similarly, the 1971 Indonesian census indicates a smaller population then expected.[6]

To build detailed estimates of future food needs on such a shaky foundation is an exercise more in arithmetic than in sound planning. However, the aggregate rate of population growth in the less developed regions, of 2.2 to 2.5% annually, gives the order of magnitude of increase in food production needed.

CALORIE REQUIREMENTS

Custom and income, as well as biological need, determine actual food consumption. Surveys of how much of which type of food a man in fact consumes can serve only as indicators of calorie requirements at the physiological level. Here, as elsewhere, there is no ought from is. To judge whether or not a diet is nutritionally adequate is to measure consumption against a set of independently derived standards. Man is an animal. What his calorie needs are is a question of physiology. A question of physiology cannot be answered by using economic or social or cultural data.

As does any mammal, man requires energy, which is measured as calories, to meet the demands of body maintenance, which is a function of body size, height and weight and surface area, of sex and ambient temperature; to meet the demands of work, a function of the work's duration and strenuousness; and to meet the demands of pregnancy, lactation, and growth. Less food is required to maintain body temperature in a warm climate than in a cold one. A population with a high percentage of young has a lower average per head calorie need than an equal population of adults because the biological mass of the former population is smaller.

Calorie requirements of man under various conditions have been estimated by FAO.[7] The basis from which all adjustments for body size, for temperature, and for work are made is the 'reference man' and the 'reference woman.' This 'reference man' appears to be a European, weighing 65 kg, leading a rather unspecified life. "On each working day he is employed 8 hours in an occupation which is not sedentary, but does not involve more than occasional periods of *hard* physical labor. When not at work he is sedentary for about 4 hours daily and may walk for up to 1½ hours. He spends about 1½ hours on active recreations and household work." This reference man is an unsuitable standard. On the basis of the studies detailed below, FAO estimates of adult total calorie needs are somewhat low, while the scale of calorie requirements for children is much too high. Furthermore, if the intensity and duration of work is the main factor in variation in calorie need, as it is, FAO uncertainty as to the actual work calorie requirements of its reference man, and the extent to which other groups differ in this respect from the reference man's work load, can lead to large and conflicting variations in calorie need estimates. However, FAO body weight and temperature adjustments have been carefully worked out and are used here.

A first step toward estimating calorie needs is to consider body weight. There are marked differences in average body weight between regions of the world and between ethnic groups. To speak of ethnic weight differences may seem to be begging the question. Is the large variation in body weights solely a result of differences in nutrition, such that, others things being equal, given adequate nutrition this variation would be eradicated? Studies of seven Asian and seven Latin American populations indicate genetic differences in body size.[8] While the evidence favors this conclusion, the question is not conclusively settled. What can be said is that adequate nutrition is needed to realize fully current genetic potential. In countries with improving nutrition, the maximum spurt of growth in the young is occurring earlier (chronologically not physiologically) without an increase in adult body weight and height; in every case current body weight differences between town and country are diminishing, both trends thus raising the average body weight and height and increasing the biomass of the population.

Bennett[9] has collected the results of some body weight studies: U.S. soldiers going to war in 1941–45 had an average weight of 70 kg, though there is a slight upward bias here; European men average 65 kg; Sudanese body weight is 57 kg; Latin Americans weigh 56 kg; and most East Asians range from 50 to 55 kg. In 1956 McFie[10] surveyed six Ugandan villages. In one village, which shared its land with pygmies (40 kg) and may have intermarried with them, men averaged 52 kg and women 48 kg. But the other five villages, with widely different food habits, showed men weighing 58 to 64 kg and women 51 to 59 kg. In 1967 The Science Advisory Committee to the President of the U.S. submitted a report of over 1,200 pages on the "World Food Problem."[8] Asian and Latin American body weight data are given in this report and are used in the calorie and reference protein need estimations in Table 7. Ashcroft et al.[11] provide a body weight series for Jamaica, which is considered representative of the Caribbean region. Meridith[12] reviews available data for a number of African countries, and Johnson[13] reports on Nigeria. The Asian and Latin American series are more reliable than the African.

A second step toward estimating calorie requirements is to consider duration and duress of working. Direct information is desired. Phillips[14] measured calorie needs of Nigerians working at various tasks. Over the whole year the average African devotes only about 4 hr per day to working his fields, ranging from periods of intense activity to almost no work. Indian[15] and Thai figures are higher and much higher again in China and the Caribbean. Phillips' subjects were aged 24 to 33 and weighed 43 to 63 kg, averaging 55 kg. In Table 5 of calorie requirements, figures for walking and sedentary activities are from Phillips, those of sleeping are from FAO 'reference man,' with adjustment for weight and temperature.

For field work, Phillips' figures, adjusted by Trowell,[16] range from 213 cal/hr for carrying a log of 20 kg, to 269 for grass cutting, 274 for hoeing, the principal agricultural activity of Africans, 360 for sawing, 372 for bush clearing, and 504 for tree felling. Very heavy work cannot be sustained for long periods. Rest pauses are necessary to preserve health. This, according to Lehmann,[17] brings calorie requirements for hard work down to 300 per hr, for the 'reference man' of 65 kg. Converting to African body weight, we take a figure of 250 cal/hr for extra calorie requirements while working.

Southern Indian[18] textile mill laborers, in their 20's, weighing an average 47 kg, used energy at the rate of 203 cal/hr, averaged over an 8-hr shift. Fox[19] shows only 165 cal/man hour equivalent for farm work, including walking to and from plots. Walking was found to require 145 cal/hr for men, 126 for women. Various farm tasks required 95 to 315 cal/hr for men, and less by body weight proportion for women. Phillips' and Trowell's results give higher figures for men of 55 kg average body weight, 184 cal/hr for walking, and 213 to 504 for various farm tasks. The high calorie demand for heavy work averages down as periods of rest and light work interspersed with the hard work are taken into account.

The adjustment of FAO's European 'reference man' to African conditions gives a requirement of 2,707 cal/day, whereas our calculations direct from African data raise this figure to 2,820 at 4 hr work per day, or 3,402 if an 8-hr day is to be worked (Table 5).

FAO scale of calorie requirements for children is much too high. Fox's estimates in Africa are much lower. His scale is the more reliable. MacArthur[20] showed that the application of FAO scales to Japan, a moderately high income country, would indicate that about one third of Japanese children lacked adequate calories.[21] FAO has based some of their principal conclusions on work done by Cullumbine in Ceylon. MacArthur pointed out what had not generally been understood before: that a number of his results were from high income families, who were consuming of their own choice and living healthy and active lives on diets considerably below the FAO scale.

Jones,[22] also analyzing the effects of family

TABLE 5

Calorie Requirements of Men Aged 20–29, Central Africa

	Hr/day	Cal/hour	Cal/day	Hr/day	Cal/hour	Cal/day
Field work[a]	4	250	1000	8	250	2000
Other active work and recreation (e.g., housebuilding, dancing)	1	250	250	1	250	250
Walking	2	184	368	1	184	184
Sedentary activities	9	78	702	6	78	468
Sleeping	8	62½	500	8	62½	500
Total			2820			3402

[a]Based on Trowell-Phillips results

(**Source:** Clark, C. G. and Haswell, M., *The Economics of Subsistence Agriculture,* 4th ed., Macmillan, London, 1970, 13.)

composition on food consumption in Maharashtra, found it impossible to substantiate the FAO standards for children. Thus, the lower standards proposed by Fox for Africa are used (Table 6). Pregnancy and lactation calorie allowances are included in the calorie requirements of children 0 to 1 years.

Some evidence from China[23] also supports the conclusion that, because of the very high allowances for children, the FAO reference standard is too high.

Using African data of Phillips, an African reference man is devised. Following FAO's method, the African body weight calorie need equation is $E = 146.4\ W^{0.73}$ at 25°C. No allowances are made for individual variability about this mean.

The African woman is estimated to work as strenuously as her European counterpart.[25] From the FAO (European) reference woman equation, an African reference woman equation is derived, by substituting the African weight and adjusting for temperature: $E = 114.1\ W^{0.73}$ at 25°C. Likewise, it is assumed that the African woman works as hard as but only three quarters as long as the African man. Her net addition of calories for work is calculated from the man/woman body weight difference (57.5/50 x 172).

These equations and the figures for net addition of calories required for each hour of work are used to estimate minimum physiological requirements in other regions of the developing world. For estimating sedentary requirements, men work 4 hr/day and women 3 hr. Work begins at 15 years, with an adjustment being made for differences in body weight between adolescent and adult. Age

TABLE 6

Children's Calorie Requirements Per Day

FAO Reference Scale				Fox (Africa)		
Age	Male		Female	Age	Male	Female
0–1		1120		0–2	700	600
1–3		1300		3–5	808	751
4–6		1700		6–10	1072	918
7–9		2100		11–15	1262	1249
10–12	2500		2400	16–20	1526	1296
13–15	3100		2600			
16–19	3600		2400			

(**Source:** Clark, C. G. and Haswell, M., *The Economics of Subsistence Agriculture,* 4th ed., Macmillan, London, 1970, 16.)

adjustments are not introduced until the ages 50 to 60 years, then for this age group sedentary calorie requirements are put at 93% for the 20 to 29 age base rate and at 86% of base rate for those 60 years and over.

The results for 15 developing regions are shown in Table 7. The figure for India of 2,100 calories per nutrition unit, reached by Sukhatme,[24] is equivalent to about 1,700 calories per head reached here.

PROTEIN REQUIREMENTS

Here, as with calorie needs, our calculations are based on human physiological requirements. Allowances for unequal distribution of food within the family and society and for disease resistance are not included. Protein requirements are usually expressed in grams/day/kilogram (g/day/kg) of body weight, with the ratio naturally much higher for children than for adults because protein is required for growth. Requirements at a given age are those estimated by Hegsted[26] (Table 8). These agree with the standards set by most other authorities. They are expressed in terms of reference protein. The amount of reference protein per gram of dietary protein varies with the actual combination of foodstuffs consumed. For India, Clark[27] has estimated 0.59 g of reference protein per gram of protein as consumed. On the other hand, Gopalan[28] sets a higher standard of reference protein for adults, 0.65 g/day/kg, though he is more favorable in his estimate of the reference/dietary protein ratio, 0.65. For Indonesia, Clark[29] has calculated a ratio of 0.64. Average per head reference protein requirements for each region are given in Table 7.

CALORIE PROTEIN INTERACTION

An ideal diet is one that, consumed in amounts satisfying calorie requirements, simultaneously meets protein and all other nutritional requirements. In undernutrition, the structure of diet is nutritionally satisfactory, but insufficient quantity is being consumed, while, in malnutrition, the structure of diet is nutritionally unsatisfactory. Numerous studies report widespread protein deficiency in many countries, particularly among children. Is this deficiency primarily a case of undernutrition or of malnutrition? The question is important, for its answer gives rise to divergent policy implications.

On this question of calorie protein interaction and the genesis of protein deficiency, Sukhatme[30] is quite certain: "If one examines the available data the conclusion is clear that what diets lack is adequate energy food which would enable active utilization of protein people do eat. . .protein malnutrition is the indirect result of inadequate energy intake. . .when the food intake is sufficient in amount the protein intake is usually satisfactory. Apparently people can have enough and more of the protein they need from the cereal/pulse diet they normally consume if only they can eat enough to meet their energy needs." Similarly, Miller and Payne,[31] McLaren and Pellet;[32] and Gopalan,[28] doing a detailed study of 15,000 preschool children from the poor socioeconomic group concludes "the protein-calorie malnutrition in poor Indian communities, which is widespread, is largely conditioned primarily by calorie deficiency." He adds, however, "this observation may not be applicable to Africa, where protein deficiency may be of primary importance." Not ideal, the diet of these preschool children was deficient in vitamin A, among other vitamins, and particularly iron, among minerals. Also of importance is the discovery that the high leucine content of millet (*Sorghum vulgare*) inhibited the metabolism of tryptophan-nicotinic acid, precipitating pellagra in human subjects and black tongue (its equivalent) in dogs, although the tryptophan content is higher than in maize and its nicotinic acid is not in a bound form. In Indonesia it has been found that groups growing and eating low protein foods, such as cassava, are aware of its inadequacy, yet they grow it because it yields greater calories per hectare than does rice and when their economic situation allows, they grow and eat the preferred food, rice.

It is well known that at any given level of protein intake the nitrogen balance is sensitive to calorie intake. Calloway and Spector[33] have reviewed the extensive literature on this subject. Up to an intake of 900 cal, no matter how much protein a man may eat, none is retained by the body. Increasing the energy value of the diet from 900 to 1,600 cal results in improved nitrogen retention at a protein intake of 40 g, but there is still a loss of some 12 g a day, which persisted through approximately 2,300 cal. "The result that whatever the protein intake, failure to consume

TABLE 7

Calorie and Reference Protein Requirements Per Day

	U.N. regions	Average[a] temp. °C	Body weight of adults (kg)[b] M	Body weight of adults (kg)[b] F	Requirements of men and women aged 20 to 29 years: Total M	Total F	Net addition each hr/day worked M	Net addition each hr/day worked F	Sedentary M	Sedentary F	Requirements per head of whole population[d] — Calories: Children[e] M	Children[e] F	Men Sedentary	Men Net addition each hr/day worked	Women Sedentary	Women Net addition each hr/day worked	Total Men working[f] 4 hr day	Total Men working[f] 8 hr day	Reference protein[g] (g)
Mainland Asia N	A1	11	55.4	49.9	2937	2122	192	172	2170	1607	204.1	178.2	619.4	57.4	488.7	53.4	1869	2099	17.44
Mainland Asia S	A1	17	50.4	45.9	2664	1940	169	152	1988	1483	198.3	173.3	571.6	51.3	445.0	47.8	1737	1942	16.51
Other East Asia	A3	13	56.8	49.3	2961	2081	191	167	2195	1581	215.0	192.5	602.4	56.1	446.3	50.1	1831	2056	17.81
Middle South Asia	B4	25	49.4	43.2	2524	1783	154	135	1908	1379	200.4	188.6	533.4	44.9	388.0	39.0	1607	1787	15.34
Southeast Asia	5	27	51.1	45.4	2547	1840	156	138	1949	1425	220.2	186.5	507.7	41.5	398.2	38.9	1595	1762	15.31
Southwest Asia	6	20	53.8	47.9	2572	1970	172	153	2064	1512	215.8	189.5	562.1	49.2	431.9	45.2	1732	1929	16.97
West Africa	*E12*	*25*	*57.5*	*50*	*2820*	*1985*	*172*[c]	*150*	*2132*	*1535*	*212.6*	*182.4*	*559.7*	*47.0*	*428.1*	*42.6*	*1699*	*1887*	*18.64*
East Africa	13	27	55.3	50.8	2716	1987	164	149	2060	1541	224.3	189.7	511.7	42.8	420.4	41.7	1643	1814	18.11
Middle Africa	14	27	56.8	56.3	2765	2142	167	160	2097	1661	186.3	164.7	581.4	47.7	517.2	50.9	1793	1984	18.67
Northern Africa	15	25	57	52	2802	2041	171	154	2118	1578	218.9	195.1	538.7	45.7	420.6	42.6	1684	1867	18.08
Southern Africa	16	22	65.2	65.3	3137	2447	194	188	2360	1883	197.3	183.1	653.4	57.4	521.4	55.9	1952	2182	21.31
Tropical South America	G18	27	49.3	51.0	2855	2033	172	152	2166	1577	208.0	187.1	565.9	47.4	438.8	44.3	1722	1912	17.64
Middle America Mainland	19	22	60.3	49.3	2953	1933	183	153	2221	1535	233.1	205.2	530.1	46.2	406.4	42.6	1687	1872	17.27
Temperate South America	20	18	65.3	57.1	3202	2261	202	177	2393	1731	157.7	142.6	814.3	73.0	614.0	66.0	2219	2511	22.63
Caribbean	21	22	61.2	53.0	2996	2101	185	161	2254	1617	226.8	205.0	436.1	46.2	522.1	45.7	1712	1897	18.45

M = Male
F = Female

a. Average mean annual temperatures are approximately estimated from examination of the maps of isotherms.

b. The results of this table depend on the reliability of body weight data. These vary from detailed studies to fairly arbitrary assumptions. Likewise, age distribution data, needed to calculate the biomass of population, depend on accurate censuses and records of vital statistics. The results of the table contain the inadequacies of the data. The following table sets out sources of body weight data (adults and children) and age distribution data. Two main sources are; for Asia and Latin Ameria *The World Food Problem* Vol. 3, Chap. 1, and *UN Demographic Yearbook 1970.* Where body weight series for several countries of a region are available, their arithmetic mean is taken as regional body weight.

Region	Body weight	Age distribution
Mainland Asia N+	Japan 1948	China[51]
Mainland Asia S	Japan 1948 (less 5 kg)	China[51]
Other East Asia	Japan 1963	Korea 1970 E
Middle South Asia	India and Pakistan	India 1970[55]
Southeast Asia	Vietnam, Burma, Malaya, Thailand	Indonesia 1964–65 E
Southwest Asia	West Pakistan	Turkey 1965 C
Western Africa	Clark and Haswell[15]	Nigeria 1963 C
Eastern Africa	Kikuyu, Masai, Uganda[12,13] Tanganyika	Kenya 1960 C and Ethiopia 1962 C
Middle Africa	Uganda (Ganda)[12,13]	Congo Dem. R. 1957
Northern Africa	Sudan[12,15] (females assumed 5 kg less)	Eygpt 1960 C and Morocco 1970 E
Southern Africa	Urban Zulus Durban@[12,13]	South Africa 1960 C
Tropical South America	Colombia, Ecuador, Bolivia, Northeast Brazil	Brazil 1970[55]
Middle America Mainland	Colombia #	Mexico 1970 C
Temperate South America	Uruguay and Chile	Argentina 1960 C
Caribbean	Jamaica[11,12]	Jamaica 1965 E

E = estimate, C = census, + China's total population assumed to be evenly distributed, half north, half south: @ data from Nigeria show urban/rural differences in body weight, which are used to modify the urban Zulu body weights: # the Middle American Mainland population is ethnically more allied to the larger bodied Colombians, both of Hispanic origin, than the smaller bodied Amerindian strain of Ecuador and Bolivia.

c. From Table 5, 250 cal/hr working, less 78 cal/hr which would have been consumed in sedentary occupation.

d. Different sections of the population weighted according to their relative numbers, so that figures can be summed directly to give average requirements per head of whole population.

e. Fox's scale of calorie requirement for children, adjusted for temperature, though not for body weight.

f. Woman's work remains at 3 hr/day in both totals.

g. Hegsted's standards of protein requirement by body weight for each age group weighted according to relative numbers of population in each age group.

TABLE 8

Calorie and Reference Protein Standards

Age	Calories[a] at 25°C Male	Female	Protein[b] gm/kg body weight/day male and female
0–1	533[c]	533[c]	1.3
1–4	781	714	0.70
5–9	1019	885	0.61
10–14	1224	1183	0.50
15–19	1473	1287	0.42
20	–	–	0.40

[a]After Fox, adjusted to different age groupings by FAO method 2.[7]
[b]After Hegsted[26]
[c]Includes allowance for pregnancy and lactation

more than 1.5 times the calories needed for basal metabolism (BMR) will result in both calorie and protein deficiency is found to hold experimentally for all age groups," so writes Sukhatme.[30] Excess protein over and above the body's need (as is the case in most developed countries) is diverted to energy production.

That protein deficiency is primarily a result of low calorie intake, and thus the body's inability to use what protein is consumed, are conclusions quite the opposite of those of Scrimshaw and his co-workers.[34] They have thought that protein is the primary limiting factor. The United Nations report, "International Action to Avert the Impending Protein Crisis,"[35] and its call to nations[36] to deal explicitly with the protein problem, recommending the promotion and production of protein foods using modern nonagricultural technology, are based on Scrimshaw's work. The conclusions arrived at here lead to different policies, and indeed simpler policies.

REQUIREMENT AND AVAILABILITY

FAO Food Balance Sheets, 1964–1966, give average calorie and (dietary) protein per head actually consumed for many countries. When the figures of available food are compared with requirement at the physiological level (Table 9), in every case average availability is greater than average requirement. Likewise, with protein, average per head consumption for developing countries as a whole is nearly 40% greater than the standards based on the most recent recommendations made by FAO/WHO.[37] Those countries where availability is only marginally greater than requirement have been marked by political incompetence.

But not everyone lives at the average; some consume far more, and some far less. It is the dispersion about this adequate average that determines the extent of hunger. Now this dispersion is primarily unequal distribution of income. As with so many situations of hunger (in developed countries as well), food is available but the individual has no money with which to buy it, or is landless and unemployed. Detailed studies of income distribution in developing countries are still few in number. Using Indian data on income distribution, Clark[27] has calculated that one quarter to nearly one third of the Indian population is consuming calories below nutritional requirements. This tallies with estimates extrapolated from nutrition surveys. Contrary to a very widespread general impression, the proportion short of protein appears to be much lower, even if Gopalan's high standards are adopted. Similar results are found in Indonesia.[29] Again, studies from Chile and Brazil reach the same conclusion. "There is a direct relationship between income and quantity and quality of food consumed among the poor classes of less developed countries. The amounts of calories and proteins obtained by poor people in these countries are inadequate to meet their physiological needs."[38]

SPENDING INCOME

As income increases with development, what proportion of income is spent on which foodstuffs determines the rate of increase in demand for food over and above that demand from population increase. Income elasticity of demand is the measure used: the proportional change in quantity of the good bought divided by the proportional change in income, price remaining the same ($dy/y/dx/x$, where y is quantity of good and x is income). Note that this is not the same as marginal propensity to consume; this is a measure of the proportion of an increment in income which will be consumed on a given commodity.

There are two types of elasticities: quantity elasticity and value income elasticity of demand for food. Value income elasticities are almost

TABLE 9

Average Calorie Intake, Total Protein and Animal Protein Intake – Asia, Africa, Latin America

Mainland Asia N + S	A1		
(standard S 1737 N 1869)			
China	2045	58.2	8.9
Other East Asia	A3		
(standard 1831)			
Korea (North)	2269	77.9	7.1
Korea (South)	2329	65.3	7.3
Taiwan	2379	58.7	16.2
Middle South Asia	B4		
(standard 1594)			
India	1964	50.6	5.8
Pakistan	1995	49.6	10.5
Iran	2029	55.2	11.7
Nepal	2033	52.0	6.7
Afghanistan	2057	65.4	7.8
Ceylon	2219	50.4	10.2
Southeast Asia	B5		
(standard 1589)			
Indonesia	1760	38.4	5.2
Philippines	1911	45.8	14.8
Vietnam (North)	2003	44.8	9.0
Burma	2011	44.1	9.2
Laos	2036	44.6	5.2
Vietnam (South)	2200	48.6	11.1
Malaysia (West)	2200	49.4	14.7
Thailand	2226	50.9	12.3
Cambodia	2231	57.7	19.1
Sabah	2434	57.7	23.0
Sarawak	2443	53.4	14.4
Singapore	2443	63.3	26.4
Southwest Asia	B6		
(standard 1730)			
Iraq	2055	58.0	13.6
Saudi Arabia	2082	58.2	9.5
Lebanon	2363	69.9	20.4
Jordan	2397	64.8	11.3
Syria	2451	69.2	11.7
Turkey	2769	78.2	14.8
Israel	2827	86.6	39.7
Western Africa	E12		
(standard 1699)			
Mauritania	1993	73.4	37.5
Guinea	2059	45.4	6.0
Upper Volta	2060	70.3	5.3
Ghana	2084	43.5	7.3
Sierra Leone	2155	49.2	9.1
Nigeria	2166	58.7	5.1
Dahomey	2173	52.2	8.0
Niger	2178	77.6	12.5
Togo	2222	51.4	7.3
Liberia	2287	41.4	8.5
Senegal	2299	64.0	21.2

Gambia	2315	62.2	42.0
Ivory Coast	2430	59.1	12.9
Eastern Africa	E13		
(standard 1643)			
Rwanda	1901	56.9	3.6
Burundi	2017	61.5	4.1
Ethiopia	2107	70.5	10.8
Mozambique	2127	40.4	4.6
Malawi	2143	58.4	3.7
Tanzania	2144	60.2	12.4
Uganda	2157	55.9	15.1
Kenya	2243	67.9	13.3
Zambia	2246	69.4	10.7
Mauritius	2343	48.9	13.3
Madagascar	2387	56.1	12.0
Rhodesia	2551	73.2	14.4
Middle Africa	E14		
(standard 1793)			
Angola	1911	39.9	9.4
Congo Democratic Republic	2036	32.7	8.9
Congo Brazzaville	2160	39.8	16.0
Central African Republic	2172	47.5	16.4
Gabon	2182	51.0	27.2
Cameroun	2228	58.9	10.8
Chad	2240	78.4	13.8
Northern Africa	E15		
(standard 1684)			
Somalia	1770	57.2	22.5
Algeria	1892	55.8	6.6
Libya	2068	53.9	11.9
Sudan	2091	58.9	18.7
Tunisia	2205	63.1	10.9
Egypt (U.A.R.)	2639	76.6	12.3
Southern Africa	E16		
(standard 1952)			
Botswana			
Lesotho			
Namibia	2372	77.0	28.3
South Africa			
Swaziland			
Tropical South America	G18		
(standard 1704)			
Bolivia	1765	45.8	12.1
Equador	1848	46.7	16.2
Colombia	2192	50.1	22.7
Peru	2271	61.0	22.6
Guyana	2291	55.1	19.6
Surinam	2365	56.3	18.3
Venezuela	2367	61.1	26.6
Brazil	2541	63.9	22.4

TABLE 9 (continued)

Average Calorie Intake, Total Protein and Animal Protein Intake – Asia, Africa, Latin America

Mainland Middle America (standard 1695)	G19			Paraguay	2732	68.1	29.8
				Argentina	2885	90.2	53.2
El Salvador	1877	47.0	14.1	Uruguay	3023	105.5	71.8
Honduras	1930	48.6	13.1				
Guatemala	1952	49.2	11.9	Caribbean (standard 1897)	G21		
Costa Rica	2234	56.7	24.6				
Nicaragua	2253	60.7	19.8	Haiti	1926	47.0	4.7
Panama	2338	62.5	24.8	Dominican Republic	2077	45.7	17.4
Mexico	2624	66.5	14.2	Jamaica	2276	59.1	26.5
Temperate South America (standard 2089)	G20			Trinidad and Tobago	2361	63.9	26.4
				Cuba	2501	62.8	27.6
Chile	2516	65.4	25.2	Puerto Rico	2531	67.3	35.5

All standards are based on men working 4 hr per day and women working 3 hr per day.
(Source of country data: FAO Food Balance Sheets, 1964-1966.)

always computed at the retail price level. Apart from the actual food component, they contain processing and distribution costs. These latter costs are the marketing margin. The value income elasticity of demand for food at retail is the weighted average of wholesale income elasticity and marketing margin elasticity.

Alternatively, quantity income elasticities may be computed as agricultural products or as food finally sold.

Accounting for all food supply flow,[39] four quantity and six value income elasticities can be measured. The four quantity points are own farm production consumed on farm (1A), own farm production marketed (2B), own country fish production and net food imports (including changes in stocks) (3C), giving total food (4E). The points for value elasticities are (A), (B), and (C), and the wholesale level (BC), marketing margin (D), retail level (BCD), giving total food (ABCD=E).

When the task is to estimate future food needs, what is wanted is the statement that aggregate food supplies must increase at this rate to provide the quantity of food to meet demand from population increase and rising incomes. This aggregate figure needs to be dissected into its components, so that demand for specific foodstuffs, at farm, at wholesale, and at retail level, may be known. For food projection purposes, then, the relevant income elasticities are value elasticities at farm-gate prices (wholesale), and quantity elasticities in terms of original commodities.

The relationship between food consumption (y) and income or total expenditure (x), may take three functional forms, called double-logarithmic, semi-logarithmic, and logarithmic-inverse, respectively.

a. $\log y = a + b \log x$
b. $y = a' + b' \log x$
c. $\log y = a'' + b''/\log x$

For the same data, each function gives a different elasticity. The semi-log function gives a value between those from the other two functions. Basu and Jones,[40] studying the relationship between real income and food consumption in a large number of economically advanced and middle- and low-income countries, after testing hyperbolae and a number of other possible mathematical relationships, concluded that the best fit to the data was obtained by a function which made food consumption vary with the logarithm of real income, the semi-log function. Consumption of cereal was best expressed by an equation containing a negative exponential, i.e., rising to a maximum at a certain specified income level and falling beyond that point. The semi-log relationship for total food implies that income elasticity must fall steadily, in inverse proportion to the quantity of food consumed, as real income rises.

A further distinction is between elasticities estimated from urban or rural data. Clark and Haswell[41] list a number of rural and urban income elasticities of demand for food, from English agricultural wage labor in 1795, 0.92, to Zambian African urban wage earners in 1947, 0.27. Noda[42] derives a stable food income elasticity of 0.2 from Japanese time series over the last 70 years. Jones[22] analyzed food budgets in Maharashtra, one of the wealthier Indian states. Measured in physiological components, income elasticities for both total calories and total protein were higher in rural than in urban households, namely 0.59 as against 0.29 for calories, 0.53 as against 0.19 for protein. This implies that the proportion of protein as well as of calories falls with income, high income elasticities for milk and pulses not being quite sufficient to balance high elasticities for sugar and oils.

The major source of elasticities is, however, FAO Agricultural Commodities – Projections for 1975 and 1985.[43] In the second volume of this study, Tables A and B give elasticities for 26 different food commodities or groups for each of the 99 countries studied.

From FAO country and commodity figures, an aggregate income elasticity for each region could be derived. Multiplying by projected aggregate population increase for each region, a region-by-region aggregate rate of, and quantity of, increase in demand for food could be estimated. Taking account of the pattern of diet particular to each region and noting the change desired for nutritional reasons, this rate and quantity of increased demand for food could be translated into rate and quantity of increase in farm production (or imports) of each foodstuff. But rather than set about this complex and doubtfully rewarding task, it is more useful to make a closer study of the FAO income elasticities of demand for food.

In his study "An Appraisal of 'Income' Elasticities for total food consumption in developing countries," Paris writes, "The main reason for underlining the particular FAO method of obtaining estimates of farm value elasticities (as well as of other commodity groups) is that such estimates may be re-used by other agencies and individuals to get their own projections of the related commodities *without realizing the non-behavioural character of such elasticities.* In fact, their character is neither behavioural nor descriptive and it is difficult to find any other meaningful aspects associated with them" (italics added).[44]

Table 10 depicts farm value income elasticities of total food as computed from FAO projections for 1975, using low and high income projections.

TABLE 10

Farm Value Income Elasticities of Total Food as Computed from FAO Projections[44]

Country	Type of Function	1975 L	1975 H	1975
India	L–L	.69	.62	.65
	S–L	.76	.68	.72
	L–I	.78	.72	.75
Pakistan	L–L	.68	.63	.65
	S–L	.72	.71	.72
	L–I	.74	.75	.75
Peru	L–L	.46	.43	.45
	S–L	.49	.47	.45
	L–I	.51	.52	.52
Morocco	L–L	.55	.54	.55
	S–L	.55	.56	.55
	L–I	.56	.58	.57
Iran	L–L	.64	.61	.63
	S–L	.68	.67	.67
	L–I	.70	.71	.71
Venezuela	L–L	.40	.38	.39
	S–L	.40	.40	.40
	L–I	.61	.42	.51
Mexico	L–L	.37	.33	.35
	S–L	.39	.34	.36
	L–I	.42	.39	.40
Chile	L–L	.42	.39	.40
	S–L	.43	.42	.43
	L–I	.45	.45	.45

L–L = double logarithmic function
S–L = semi-logarithmic function
L–I = logarithmic-inverse function
L = low income projection
H = high income projection

Table 11 shows value and quantity elasticities for urban and rural populations, for cereals in India, for a number of food commodities in Venezuela, and, quantity income elasticities, urban and rural, in the Philippines, as compared with FAO figures.

As seen in the tables and from the results of Paris's study, "FAO income elasticities for individual commodities or groups might be subject to an upward bias. As a consequence, the farm value income elasticity of total food would be similarly overestimated."[45]

When the bias of income elasticities of demand for food is compounded with the uncertainty of

TABLE 11

Value and Quantity Income Elasticities in Venezuela, India, and the Philippines, for Selected Commodities, Compared With FAO

	Rural		Urban		FAO
Commodity Venezuela, 1962[53]	Value elas-ticity	Quanti-ty elas-ticity	Value elas-ticity	Quanti-ty elas-ticity	Quanti-ty elas-ticity
1. Rice	.59	.40	.72	.19	.5
2. Wheat flour	.54	.38	.71	.31	
3. Wheat bread	.60	.28	.72	.39	.4
4. Spaghetti, etc.	.56	.32	.71	.18	
5. Potatoes	.58	.34	.73	.34	
6. Manoic	.51	.11	.71	.05	.2
7. Sugar (refined)	.63	.38	.72	.29	
8. Crude sugar	.50	−.15	.72	−.16	.3
9. Bananas	.52	.24	.71	.22	.3
10. Beef	.63	.33	.68	.35	.7
11. Pork	.50	.35	.69	.26	.5
12. Other meat	.48	.20	.68	.48	.5
13. Fish	.67	.47	.78	.20	.3
14. Eggs	.64	.34	.66	.24	.5
15. Natural milk	.60	.23	.57	.28	
16. Pasteurized milk	.78	.55	.69	.50	.4
17. Powdered milk	.55	.43	.70	.35	
18. Butter	.52	.24	.70	.50	1.0
19. Vegetable oils	.57	.32	.66	.40	.5
India Household Budget Survey Round – Cereals[52]					
4th	.71	.46	.31	.16	
5th	.59	.38	.37	.22	
6th	.65	.49	.40	.21	
7th	.52	.31	.30	.07	
10th	.62	.49	.32	.14	

Philippines, 1960 – Quantity Income Elasticities[54]

Commodity	Manila L-L	Urban L-L	Rural L-L	FAO
1. Rice	.001	.120	−.149	.5
2. Wheat (bakery)	.367	.396	.605	
Wheat (noodles)	.408	.446	.456	.6
3. Starchy roots	.211	.233	−.069	.1
4. Pork	.380	.413	.212	
5. Beef (fresh)	.555	.380	.124	
6. Beef (processed)	.287	.572	.303	1.1
7. Poultry	.176	.393	.258	
8. Fish	.153	.272	.329	.7
9. Milk (fresh)	.649	.809	−.022	
10. Milk (canned whole)	1.588	1.277	.406	1.5
11. Milk (canned filled)	.464	.317	.303	
12. Vegetable oils	.265	1.530	.077	2.0

population projections, the quite laborious task of calculating rate and quantity aggregate world food demand is not matched by a worthwhile result. Such a figure is, as Paris stresses, nonbehavioral, and not a basis for political and economic and technical action aimed at increasing food supplies.

POLICY IMPLICATIONS

Food Supply Fertility Linkage

It has been an assumption of this essay, as it is of many others, that population growth is an independent variable with respect to food needs at the customary level. The assertion that people on low protein intakes are more fertile is mere myth. But beyond the solely biological level, this question arises. Is there feedback from an individual's or group's knowledge that its level of nutrition is adequate and that food supplies are secure, to fertility? Indirect linkages between food supply and fertility are known; child morbidity and mortality and the incidence of tuberculosis in a population are correlated with nutrition levels. The willingness to move from agricultural to other occupations, which are often associated with lower fertility rates, is, as our work is showing, highly correlated with level and surety of food supply. However, with current knowledge, this remains an open question.

Quantity Before Quality – The Peasant Is No Fool

Rapid population increase evidently calls for a greater production of food. Increasing income calls for a further added increase. Because the widespread protein deficiency found in many countries is largely precipitated by low calorie intake, plans of agricultural development which do not acknowledge this fact are misconceived. Thus, to concentrate scarce material resources, and the even more scarce resource of administrative ability and imagination, of a developing country upon the production and promotion of protein from unconventional sources is to leave the root cause of hunger and deficiency disease festeringly present. Efforts need to be concentrated on increasing the quantity of food available. Of course, we are not urging the continuance of poor quality diets, simply that clinical signs of malnutrition are not evidence in the first instance that the structure of diet is inadequate.

What is often not recognized, either by local planners and agricultural advisers, or by foreign observers[46] on development, is the distinction between illiteracy and stupidity. Although often unable to read and write, the peasant is no fool, either as a farmer or in knowing what makes his family and himself healthy. There is a modernity permeating his tradition.[47] The reported resistance of some village farmers to some new agricultural techniques is likely to be their well-founded albeit inarticulate knowledge that the advice did not treat a root cause. High-yielding varieties of rice, wheat, and other crops are sought after far beyond currently available supplies of seed and fertilizer.

Income to Buy Food

The average supplies of food are greater than the average demand for food, yet hunger is common. Inequalities in distribution of income place a substantial proportion of the population below the level of nutritional requirements. The poor are hungry because they are poor (this is true in developed countries also). Thus, raising incomes is a condition, necessary but not sufficient, of eradicating hunger.

Increased agricultural productivity allows the farmer both to consume more of his own produce and to send more to market. His imputed income – that saved by not having to buy food – thus increases. In rural areas, landless agricultural laborers are a large, depressed, exploited group. Evidence from India[48] shows a decline in their real wages to below what their employers are gaining from that proportion of production attributable to their labor, that is, to below their marginal labor productivity.

Food at Low Prices

As economic development occurs, the terms of trade between the agricultural and other sectors go against agriculture with respect to output, but not necessarily with respect to income. This means that the amount of industrial goods a unit quantity of agricultural output can purchase becomes less. It does not follow that farmers' incomes decline absolutely or that, relative to income in the nonagricultural sectors, farmers are worse off. When farmers see they are getting a lower relative price for their produce, there is political demand for support prices. To yield to this pressure is a most dangerous political error. A cheap food policy is another condition of eradicating hunger.

Employment to Get Income

Finding a job is difficult enough. Employment as a means of getting income is jeopardized when high food prices lead to demand for high money wages. Entrepreneurs are more likely to turn to nonlabor intensive methods when faced with demand for such wages. It is the poor who most need jobs, and it is the poor who most benefit from a cheap food policy.

Transport to Distribute Food

The number of people in cities is increasing rapidly. To feed these people food must be transported from country to town.[49] With processing and distribution costs added, retail food prices are nearly double farm-gate, or rather, paddy-bund prices. A transport and communication system is necessary to get food to urban markets; an efficient transport system helps to minimize marketing costs.

CONCLUSION

Population increase, change in age structure, heavier body weights, longevity, rising incomes, and desire for variety in diet combine to make the demand for food. Careful and thorough study shows there is no lack of physical resources or technological knowledge needed to produce food in quantity and quality to meet current and projected demand for food. That it can be done is not in doubt.[50] Whether or not it may be done is a social and political question. However, this question is beyond the brief of this study, although not beyond the concern of its authors.

REFERENCES

1. *United Nations Population Studies,* No. 49, September, 1971.
2. Population Index, 37, 3, 1971: 37, chart, 1971: 36, 3, 1970: 35, chart, 1969, Office of Population Research, Princeton University, Princeton, N.J.
3. **Borrie, W. D.,** *The Growth and Control of World Population,* Weidenfeld and Nicolson, London, 1970.
4. **Bourgeois-Pichat, J.,** Essai sur la mortalité biologique de l'homme, *Population,* 7, 1952.
5. *United Nations Demographic Yearbook 1970,* 10.
6. **Sundrum, R. M.,** First glimpses of the 1971 Census, *Bull. Indonesian Econ. Stud.* , 8(2), 93, 1972.
7. Food and Agricultural Organization, Calorie Requirements, Report of the Second Committee on Calorie Requirements, FAO Nutritional Studies, No. 15, 1965.
8. United States President's Science Advisory Committee, *The World Food Problem,* Vol. 3, The White House, Washington, D.C., May, 1967, Chap. 1.
9. **Bennett, M. K.,** *The World's Food,* Harper, New York, 1954.
10. **McFie, J.,** Uganda Protectorate Nutrition Surveys, A comparison of the health of six villages consuming different types of food, 1965, 23.
11. **Ashcroft, M. T., Ling, J., Lovell, H. G., and Miall, W. E.,** Heights and weights of adults in rural and urban areas of Jamaica, *Br. J. Prev. Soc. Med.,* 20(1), 22, 1966; **Ashcroft, M. T. and Lovell, H G.,** *J. Trop. Geogr. Med.,* 16, 346, 1964.
12. **Meridith, H. V.,** *Child Develop.,* 39, 315, 1968; 41,551, 1970. *Adv. Child Develop. Behav.,* 6, 153, 1971; *Monogr. Soc. Res. Child Develop.,* 34(1), 34(7), 1969.
13. **Johnson, T. O.,** Height and weight patterns of an urban African population sample in Nigeria, *Trop. Geogr. Med.,* 22, 65, 1970.
14. **Phillips, P. G.,** The metabolic cost of common west African agricultural activities, *Trop. Med. Hyg.,* 57, 12, 1954.
15. **Clark, C. G. and Haswell, M.,** *The Economics of Subsistence Agriculture,* 4th ed., Macmillan, London, 1970, Chap. 1, 8.
16. **Trowell, H. C.,** Calorie and protein requirements of adult male Africans, *East Afr. Med. J.,* 32, 156, May, 1955.
17. **Lehmann, C.,** in *FAO Calorie Requirements,* Report of the Second Committee on Calorie Requirements, FAO Nutritional Studies, No. 15, 57, 1965.
18. **Banerjea** et al., *Indian J. Med. Res.,* 47, 657, 1959.
19. **Fox,** A study of energy expenditures of Africans engaged in various rural activities, London University Ph.D. thesis, 1953.

20. **MacArthur, M.,** *J. Roy. Stat. Soc.,* 127, 392, 1964.
21. Nutritional status – Japan, *Nutr. Rev.,* 275, October, 1969.
22. **Jones, G. T.,** *Farm Economist,* 10(11), 1965.
23. *China Quart.,* various dates 1961-3; see **Clark, C. G. and Haswell, M.,** *The Economics of Subsistence Agriculture,* 4th ed., Macmillan, London, 1970, 18.
24. **Sukhatme, P. V.,** *J. Roy. Stat. Soc.,* Series A, 124, 463, 1961.
25. **Clark, C. G. and Haswell, M.,** *The Economics of Subsistence Agriculture,* 4th ed., Macmillan, London, 1970, 13, 14.
26. **Hegsted, D. M.,** Theoretical estimates of the protein requirements of children, *J. Am. Dietet. Assoc.,* 33, 225, 1957; quoted in Altschul, A. A., *Proteins,* Chapman & Hall, London, 1965.
27. **Clark, C. G.,** The extent of hunger in India, *Economic and Political Weekly* (Bombay), 7(40), September 30, 1972.
28. **Gopalan, C.,** Some recent studies in the nutrition research laboratories, Hyderabad, India, *Am. J. Clin. Nutr.,* 23, 33, 1970.
29. **Clark, C. G.,** Calories and proteins in Indonesia, *Bull. Indonesian Econ. Stud.,* 8(2), 98, July, 1972.
30. **Sukhatme, P. V.,** Protein strategy and agricultural development, *Indian J. Agric. Econ.,* 28, 1, 1972.
31. **Miller, D. S. and Payne, P. R.,** *Proc. Nutr. Soc.,* 28(2), 255, 1969.
32. **McLaren, D. S. and Pellet, P. L.,** *World Rev. Nutr. Dietet,* 12, 43, 1970.
33. **Calloway, D. H. and Spector, H.,** *Am. J. Clin. Nutr.,* 2, 405, 1954.
34. **Scrimshaw, N. S.,** *Arch. Environ. Health,* 18, 1, 51, 1969.
35. United Nations, International Action to Avert the Impending Protein Crisis, a report to the UN Committee on Application of Science and Technology to Development, 1968.
36. United Nations General Assembly Resolution No. 2416 (XXIII).
37. FAO/WHO Rep. Committee on Nutrition, 1970.
38. United States President's Science Advisory Committee, *The World Food Problem,* Vol. 3, The White House, Washington, D.C., May, 1967, Chap. 2.
39. **Stevens, R. D.,** Elasticity of Food Consumption Associated with Changes in Income in Developing Countries, United States Department of Agriculture, ERS-Foreign-23, 1965.
40. **Basu, D. and Jones, G. T.,** *Farm Economist,* 8(9), 8(10), 1957.
41. See, **Clark, C. G. and Haswell, M.,** *The Economics of Subsistence Agriculture,* 4th ed., Macmillan, London, 1970, 179, for detailed references.
42. **Noda, T.,** quoted by Johnston and Mellor, Food Research Institute Studies, November, 1960, in Japanese, 1959. Noda (personal communication) using new data has shown that pre-1921 income elasticity of demand for food is also 0.2.
43. FAO Agricultural Commodities – Projections for 1975 and 1985, 2 Vols., Rome, 1967.
44. **Paris, Q.,** An appraisal of "income" elasticities for total food consumption in developing countries, OECD, Paris, 1970, 17.
45. **Paris, Q.,** An appraisal of "income" elasticities for total food consumption in developing countries, OECD, Paris, 1970, 45. See also, **Noda, T.,** Comparisons of level of living in Japan and selected Asian countries, *Rural Econ. Prob.,* 4, 61, Tokyo, 1968, and **Usher, D.,** Rich poor countries, a study in problems of comparisons of real income, *Inst. Econ. Affairs,* London, 1966.
46. **Myrdal, G.,** *Asian Drama, An inquiry into the Poverty of Nations,* Vol. 1, Penguin Book A 981, Middlesex, England, 1968, 72. (For a criticism of Myrdal, see **Geertz, C.,** *Third World Illusions Myrdal's Mythology,* Encounter, London, July, 1969).
47. **Rudolph, L. and Rudolph, S.,** *The Modernity of Tradition: Political Development in India,* University of Chicago Press, Chicago, 1967.
48. **Krishnaji, N.,** Wages of agricultural labor, *Econ. Polit. Week.,* (Bombay), 1-143, September, 1971.
49. United States President's Science Advisory Committee, *The World Food Problem,* Vol. 2, The White House, Washington, D.C., May, 1967, Chap. 11.
50. **Clark, C. G.,** *Population Growth and Land Use,* Macmillan, London, 1968.
51. **Clark, C. G.,** La population de la chine depuis 1915, *Population,* 21, 1191, 1966.
52. **Biskas, A. K. and Bose, D. W.,** Consumption projections of selected items over the period of the third five year plan, published in Papers on National Income and Allied Topics, Vol. 11, Rao, V.K.R.V., et al., eds., Asia Publishing House, 1962, 43, quoted in Paris, Q., An appraisal of "income" elasticities for total food consumption in developing countries, OECD, Paris, 1970.
53. From information given in Consejo de Bieaster, Rural, Long term projections of supply and demand for selected agricultural commodities, Caracas, 1966, in Paris, Q., An appraisal of "income" elasticities for total food consumption in developing countries, OECD, Paris, 1970.
54. USDA-ERS, The Philippines – long term projections of supply and demand for selected agricultural products, Washington, 1961, quoted in Paris, Q., An appraisal of "income" elasticities for total food consumption in developing countries, OECD, Paris, 1970.
55. United States President's Science Advisory Committee, *The World Food Problem,* Vol. 2, The White House, Washington, D.C., May, 1967, Chap. 1.

EXPANDING FARM PRODUCTION: EXTENDING THE AREA OF SOILS USED

Charles E. Kellogg

TABLE OF CONTENTS

Introduction . . . 79

The Nature of Agriculture . . . 79

Town and Country . . . 80

Accelerated Soil Study . . . 81

Development and Spread of Technology . . . 84
  Land Clearing . . . 85
  Assistance to Farmers on New Lands . . . 85

Why So Much Potential Arable Land Is Not Used . . . 85

References . . . 89

INTRODUCTION

Food production from the soils of the world can be increased enormously in three principal already proved ways.

1. A great unrealized potential exists on the responsive soils already being used for field, horticultural, and industrial crops and the forage for domestic animals. Unhappily, some soils are now being used for farming that do not respond to fertilizers, water control, and genetically improved varieties of plants and breeds of animals; yet most do. Generally speaking, most soils improve under good farming systems over the natural soils before farming. But many thousands of contrasting kinds of soil are used that require different combinations of practices for harvests that give good labor incomes to farm people.

2. The total area of potentially arable soils is more than double the total area now being farmed. The largest of such areas are in Africa and South America, although North America, the Soviet Union, Australia, parts of Southeast Asia, and some of the Pacific and other islands have good unused soils. By the "accidents" of migration and history, many of these areas were passed by for farming. With market incentives, Canada and the U.S. together could increase their cultivated acreage by some 175 million hectares or more.

3. Under many systems now in use, great wastes during production, harvesting, storage, and processing could be enormously reduced. Such reductions in the U.S. and other advanced countries took place gradually during the latter part of the 19th century and with rapid acceleration since about 1935.

THE NATURE OF AGRICULTURE

To improve the harvests in many existing farming areas, and especially to develop new arable soils as people need the products from farming, the agricultural services – infrastructure – must be improved. By the term "agriculture," in contrast to "farming," we include all the industrial, transport, processing, supply, financial, research, and advisory services, as well as farming itself.

Under good modern systems of agriculture, the total work force required is many times greater than that in farming alone. In the U.S. about 4% of the total national labor force works on farms, yet around 30 to 34% of the labor force works in agriculture, including farming. Most of this labor force works in towns and cities. They store, transport, and process the products. They make the chemicals, machines, tools, fencing, pipe, and all the many other items used by farmers, as well as performing many other services. When I was a boy on a Midwest farm, we produced all our own power – hay and grain for the horses and oak trees for the stoves. Now this is nearly all supplied by oil and electric companies.

TOWN AND COUNTRY

Agriculture probably began independently in several parts of the world. Very early, no doubt, most people in a village were engaged in food gathering. Yet as time went on, not all people actually were cultivators or herdsmen. Some became skilled at making tools of wood, stone, and metal, while others specialized in making cloth and leather goods. Early natural and social science began in these villages. Thus technology gradually developed.

Trade followed, first with beasts of burden and canoes and later with boats for both light and heavy transport. Cities developed with concentrations of artisans and merchants. Nearly all cities were located near oceans or navigable streams and lakes. Science began to help both invention and the great explorations.

Later came the industrial revolution. Steam added enormous power to the workman's arm, but it could not be transported far, so the families of workmen were crowded together in the great cities. Since the levels of oceans and streams widely fluctuated during the three million years of Pleistocene, the land near the sites of these cities was alternately flooded and gullied. The soils are highly variable in short distances with many combinations of clay, sand, gravel, and muck. In most of the old port cities, it is costly to have good construction sites.

Roughly 150 to 200 years ago, the industrial revolution began to affect agriculture. Machines such as the cotton gin threw thousands of farm hands out of their jobs and many went to the port cities to find employment. Gradually this process accelerated. The equivalent of many farm jobs moved to cities. At the beginning of World War I most Americans still lived in the country; at its end the majority lived in cities. And the process has continued to accelerate.

Now we have these terrible overcrowded cities with no places for children to play except in the streets. Crime increases and so does noise and smog as the buildings are made higher.

Perhaps worst of all, it has separated so many of us into "rural" and "urban" people, even within agriculture. The very word "rural" suggests backwardness to many. Moreover, no one knows what to do about the old port cities.

Certainly we should not continue to crowd the cities and spread out the crowded suburbia around them. What we need are several hundred more smaller cities in the U.S. as centers for country trade areas.[1] Now good highways are being built and more can be. Away from the oceans and big rivers are abundant good sites for cities to service farming, forestry, mining, manufacturing, etc. within a trade area. Country people need good health centers, libraries, colleges, stores, and other services. Industries for making machines, chemicals, and other inputs for farmers and processing plants for farm, forestry, and other local resources can be built near these towns without pollution. They can be planned to have adequate places for young people. People could have good jobs near their homes. Farming itself could be much better served with storage, processing, and other essential services.

Increasingly local leadership, along with labor and business leadership, is realizing the potentials of town-and-country development in several countries.

This is greatly emphasized because of the near tragedies that lie ahead in many less-developed countries if they go forward improving their farming and developing the new arable soils that are likely to be needed without more small cities. If all manufacturing is concentrated in the big port cities, the present villagers that make and repair tools such as carts and plows and those who make cloth and shoes will need to move away to get jobs. With modern and efficient farming, a high percentage of the existing cultivators will become redundant and will need other jobs, including those in the industrial sectors of agriculture. Many villagers who go from the village to the big city will be much worse off than they were.

Most of these needs can be foreseen especially in the development of the new areas for farming. With proper soil surveys, the responsive soils can be selected and the others left with their natural cover.

Such town-and-country development needs the pooled skills of all aspects of agriculture, including its essential infrastructure. The essential local leadership will need technical assistance in engineering, economics, law, forestry, soil science, and many other fields. Priority should be given to those areas that have good soils for farming *and* other potential resources, such as forestry, mining, and hydroelectric power, to share in the cost and use of transport and the other essential common services.

ACCELERATED SOIL STUDY

Study of the soils of the world had been accelerating in many countries since before 1900. Based on earlier soil surveys and the pressing need, in 1895 the 53rd Congress of the United States authorized the Soil Survey in the Agricultural Appropriation Act for Fiscal Year 1896. After a few years, nearly all soil surveys were made cooperatively with appropriate state agencies, especially the land grant universities. Progress was gradual and the kinds of applications steadily increased. Now in the U.S. more of the funds used for soil surveys are to help guide the planning of pipelines, highways, and towns than for guiding farm and forest uses, important as those are.

With World War II, soil maps, with interpretations for several purposes, were urgently needed for the war effort and later to help guide development programs abroad. All soil maps and systems of soil classification had to be studied. In areas lacking soil maps, estimated soil maps were made from studies of all available data on climate, vegetation, geology, relief, and age of the landforms. The same combinations of these five factors lead to soils that are alike in their characteristics and responses to management or manipulation.

In 1951, a start was made to improve the system of soil taxonomy again. This new system, to be published by the Soil Survey, U.S. Department of Agriculture, should be available in 1973. Fortunately, soil scientists in many other countries helped with this task. On the basis of the literature and travel notes of many soil scientists, it was possible to develop a working soil map of the world at a scale of 1:1,000,000. (This means 1 cm on the map for 1,000,000 cm or 10 km on the ground.) This map makes possible relatively good estimates of the nature and potential of areas of responsive soils in the world.[2] Although of great usefulness, this map is not yet published. The estimates given in this paper and the very small-scale maps in Figures 1 and 2 are based on this manuscript map.

FAO and UNESCO have had an international committee of soil scientists working on a general soil map of the world at an approximate scale of 1:5,000,000. The first section of this to be printed was in 1971 from Rome – Volume IV for South America.[5] The system of nomenclature is a general compromise among several national systems. But for the soil units shown on the map, estimates are given of the climate, vegetation, landform, and lithology of parent material, together with general statements on prospects for useful kinds of crops, grasses, and trees.

The map will be useful for giving a general idea of the kinds of soil to an experienced soil map reader, familiar with soil terms and with a good hand lens for the areas with complex patterns in relation to the small scale.

With close international study, good soil maps permit the transfer of the results of both experience in soil use and research within countries and between countries and continents by specific kinds of soil. This kind of study enormously helps to avoid the very costly and now unnecessary trial-and-error methods of selecting responsive soils for use, or, to turn the problem around, of selecting rewarding systems of use for known kinds of soil.

With modern soil surveys and related soil study, it is no longer necessary to take chances in the development of new lands for farming that may result in wasted efforts, nor should arbitrary sizes of holdings be established with the same number of acres or hectares. To give each family 20 or 40 hectares is bound to lead to injustice. Instead, by developing reliable average productivity indices for

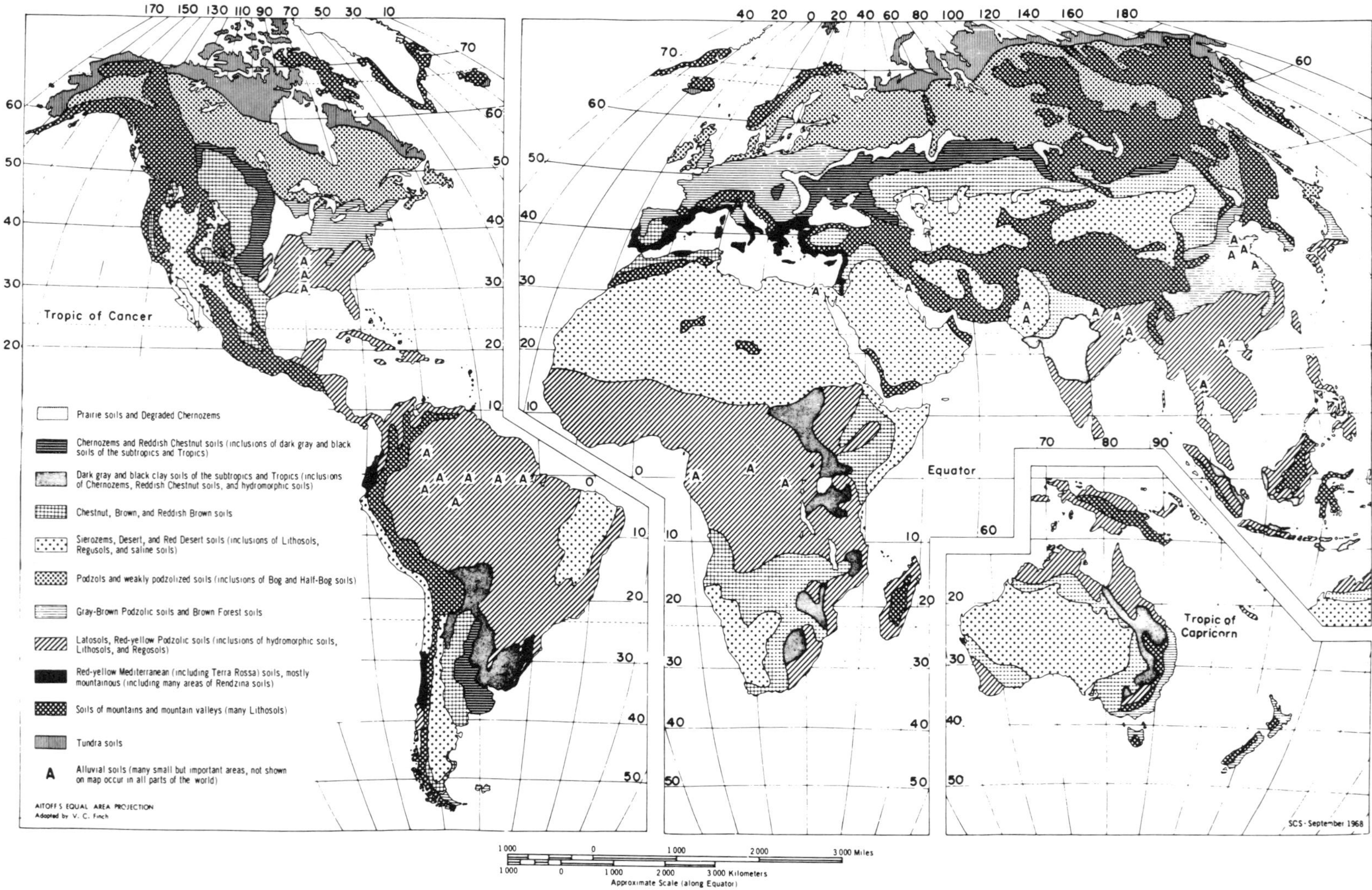

FIGURE 1. A small-scale soil map of the world based on the soil classification current in the U.S. from about 1950 to 1965. (For detailed descriptions of the map units, see Reference 2.)

SOILS OF THE WORLD
Distribution of Orders and Principal Suborders

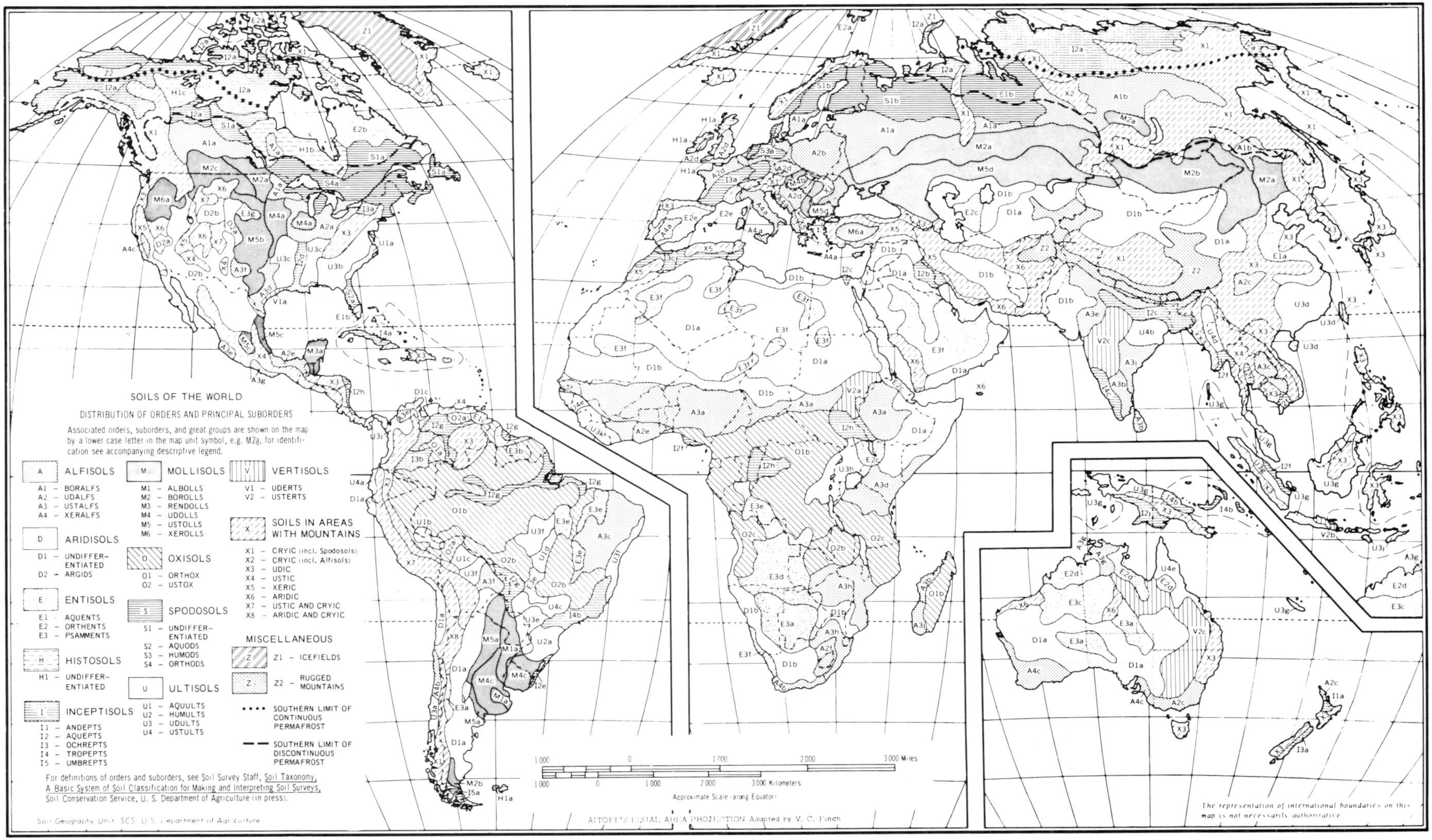

FIGURE 2. A small-scale soil map of the world based on the current system of soil taxonomy in the U.S. (For detailed descriptions of the soil units, see Reference 3.) (Courtesy Soil Survey, U.S. Dept. of Agriculture.)

the crops to be grown, by kinds of soil, such figures can be adjusted up or down so that each parcel has about the same potential productivity. Thus, some holdings may need to be larger or smaller than the average.

Then, too, the beginning plan for new land settlement should be in accord with the skills of the settlers, as they cannot be expected to learn new skills suddenly. Also, some commonly work harder than others, so not all land should be allocated at the beginning, so as to increase the sizes of holdings as skills develop. With cooperative development, rather than individual property holdings, these adjustments can be made within the cooperative.

At the same time that a new land development or land reform scheme is planned, plans need to be made for the location of small towns or villages, roads, and other common services. Not all these services need to be started at once, but they do need to be in the plan. Soil surveys are very helpful for the location of towns and highways. Some kinds of soil highly useful for farming are not suitable as foundations for buildings, roads, airports, and other structures.

DEVELOPMENT AND SPREAD OF TECHNOLOGY

Since the industrial revolution, most farming in all the advanced countries has had enormous inputs of chemicals, machines, and other supplies from industry. For example, in their natural condition, the soils of Florida would produce very little food. The Indians there lived mainly on foods from the sea. But by the application of modern principles of water control, plant and animal breeding, fertilization with both the primary and secondary plant (and animal) nutrients, controls of insects, diseases, and weeds, Florida now has highly successful farming. Yet without a vigorous industrial sector in agriculture to supply the essential inputs, progress would have been slow indeed.

The spread of modern farm technology to the less-developed countries also depends on agricultural industries. But, as in Florida, kinds and varieties of crops and practices adapted to the local kinds of soil, as managed, must be used.

Fortunately, enough examples of good systems for many kinds of tropical soils suggest that *combinations* of practices can be developed and taught to farmers. Yet there are no easy panaceas.

The principle of interactions must be carefully observed in this process of developing new soils or improving the harvests on old ones.

Every hectare in the world with a good harvest for the labor and inputs used has at least four aspects of soil management in proper relationship to one another and to the local kind of soil:

1. The rooting zone in the soil has an adequate depth for the crop roots and contains both air and moisture as the plants require. This commonly means water control – runoff control, irrigation, drainage, or some combination of these.
2. The soil has a balanced supply of plant nutrients, considering original supplies, crop residues, legumes in rotations, manure, compost, fertilizer, or some combination of these.
3. The kinds and varieties of crops are those with the genetic potential to respond to good soil management within the limitations of temperature, length of day, and water management potentials.
4. The farmer has adequate systems for protecting his crops against weeds, insects, and diseases.

If any one of these critical aspects is omitted, the farmer is apt to get little return from his labor and cost for all the others. In special situations he may also need protection against storms from the ocean, mountain torrents, or fire.

The observance of the principle of interactions leads to specific groups or practices, or "package programs," for each kind of soil. A "package" for one kind of soil may not work at all on another kind. And the "package" used must be within the skill of the cultivator with advisory assistance.

Water control methods have been improved a great deal within the past 30 to 40 years. Taking the world as a whole, most crops receive their moisture from the water that falls as rain. With well-designed earthen terraces at a slight angle to the contour, the water can be slowed down so that a good proportion of it soaks into the soil. Such conservation of water may permit two crops to grow in successive seasons on the same field in warm countries, including one in the dry season from the stored water in the soil. The services of a skilled engineer are required to lay those out accurately for the best results, as well as for proper irrigation and drainage systems where needed.

Both the nature of the soil and the rainfall patterns need to be taken into account.

Fertilizers are now widely used except in remote areas without transport where only manure and compost, made partly at least from plants with high protein leaves, can be available. Especially on soils already being farmed, for fertilizer applications a simple soil laboratory is helpful for tests to indicate the requirements for balanced plant nutrients, along with a few trials in fields.[4] It is highly important to know the local kinds of soil because similar test results on contrasting kinds of soils lead to different recommendations and by knowing the names of the soils, use can be made of results from other developed farming areas having the same kinds of soils.

Control of soil erosion is important, especially on soils with low rates of infiltration of water or wherever running water is concentrated, as at a poorly located terrace outlet. Actually, soil erosion control goes back primarily to runoff control.

Control of soil blowing is important on soils where winds are strong and the soil is left uncovered in dry seasons after harvest or with overgrazing. Newer methods for "mulch" or minimum tillage help control both soil erosion and soil blowing, although the practices vary in the two unlike situations.

Land Clearing

A high proportion of the unused but potentially arable soils of the world that are not used for farming require clearing of the forest, as did most of those in the eastern part of the U.S. and in Western Europe. By hand with axes this is slow arduous work, especially in the humid tropics. Even clearing with bulldozers is expensive and leaves the soil in poor condition.

In recent years with very heavy machines, the costs of clearing have been reduced greatly, say from around $750 to $1,200 per hectare to about $160 dollars or less. This does not include any additional road construction for access to the area. The soil is left in better shape for use, with the old roots remaining in the soil.

In some systems the trees are pushed over with a huge steel frame and the wood crushed. In other systems the trees are cut off at the ground level with a steel blade pushed by a powerful crawler-type tractor (Figure 3). The very large ones are split with a "stinger" and taken out, piece by piece (Figure 4). The logs and brush are piled for burning (Figure 5). In areas with no dry season, some oil may be necessary to start the burn.

After the wood is removed, the area is gone over with a heavy cutaway disc. Each disc is controlled by a heavy spring that allows it "to jump" the stumps. By going once each way with this tool, sprouting is low. With this finished, any necessary ditches or terraces are made and the soil is ready for planting after the required fertilizers are used.

Assistance to Farmers on New Lands

The major points in soil management in which farmers need good advisory (or extension) help have been outlined. In many new areas, much useful information can be had from a good soil survey, which is essential anyway to avoid soils unresponsive to known management systems. Not all local soils in the world have been studied, but a very high proportion of them have been. So after the soil survey is made, experienced soil scientists can suggest where similar kinds of soil have already been studied and put to use. The results of research and of the experience farmers have already had are extremely valuable to the development of a new area.

WHY SO MUCH POTENTIAL ARABLE SOIL IS NOT USED

As we pointed out at the start, less than one half of the potentially arable soils of the world are used for crops. These unused soils are widely scattered in both large and small areas. The total area of potentially arable soils in the world approximates 3.16 billion hectares of which about 1.37 billion hectares are in use.

We have made some estimates by large regions, not counting the continent of Australia and the many large and small islands.

Africa has a potential of about 733 million hectares of which around 125 million are cultivated. The Zaire River (Congo) Basin alone has enormous potentials.

South America uses a bit over 77 million hectares out of a total potential of around 648 million.

North and Central America could increase farming on about 267 million hectares. Roughly

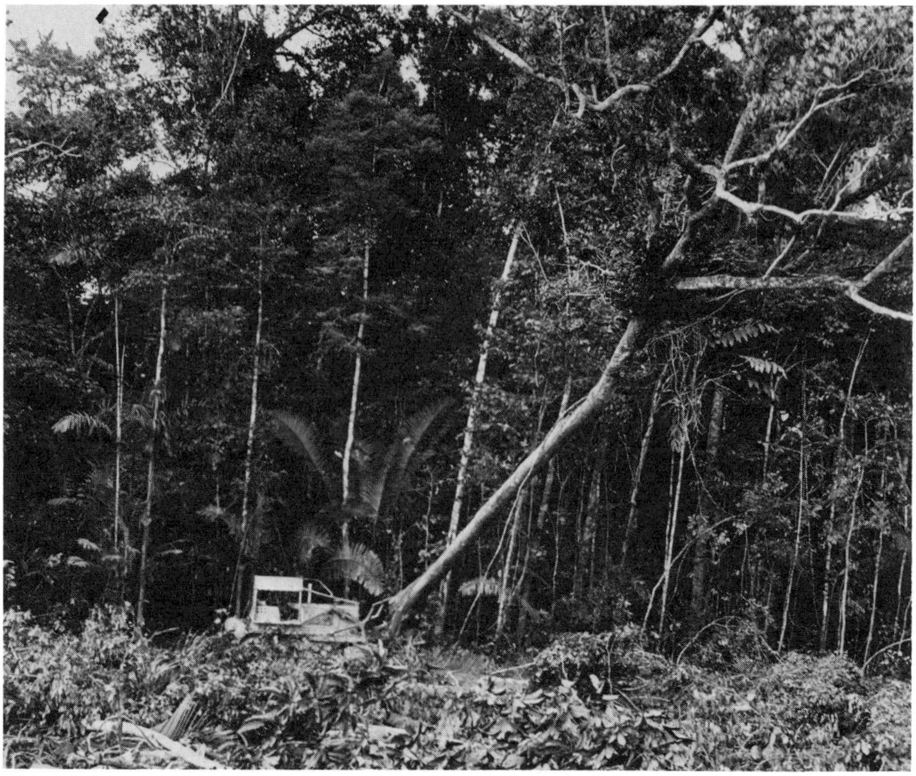

FIGURE 3. Cutting a tree in the tropical rain forest at ground level. (Courtesy of Rome Industries.)

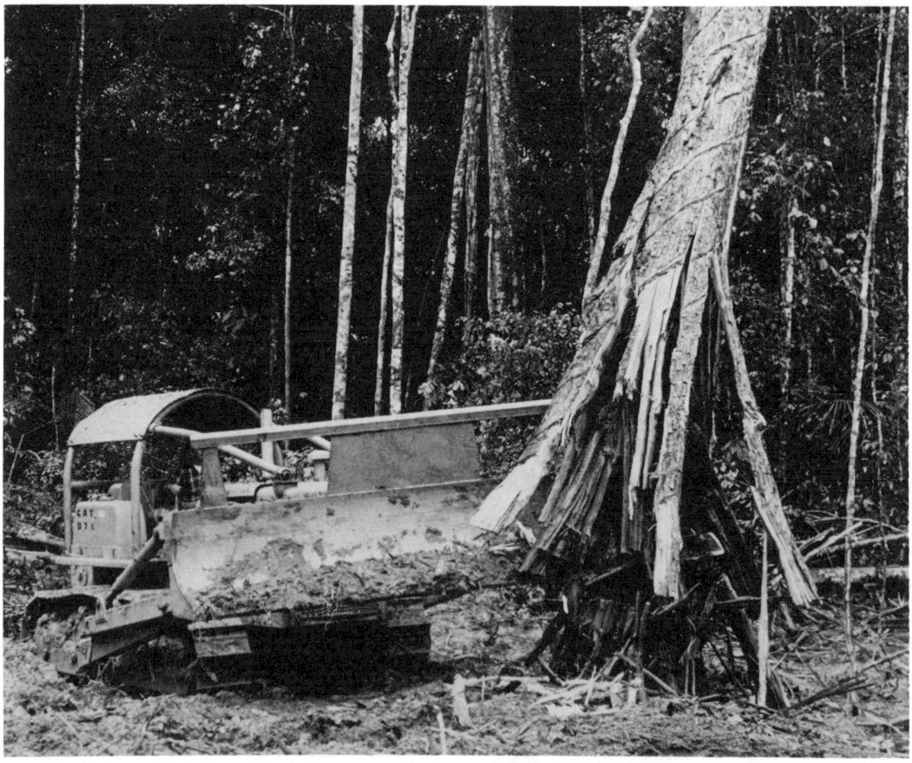

FIGURE 4. "Stinger" on blade splits large tree in tropical forest. The tree is split into three to five pieces and each removed separately. (Courtesy of Rome Industries.)

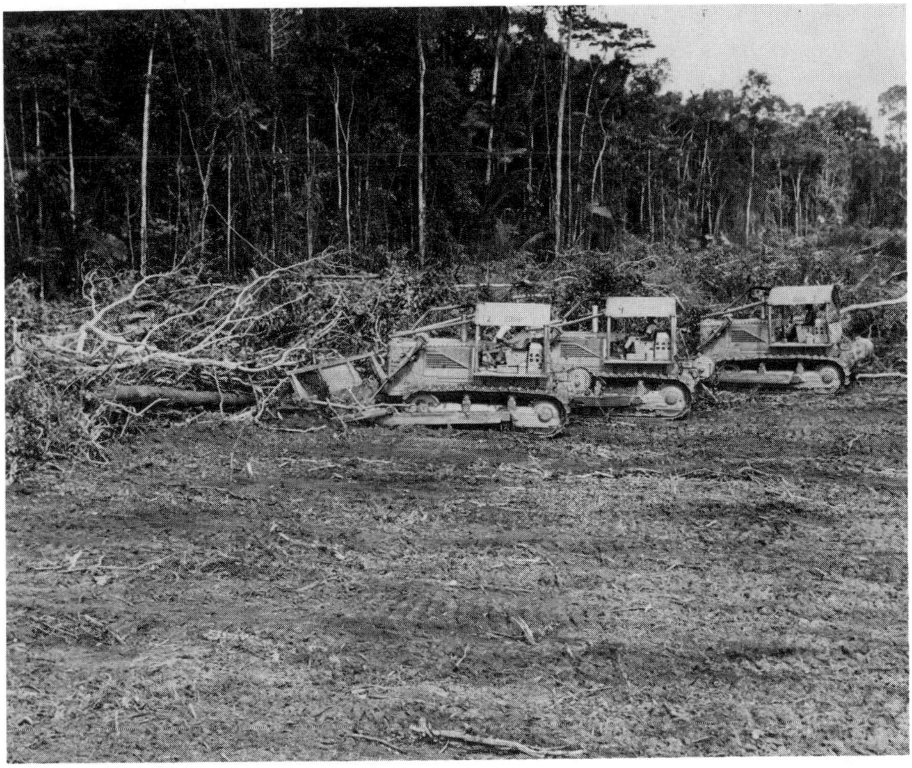

FIGURE 5. Piling brush and logs after cutting trees in tropical rain forest. (Courtesy of Rome Industries.)

one third of this is in the U.S. With the new practices available since about 1940, much of this in the U.S. and Canada would have been brought into use had market outlets been available.

Europe west of the Soviet Union could increase by about 20 million hectares. But much of this may be offset by needs for highways, airports, towns, and recreational areas.

The Soviet Union could increase by around 109 million hectares. If farming and other agricultural practices continue to improve, this estimate may turn out to be too low.

China could probably increase its farm land area a little with need and if their practices continue to improve.

Southeast Asia could increase by about 84 million hectares.

These estimates assume no extensive schemes for desalinization of sea water to supplement existing supplies of water from rain, groundwater, and surface streams. On the whole, the author believes the figures are conservative, considering the continual improvements in farm technology – fertilizers, tillage, plant varieties and protection, and methods of water control. The outlook for better animal husbandry is also good. But, of course, all of this requires much work.

Early accidents of migration have had a great deal to do with the heavy concentrations of the good soil not used for farming in Africa and South America. During the last three million years, the northern areas, and some of the most southern ones, had great continental glaciers. During the glacial periods the presently dry areas in North Africa and the Near East were moist.

After the last glaciation, some 10,000 years ago, many people of the Mediterranean region migrated north, following the retreating glaciers, rather than south. With the great discoveries many also migrated to North America and fewer to South America. Africa was explored, with gradual European settlement mainly in the southern part.

Thus, many potentially arable soils were passed by, especially in Central and South America and in Africa. Then too, the heavy tropical rainforest was not easy to clear with simple tools. But now railways and highways for heavy transport are not available for carrying supplies to farmers or for shipping out their products. As with other soils, fertilizers are needed for good harvests of most field, horticultural, and industrial crops. Much new technology to control pests in tropical areas had to be learned. Although the rainy tropics have many advantages, pest and weed controls are difficult because of the absence of either dry or cold seasons, which have therapeutic effects on weeds and other pests. Also plant geneticists have had to develop new varieties of many familiar food crops to accommodate to the short days of the tropics.[6] Great progress has already been made with several cereal crops, rubber, African oil palm, and many others.

Scientific study of these kinds of soil and the technology needed for their effective use has advanced enormously during the past 30 to 40 years. Many tropical soils have been producing well for a long time where there has been an adequate infrastructure, especially near seaports.

The present chief limitation to bringing in new soils is an inadequate infrastructure, including heavy transport and the other common services.

Recently, a few have exaggerated enormously the hazard of "laterite" in tropical soils. In many spots the soils are underlain by doughy laterite that hardens irreversibly if exposed to the sun and rain by removal of upper soil above the laterite, now called by the more specific term, "plinthite."[3] Such crusts can be seen here and there in most tropical or former tropical areas. A few tiny examples can be seen in southern and central parts of the U.S. In some places the doughy laterite is exposed and cut into bricks that harden (Figure 6). For a good explanation of laterite see Reference 7.

In modern times, no development should be undertaken without a soil survery to avoid not only laterite near the surface, but also many other soil conditions that can lead to failure.

Among the worst are the acid-sulfate soils, formerly called "cat clays," commonly found in ill-drained places near the sea where hurricanes have carried salty sea water onto them. The sulfates from the sea water are reduced to sulfides by the wet condition and the presence of organic matter. The sulfides form new minerals with potassium and other elements. So long as the soil remains wet, nothing special happens. But if such soils are drained, sulfuric acid forms. In clayey materials the pH may be so low that enormous amounts of lime may be required, so much as to upset the balance among the plant nutrients.

A few of them have been used for rice, as years

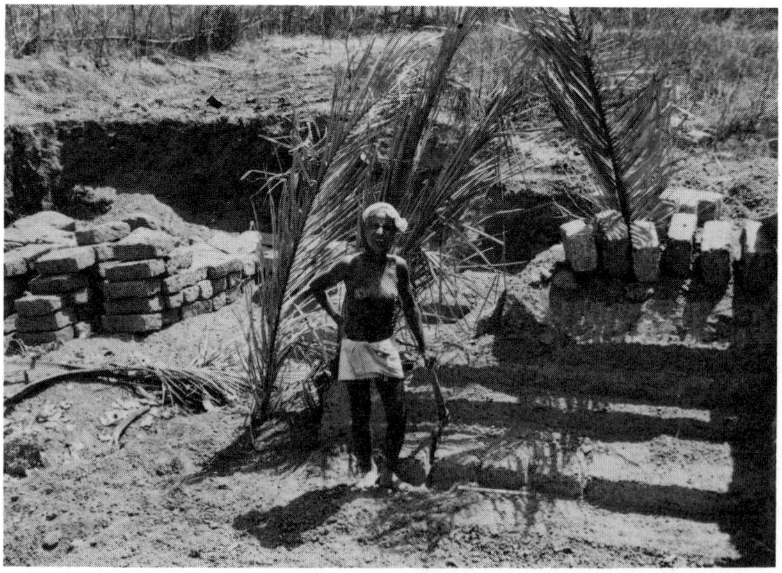

FIGURE 6. In Kerala State, India, a man rests while cutting the doughy laterite into potential bricks. After these are exposed to sun and rain a few months, they harden irreversibly into excellent building bricks.

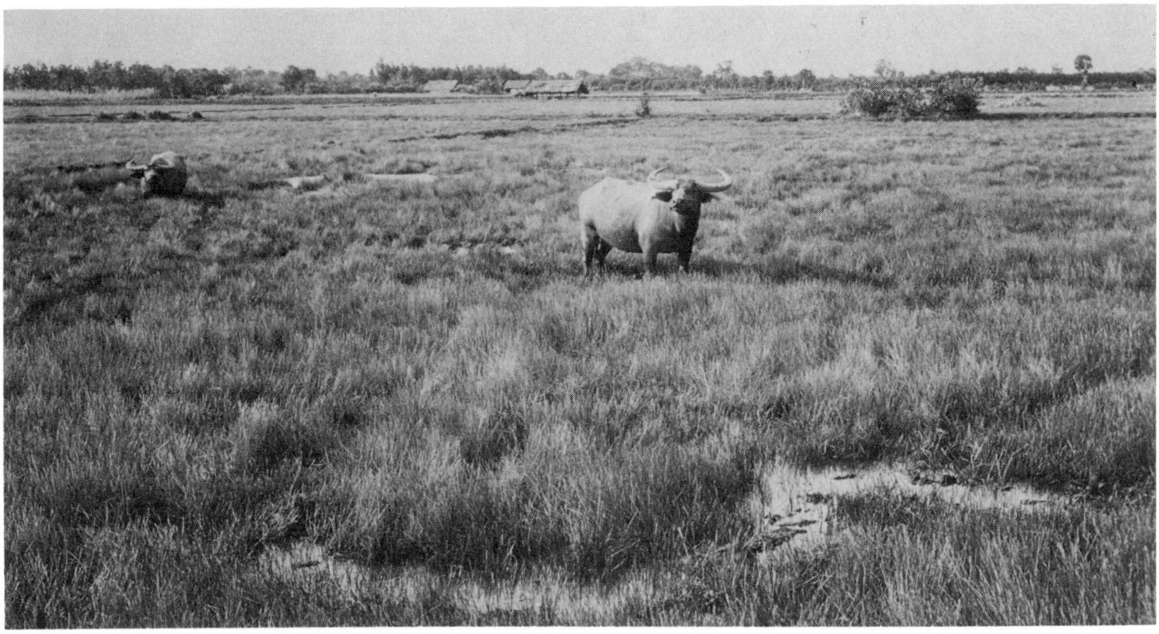

FIGURE 7. A typical acid sulfate clayey soil with rushes in the delta of the Mekong River not far from Saigon.

ago along the Atlantic Coast south of Charleston, S.C., by keeping the soil wet except during a harvest about every other year. Yields were low under such conditions. Some can be reclaimed if the soils are not too extremely acid and are kept wet except during harvest (Figure 7).

In crowded areas many potentially erosive hilly lands are used without damaging erosion by building high stone-wall terraces. Much hand labor is required for this.

The author is not advocating that all these billions of hectares of soils should now be developed; but they could be, and some should be. Of course, it would take hard work as it did where many people are now farming. Now better kinds of food crops with adequate protein and vitamins are available for planting.

REFERENCES

1. **Kellogg, Charles E.**, Town-country planning, in *1971 Yearbook of Agriculture,* U.S. Department of Agriculture, Washington, 1971, 28.
2. **Kellogg, Charles E. and Orvedal, A. C.**, Potentially arable soils of the world and critical measures for their use, in *Advances in Agronomy,* Vol. 21, Academic Press, New York, 1969, 109.
3. Soil Survey Staff, Soil Taxonomy: A Basic System of Soil Classification for Making and Interpreting Soil Surveys, Soil Survey, U.S. Department of Agriculture, Washington, 1973.
4. **Ignatieff, V. and Page, H. J.**, Eds., *Efficient Use of Fertilizers,* 2nd ed., FAO Agricultural Studies No. 43, Rome, 1958, 355.
5. FAO-UNESCO, *Soil Map of the World, Vol. IV. South America,* Rome, 1971, 193.
6. **Jurion, F. and Henry, J.**, *Can Primitive Farming be Modernized?* INEAC, Brussels, 1969, 457. (Original edition in French, 1967.)
7. **Alexander, L. T. and Cady, J. G.**, *The Genesis and Hardening of Laterite in Soils,* Tech. Bull. No. 1282, U.S. Department of Agriculture, Washington, 1962, 90.

INCREASING CROP YIELDS: TECHNICAL MEASURES FOR INCREASING PRODUCTIVITY

G. F. Sprague

TABLE OF CONTENTS

Introduction . . . 92

Soil Management . . . 92
- Plant Nutrients . . . 93
  - Nitrogen . . . 93
  - Phosphorus . . . 93
  - Potassium . . . 94
  - Secondary Elements . . . 94
    - Calcium . . . 94
    - Magnesium . . . 94
    - Sulfur . . . 95
  - Micronutrients . . . 95
- Organic Matter . . . 95
- pH . . . 96
- Fertilizer Requirements and Response . . . 97
- Water Management . . . 98

Production Practices . . . 99
- Tillage . . . 99
  - Soil Tilth . . . 99
  - Crop Residues . . . 99
- Weed Control . . . 100
- Time of Planting . . . 100
- Population Densities . . . 101
- Disease Control . . . 102

Crop Improvement . . . 103
- Self-pollinating Species . . . 103
- Cross-pollinating Species . . . 104
- Population Improvement . . . 105

Infrastructure . . . 106

References . . . 107

INTRODUCTION

All plants require light, water, nutrients, and heat for growth and reproduction. Species differ in their requirements for each of these. Thus, through evolutionary processes, different types of plants have assumed dominance within certain climatic or ecological zones, e.g., mosses and lichens in the tundra, xerophytic types in very dry areas, grasses in areas with somewhat greater and more uniform rainfall distribution, and rain forest vegetation in the humid tropics. Within each such ecological zone the characteristic species reach their greatest diversity and productivity. The ancestors of our cultivated crops and the currently used cultivars also require certain combinations of environmental factors which delimit the areas where commercial production is economic.

The same climatic factors (temperature, rainfall amount and distribution, etc.), in combination with the characteristic of the parental rock, have had an important influence on the derived soils, their physical and chemical properties, organic matter content, pH, and other important attributes.

Improvement in production capacity may be realized only through minimizing the effects of currently limiting constraints. The type and magnitude of the limiting constraint may vary for each climate-soil combination but will certainly involve, to some degree, each of the following: soil management, production practices, and improved genetic materials. This topical subdivision is highly artificial; any change in one has a marked influence on the remaining two. Single improvements in each area may lead to yield improvement, but the interrelations are such that the combined effect of improvements in two or more areas is much greater than the sum of the single substitutions. This is the basis for the "package" approach used so effectively for wheat, rice, and corn.

SOIL MANAGEMENT

The objective of soil management is to provide conditions for plant growth which will be optimum for a crop or sequence of crops of local interest under a particular set of soil and environmental constraints. Such a system may not provide optimum conditions for a different group of crops or under different climatic conditions. Soils having good water infiltration rates and high storage capacities can and should be managed quite differently than soils with low water holding capacity. For these and other analogous reasons, soil management practices cannot be reduced to a series of specific processes and rules of universal applicability. Rather, soil management consists of devising practices suitable for a given set of soil and climatic conditions to effect the desired crop response. The greater the crop response desired, the greater will be the need for modification of current practices.

Soils provide the water and nutrients required for plant growth although limited quantities of nutrients can be supplied through foliar application. Each unit of dry matter produced requires the utilization of several hundred units of water plus varying fractional units of the several required nutrients. Thus, the demands upon the soil vary with the level of productivity, current or desired.

Under the "Milpa" (slash and burn) system of primitive agriculture, many of the required nutrients are provided by the ash of the burned material. Nitrogen, of course, is lost in the burning process and must be provided by the decomposition of soil organic matter. Planting is done among the stumps and partially burned debris. Two or three crops may be produced before yields decline. The land is then left to revert to native vegetation. The period of fallow varies with the local pressure for land. Yields under this system are low and nutrient demands correspondingly limited. Any crop residues harvested are used for building material or fuel, and only very limited quantities are returned to the soil directly or in the form of animal manure. Even when large quantities of crop residues are available, the primitive tools of the traditional farmer are inadequate for their effective incorporation. Thus, the Milpa system is essentially a fertility mining operation with very definite limitations on the level of productivity which may be achieved.

A much higher level of management was in use in the U.S. Corn Belt prior to 1945. Essentially no nitrogenous fertilizer was used on corn. Attempts were made to supply this needed nutrient through crop rotation, the use of green manure crops, and the extensive use of farm manure. Under this system, average corn yields seldom exceeded 40 bushels per acre. Current average yields, in excess of 90 bushels per acre, have been achieved only as greater attention has been given to all phases of management, including increased use of chemical fertilizers, primarily nitrogen, phosphorus, and potassium.

These illustrations are presented to emphasize that any management system has an inherent productivity ceiling. Only as the limiting factors are recognized and corrected do new levels of productivity become possible.

Soils differ widely in their inherent fertility and therefore in their ability to supply the essential elements required for crop growth. Sandy soils may be deficient in most of the required elements. Effective use of such soils requires the addition of all needed elements. Finer textured soils, unless strongly leached, may possess most of the essential elements in quantities required for modest yields. Even such soils require the addition of one or more elements if high average yield levels are to be achieved.

Plant Nutrients

Plant nutrients may be divided into three classes: major elements (nitrogen, phosphorus, and potassium), secondary elements (calcium, sulfur, magnesium, and chlorine), and the micronutrients (iron, copper, manganese, boron, zinc, and molybdenum). This classification is based largely on the amounts required for satisfactory growth; all are essential. About 50 to 100 lb of supplemental nitrogen may be required for optimum growth, whereas an ounce of molybdenum may be adequate. Inadequate amounts of either will seriously limit yields.

Nitrogen

The most commonly limiting nutrient is nitrogen, which is required in rather large quantities. Nitrogen is a constituent of all proteins and of the nucleic acids which control growth and reproduction. Leguminous plants can make use of atmospheric nitrogen by means of the symbiotic bacteria which inhabit their roots. All other plants obtain most of their required nitrogen from the soil, but small amounts of NH_3 may be absorbed by leaves. Absorption is usually in the form of the NO_3 ion, less commonly by NH_4 ion. After absorption, nitrate is rapidly reduced ($NO_3 \rightarrow NO_2 \rightarrow NH_3$) and the ammonia combines with keto-organic acids to form amino acids. These are then ordered in specific sequences to form various types of metabolically active (enzymes, etc.) or storage proteins.

Nitrate is highly soluble and under conditions of moderate to heavy rainfall may be leached from the soil unless utilized either by plants or the soil microflora. The major fraction of nitrogen in soils exists in the organic form. Soils may be low in organic matter because of their physical structure, texture, rainfall amounts and distribution, temperature, and, of course, native vegetation or past management practices. The nitrogen of organic matter is not directly available to plants. To become available it must be mineralized. Mineralization is a complex process involving microbial action as the primary agent. The general sequence involves the steps: organic nitrogen $\rightarrow$ ammonia $\rightarrow$ nitrite $\rightarrow$ nitrate. The first step is normally the rate-limiting one and can be performed by a wide variety of organisms. The changes from ammonia to nitrite or nitrite to nitrate can be effected by a much more limited group of autotropic organisms.

Soil organic nitrogen is rather resistant to microbial attack and is changed to inorganic at a rate of only 1 or 2% annually. Thus, nitrogen released from organic matter is usually inadequate to supply nitrate in the amount required for satisfactory yields. Stated in reverse, if a crop is dependent upon organic nitrogen to satisfy its nitrate requirements, yields will tend to be low. Where crop residues are not returned to the soil, organic matter decreases and the nitrate-supplying power still further reduced.

The greatest damand for nitrogen is during the rapid growth phase. Nitrogen deficiency is expressed as a marked reduction in plant growth with a general chlorosis. At later growth stages the older leaves turn yellow and die. This type of symptom expression was long interpreted as drought injury.

Phosphorus

Phosphorus is required for both growth and reproduction. It is an important constituent of the nucleus and is involved in many energy transfer reactions essential for growth. For these reasons phosphorus concentration is much greater in young than in older tissues. Even in mature tissue, however, large differences in phosphorus content occur. Concentration within the plant varies with the available supply and with crop yield. Low yields are associated with low phosphorus content, while greater yields of the same crop species remove much greater quantities of phosphorus from the soil.

Soils differ greatly in phosphorus content and in the availability of this phosphorus for plant growth. Phosphorus may occur as salts of calcium, iron, and aluminum or as organic phosphates. The type and amount of these fractions vary with soil type, pH, and past management practices. Only a small fraction of the total phosphorus is soluble and immediately available for plant growth. Sizeable fractions of applied phosphatic fertilizers may become bound (adsorbed) and thus not immediately available. Both applied fertilizers as well as the natural forms of phosphate gradually release phosphate in a soluble form.

Phosphate mobility within soils is quite limited; the portion available for growth is probably limited to that in solution within a few centimeters of the growing root.

Phosphorus deficiency symptoms differ rather widely among crops. In some the plants develop a strong purple or bronze coloration. In other species deficiency may be expressed primarily as a marked reduction in plant size and delay in maturity.

Potassium

Potassium is required for the production of sugars, starch, protein, cell division, and growth. It also contributes to stalk strength and the desirable color of some fruits and vegetables. Potassium is not firmly bound and is highly mobile within the plant. Plants differ greatly in their potassium requirements; e.g., a 100 bushel maize crop requires about 65 lb of potassium, while the requirement for alfalfa or sweet clover may be twice as great. Potassium demands vary with the stage of plant growth and are particularly heavy preceding flowering and early fruit development (Figure 1).

Most soils contain large quantities of potassium with the exception of peats, mucks, and acid sandy soils. Potassium exists in the soil in a number of forms, some readily soluble and others highly insoluble. A large proportion may occur as high-potassium minerals in the silt and sand-sized fractions or as clay-sized mica particles. Some of the soluble potassium supplied in fertilizers may become bound by the clay-like particles but becomes rather readily available if the soluble fraction is depleted by crop growth.

If the initial supply of potassium is limited or becomes depleted by heavy cropping and removal of residue, reductions in yield can be quite drastic. Deficiency symptom expression varies among crop species but seems generally to be first evident around leaf margins and on older leaves because potassium is readily translocated to areas of new growth. Deficiency symptom expression varies among the crop species and no detailed description will be attempted here.

Secondary Nutrients

Calcium

Consideration of the role of calcium compounds in soil management is often limited to its use as an amendment to correct soil acidity. This may be of great importance in increasing availability of certain nutrients in acid soils and in promoting microbial activity. However, calcium is also an essential element.

Calcium is a compound of cell walls and therefore essential for cell division and elongation. It also functions in regulating cell permeability and acidity and thus has a direct or inherent influence on all cell reactions and processes.

Magnesium

Magnesium is a constituent of the chloroplast molecule and plays an important role in many biosynthetic pathways. In some crops at least, efficiency or inefficiency of magnesium adsorption or translocation appears to be under rather simple genetic control.

Magnesium interacts strongly with potassium in such a manner that the K:Mg ratios become of great importance in both plant and animal nutrition. A serious imbalance can lead to a

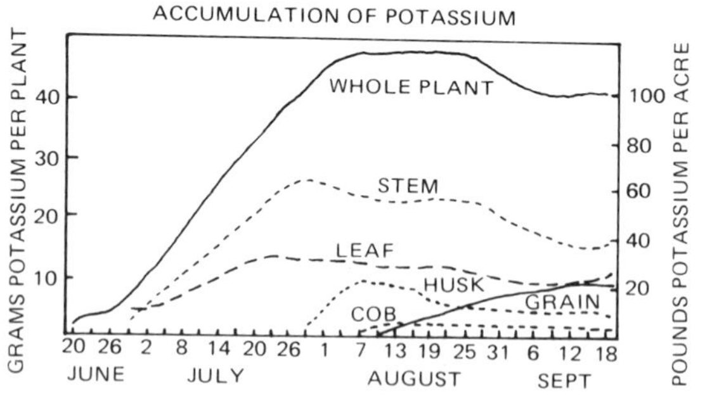

FIGURE 1. Graph showing potassium accumulation in corn for the whole plant and plant parts. Potassium accumulation and distribution will vary among species but normally reaches its maximum at the time of flowering. (From *Advances in Corn Production*, Iowa State University Press, Ames, 1966. With permission.)

nutritional disorder in cattle known as grass tetany. This condition is often characterized by a reduced level of magnesium in the blood serum.

Magnesium deficiency gives rise to a characteristic chlorophyll striping pattern. This condition can be readily corrected through use of dolomitic limestone or the use of epsom salts (magnesium sulfate) or special magnesium-supplying compounds used either as a plant spray or as a soil additive.

Sulfur

Plants of the lily and crucifer families have high sulfur requirements. Sulfur is found in proteins and some of the growth regulators as well as certain of the oil glycosides. Two of the essential amino acids, cystine and methionine, contain sulfur. Sulfur has an influence on several important processes (protein synthesis, chlorophyll formation, and carbohydrate metabolism) and also plays a role in legume nodulation.

Sulfur deficiency symptoms parallel rather closely those for nitrogen. The sulfur-nitrogen balance is of importance. Where both nutrients are supplied primarily by the decomposition of organic matter, sulfur requirements will be adequately met. When additional nitrogenous fertilizers are used, the sulfur supply may rapidly become inadequate.

Sulfur requirements may be satisfied in most areas through the use of superphosphate and ammonium or potassium sulfate fertilizers. The increasing use of high-analysis fertilizers (concentrated superphosphate, ammonium nitrate, urea, etc.) may eventually lead to widespread sulfur deficiencies.

Micronutrients

Iron, zinc, manganese, copper, boron, and molybdenum are each essential for normal growth but each is required in only small amounts. In many cases deficiencies arise due to insolubility rather than through lack of presence in the soil. Availability is influenced by pH and by soil organic matter (see Figure 2).

Even in soils where these nutrients are adequate or marginally adequate, sustained increases in agricultural productivity will eventually lead to a deficiency situation. Blanket applications of this group of nutrients may result in more damage than benefit due to antagonistic or precipitation reactions. Micronutrient needs may best be met through spray applications or fertilizer incorporation as chelates or other forms that resist fixation after the specific needs have been clearly identified.

Organic Matter

Soil organic matter is a complex mixture of plant and animal remains in various stages of decomposition. Due to its origin, organic matter is chemically complex, but three major classes of constituents make up the bulk of the mass: polysaccharides, lignin, and protein.

Soils differ greatly in organic matter in their undisturbed state. The type and distribution are related to such factors as soil microbial population, temperature, rainfall, soil characteristics, native vegetation, or management practices. In forests much of the organic matter is derived from leaf fall and tends to be concentrated in the upper few inches of the soil surface. In grassland areas much of the organic matter is derived from the fibrous root system and is, therefore, distributed throughout a considerable depth. Cultivation normally leads to a decrease in organic matter, the extent of this decrease varying with environmental conditions and the management system used.

Raw plant residues are high in carbon and relatively low in nitrogen. In the process of decomposition the nitrogen percentage tends to increase, as nitrogen is an important constituent of microbial cells. In the process some of the nitrogen is mineralized and therefore available for plant growth. Much of the soluble nitrogen of the soil has its origin in this process.

Organic matter contains less phosphorus than nitrogen, but it may account for a sizeable fraction of the total phosphorus present. In the early stages of decomposition, phosphorus will be immobilized but as decomposition proceeds the inorganic phosphorus is increased, some of which becomes available for growth.

Organic matter also contains small amounts of the secondary and micronutrient elements required for growth. In the decomposition process nutrients such as iron, boron, manganese, etc. may be retained in forms available for growth.

Organic matter has some effect on soil reaction but a much greater effect on buffering capacity and therefore a marked effect on the availability of many of the nutrients.

The best known influence of organic matter is on soil tilth. In heavy soils, organic matter

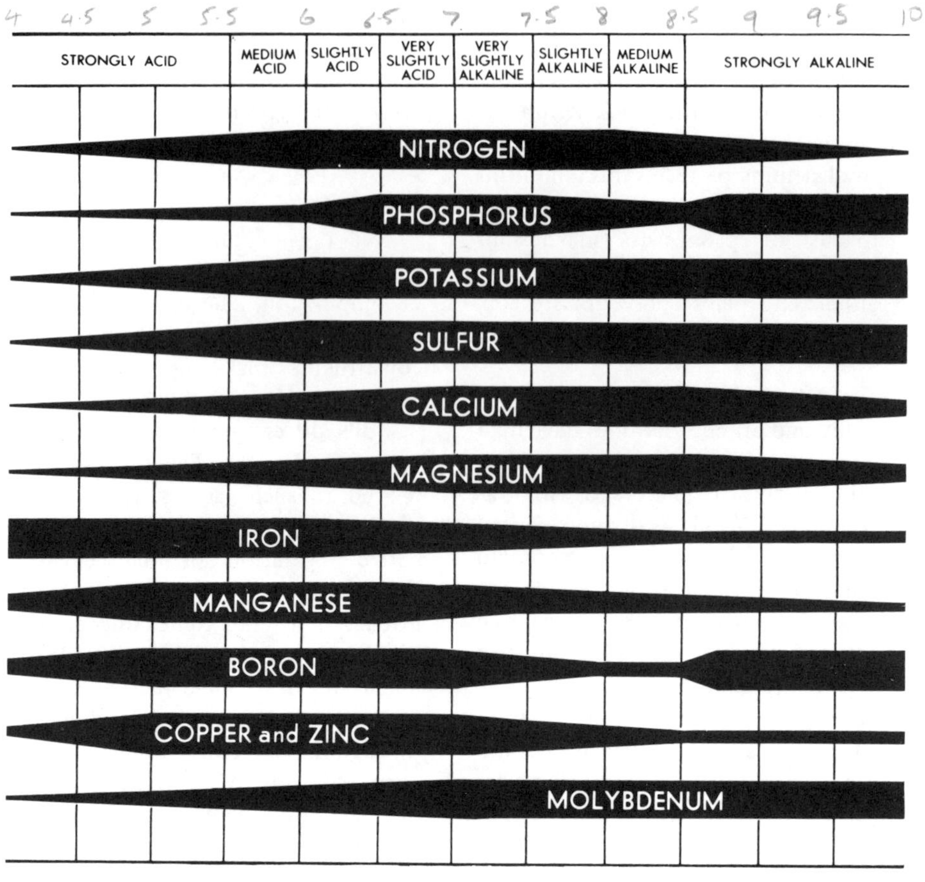

FIGURE 2. The influence of soil pH on the relative availability of certain nutrients. Availability of the above nutrients decreases as the width of the bar decreases. (From The Fertilizer Institute, Washington, D.C. With permission.)

increases the rate of water infiltration, thus reducing run-off and erosion. Aeration is increased providing a better medium for root growth. In sandy soils organic matter increases water holding capacity and reduces leaching of the more soluble nutrients.

In primitive agricultural systems organic matter tends to be low. As a consequence, water absorbing and holding capacity tends to be low and the nutrient supply diminished. Crop residues are seldom returned to the soil, so under continuous cultivation the favorableness of the soil microclimate gradually deteriorates. Where manure is returned to the soil, distribution tends to be concentrated close to the villages.

Incorporation of crop residues poses a very serious problem to the small cultivator. His hand operations or the bullock plow are poorly suited to the incorporation of bulk materials whether these be crop residues or meadow or green manure crops.

pH

The pH of the soil is of importance for two main reasons: (1) Many plants can be grown successfully over a wide range while others do best over a narrow range, some favored by moderately acid, others by a neutral pH and (2) pH has a marked effect on the solubility or availability of many soil nutrients (Figure 2). When soil pH is high (above 9.0) phosphorus availability is also high, but iron, zinc, and manganese may become relatively unavailable. Conversely, when the pH is below 5.0, the concentration of manganese and aluminum may reach toxic levels and molybdenum may become limiting.

In temperate areas heavy periodic applications of lime may be made to maintain soil pH within certain desired limits. The resulting improvement in crop production is a complex phenomenon involving not only the addition of calcium as an essential nutrient but changes in solubility of other elements and changes in the soil microflora.

In the highly leached lateritic soils characterized by high acidity, low organic matter, and low base exchange capacity, heavy applications of lime may be detrimental. In these highly leached soils only small quantities of lime are required to bring about marked changes in soil pH values.

Fertilizer Requirements and Response

All plants require the same major and minor elements for satisfactory growth. The amounts of nutrient elements removed from the soil, however, vary rather widely among plant parts (stover vs. grain) and among plant species. Obviously, the amount of nutrients removed from the soil also varies with the yield level attained.

Various procedures have been used to estimate needs. These have included chemical analyses of both soil and plant parts, soil extractions with various solvents to estimate available nutrients, tissue tests and nutrient deficiency symptoms, and finally replicated field tests. Each of these approaches has provided useful information but only the latter provides information suitable for management recommendations.

Chemical analyses of soils have been used to determine the total amounts of the various elements of interest. Similarly, plant analyses have provided data on composition at various growth stages and at maturity. It was early recognized that the total amount of a given element in the soil provided an inadequate guide as to the availability of the element for plant growth. Accordingly, extensive research was performed to develop mild extraction procedures which would correlate with plant availability. Considerable progress has been made, but unfortunately each soil group has distinctive properties such that extraction methods suitable for an acid soil may be quite inappropriate for neutral or alkaline soils. When suitable extraction methods are available for a given soil, the results obtained correlate rather well with both pot and field response. Because of this relation, soil testing laboratories are being widely used to estimate fertilizer needs and response.

Deficiencies of certain elements produce characteristic symptoms. Nitrogen deficiency may be expressed as a general plant chlorosis or by a characteristic yellowing and dying of the older leaves. Sulfur or iron deficient plants may also exhibit chlorosis, but the patterns for each are somewhat different. Drought, poor drainage, insect attack, and certain diseases may cause effects paralleling certain deficiency symptoms. Plant appearance alone, therefore, is not an infallible guide to nutrient status. Where minor or micronutrient deficiencies are suspected, the only completely satisfactory approach is to resort to pot or field experiments. The suspected element or elements are applied to the soil or as plant sprays to establish whether the suspect condition can be corrected. In such tests, several levels of application are desirable. Tissue tests are often useful as a diagnostic tool in indicating nutrient status. Such information, however, becomes available too late in the development of annual crops to apply any corrective measures.

Field experiments provide the best approach to evaluate nutrient needs and responses. FAO has conducted a very extensive series of fertilizer trials in many of the developing countries. Only a single level of application of each nutrient was involved. This type of survey data may be very useful in delineating areas where certain nutrients are adequate, but more refined tests are required to evaluate desired levels of application and to reveal important interaction effects.

An assessment of the economic value of fertilizer use requires field experiments involving graded levels of each of the major nutrients plus basal applications of lime and all micronutrients suspected to be of importance. Such replicated field trials must be repeated over both time and area to provide information suitable for general recommendations. The average yield response data obtained will be rather highly specific for the crop involved, the soil type, and the climatic conditions. Initially such tests should involve at least three or more levels of each major nutrient, as interactions may be of great importance. Response curves may be developed for each nutrient separately, but such data have value only when it is known that other elements are not limiting. Thus, meaningful fertilizer recommendations for any given locality must be based on the accumulation of a very considerable body of research information.

Ibach and Adams[7] have presented extensive data based on response curves and field experience for a series of crops within each of the crop reporting districts of the U.S. A selected sample of these response data estimates for corn from areas having roughly comparable levels of fertilizer use is presented in Table 1.

These response estimates cannot be extrapolat-

TABLE 1

Estimated Fertilizer Rates and Yield Responses for Corn for Two Selected Agricultural Subregions in the U.S.[7]

Georgia ASR 15				Iowa ASR 57			
N	P	K	Yield	N	P	K	Yield
0	0	0	16.0	0	0	0	50.0
30	4.4	16.6	34.3	40	10.0	35.0	69.3
60	8.7	33.2	49.7	80	20.7	45.0	79.0
90	13.1	49.8	60.5	120	29.3	58.3	85.3
120	17.5	66.4	67.5	160	36.0	75.0	88.4
150	21.8	83.0	72.0	200	36.0	75.0	89.3

ed to other regions having different soils, climates, and farming systems, but they do illustrate several broad generalities. The first is that the proportional yield response decreases with each added increment of a nutrient. Second, the initial yield response is much greater on soils of low than of high fertility. Third, the phosphorus and potassium ratios listed are those considered appropriate for the selected levels of nitrogen. In other regions having various soil types or management systems quite different phosphorus:potassium ratios may be required in the fertilizers applied.

The estimates presented in Table 1 and other very extensive experimental data serve to emphasize that balanced fertilization is essential to increased productivity. The levels of nutrients to be used and their ratios will depend upon local conditions and the increased yield level desired.

Water Management

One of the important aspects of soil management is the efficient use of the available water supply. Each of the mineral elements required for plant growth is absorbed by roots from the soil solution. Although the actively growing plant has a high water content, only a small fraction of the water absorbed by roots is retained, most being translocated to the leaves where it is lost through transpiration. Water movement through the plant is required for internal transport (minerals, sugars, amino acids, etc.) and loss through transpiration may provide an effective cooling system. When water lost through transpiration exceeds that absorbed by the roots, wilting occurs. If wilting persists for short periods, yields may be drastically reduced and if prolonged, death will result.

An excess of soil water may be as damaging as a deficiency. Roots of most crop plants will not develop or function efficiently in waterlogged soils.

Crop plants vary in the time of peak water use and their total seasonal demands for water. Demand is lowest during the early growth stages and increases with plant development and the length of the growing season.

Where total rainfall is limited or its distribution erratic, management practices must be adopted which will most effectively utilize the limited supply. Three alternatives are available: (1) the use of tillage practices which permit a higher rate of water absorption, (2) the use of fertilizer regimes, population densities, and crop maturities suitable for a limited water supply, and (3) adjusting the choice of crop or time of planting to the anticipated time of rainfall. These topics will be covered in more detail in the section on production practices.

Large areas of the world are unproductive due to inadequate or erratic rainfall distribution patterns. Some of this land could be made highly productive if adequate water resources could be made available through use of tube wells or impounded water. Many irrigation schemes have been established solely on the basis of availability of water with quite inadequate attention given to either water use or to drainage. It has been estimated that some 18% of the cultivated lands in the Indian Plains have been damaged by waterlogging or salt accumulation. The loss in productive area is increasing by 0.2 to 0.4% per year.

No irrigation project should be established unless the plan encompasses a comprehensive land-water-drainage scheme. Attention must also be given to social, political, economic, and health aspects. Due to the large investments required in any water delivery and drainage system, planning must be on an area rather than on an individual farm basis.

Quality of the water available poses certain restrictions on its effective use. If the water carries excess silt or sand, settling basins may be required to avoid clogging of the water transport system. Where salt concentration is high, periodic heavy irrigations will be required to avoid toxic concentrations of salt near the soil surface. Information will also be required on the amount of water needed to grow a crop, the water holding capacity of the soil, and the periods of greatest water demands by the growing crop. Each of these factors will have a bearing on the required frequency of irrigation and the most effective utilization of the water available.

PRODUCTION PRACTICES

Crop production is concerned with the effective utilization of the nutrient and water resources available within the constraints imposed by the light and temperature regimes. The first two can be modified within wide limits, while the second two are relatively fixed. Some accommodations to light and temperature are possible, however, through time of planting and crop maturity adjustments and through modification of planting densities.

The traditional system of mixed plantings involving both tall- and short-statured materials (maize, sorghum, millet and ground nuts, cowpeas, etc.) tends to minimize both water and light problems. The different crops may make their heaviest seasonal demands for water at different periods and the short-statured plants tend to give complete ground cover, thus reducing evaporation from the soil.

Improvements in production practices and in soil management are strongly complementary. One cannot effectively measure response to fertilizer applications without plant population densities sufficiently great to effectively utilize the fertilizer applied. Similarly, one cannot expect to obtain meaningful estimates of the optimum planting dates if the yield level of all comparisons is established by a nutrient or water deficiency.

Tillage

The general term tillage is used to describe operations with one or several types of implements to achieve one of three objectives: (1) to modify soil tilth, (2) to incorporate or utilize crop residue, or (3) to control weeds. Each of these functions is a necessary part of an efficient farming operation.

Soil Tilth

Soils that have been under cultivation for long periods of time tend to lose structure. With loss of structure there may develop a tendency for surface crusting which lessens the rapidity of water penetration, decreasing the supply available for growth and increasing the likelihood of either sheet or gully erosion. Plowing, or some comparable operation, breaks this surface layer and permits more rapid and extensive water penetration.

Some soils, because of continuous plowing at the same depth or because of natural soil-forming processes, develop a hard-pan just below the normal tillage zone. This presence of such a layer limits both water penetration and root growth. This layer can best be broken when the soil is somewhat dry and therefore more frangible. The effects of such treatment may be rather short-lived, the impermeable layer rapidly re-forming. Power requirements for such an operation are great and well beyond the capabilities of a hand or bullock-based agriculture. Use of some of the deep-rooted legumes may be somewhat beneficial in opening channels through this hard layer, but such legume types are not available for all ecological zones. If the situation cannot be corrected in some manner, it will continue to limit the level of agricultural productivity which may be achieved.

Excessive tillage reduces soil tilth. To minimize this harmful effect many types of minimum tillage systems have been developed and are used rather extensively within the U.S. These range from a slight reduction in the number of operations performed (plowing, discing, harrowing) to plowing and planting in a single operation. The main impetus for simplifying seedbed preparation has been to reduce costs rather than to increase productivity.

Crop Residues

Crop residues contain an appreciable fraction of the mineral elements removed from the soil. If these are returned, the net loss in nutrients is limited to that contained in the grain. If the entire crop is removed, the usual procedure in a primitive agriculture, mineral losses are proportionately greater. Unless nutrients are replaced through use of manures or chemical fertilizers, farming becomes essentially a fertility mining operation.

In the temperate zones, crop residues or their by-products are normally handled in one of two ways: incorporated in the soil by some tillage operation (usually plowing) or left on the soil surface as a mulch. Either system accomplishes somewhat the same objective, but decomposition and contribution to the nitrogen, phosphorus, sulfur, and other cycles may be much more rapid with plow incorporation. When the residue is left on the surface, planting and subsequent operations are done through the mulch. The mulch has a desirable effect in increasing water penetration, reducing evaporation from the soil surface, and maintaining a somewhat lower soil temperature. This later factor may not always be desirable during seedling emergence and early growth stages.

Weed Control

It has been estimated that the annual loss from weed competition in the U.S. is in excess of $2.5 billion. This is in spite of the $2.5 billion spent for herbicides used for weed control. Loss estimates are not available for the developing countries, but it appears reasonable to assume that their proportionate losses would be even greater.

Weeds may be controlled most effectively just before or just after they emerge from the soil. Two main control methods are available: cultivation including hand hoeing and the use of selective herbicides. Cultivation at about the time of seedling emergence can be effectively done with such implements as the rotary hoe, the spike-tooth harrow, or the spring-tooth weeder. Since most annual weeds germinate within the surface inch of soil, they can be easily killed with little or no damage to the root system of the crop which is deeper and stronger. Soil conditions and travel speed are important factors in the efficiency of weed kill.

If weeds persist beyond the seedling stage in row crops, cultivation with either a shovel or sweep implement may be employed. Such implements are not generally available at the small farm level and the only alternative is hand hoeing. Weeds will continue to germinate following each rain until a closed canopy develops. Thus, any mechanical type of control may have to be repeated several times to effect adequate control.

Tremendous progress has been made in recent years in the development of highly selective herbicides which will kill certain types of weeds and leave the crop relatively undamaged. Due to their specificity, the selection and correct use of the appropriate herbicide become of the utmost importance, e.g., a herbicide suitable for corn might be disastrous if applied to soybeans.

Herbicides can be applied either before or after crop emergence. Preemergence herbicides are applied at planting time or at any intervening period before crop emergence. Soil type will influence the rate of application required and rainfall may affect the efficacy of the treatment. Heavy rains may wash the chemical below the soil layer where weed germination normally occurs.

Postemergence applications are usually applied as sprays. In early growth stages the entire soil area is covered, crop as well as weeds. At later stages the spray is usually "directed," i.e., the intra-row is protected or shielded with the main concentration of the spray directed to the inter-row area. Here, again, specificity becomes an important factor in the choice of the most suitable herbicides.

No single method of weed control may be completely successful on all soils under all climatic conditions. Effective weed control, therefore, may require the judicious use of both cultivation and herbicides.

Time of Planting

Crops vary in their temperature requirements for germination and their rates of development during early growth stages. The small grains (wheat, oats, barley) germinate at low temperatures and cool weather favors tillering. Sorghum, on the other hand, requires a much higher temperature for germination and cool weather retards growth.

Within the limitations posed by such crop specificities, it appears to be generally true that early planting is desirable. Extensive data are available from studies in the U.S. indicating a substantial reduction in yield for each week of delay in planting. Data from other areas of the world are in general agreement. Such yield depressions are influenced but little by the fertilizer regime or management system employed.

Adequate explanations for this early planting response may be as varied as the specificities of the crops involved. Environmental-genetic interactions influencing the critical stages of germination, flowering, and maturity are doubtlessly involved. In the small grains low temperatures at the time of germination and early growth are favorable for tillering and for the satisfaction of any cold requirement. Later plantings result in a delay in flowering and maturity, although part of the delay in planting is offset by more rapid growth. Nevertheless, any delay may bring the plant into flower and ripening under less favorable conditions of either moisture or temperature.

Successive delays in time of planting corn or sorghum are also associated with progressive reductions in yield. The early planting effect has been ascribed to an early season, increased nitrate supply, and to more favorable conditions of soil aeration. If increased nitrate availability were involved, proper fertilization should minimize the time-of-planting response. This appears not to be generally true. Soil aeration has also been suggested as a contributing factor. Soil aeration is usually at a maximum in early spring, as successive rains have not decreased soil pore space. With heavy rains the soils may become waterlogged, providing less favorable conditions for root development. Soil aeration may be a factor under some conditions, but this can hardly supply the sole explanation. The delayed-planting effect is noticeable even under conditions where water-logging is never a problem. Conditions at flowering and kernel development may be of equal importance, but a completely satisfactory explanation is still to be devised.

It has been the general observation that the highest yields are obtained from genotypes which most fully utilize the entire growing season. This generalization, however, must be modified in accordance with seasonal conditions. If the rainfall distribution is such that periodic droughts are expected at a certain period, either planting date or plant maturity should be adjusted so that the drought probability is least during some critical stages of growth.

Where two or more crops are to be planted in succession, each crop must have a prescribed maturity to make the scheme economic. Here the objective may well be to achieve the maximum economic productivity per season. Each crop may be of a shorter growth duration period than desirable for maximum yield but the total yield of the combination may be greater than for any single crop.

Population Densities

In traditional agriculture, plant stands are usually sparse and often involve the intermingling of two or more crops. This system is based on long experience and doubtlessly resulted from the fact that water and nutrients were often yield limiting. Sparse stands made minimal demands on the soil for either water or nutrients. Several crops provided additional food insurance as the demands of the individual crops would seldom be simultaneous. Such a system of farming would likely minimize the destructive effects of disease and insect pests, but would probably increase the severity of the weed problems.

The optimum plant density under any set of environmental conditions involves the interaction of several variables, the most important of which are fertility level, water supply, and the rapid development of a closed canopy. The fertility needs may be satisfied, within certain limits, by the use of chemicals. Water relations are characteristic of an ecological zone and less readily modified. Where water availability (rainfall amount and distribution, plus stored moisture) is the factor limiting plant development and yield, fertilizer applications must be adjusted accordingly and total light interception will be less than optimum.

We have previously stressed that the proper fertilization of crops is related to the expected or desired yield level. If water availability is the limiting factor, overfertilization must be avoided. Otherwise, the stored water reserves may be exhausted before the crop reaches the flowering and seed development stage. A limited moisture supply may be used most effectively by growing a very early variety and by the proper adjustment of planting density, i.e., sparse planting. Under such conditions, a closed leaf canopy cannot be achieved and large amounts of water will be wasted through evaporation from the soil surface.

Where the water supply is adequate, planting densities may be increased accordingly. Under such conditions, the rapid development of a closed canopy will permit more effective use of both fertilizer and light.

Only within the last several years have the close relations between optimum densities, plant genotypes, and fertilization rates been fully appreciated even within the temperate zones. As a result of this appreciation, new varieties have been developed, the fertilization rate has increased several-fold, and planting rates doubled for maize within the central U.S. Fertilization rates for small grains within the same area have been more restricted because of the tendency of heavy nitrogen fertilization to induce lodging. This difficulty is being overcome through the development of short-statured wheats and rice which have the capacity to give economic responses to increased fertility levels.

Ability to respond to increased fertility appears to be a genetic trait. Not all short-statured types can make effective use of increased fertility. Similarly, many maize hybrids of normal stature show little yield response to increased levels of nitrogen. Those unable to respond effectively have been dropped from commercial production.

Planting densities under the hand operation or bullock system of farming are consistently low. This is due in part to custom, but is a reflection of low fertility, poor management practices, and unresponsive genetics material. Substantial increases in productivity cannot be achieved without a drastic change in all aspects of the total production system.

Disease Control

The control of plant disease may involve a number of aspects; these include avoidance or exclusion, eradication, protection, disease resistance, and therapy. These are not all equally applicable under any given set of conditions.

Avoidance and exclusion include such factors as quarantine measures to prevent introduction of a new parasite. This is the main purpose of strict quarantine measures imposed by many countries. If such measures are so strict as to completely exclude new and valuable germ plasm, they may be self-defeating. In any effective quarantine system, provision must be made for the introduction of new plant materials under some system of isolation or control to insure their freedom from destructive diseases not known to exist within the area. Some measure of avoidance may also be attained through a proper selection of growing site or time of planting. These measures fall within the crop management aspect and relate to the adaptation of crops to specific ecological sites. Certain crops would not be grown in areas where heavy disease infection is expected unless adequate measures are available.

Eradication of a pathogen is seldom feasible except under very special circumstances. Greenhouse soil may be fumigated or sterilized to eliminate various soil-borne organisms or nematodes; similarly, seedbeds may be appropriately treated to eliminate infestations of various parasites. Alternate hosts or weed hosts may be eliminated to minimize infestations but complete eradication is seldom, if ever, achieved.

Some degree of protection may be achieved through the proper handling of crop residues and through crop rotation. When these measures prove inadequate, reliance must be placed on an appropriate fungicide. Fungicides may by applied as seed treatments, dusts, or sprays, depending upon the characteristics of the pathogen involved and the stage of plant development at the time of onset of the disease. Depending upon climatic conditions and the growth stage of the plant, one to several herbicidal applications may be required. The control measures used must be economic; complete control is seldom feasible. Fungicides tend to be highly specific; a chemical effective for the control of mildew may be completely ineffective against rust. Choice of fungicides, therefore, is dependent upon the proper identification of the pathogen, knowledge concerning its life cycle, and the most vulnerable point in its development history.

Close cooperation has existed for many years between the crop breeders and the plant pathologists. As a consequence, great progress has been achieved in the development of plant types resistant to certain pathogens or to specific races within pathogenic species. The rusts of cereals provide a useful illustration. The commercial life span of such resistant types, however, may be relatively short. Previously resistant varieties eventually become susceptible. This susceptibility is not due to the variety running out as is commonly assumed. Rather it is due to the origin of a new race or races of the pathogen which have an altered pattern of infectivity. Plant pathogens are as susceptible to evolutionary forces (mutation and natural selection) as are the host plants. Since pathogen population sizes are tremendous, the production of mutant forms is a common event. Survival of such mutant forms is dependent upon their adaptation to local environment and their increased capacity for infectivity of the host plant. If there is a high concentration of a given host, genotype conditions are favorable for the rapid increase and spread of any new, adapted mutant form. Given that the useful life span of a resistant host variety may be short, the commercial use of such resistance as is available may be much more economical than repeated (within seasons and over years) applications of fungicides.

Progress is being made in disease therapy. At the present time, however, only a few plant diseases can be cured after they become established. Effective control is still largely dependent upon methods which prevent or limit the spread of disease infestations.

The principles outlined for the control of plant pathogens are equally applicable to insect pests. Much less work has been done on the development of host resistance to insect attack than on plant diseases, but much progress has been achieved in recent years. Notable examples are resistance to the Hessian fly, the first brood of the European corn borer, to aphids and weevils in alfalfa, and to the sorghum shoot fly. The development of types resistant to other insect pests should be equally feasible if the necessary research is undertaken on an adequate scale.

CROP IMPROVEMENT

The objective of crop improvement is to develop adapted varieties with a high yield potential, the maximum possible resistance to the major insect and disease pests of the region and possessing the various characteristics making for local acceptability. The native varieties have been selected for centuries, naturally and by man, to survive under adverse cultural environments. Under such conditions the locally used types have often lost the capabilities to respond to more favorable management practices.

In the establishment of a new breeding program several developments are necessary: (1) a survey of the locally grown types to establish the range in maturity, resistance to disease and insect pests, and other attributes of local importance, (2) extensive introduction of types from other areas of the world having similar ecological conditions, (3) a study of wild relatives, local or introduced, to establish whether these may serve as sources of resistance to local pests, and (4) the establishment of a series of priorities for the most effective utilization of the manpower and financial resources available. These priorities will be dependent upon the uses for the crop (food or feed) and an assessment of where the greatest gains may be made with the least effort. Crop breeding, of course, must involve cooperation with other related disciplines such as entomology, pathology, soil scientists, and production specialists.

The development and evaluation of new varieties must be done under conditions of favorable fertility and management. Yield increases obtainable with improved varieties grown under traditional management systems will normally be rather small. Fertility and management may be the factors limiting yield rather than the genetic potential of the crop. This is well illustrated by a series of factorial trials with maize grown in Kenya. The factors involved included six contrasts: hybrid vs. local seed, early vs. normal time of planting, traditional weed vs. clean cultivation control, heavy vs. normal plant populations, 56 lb vs. 0 P_2O_5, and 79 lb vs. 0 NO_3.

Substantial improvements in yield were achieved through single factor substitutions. In decreasing order these were hybrid seed, early planting, increased plant population, and weed control. Gains from either nitrogenous or phosphatic fertilizer were not economic as single factor substitutions. Interactions were highly profitable. Some of the possible contrasts have proven to be a very effective field demonstration extension tool (Figure 3).

The yield figures at the top of the diagram are those for the traditional system of corn production. The right-hand box gives yield and cash-input costs when three changes are made in the traditional system: early planting, increased stand densities, and clean weeding. The left-hand box gives comparable figures for the substitutions involving sizeable cash outlays. When cash is limited, greater economic gains may be achieved through use of the low cost substitutions. The interaction effects among substitutions, however, were such that the greatest economic returns could be achieved when all the new practices were used in combination. In this series of experimental trials, yield increases of approximately 400% were obtained.

Additional information on increased productivity achieved through improved varieties and management practices is illustrated in Table 2. The yields of the individual crops listed have increased approximately two- to fourfold in the last 40 years. Even greater increases should eventually be possible in the developing countries as they are starting from a relatively lower base.

Historically, plant breeding has been divided into two separate procedural operations based on the reproductive characteristics of the species: the primarily self-pollinating and the primarily cross-pollinating species. With the advent of commercial hybrids, differences in flowering behavior are becoming progressively less important in the design of breeding programs.

Self-pollinating Species

In the land races of the self-pollinating species genetic variability exists within and among the commonly grown cultivars. Improvement characteristically involves two sequential procedures. The first involves selection among

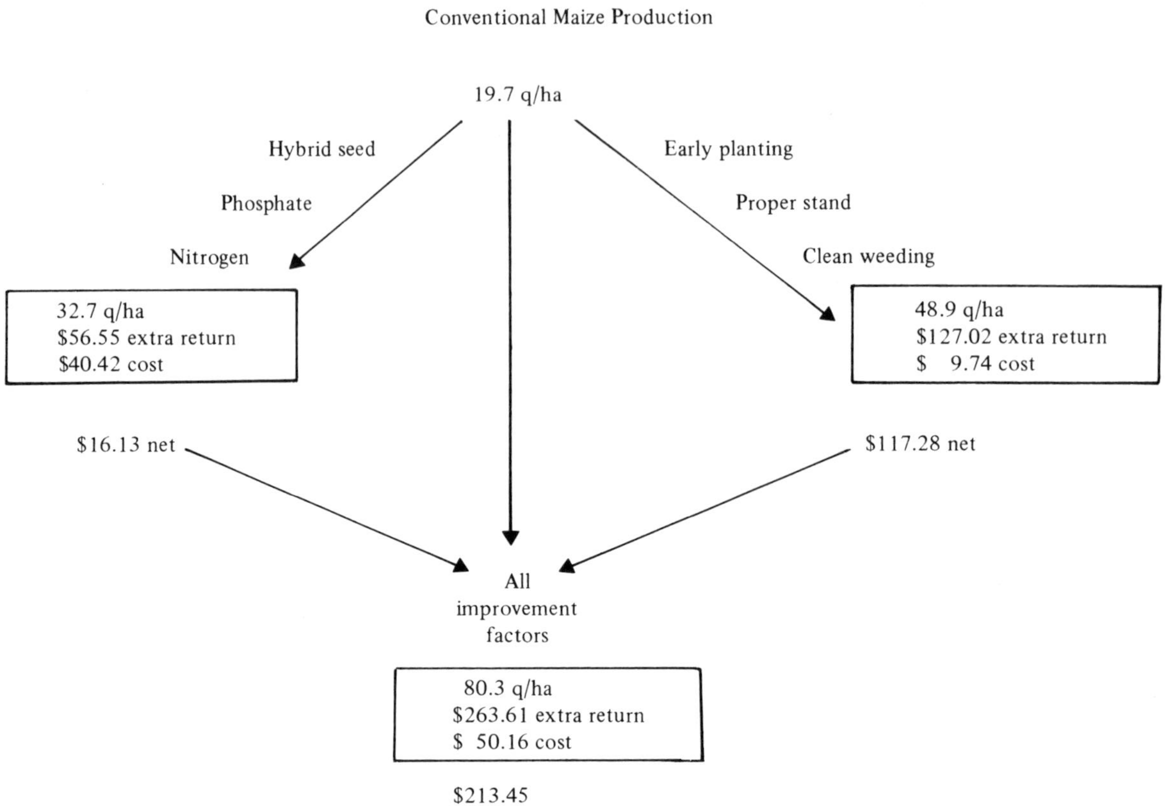

FIGURE 3. Economic benefits from three combinations of improved management practices used to achieve increased corn production in Kenya. (Data from Fourth Annual Report, Major Cereals in Africa Project.)

TABLE 2

U.S. Average Yields of Selected Crops for the Years Indicated

Crop	1930	1950	1970
Wheat	8.5	9.9	16.7
Corn	11.5	21.1	40.2
Rice (rough)	20.9	23.7	45.6
Potatoes	65.7	152.6	228.0
Soybeans	7.8	13.0	16.1

All yields expressed as cwt/A. Agricultural Statistics, U.S. Department of Agriculture.

local and introduced types. The improvements may be modest or substantial, depending upon the level of genetic variability initially present. Such selection and evaluation, while a very essential first step, are quite unlikely to isolate types having the entire array of characteristics desired.

New combinations of traits are possible only through selection among progeny of carefully selected parental types. One strain of wheat may possess desirable yield and processing characteristics but be highly susceptible to some important pathogen. A second strain may possess resistance to the disease in question but be less desirable in yield or processing characteristics. The two varieties are crossed artificially and selection practiced among their segregating progeny for those individuals which possess the desirable characteristics of both parents to the highest degree. Any superior types isolated may be released for commercial production and at the same time may be used as parents in a new cycle of improvement. This entire process may require eight to ten plant generations, depending upon the complexity of the evaluation criteria involved.

Cross-pollinating Species

Several procedures have been used in the improvement of the cross-pollinating species. These include (1) mass selection, (2) inbreeding and hybridization, and (3) the development of improved populations and the use of these either directly or in interpopulation hybrids.

Mass selection, as it has commonly been used, is very effective in modifying maturity, grain characteristic, and plant type, but rather ineffective in increasing yield. This apparent limitation resulted from an inadequate understanding of genetic variability and of the inadequate field plot techniques used for estimating yield differences. In the period 1910 to 1920, mass selection for yield was considered an ineffective breeding procedure and attention was concentrated on inbreeding and hybrid development. At a later date, however, when better field designs and adequate replication were used, mass selection has been shown to be an effective method.

When any cross-pollinating species is inbred, the resulting lines exhibit variability for all phenotypic traits: vigor, plant height, disease and insect resistance, and other traits. With further inbreeding these characteristics become stabilized in a true breeding condition. At this point they are genetically comparable to a pure line of a self-pollinating species except that they exhibit a much greater reduction in vigor compared to the parental form.

Inbreeding performs one essential function: it separates an extremely variable parent or population into a series of discrete and reproductive forms. On an average, intercrosses among this diversity of forms will lead to no increase in yield; such random intercrosses merely reproduce the average performance of the parental source. Increases in yield are only possible through the identification of certain hybrid combinations which have superior yielding ability.

The development of inbred lines, therefore, must be accompanied by extensive and detailed performance (yield, pest resistance, quality, etc.) trials, repeated over time and area to sample the environmental conditions to which any commercial product will be exposed. The inbred lines may be evaluated in paired combinations (single-crosses) or in top-crosses (inbred x variety). The latter procedure is better suited to the handling of large numbers because of the reduced testing load required. Under either testing procedure a large proportion of the lines can be discarded. The lines remaining are then evaluated in single-cross hybrids. Single-cross performance data may then be used to predict double-cross performance.

The saving in cost and field facilities through use of the preliminary top-cross test and double-cross prediction is very substantial. If 50 lines are available, all possible single-crosses among these would total 1,225. The same 50 lines could be evaluated as 50 top-cross entries. The same 50 lines could be combined to produce nearly 690,000 double-crosses. Prediction of double-cross performance from single-cross data would permit discarding of a very large proportion of these possible combinations. Combinations predicted as superior would still need to be produced and subjected to extensive field evaluation to identify the very few which are worthy of commercial production. This system of breeding was responsible for the hybrid maize development within the U.S. The transition from open-pollinated varieties to hybrids required 10 to 15 years within the Corn Belt area and a somewhat longer period in other areas where maize was not a major crop. Yield increases from this single trait substitution have been estimated at 25 to 35%. Since that time, still better hybrids have been developed and these in combination with increased use of fertilizers, thicker planting densities, and more adequate weed and pest control have led to still further yield increases. Average yields for the 1968–1972 period have been approximately four times as great as for the pre-hybrid era.

Hybrids of sorghum, wheat, and other self-pollinating crops are developed following the same general pattern as sketched for maize. The production of such hybrids depends upon the use of cytoplasmic male sterility as a pollination control mechanism in the seed field. Evaluation of new lines is greatly simplified, as these are evaluated in combination only with cytoplasmic male sterile stocks. The hybrids of commerce then are equivalent to single-crosses of maize.

In spite of the tremendous progress made in the development and utilization of hybrids, an increasing number of scientists are of the opinion that much more efficient breeding procedures are now available. These new methods are the outgrowth of extensive studies dealing with quantitative genetics and the efficiency of breeding schemes.

Population Improvement

The new procedure has been given the general designation population improvement and makes use of one or more of the several recurrent selection schemes. Basically the system involves the formation of two or more broad-based populations. These are developed to include all, or as many as possible, of the characteristics required for acceptable performance in a given ecological zone. After such populations have been stabilized through a series of random-mating generations, they are subjected to some type of recurrent selection. The details of the several possible systems cannot be discussed here, but all depend upon the fact that when large numbers of genes are segregating the frequency distribution is essentially normal. Superior individuals are identified on the basis of either individual or test-cross progeny performance. Such individuals are then recombined to form a new population for further improvement. The selection practiced brings about successive changes in gene frequency which are expressed as improved population performance. The selection practiced may involve yielding ability, pest resistance, chemical composition, or any other attribute for which adequate screening tests may be devised.

Extensive data now available attest to the efficiency of this general breeding method. Populations have been improved as has also their performance in interpopulation hybrids. This breeding scheme has been partially responsible for the very rapid progress made in the Kenya corn program (see Figure 3).

The method is well suited to the needs of the developing countries. The improved products may be used directly or as interpopulation hybrids. The development time may be considerably less than for a conventional inbreeding-hybridization program. The demand for trained manpower at both the breeding and seed production levels is also materially reduced. As progress is realized and the general level of productivity increases, the improved populations may be utilized as sources of inbred lines to achieve still higher yield levels. The method thus permits progress toward both short- and long-range goals. With appropriate modifications, this system is equally applicable to the self-fertilizing species where genetic mechanisms are available to enforce random-mating.

INFRASTRUCTURE

In the developed countries the very elaborate infrastructure that serves agriculture has been in operation so long and functions so effectively that the essential role played and even its existence are taken for granted. Sustained improvement in agricultural productivity within the developing countries can be achieved only with the development of an adequate supportive infrastructure. In its absence, research accomplishments in developing improved soil management and production practices and improved plant materials will be largely ineffective.

The necessary infrastructure must provide the following: (1) a system for seed production and distribution; (2) timely, adequate, and locally available supplies of fertilizers, herbicides, and pesticides; (3) a system for the storage, transportation, and marketing of production in excess of family needs; (4) credit adequate to provide for all needed cash inputs and a price structure which will permit a reasonable return on cash or labor inputs; and (5) an effective extension service.

Adequate seed production and distribution systems are lacking in most of the developing countries. As a consequence, improved varieties have had only limited distribution, their potential for increased productivity has not been fully realized, and seed stocks soon become badly contaminated. If plant breeding is to receive support in any program to achieve increased agricultural productivity, both funds and labor will be largely wasted unless adequate provision is made for the maintenance and distribution of the improved types.

The effective use of fertilizers requires that application be timely and that the proper formulations are available. Advance planning is required to assure that the needed materials are available locally well in advance of the planting season. Similarly, herbicides and pesticides must be applied at the proper time if they are to be effective and economical.

Although losses from insects and rodents have been great, home storage has been adequate to support a subsistence population. As production increases beyond family or local needs, a market must be established to provide incentive for a sustained increase in productivity. Where yield levels are subject to the vagaries of the weather some reserve storage capacity becomes highly desirable.

Substantial increases in agricultural productivity require cash inputs for seed, fertilizer, and pesticides. Additional seasonal labor may also be required. If the price received for this increased production does not cover all costs plus a reasonable profit, a sustained production greater than the subsistence level will not be achieved.

One of the key elements in any push for increased productivity is an effective extension service. Most of the past extension efforts in the developing countries have been of limited value due to the general lack of research information and the generally unfavorable economic situation. If, however, research efforts permit the assembling of a productive, economic package of practices, comprehensive extension efforts will be required to speed general acceptance.

REFERENCES

1. **Aldrich, S. R. and Leng, E. R.,** *Modern Corn Production,* The Farm Quarterly, Cincinnati, 1965.
2. **Aldrich, S. R.,** *Modern Soybean Production,* The Farm Quarterly, Cincinnati, 1970.
3. **Black, C. A.,** *Soil-Plant Relationships,* John Wiley & Sons, New York, 1957.
4. **Buol, S. W., Hole, F. D., and McCracken, R. J.,** *Soil Genesis and Classification,* Iowa State University Press, Ames, 1973.
5. **Chandler, R. F., Jr.,** *Rice Breeding,* International Rice Research Institute, Los Banos, Philippines, 1972.
6. **Cooke, G. W.,** *Fertilizing for Maximum Yield,* Crosby Lockwood and Son, LTD., London, 1972.
7. **Ibach, D. B. and Adams, J. R.,** Crop Yield Response to Fertilizers in the United States, Statistical Bulletin 431, U.S. Dept. of Agriculture, Economic Research Service and Statistical Reporting Service, Washington, D.C., 1964.
8. **Mitchell, R. L.,** *Crop Growth and Culture,* Iowa State University Press, Ames, 1970.
9. **Pawley, W. H.,** Possibilities of Increasing World Food Production, FAO Basic Study No. 10, Rome, 1963.
10. **Pierre, W. H., Aldrich, S. A., and Martin, W. P.,** Advances in Corn Production: Principles and Practices, Iowa State University Press, Ames, 1966.
11. **Poehlman, J. M.,** *Breeding Asian Field Crops with Special References to Crops of India,* Oxford and IBH Publishing Co., New York, 1969.
12. **Quisenberry, K. S.,** Wheat and Wheat Improvement, Monograph No. 13. American Society of Agronomy, Madison, Wisc., 1967.
13. **Russell, E. W.,** *Soil Conditions and Plant Growth,* John Wiley & Sons, New York, 1961.
14. **Sprague, G. F.,** *Corn and Corn Production,* Academic Press, New York, 1955.
15. **Sprague, G. F.,** *Hunger Signs in Crop Plants,* 3rd ed., David McKay Co., New York, 1964.
16. **Thorne, D. W. and Peterson, H. B.,** *Irrigated Soils, Their Fertility and Management,* 2nd ed., Blakeston, New York, 1964.
17. Anon., *Maximum Crop Yields – The Challenge,* Am. Soc. Agron., Special Publ. Series No. 9, Madison, Wisc., 1967.
18. Anon., Soils, *The 1957 Yearbook of Agriculture,* U.S. Department of Agriculture, Washington, D.C., 1957.
19. Anon., *Soil Testing and Plant Analyses,* Special Publications I and II, Soil Science Society of America, Madison, Wisc., 1967.

INCREASING CROP YIELDS – RELATIVE POTENTIAL OF SPECIFIC CROPS BY REGION AND/OR COUNTRY

C. A. de Vries

TABLE OF CONTENTS

Crops in Man's Food Supply 110

Crop Yield Increases in the Past 110
  Yield Increase Compared to Farmed Area Increase 110
  Yields and Yield Increases by Region 110
  Yields and Yield Increases by Country 113

Potential Yields 113
  Factors Determining Crop Yields 113
  Potential of Cereals, Root Crops, and Legume Crops 120
  Future Potentials 123

Expected Yield Increases 123
  Acknowledgments 124

References 125

CROPS IN MAN'S FOOD SUPPLY

By far most of the world's food consumption is derived directly from crops, while the remaining part, consisting of animal products, indirectly also originates from plants.

Quantitatively, people need carbohydrates and/or fats, which provide energy measured as calories, as the main food items supplemented by proteins, vitamins, and minerals.

The main crops providing calories are cereals and root crops. They are also important in supplying minerals, vitamins, and proteins; however, the last two items are not provided in sufficient quantity. Proteins have to be supplemented either from animal products or from the far less expensive grain legume crops, and vitamins from vegetables and fruits.

If average daily requirement per capita can be assumed to be about 2,500 kcal provided by carbohydrates or fats, and 70 g proteins, together with minerals and vitamins,[5] and if all these nutrients could be derived from crops, as is theoretically possible and practiced by vegetarians all over the world, then an average person would need per day about 600 g cereals (partly replaced by root crops and oil crops), 100 g pulses, and 250 g vegetables and fruits. This means that, on the average world yield basis of today (see Table 2), about 1,200 m^2 for cereals, 360 m^2 for pulses, and 40 m^2 for vegetables and fruits, totaling 1,600 m^2, would be needed per person per year. This means that about 1 hectare (ha) is needed for every six persons.

In many countries such as China, India, Indonesia, and Nigeria, the total animal protein intake per day is less than 10 g, exactly 7.9, 5.6, 5.2, and 8.4 g, respectively, as compared to 71.5 g per day in the U.S.[22] Total world area planted to cereals, root crops, pulses, oilseeds, and vegetables is about 1 billion ha. With a world population of 3.7 billion people, this means that 1 ha is available for nearly four persons.[22] If, however, all people could have the same animal protein intake as in the U.S., then a far bigger area would be needed since only 10 to 15% of the plant calories are actually available to men when taken as animal food.[2]

CROP YIELD INCREASES IN THE PAST

Yield Increase Compared to Farmed Area Increase

For many centuries, people grew the food they needed for their own family and society. The world population up to the 19th century increased slowly, so food production did not need to increase much either. When local population numbers temporarily increased, food production was increased by enlarging the cultivated area, not by increasing yields. Crop yields were stable, assumably between 0.4 and 1.2 tons of dry matter per ha, depending on local soil fertility, climate, and local agricultural methods. Population, therefore, determined the size of food production; on the other hand, the maximum cultivatable area limited food production, often diminishing population by extensive bad harvests caused by unfavorable weather, attacks of pests and diseases, or deterioration of soil fertility.

During the last century, the world population sharply increased, first in Europe and North America and in the last decades in other regions. In many areas, most of the easily cultivatable land was farmed rapidly. Presently in most areas a further increase in food production has to be realized more and more through an increase in yield rather than through an increase in acreage, as shown in Table 1. If not, future bad harvests will diminish population on a much larger scale than in the past.

The four most important cereals cover about 70% of the total area planted to cereals, root crops, and pulses. Table 1 shows that the major part of the increase in world production of the four mentioned cereals came during the last two decades through yield increase rather than through area increase. In regions of western Europe and North America, where an explosive population increase started first, the area sown with the most important cereals – wheat in western Europe and wheat and corn in North America – even decreased. In the other regions, yield increases also play an important part, and their role in food production increase is growing year by year.

The data in Table 1 for root crops show the same picture if we consider that potatoes are grown mainly in Europe and North America, and cassava, sweet potato, and yam mainly outside these regions.

In North America, the considerable decrease in area sown with wheat and corn resulted in a surplus of arable land. Because of a sharp increase in demand for animal products, both in North America and in western Europe, a major part of the surplus area was destined to soybean and sorghum cultivation. In these areas the habit of eating relatively large amounts of animal products originated in a time when there was plenty of land, while the further increase in the consumption of animal products is related to an increase in income.

Summarizing, we may expect the following evolution in crop production. As long as population numbers increase and good soils are still available, food production increase is going to be practiced mainly by extending the cultivated area. If suitable uncultivated soils are not available, the only possible means to increase food production is through yield increase; in the first instance, this is done through labor increase per hectare, often until the marginal labor productivity is near zero. These two traditional methods of increasing food production can be practiced by local society itself. Further yield increases, however, are only possible through increases in know-how, which has to come from outside, and in capital investment; otherwise, either land that should not be cultivated may be farmed, e.g., wooded steep mountain slopes, the farming of which may result in an increasing danger of floods; or lands may be cultivated too often, resulting in a decrease in soil fertility, lower yields, and in ever shorter fallow periods.

Yields and Yield Increases by Region

Table 2 shows that during the last 20 years in all regions substantial yield increases were achieved for the most important cereals and root crops with a few exceptions, that is, rice in Latin America and wheat and sorghum in the Near East. The average world yield increases were highest for cereals, followed by root crops and by legume crops, namely, 60, 26, and 21%, respectively. Sorghum was the only food crop of which the average world yield doubled within the last 20 years.

What is the reason that yields of cereals increased more than those of root crops and pulses? Is it because consumer demand for cereals

TABLE 1

Yield Increase Compared to Farmed Area Increase Between 1950* and 1970* in Percentage

	World		Western Europe		U.S.S.R.		North America		Latin America		Near East		Far East		Africa		Oceania	
	Area	Yield	Area	Yield	Area	Yield	Area	Yield	Area	Yield	Area	Yield	Area	Yield	Area	Yield	Area	Yield
Cereals																		
Wheat	25	52	- 1	77	51	64	-31	77	8	35	71	12	65	54	33	40	67	6
Rice	31	39	*29*	*7*	*148*	*154*	*3*	*97*	136	1	43	54	29	38	30	43	*79*	*90*
Corn	23	61	11	170	-12	118	-19	104	84	31	14	49	79	46	62	40	18	62
Sorghum + millet	20	67	*6*	*219*	-20	102	92	165	390	120	61	- 3	15	38	23	27	*560*	*29*
Root crops																		
Potato	0	23	-24	33	- 6	24	*-13*	*56*	42	37	*116*	*41*	66	28	36	37	*- 8*	*87*
Cassava	42	27	–	–	–	–	–	–	82	23	*29*	*26*	63	29	22	21	*38*	*35*
Sweet potato + yam	66	28	*-62*	*11*	–	–	*-67*	*93*	*9*	*47*	*57*	*81*	13	9	31	11	*80*	*- 6*
Legume crops																		
Soybean	121	32	*128*	*92*	*126*	*47*	231	28	3283	8	*1184*	*132*	14	3	*72*	*49*	–	–
Groundnuts	57	15	*-35*	*28*	*-88*	*135*	*-35*	*136*	203	27	*716*	*19*	67	15	51	18	*293*	*-13*
Dry beans	48	14	- 3	18	*-72*	*229*	*-11*	*17*	91	6	*11*	*35*	81	18	47	31	*400*	*-43*
Dry peas	32	41	*-28*	*29*	150	131	*8*	*46*	*45*	*-17*	*67*	*159*	1	26	*5*	*10*	*21*	*21*
Chick peas	- 2	23	*-49*	*43*	–	–	–	–	*58*	*8*	*30*	*11*	- 3	25	*36*	*13*	–	–
Cow peas	100	6	*600*	*-19*	–	–	*-79*	*42*	–	–	*167*	*49*	*13*	*-26*	123	13	*34*	*0*

Areas less than 1 million ha in italics. (Source: FAO, Production Yearbook 1971).

*Figure for 1950 are 5-year averages (1948-52), figures for 1970 are 3-year averages (1969-1971).

TABLE 2

Yields in 100 kg/ha and Yield Increases of Food Crops Between 1950* and 1970* by Region

	World			Europe			North America			Latin America		
	1950	1970	%	1950	1970	%	1950	1970	%	1950	1970	%
Cereals												
Wheat	9.9	15.0	52	10.9	17.4	60	11.6	20.5	77	10.5	14.2	35
Rice	16.3	22.6	39	34.0	41.8	23	25.6	50.4	97	17.0	17.1	1
Corn	15.8	25.5	61	12.6	32.2	156	24.9	50.7	104	10.8	14.2	31
Sorghum	5.7	11.9	109	9.6	28.2	194	12.6	33.4	165	10.3	20.4	98
Millet	4.3	6.2	44	4.7	9.3	98	–	–	–	7.6	9.1	20
Barley	11.3	17.9	58	12.2	21.8	79	14.5	23.0	59	10.5	10.4	–1
Oats	11.4	17.6	54	11.5	19.2	67	12.7	19.0	50	10.4	11.8	13
Rye	9.6	15.3	59	10.0	15.7	57	7.9	15.0	90	7.3	6.3	–14
Root crops												
Potato	109	134	23	117	147	26	155	242	56	59	81	37
Cassava	74	94	27	–	–	–	–	–	–	111	136	23
Sweet potato + yam	68	87	28	146	162	11	59	114	93	62	91	47
Legume crops												
Soybeans	10.0	13.2	32	4.5	6.7	49	14.3	18.3	28	12.0	13.0	8
Groundnuts	8.2	9.4	15	10.8	17.9	66	9.2	21.7	136	9.4	11.9	27
Dry beans	4.4	5.0	14	2.3	2.9	26	11.9	13.9	17	5.6	5.9	5
Dry peas	8.5	12.0	41	8.7	16.0	84	12.2	17.8	46	8.3	6.9	–17
Chick peas	5.3	6.5	23	4.3	6.2	43	–	–	–	7.2	7.8	8
Lentils	5.3	6.3	19	4.8	9.4	96	6.7	12.9	93	8.2	6.3	–23
Pigeon peas	5.8	6.8	17	–	–	–	–	–	–	5.7	7.4	30
Cow peas	3.5	3.7	6	10.0	8.1	–19	4.3	6.1	42	5.0	–	–
	Near East			**Far East**			**Africa**			**Oceania**		
	1950	1970	%	1950	1970	%	1950	1970	%	1950	1970	%
Cereals												
Wheat	9.2	10.3	12	7.8	12.0	54	6.0	8.4	40	11.3	12.0	6
Rice	23.6	36.3	54	14.4	19.9	38	10.4	14.9	43	31.1	59.2	90
Corn	15.1	22.5	49	8.2	12.0	46	7.8	10.9	40	18.0	29.2	62
Sorghum	10.9	11.2	3	3.8	5.0	32	6.2	8.1	31	13.4	17.4	30
Millet	6.4	6.8	6	3.8	5.4	42	4.9	6.7	37	10.0	9.0	–10
Barley	9.5	9.9	4	10.9	13.3	22	6.8	8.7	28	12.2	11.8	–3
Oats	10.5	13.1	25	9.8	9.4	–4	7.0	4.9	–30	7.0	10.4	49
Rye	10.1	11.5	14	9.4	13.5	44	4.1	3.7	–10	4.3	4.5	5
Root crops												
Potato	87	123	41	80	102	28	51	70	37	102	191	87
Cassava	62	78	26	70	90	29	62	75	21	83	112	35
Sweet potato + yam	47	85	81	93	101	9	65	72	11	108	102	–6
Legume crops												
Soybeans	10.0	23.2	132	7.3	7.5	3	4.9	7.3	49	–	6.7	–
Groundnuts	9.1	10.8	19	7.4	8.5	15	6.7	7.9	18	10.0	8.7	–13
Dry beans	9.4	12.7	35	2.9	3.4	17	5.3	6.9	30	6.4	5.7	–11
Dry peas	5.0	12.9	158	6.7	8.4	25	6.6	7.2	9	13.8	16.7	21
Chick peas	7.5	8.3	11	5.2	6.5	25	5.3	6.0	13	–	–	–
Lentils	8.2	8.2	0	4.6	5.0	9	5.3	5.8	9	–	–	–
Pigeon peas	–	–	–	5.9	6.9	17	3.9	4.8	23	–	–	–
Cow peas	7.5	11.2	49	8.2	6.1	–26	3.2	3.6	13	5.0	5.0	0

(**Source:** FAO, Production Yearbook 1971.)

*Figure for 1950 are 5-year averages (1948-52), figures for 1970 are 3-year averages (1969-1971).

increased most? No, in fact there is little difference in the relative increase of consumer demand for cereals, root crops, and pulses, but in absolute figures, cereals take by far the biggest share in food crop production. This may be the reason that more research work was and still is being devoted to cereals than to other crops, and that activities of extension services are more directed to distribute know-how about cereals than about root crops. In some cases, however, people have a relative preference for root crops. Both cereals and root crops supply calories and serve as staple food. The need for staple food increases with population increase. However, in case no virgin land is available, marginal labor productivity reaches zero, and know-how and capital are insufficiently available, only one possibility to increase production per hectare is left to cereal growers, namely, to switch from cereals to root crops, which have a higher output in calories per hectare.[32] From experience, farmers are often aware of this. This can be observed in densely populated areas with low per capita income, such as Kerala State in India, central Java in Indonesia, and eastern Nigeria. In the past, cereals were partly replaced by potatoes for the same reason in western Europe.

Table 2 shows that among the cereals, millet had the lowest average world yield, while corn had the highest; actually, corn yielded four times greater than millet. In climates where both crops can be grown, e.g., in east Africa, a tendency to shift from millet to corn can be observed. In areas where irrigation facilities become available, often a shift is observed from sorghum or millet to rice, and in the high altitude areas or in the cooler season to wheat.

In the most densely populated region, the Far East, average yield of sorghum lags far behind that of the other cereals. Sorghum, because of its lower water requirement, is usually grown on land where rainfall is too low for other crops. To produce 1 kg of dry matter, millet and sorghum need 250 to 300 kg water, while corn needs about 350 kg, and rice and beans about 700 kg.[6] However, although sorghum grows where other crops do not, yields are necessarily low under prevailing conditions.

Yields and Yield Increases by Country

Table 3 presents yields and yield increases of the most important cereals, root crops, and legume crops in the various countries. The differences in yields between the countries are very large. As an example it may be observed that the highest and lowest average yields in 1969 – 71 were for wheat 46.0 quintals (100 kg) in the Netherlands, and 2.3 quintals in the Libyan Arab Republique; the respective figures for rice were 70.4 in Australia and 8.0 in Mali and Uganda; for corn 71.1 in New Zealand and 3.2 in Botswana; and for sorghum 41.7 in Egypt and 2.7 in Botswana.

POTENTIAL YIELDS

Factors Determining Crop Yields

In the near future, the world population most likely will increase sharply and double within a few decades, demanding a large increase in food production. Moreover, because a major part of the world population lives on a low food intake of about 2,000 kcal per person per day in the developing countries, as compared to about 3,000 kcal in Europe and North America,[22] an increase in income will also cause an increase in food demand per capita.

As explained in the former section, an increase in food production has to be realized more and more through yield increases. We observed substantial yield increases in the recent past. Can we ever continue to increase crop yield? Or is there a limit? If so, where is that limit? In other words, what is the potential crop yield and is this different for the various crops?

The yield of a crop depends on several factors which will be discussed.

1. As is well known, a good soil in which plant roots can easily penetrate, sufficient nutrients and water in the soil, and an average daily temperature of at least 10°C are preconditions for high crop yields.

The acreage of cultivatable soils on earth is, in general, a limiting factor, of which the potential has been dealt with in other chapters.

Although only about 5 to 10% of plant dry matter consists of elements taken from the soil, the lack of plant nutrients is often responsible for very low yields. However, the quantity of plant nutrients can be influenced rather easily. Whether the large quantity of fertilizer required for high yields will be applied is, besides a matter of know-how, mainly a matter of remuneration, and, therefore, depends particularly on a favorable price ratio between the harvested food crop and the fertilizer. In general, farmers react very sharply

TABLE 3
Yields in 100 kg/ha and Yield Increases by Country

	Wheat			Rice			Corn			Sorghum			Potato			Cassava		
	1950	1970	%	1950	1970	%	1950	1970	%	1950	1970	%	1950	1970	%	1950	1970	%
EUROPE																		
Albania	9.5	14.4	52	18.8	33.0	76	8.8	19.0	116				62	115	85			
Austria	17.1	32.7	91				20.5	55.5	171				130	255	96			
Belgium	32.2	40.9	27				43.3	50.5	17				235	296	26			
Bulgaria	12.4	28.0	126	29.7	38.1	28	9.8	40.3	311	11.3	25.8	128	86	122	42			
Czechoslovakia	19.0	30.7	62				18.6	40.3	117	10.0	29.6	196	113	157	39			
Denmark	36.3	45.6	26										193	237	23			
Finland	15.4	24.2	57										152	161	6			
France	18.3	36.3	98	36.1	42.1	17	13.6	50.6	272	15.0	36.9	146	122	224	84			
Germany Fed. Rep.	26.2	41.4	58				22.8	50.4	121				211	272	29			
Germany Dem. Rep.	26.3	35.9	37				20.5	25.9	26				161	177	10			
Greece	10.2	17.8	75	31.4	49.3	57	9.2	29.6	222	7.4	10.0	35	110	123	12			
Hungary	13.8	26.4	91	25.1	20.9	-17	17.7	35.9	103	11.9	16.0	34	68	113	66			
Ireland	22.6	41.8	85										211	273	29			
Italy	15.2	23.9	57	48.5	49.8	3	18.4	46.4	152				70	132	88			
Luxembourg	18.4	30.7	67										172	268	56			
Malta	12.4	15.5	25										58	67	15			
Netherlands	36.6	46.0	26				33.0	40.7	23				251	354	41			
Norway	20.6	31.2	52										197	245	24			
Poland	12.5	23.9	91				10.0	24.5	145				115	178	54			
Portugal	7.2	10.0	39	41.6	45.1	8	8.6	13.5	57				122	112	-8			
Azores	16.3	21.6	32				38.8	23.5	-40				74	94	27			
Madeira	7.1	8.5	20										52	78	50			
Romania	10.2	16.8	64	22.3	24.2	9	8.1	22.9	182				79	81	3			
Spain	8.7	12.7	46	48.6	60.2	24	15.5	34.3	121	7.3	34.3	370	93	131	41			
Sweden	21.0	38.1	82										137	240	75			
Switzerland	26.6	35.0	31				32.2	59.0	83				184	324	76			
U.K.	27.2	42.1	55										190	269	41			
Yugoslavia	11.9	24.6	107	22.6	42.8	89	13.4	30.8	130				65	91	41			
U.S.S.R.	8.4	13.8	64	14.5	36.8	154	13.1	28.5	118	8.9	12.5	41	94	116	24			
AFRICA																		
Algeria	6.2	6.4	4	30.8	25.6	-17	9.1	9.5	4	6.9	9.4	37	92	55	-40			
Angola	9.3	9.0	-3	10.0	13.8	38	7.1	9.2	29				51	63	24	107	133	24
Botswana							0.9	3.2	256	1.9	2.7	44						
Burundi	6.8	11.9	75	14.3	27.3	91	8.8	10.7	22	11.2	9.6	-14	96	59	-38	82	86	5
Cameroon				8.8	11.7	33	10.1	10.6	5				11	26	139	115	49	-57
Cape Verde							5.0	6.0	20									
Central African Rep.				4.7	9.6	104	7.1	7.7	9							47	50	6
Chad	12.3	18.1	47	11.8	10.0	-15	7.3	17.5	140							96	32	-67
Comore Isl.				10.0	13.3	33	10.2	10.6	4							21	36	71
Congo				5.8	9.4	62	5.0	6.3	26							71	41	-41
Dahomey				1.9	27.7	1356	4.6	5.8	26							49	65	33
Egypt	18.4	26.5	44	37.9	53.2	40	20.9	38.9	86	27.1	41.7	54	147	167	14			
Equat. Guinea																18	28	56
Ethiopia	5.5	7.7	40				7.5	10.9	45				50	53	7			
Gabon				6.0	17.1	185	6.6	10.6	61							50	27	-46
Gambia				18.8	18.5	-1	12.6	5.7	-55							40	53	33
Ghana				11.5	12.6	9	11.8	10.1	-14	5.9	6.0	1				77	94	22
Guinea				6.1	13.5	121	14.2	12.4	-13							39	150	285
Ivory Coast				5.1	10.7	110	3.5	7.5	114	5.8	5.1	-12				49	33	-33
Kenya	10.7	14.0	31	15.0	51.1	240	12.7	13.2	4				37	37	-1	70	67	-4
Lesotho	10.1	7.2	-28				7.1	6.2	-13	8.8	7.4	-16						
Liberia				6.8	8.1	19	6.7	–	–							72	65	-10
Libyan A. Rep.	0.9	2.3	159				8.2	9.4	15				100	62	-38			
Madagascar				15.6	20.1	29	8.4	10.3	23	–	6.4	–	36	67	85	44	66	50
Malawi				5.4	11.1	106	9.0	10.1	12	4.8	–	–	25	32	28	73	288	295
Mali	10.0	13.3	33	8.2	8.0	-2	6.0	8.2	37							100	155	55
Mauritania							6.3	5.5	-13									
Mauritius				19.3	44.5	131	16.6	19.5	17				75	148	98	59	58	-2
Morocco	6.1	9.7	59	38.9	52.1	34	5.8	8.4	44	4.9	8.5	73	79	107	35			
Mozambique	6.2	10.0	61	10.0	18.8	88	7.1	10.0	41	7.6	8.2	8	39	64	64	44	49	11
Namibia	12.7	10.0	-21				5.5	3.8	-31	7.3	3.3	-55						
Niger	4.8	11.3	135	6.6	24.3	268	6.9	5.7	-17	5.9	5.5	-7				30	69	130
Nigeria				14.6	17.8	22	8.9	11.1	25	6.5	8.8	35				58	66	14
Port Guinea				13.6	10.9	-20										52	62	19
Réunion							9.4	11.3	21				37	85	130	105	75	-29
Rhodesia	7.8	33.3	327	10.4	–	–	7.1	22.5	216	3.5	7.4	111	65	112	72			
Rwanda	7.9	8.9	13	–	20.1	–	10.1	11.3	12	11.1	10.3	-7	83	72	-14	80	120	50
São Tomé Pr.																100	100	0
Senegal				9.0	13.4	49	9.5	8.5	-10				133	89	-33	19	40	111
Seychelles																59	62	5
Sierra Leone				8.7	13.6	56	10.1	6.1	-40	16.5	17.1	4				25	31	24
Somalia							8.9	4.8	-46							94	109	16
South Africa Rep.	6.0	10.8	80	15.7	–	–	8.1	12.0	48	6.4	11.2	75	40	121	202			
Sudan	11.8	10.5	-11	–	10.8	–	10.0	7.2	-28	7.3	7.9	8	100	118	18	62	78	26
Swaziland				–	25.7	–	24.2	6.3	-74	2.2	3.0	38	62	27	-56			
Tanzania	5.6	12.4	121	12.8	11.6	-10	6.3	6.0	-4	8.4	11.9	42	30	35	18	34	53	56
Togo				6.8	8.4	23	3.5	4.9	40							51	78	53
Tunisia	4.9	5.5	13							3.1	3.3	6	94	195	107			
Uganda				12.0	8.0	-33	10.0	11.2	12	7.4	12.0	62	51	50	-3	66	86	30
Upper Volta				8.7	8.6	-1	5.3	6.2	17	4.5	5.3	17				49	161	229
Zaire	8.7	10.0	15	10.0	10.3	3	9.6	10.6	10				60	66	10	91	125	37
Zambia	7.1	20.0	182				6.6	25.0	278				39	88	126	34	31	-9

TABLE 3 (Continued)

	Sweet potato and yam			Soybean			Groundnuts			Dry beans			Dry peas		
	1950	1970	%	1950	1970	%	1950	1970	%	1950	1970	%	1950	1970	%
EUROPE															
Albania										3.1	8.2	165			
Austria										13.6	20.1	48	14.5	22.5	55
Belgium										17.9	24.1	35	25.8	30.3	17
Bulgaria				6.7	10.5	56	10.2	11.4	11	4.8	11.1	131	7.6	15.1	98
Czechoslovakia										15.1	10.3	-32	12.3	15.7	28
Denmark															
Finland													14.1	16.8	19
France										7.5	12.9	72	15.2	31.9	110
Germany Fed. Rep.										13.5	29.1	116	14.3	22.5	57
Germany Dem. Rep.										10.5	13.6	30	13.2	17.0	29
Greece							17.4	22.3	28	7.7	15.6	103	5.6	10.5	87
Hungary				5.1	7.1	39				6.1	6.2	1	9.4	14.0	49
Ireland															
Italy	125	176	41	14.0	20.6	47	18.0	22.5	25	2.9	9.0	211	6.3	12.2	94
Luxembourg															
Malta															
Netherlands										22.1	25.4	15	27.6	33.8	22
Norway													20.1	25.0	24
Poland										13.3	14.9	12	11.0	12.3	12
Portugal	136	75	-45							1.4	1.4	0			
Azores										4.0	4.1	2			
Madeira										–	4.0	–			
Romania				3.9	11.0	183				3.7	7.8	110	7.7	13.5	76
Spain	148	132	-11				16.2	17.8	10	7.4	12.9	74	5.3	8.7	65
Sweden										17.5	16.4	-6	15.2	19.3	27
Switzerland															
U.K.													18.5	30.5	65
Yugoslavia				5.2	11.3	117	9.4	12.4	32	7.0	10.5	50	10.0	10.5	5
U.S.S.R.				4.3	6.3	47	2.4	5.6	135	5.4	17.8	229	6.9	16.0	131
AFRICA															
Algeria	100	–	–							6.2	5.5	-11	5.2	4.5	-13
Angola	57	82	44				6.8	6.8	0	8.9	5.4	-39			
Botswana							–	9.9	–						
Burundi	68	60	-12				4.7	12.5	166	6.4	12.2	91	5.8	8.0	37
Cameroon	39	34	-13				7.1	9.5	33	3.0	4.5	50			
Cape Verde															
Central African Rep.	73	29	-60				3.3	8.2	148						
Chad	64	43	-33				6.4	7.2	12						
Comore Isl.	10	100	900												
Congo	60	50	-17				3.3	10.0	203						
Dahomey	67	81	21				2.9	6.2	114	2.1	3.2	52			
Egypt	136	209	54				17.0	19.9	17	7.6	17.4	129	13.1	12.9	-1
Equat. Guinea	40	39	-3												
Ethiopia	40	43	8	5.4	6.0	11	6.0	5.6	-6	7.0	7.7	10	8.3	9.4	13
Gabon	20	15	-25				10.0	–	–						
Gambia							6.7	7.9	17						
Ghana	76	94	24				7.7	7.2	-7						
Guinea	26	68	126				5.9	8.4	42						
Ivory Coast	59	76	29				4.4	8.0	83	3.5	4.0	14			
Kenya	75	84	12				5.0	5.7	15						
Lesotho										3.4	2.9	-16	9.8	7.7	-22
Liberia							5.0	6.1	22						
Libyan A. Rep.							15.5	21.0	35				6.5	13.3	105
Madagascar	32	58	81				7.7	10.0	29	6.9	8.4	22			
Malawi	17	21	24				–	7.3	–	5.6	5.5	-1			
Mali	58	96	66				5.1	5.4	6						
Mauritania	10	10	0												
Mauritius	60	106	77				13.2	22.4	70						
Morocco										4.3	5.9	37	5.8	6.5	12
Mozambique	46	53	15				5.4	6.1	13						
Namibia															
Niger	75	77	3				5.0	7.5	51						
Nigeria	76	75	-1	5.3	8.7	65	7.1	9.0	27						
Port Guinea							7.1	7.2	1						
Réunion	50	120	140				8.1	10.0	23	7.9	17.5	122			
Rhodesia	25	32	28	–	6.0	–	4.2	7.3	73	2.6	4.9	87			
Rwanda	68	60	-12	4.6	7.3	59	4.6	8.3	81	6.4	8.9	40	7.0	8.4	20
São Tomé Pr.															
Senegal	49	67	37				8.2	7.9	-4						
Seychelles															
Sierra Leone	26	27	4				7.9	6.5	-18	5.0	6.6	33			
Somalia	100	100	0				9.0	10.0	11	2.7	5.0	85			
South Africa Rep.	34	40	18	4.6	3.9	-16	5.7	9.6	68	4.6	6.7	46	7.9	11.3	43
Sudan	13	16	23				5.1	9.1	78	8.5	11.5	35			
Swaziland	44	42	-5							5.0	4.0	-21			
Tanzania	30	78	160	5.1	4.0	-22	10.6	6.1	-43	5.1	5.5	8	2.6	2.8	8
Togo	52	89	71				5.8	4.0	-31	2.1	3.2	51			
Tunisia															
Uganda	51	59	16	3.6	6.4	78	10.6	9.4	-11	5.0	6.2	23	5.0	4.0	-20
Upper Volta	111	31	-72				3.1	5.0	60						
Zaire	62	66	6	5.0	10.0	100	6.2	7.4	19				5.6	6.2	11
Zambia	50	65	30				5.1	9.6	88						

TABLE 3 (Continued)

	Wheat			Rice			Corn			Sorghum			Potato			Cassava		
	1950	1970	%	1950	1970	%	1950	1970	%	1950	1970	%	1950	1970	%	1950	1970	%
N. AND CENT. AMERICA																		
Barbados							9.8	17.7	81							101	267	164
Bermuda													101	151	50			
Br. Honduras				20.5	18.9	-8	8.1	13.9	72									
Canada	12.8	18.2	42				32.0	50.3	57				127	192	51			
Costa Rica				14.2	20.2	42	13.2	13.5	2	–	16.4	–	54	95	75	45	27	-40
Cuba				17.4	23.5	35	8.8	9.6	9	8.5	11.5	35	86	133	54	33	67	103
Dominican Rep.				15.9	25.0	57	10.2	17.1	68				98	153	56	84	120	43
El Salvador				16.9	36.0	113	10.5	16.5	57	12.4	11.7	-5	33	67	102	28	80	186
Guadeloupe							6.5	20.4	214							114	130	14
Guatemala	6.0	10.7	78	11.8	16.9	43	8.1	10.2	26	6.1	9.8	60	30	60	101	30	31	3
Haiti				10.0	10.8	8	7.5	8.1	8							35	45	29
Honduras	5.8	6.7	16	16.4	16.3	-1	7.3	9.0	23	8.3	14.9	80	18	28	57	34	36	6
Jamaica				20.2	16.1	-20	7.7	11.9	55				21	75	259	36	23	-36
Martinique																		
Mexico	8.8	28.1	219	17.9	25.4	42	7.5	12.0	60	–	26.0	–	45	110	145			
Neth. Antilles										14.7	15.0	7						
Nicaragua				13.9	22.5	62	10.3	9.0	-13	14.2	10.9	-23	36	40	11	35	42	20
Panama				13.3	13.4	1	9.6	8.7	-10				59	58	-1	100	63	-37
Puerto Rico				–	–	–	8.9	9.7	9							25	35	40
Trinidad Tob.				25.1	16.7	-33	21.6	18.8	-13							83	111	34
U.S.A.	11.2	21.4	91	25.6	50.4	97	24.9	50.7	104	12.6	33.4	165	161	254	58			
South America																		
Argentina	11.5	13.4	17	29.9	39.4	32	16.3	22.3	37	9.5	19.2	102	63	116	84	148	113	-24
Bolivia	6.1	7.0	15	15.3	14.9	-2	13.9	13.1	-6				45	69	53	192	123	-36
Brazil	7.4	9.9	34	15.8	14.3	-9	12.6	14.0	11				48	71	49	130	146	12
Chile	11.9	17.6	48	29.5	25.8	-12	14.2	30.7	116				96	93	-3			
Colombia	7.1	13.3	87	19.3	31.2	62	10.3	11.7	14	–	23.1	–	95	102	7	54	80	48
Ecuador	4.2	9.3	121	17.7	22.9	29	7.2	7.13	-1				40	79	97	16	100	525
Fr. Guiana																99	80	-19
Guyana				22.2	15.1	-32	9.2	15.5	68							100	120	20
Paraguay	6.7	9.4	40	18.5	22.4	21	12.1	13.2	9	7.5	15.6	108	47	43	-8	151	140	-7
Peru	9.2	9.2	0	37.2	41.7	12	14.4	16.4	14	–	29.9	–	57	61	7	102	129	26
Surinam				29.4	33.1	12	14.3	21.8	52							16	85	431
Uruguay	8.9	12.2	37	31.3	38.7	24	6.1	8.0	31	5.4	11.3	109	40	60	50			
Venezuela	5.2	3.8	-28	11.4	18.8	65	9.8	11.5	18	–	18.0	–	24	84	249	37	82	122
OCEANIA																		
Australia	11.2	11.8	5	46.6	70.4	51	17.6	25.2	43	13.3	17.4	31	92	174	89			
Br. Solomon																		
Fiji				15.3	18.0	17										79	125	85
Fr. Polynesia																74	178	141
New Caledonia							11.5	13.3	16				115	82	-29	46	47	2
New Guinea																		
New Zealand	27.3	31.8	16				36.1	71.1	97				158	251	59			
Pacific Islands																102	100	-2
Papua																		
ASIA																		
Afghanistan	8.5	10.5	24	18.4	17.3	-6	10.0	13.7	37									
Brunei				16.6	22.2	34										151	53	-65
Burma	2.9	5.5	91	14.6	17.0	16	4.5	5.4	21				36	45	26			
Ceylon				14.2	26.3	85	5.1	8.0	57	5.9	7.0	18	21	94	346	32	59	84
China P. Rep.	6.9	–	–	21.7	–	–	14.7	–	–				64	–	–			
Cyprus	6.4	12.5	96										96	160	66			
Hong Kong				22.9	20.7	-10												
India	6.6	12.3	86	11.1	16.7	51	6.5	11.5	76	3.8	4.9	28	68	86	27	54	148	174
Indonesia				16.1	20.9	30	7.6	9.6	26				37	–	–	78	73	-6
Iran	9.0	7.4	-17	19.3	28.6	48	10.6	14.0	32	8.7	10.0	15	100	52	-48			
Iraq	4.8	5.6	17	11.6	22.9	98	6.8	11.7	72	10.0	11.5	15	62	120	94			
Israel	6.6	14.2	116				9.8	47.1	381	5.6	27.9	398	159	260	64			
Japan	18.5	24.5	33	42.5	54.8	29	14.3	28.1	96	11.8	11.4	-3	117	214	83			
Jordan	7.0	7.0	0							6.7	12.0	80	69	77	11			
Khiner Rep.				9.7	14.4	49	15.1	13.4	-11							122	108	-11
Korea D.P.R.	6.4	–	–	29.4	–	–	13.4	20.9	56	7.6	–	–	58	63	9			
Korea Rep.	14.6	23.2	59	36.2	46.0	27	5.7	14.3	151	4.2	6.7	60	71	110	55			
Laos				7.4	13.6	83	6.8	6.2	-8				82	55	-33	100	100	0
Lebanon	7.3	8.1	11				18.9	12.8	-32	10.0	5.9	-41	80	95	18			
Malaysia Sabah				11.5	21.1	83	12.3	7.5	-39							74	110	49
W. Malaysia				19.3	27.9	45	12.6	18.5	47							150	160	7
Mongolia	5.1	5.9	16										61	68	11			
Nepal	9.1	11.6	28	19.0	19.4	2	18.0	16.8	-7				40	56	40			
Pakistan	8.7	11.1	27	13.8	17.2	25	9.8	10.6	8	4.7	5.9	25	83	97	17			
Philippines				11.8	17.1	45	7.2	8.4	16				19	63	232	59	54	-8
Port Timor				15.0	17.5	17	8.7	9.9	14							26	20	-23
Ryukyu Isl.				18.3	29.9	63							131	221	69	112	–	–
Sarawak				10.3	11.6	12												
Saudi Arabia	13.7	15.0	9	10.5	23.6	125				10.0	10.4	4						
Singapore																119	113	-5
Syrian A.R.	7.7	6.6	-14	22.9	17.9	-22	13.2	14.2	8				93	108	16			
Taiwan	9.6	21.3	122	23.2	38.2	65	14.1	25.6	82	2.7	16.2	499	27	115	325	106	125	18
Thailand				13.1	19.6	49	9.1	26.3	189	–	21.3	–	–	64	–	188	152	-19
Turkey	10.0	12.6	26	35.1	38.3	9	12.5	15.8	26				77	124	61			
Vietnam D.R.				12.5	19.6	57	11.1	11.4	3							44	73	66
Vietnam Rep.				13.6	22.2	63	12.1	10.8	-11				108	200	85	99	71	-28
Yemen Ar. Rep.	10.4	10.7	3				12.0	13.8	15				57	51	-11			
Yemen P.D.R.	16.4	17.0	3															

TABLE 3 (Continued)

	Sweet potato and yam			Soybean			Groundnuts			Dry beans			Dry peas		
	1950	1970	%	1950	1970	%	1950	1970	%	1950	1970	%	1950	1970	%
N. AND CENT. AMERICA															
Barbados	83	100	20												
Bermuda															
Br. Honduras															
Canada				15.8	18.5	17				12.9	15.7	22	12.1	13.6	12
Costa Rica										4.1	9.1	123			
Cuba	29	40	38				9.0	10.0	11	5.3	6.5	23			
Dominican Rep.	86	107	24				6.6	10.1	53	8.9	8.9	0			
El Salvador										8.1	12.1	50			
Guadeloupe	136	100	-26												
Guatemala										4.7	3.8	-19			
Haiti	50	48	-4				1.7	2.2	29	6.5	6.3	-3			
Honduras	27	23	-15							4.4	5.0	14			
Jamaica	41	48	17												
Martinique															
Mexico	56	100	79	–	17.3	–	11.9	12.5	5	2.6	5.1	96	5.8	6.8	18
Neth. Antilles															
Nicaraqua										7.2	8.1	13			
Panama	102	121	16							5.4	2.9	-46			
Puerto Rico	31	46	48							4.6	5.9	29			
Trinidad Tob.	72	78	8												
U.S.A.	59	115	95	14.3	18.3	28	9.2	21.7	136	11.8	13.8	17	12.3	19.0	54
South America															
Argentina	100	99	-1	8.3	12.6	52	9.5	10.8	14	9.6	8.3	-14	12.4	9.7	-22
Bolivia	37	75	103				11.6	15.0	30	8.3	6.7	-19	5.4	9.0	67
Brazil	80	118	48	13.0	12.1	-7	10.0	12.9	29	6.8	6.3	-7			
Chile										9.2	11.1	21	8.2	7.3	-11
Colombia	108	115	6	12.5	20.2	62				5.3	6.2	18	5.8	5.9	2
Ecuador	51	26	-49				4.6	7.3	59	8.9	4.6	-48	6.6	6.2	-6
Fr. Guiana	70	143	104												
Guyana	27	35	30												
Paraguay	93	107	15	–	15.4	–	8.7	8.1	-7	8.3	6.6	-21	8.3	6.6	-20
Peru	77	130	69	–	11.1	–	13.1	13.8	5	9.1	8.0	-12	11.5	7.9	-31
Surinam							7.5	10.3	37						
Uruguay	46	57	24				6.3	7.2	14	4.7	5.0	6			
Venezuela	36	90	150				9.0	7.3	-19	5.7	4.3	-25	5.5	5.5	1
OCEANIA															
Australia	81	57	-30	–	7.5	–	10.3	8.8	-14	6.4	5.7	-11	10.9	10.2	-7
Br. Solomon	105	98	-7												
Fiji	104	74	-29												
Fr. Polynesia	100	108	8												
New Caledonia	64	82	28												
New Guinea	94	74	-21				6.4	4.7	-26						
New Zealand	125	150	20										17.6	22.7	29
Pacific Islands	71	46	-35												
Papua	82	44	-46												
ASIA															
Afghanistan															
Brunei	80	71	-11												
Burma							5.6	7.8	39	6.2	7.4	19	4.0	7.1	78
Ceylon	24	46	92				–	9.2	–	3.6	5.0	39			
China P. Rep.	64	–	–	8.1	8.0	-1	13.5	12.4	-8	6.3	7.0	11	9.1	9.5	4
Cyprus										7.7	7.2	-6			
Hong Kong	44	90	105												
India	61	70	15				7.3	8.0	9	2.2	2.8	29	6.8	8.4	24
Indonesia	67	85	27	7.1	7.0	-1	9.9	12.0	22						
Iran				–	31.0	–				10.0	11.4	14			
Iraq										5.3	6.7	26			
Israel							34.0	38.2	12				1.5	8.8	485
Japan	151	199	32	10.8	12.8	19	12.9	20.4	58	10.3	12.4	20	11.3	11.9	5
Jordan															
Khmer Rep.	148	84	-43	6.8	8.7	28	6.2	9.5	54	5.2	6.4	23			
Korea D.P.R.	61	79	30	5.6	–	–									
Korea Rep.	116	168	45	5.6	7.8	39	4.5	11.8	162	4.9	6.2	27	5.5	6.2	13
Laos	50	68	36				6.4	8.7	36						
Lebanon	125	188	50				7.6	10.8	42	17.4	12.6	-28	16.0	12.1	-24
Malaysia Sabah	84	66	-21												
W. Malaysia	105	156	49				8.0	17.0	113						
Mongolia															
Nepal															
Pakistan	85	102	20				7.3	15.4	111	5.4	6.5	20			
Philippines	41	54	32	6.7	8.3	24	7.2	5.1	-29	6.3	4.8	-24			
Port Timor	38	41	8							6.3	7.7	22			
Ryukyu Isl.	88	277	215	6.9	7.5	9									
Sarawak															
Saudi Arabia															
Singapore	101	100	-1												
Syrian A.R.							14.5	17.9	23	8.2	12.4	52	9.2	8.5	-8
Taiwan	91	151	66	6.0	15.0	151	7.1	13.5	90	5.7	9.5	67			
Thailand	70	63	-10	8.0	9.4	17	9.5	15.9	67	7.5	10.9	45			
Turkey				8.8	11.7	33	19.0	25.0	32	10.1	13.4	33	5.9	11.1	88
Vietnam D.R.	30	47	57	2.9	4.9	69	8.3	9.6	15	3.0	2.5	-17			
Vietnam Rep.	55	67	22	5.0	10.1	102	5.9	10.8	83	4.6	7.0	52			
Yemen Ar. Rep.															
Yemen P.D.R.															

(Source: FAO, Production Yearbook, 1971.)

to this price ratio when deciding whether to increase production. For instance, much of the high increase in rice production in Japan during the last decades was due to a favorable rice-fertilizer price ratio, while this was much less favorable for the farmers in India and Indonesia, where rice yield increase was much less.

The availability of sufficient water depends on rainfall and rainfall distribution. Where rainfall is insufficient, additional water can be applied by means of irrigation, but the costs involved may differ greatly from place to place. Often the possibility of irrigation cannot be realized by the individual farmer but only through expensive projects, such as dams, irrigation canals, drainage systems, etc. In a major part of the arid and semiarid areas, water is insufficiently available or the source of irrigation water is too far away from the fields, resulting in an unfavorable input-output price ratio.

The optimum day temperature for maximum plant growth differs with crop species and ranges roughly between 15 and 35°C, e.g., maximum photosynthesis of corn and sorghum is at 30 and 40°C, respectively.[17] Temperature can be influenced by men but only at very high costs, which are at the moment only remunerative in some areas for the production of high quality vegetables as, for instance, is practiced on a large scale in hothouses in the Netherlands.

2. Although the carbon dioxide concentration of the air is very important, as about 90 to 95% of the plant dry matter is formed from CO_2, it may be considered as a given quantity. Its concentration does not differ widely from place to place, averaging about 0.03% in the atmosphere. Because of the high costs, just as with temperature, it is not likely that people will increase the CO_2 concentration to increase crop yields, unless food prices would rise very steeply. In hothouses for vegetable production, however, where temperature is increased, "fertilizing" the air with CO_2 also appeared very successful.[19]

3. When the availability of nutrients and water is optimal, sunlight, or the visible part (approximately 50% of total solar radiation), is the ultimate factor determining plant growth, if temperature is not a limiting factor. Sunlight provides the energy required to convert CO_2 from the air (and for a small part from the soil) with water and nutrients from the soil into the dry matter of the plant, providing food elements, namely, carbohydrates, fats, proteins, vitamins, and minerals. The intensity of sunlight, influencing crop yield, differs widely with the sun's altitude, and also with season at high latitudes. In the tropics, high intensity of sunlight and high temperature make it possible to grow crops throughout the year. Depending on the growth duration of the crop and the time required for soil preparation, two to four crops per year can be grown. Generally, in regions in higher latitudes, only one crop can be grown, limited to the summer season. Therefore, potential yields per year differ widely with the latitude of the regions.

In principle, light intensity can also be influenced by man, but costs may be regarded as prohibitive in food crop cultivation. Only when food prices could rise to a very high level and energy prices become very low, could it become a payable proposition, in combination with increasing temperature and CO_2 concentration. But in such an environment of artificial light, even soil would not need to be a limiting factor, as the gardens, with natural or artificial soil, could be stored on floors, as in a high-rise apartment building.

Although in this way the crop area could be increased almost unlimitedly, in practice hundreds of millions of people envisage food shortages due to lack of know-how and capital and fear harvest failures caused by droughts or floods.

4. Efficient farming for higher yields has led to monocultures and "monovarieties," enlarging the danger of heavy attacks of pests and diseases. In general, man can limit the damage to a great extent by controlling these pests and diseases with mechanical, chemical, or biological means and by breeding resistant varieties.

5. All plants produce dry matter, but some are more efficient than others. With regard to photosynthetic efficiency, it seems that plant species roughly can be divided into two categories often called efficient and nonefficient, or C_4 and C_3 species. The most important differences are that efficient species have much less photorespiration,[9] a much lower water requirement, and a higher optimum temperature.[6] Of the food crops mentioned in this section, only corn, sorghum, and several millets (*Panicum miliaceum, Eleusine coracana,* and *Setaria italica*) belong to the efficient species.[16] These species are particularly efficient under conditions of high light intensity and high temperature. Therefore, for the

tropics and subtropics it could be an important factor with regard to crop yields. In higher latitudes, e.g., in the Netherlands, no great differences between efficient and nonefficient species were found.[27]

Under a totally clouded sky, light intensity is about 20% of that of a perfectly clear sky. However, photosynthesis of a crop on such an overcast day is about 50% of that on a clear day.[36] In species with narrow and more erect leaves, such as the cereals, light is more evenly distributed over the various layers of leaves than in species with broad horizontal leaves, such as most root crops and pulses. With increasing light intensity, marginal photosynthesis decreases to zero at the light saturation point. This point differs for various species.

Also, there is a large difference in the part of dry matter produced which is fit for human consumption. For root crops, pulses, and cereals, the maximum percentage of edible dry matter produced may roughly be as high as 80, 50, and 40, respectively.[32,33] The explanation for this difference between crop species may be that root crops such as potatoes do not need a strong stem to support the edible part. Therefore, yields per unit of area and time may be increased by choosing root crops instead of cereals or legume crops.[32]

6. Within the species there is a great difference in dry matter production between varieties. Therefore, by means of breeding, one can try to obtain varieties with the most favorable characteristics.[30]

Varieties differ, particularly in response to nutrients. For highly fertilizer responsive cereal varieties, plants were bred with a short stiff stem in order to prevent lodging.

As in low light intensity conditions, relatively more light is used for dry matter production; yields could be increased by breeding varieties with the most favorable leaf position with regard to solar radiation.

Since the length of daylight differs widely between latitudes and many varieties are very susceptible to day length with respect to vegetative and generative growth (photoperiodicity), breeding should be directed to the most suitable varieties with regard to local day length.

As the photosynthetic processes are conducted mainly in the leaves, the leaf area per unit area of land (i.e., the leaf area index, LAI) is closely related to the dry matter yield of the food crops, and therefore also a subject for breeding.[35] The optimum LAI, however, varies also with crop species.[8]

A major limitation to high yields of annual crops is the length of time required from sowing until the leaf area is optimum, during which time a large proportion of the sunlight is not intercepted by the crop. Therefore, breeding may also be directed toward varieties which quickly develop their leaves and then stop extending leaf area, maintaining a fresh green photosynthetically active canopy of leaves for as long as possible. With such varieties, farmers can determine the plant spacing which is optimal for light conversion. However, photosynthetic efficiency decreases with increasing leaf age. Therefore, short duration varieties often have a higher yield per unit of time than long duration varieties.[20,21,25]

Varieties may also differ greatly in dry matter distribution. The grain/straw ratio of 40 rice varieties varied from 0.1 to 1.6.[29] During the last half century, improvement of the grain/straw ratio was an important factor in breeding.[12]

Where one or more of these factors (soil, nutrients, water, temperature, light, pests and diseases, etc.) is limited, varieties most adapted to these local conditions should be bred; for instance, under water stress conditions, breeding can be directed to drought-resistant varieties.

If in the course of time, know-how increases or price ratios change, breeding targets also have to be adapted to the new circumstances.

7. To produce the highest possible yield, agricultural techniques have to be used that utilize the above-mentioned factors optimally, individually, and in combination. The most suitable practices are found through experience and research, while the results of research have to be distributed by agricultural extension and education. However, the extent to which this know-how is practiced by the farmers is largely determined by the input-output price ratios and the availability of capital or credit.

The big differences in crop yields between various countries, as shown in Table 3, are mainly due to lack of both know-how and capital. These are the main limiting factors of today. Large yield increases are possible by supplying both.

Potential of Cereals, Root Crops, and Legume Crops

If the factors mentioned above are optimal, i.e., good soil, sufficient nutrients and water, normal temperature and CO_2 concentration, and absence of pests and diseases, the production of dry matter of a crop is mainly determined by photosynthesis, and thus by the intensity of sunlight and by the photosynthetic efficiency of the crop concerned.

On clear days, sunlight or solar radiation varies between 600 and 700 cal/cm^2 per day near the equator, reaches a maximum of 800 near latitude 30°, and exceeds 700 in greater latitudes during summer. An average cloudiness between 0.5 and 0.8 during summer in western Europe and throughout the year in the humid tropics decreases the radiation to an average of 300 to 400, but in western U.S., the Near East, Australia, and other relatively cloudless regions in middle latitudes, mean radiation is between 550 and 700 cal/cm^2 per day throughout the summer. About 50% of this total radiation consists of visible light and is available for photosynthesis.[3]

TABLE 4

Mean Monthly Global Solar Radiation in cal cm^{-2} day^{-1}

Region	May	September	December
Europe	400	250	50
North America	500	450	200
Near East	600	450	200
Far East	500	450	300
Latin America	400	500	500
Africa	450	500	500
Oceania	400	500	500

(After Ashbel, 1965[4])

Generally, it is accepted that approximately 10 quanta of light energy (Einsteins) are used for the conversion of 1 mol CO_2 into carbohydrate.[7] Of these 10 light quanta, or about 520 cal from the incident visible radiation range, only 105 cal are stored in the dry matter produced. Therefore, the maximum gross photosynthetic efficiency is expected to be 105:520 = 20%.[7]

Due to respiration that ranges from 25 to over 50% of gross photosynthesis, maximum net photosynthesis is 10 to 15%. In experiments under low light intensity, a photosynthetic efficiency of 15% was indeed observed during a short period. Under higher light intensity, CO_2 diffusion rates become a limiting factor and reduce photosynthetic efficiency. Under normal light, the highest efficiencies observed in a closed crop canopy were 7 to 8%.

Due to the juvenile stage of the crop, during which a major portion of incident radiation is not intercepted by leaves, and due to the decreasing efficiency of the older shaded leaves, maximum photosynthetic efficiency during the entire growth period under optimal conditions observed was 2 to 2.5% for nonefficient crops, such as rice, and 3 to 3.5% for efficient crops, such as sugar cane.[26]

Based on these findings, a method was developed to calculate the potential yield of crops for different latitudes,[36] while specified calculations were made for rice[18] and for potatoes.[25] In the latter case, a method was developed to calculate the potential yield even when water supply was not optimal.

For a few modern rice varieties, maximum photosynthesis was determined as well as the relation between photosynthesis and varying incident visible radiation. Based on these data, the expected yields in different latitudes and various seasons were calculated.[18] Field experiments showed that the method of calculation was quite reliable.

Figure 1 shows that with the high yielding varieties of today, potential yields per crop range, depending on rate of cloudiness, between 6 and 14 tons per ha near latitude 40° during summer and between 6 and 10 tons per ha near the equator throughout the year. However, near latitude 40° only one crop per year is possible, while roughly between 20° northern latitude and 20° southern latitude, two to three rice crops are possible.[18]

In practice, these yields will not be achieved on a large scale because perfect soil preparation,

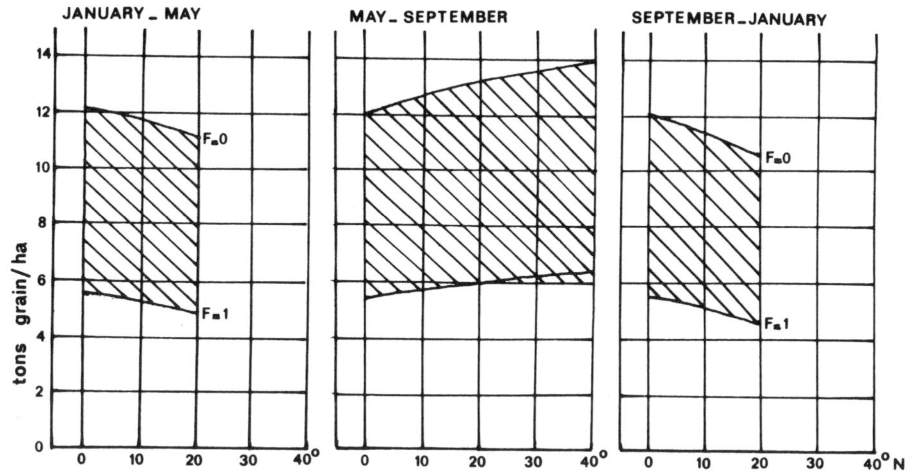

FIGURE 1. Ranges of potential rice yields for a modern nonlodging variety with a constant growth cycle at different latitudes and in different seasons. F is the fraction of the daytime when the sky is overcast. (From van Ittersum, A., *Neth. J. Agric. Sci.,* 20, 1, 1972. With permission.)

nutrition, weed control, irrigation and drainage, control of pests and diseases, harvesting, etc. are generally uneconomic. Besides presenting an estimate of the potential yields, Table 5 also gives figures for target yields. Target yields are based on the assumption that 65 to 75% of the potential yield must be obtainable on a large scale and under good weather conditions.

As stated before, in temperate climates dry matter production of cereals, root crops, and legume crops does not differ very much.[14,27] Under optimal conditions, an average growth rate of about 200 kg of dry matter per ha per day was observed for the period of a closed green crop canopy.[36] This was about the same as observed in the tropics for rice.[18] In the tropics, growth rates

TABLE 5
Potential Yields in Tons and Calories of Grain, Roots, or Tubers per ha per Year

Food crops	Edible part percent	Kcal per 100 g	Temperate regions (one crop): Potential Tons	Temperate: Target Tons	Temperate: Target Kcal x 10^6	Tropics (per year): Potential Tons	Tropics: Target Tons	Tropics: Target Kcal x 10^6
Cereals								
Wheat	100	344	12	9	31.0	25	18	61.9
Rice	70	354	12	9	22.3	30	20	49.6
Corn	100	363	15	11	39.9	38	24	87.1
Sorghum + millet	90	355	15	11	35.2	40	26	83.1
Root crops								
Potato	85	75	100	65	41.4	140	80	51.0
Cassava	83	153	—	—	—	100	65	82.5
Sweet potato + yam	87	109	80	50	47.2	160	100	94.8
Legume crops								
Soybean	100	382	9	7	26.7	20	15	57.3
Groundnuts	70	579	12	9	36.5	30	20	81.1
Dry beans	100	339	8	6	20.3	18	12	40.7
Dry peas	100	337	8	6	20.2	18	12	40.4

were observed up to twice as high[38,40] only for the photosynthetic efficient crops (corn, sorghum, and millet) grown under high light intensity.

The potential yield figures in Table 5 are yields which are thought to be obtainable with modern varieties under optimal conditions as far as water and nutrient supplies are concerned. Under exceptional conditions, e.g., a perfectly clear sky during the entire growth period (no exception in arid areas), these yields can even be surpassed.

In the tropics the cultivation of wheat and particularly potatoes is, in general, restricted to high altitude areas or to the cooler season.

The potential yields of the legume crops, other than soybean and groundnuts, and for the root crops, other than potatoes, are unfavorably influenced by the fact that up to now less research in breeding high yielding varieties and in optimal agricultural practices has been done than for cereals such as wheat, rice and corn.

Cassava yields per year are considered to be relatively small because of the long growth period and the unfavorable edible/nonedible dry matter distribution pattern, although exact figures concerning the last factor were not available.

Except for cassava and yam, growth periods of the crops were supposed to range in the tropics between three and five months, and in the temperate zone between four and six months, not including the winter period.

However, to what extent are these potential yields realistic? Figure 2 presents calculated wheat yields and yields obtained in experiments in the Netherlands since 1965. Table 6 presents the highest yields of the most important food crops already realized.

For instance, the potential yield of 12 tons per

TABLE 6

Realized Record Yields in tons/ha

Crops	Yield	Reference
Wheat	14.0	11
Rice	14.0	10
Corn	20.0	11
Sorghum	22.0	11
Potatoes	100.0	37
Cassava	77.0	41
Sweet potatoes	41.0	24
Yam	45.0	13
Soybean	4.5	39
Groundnuts	10.0	15

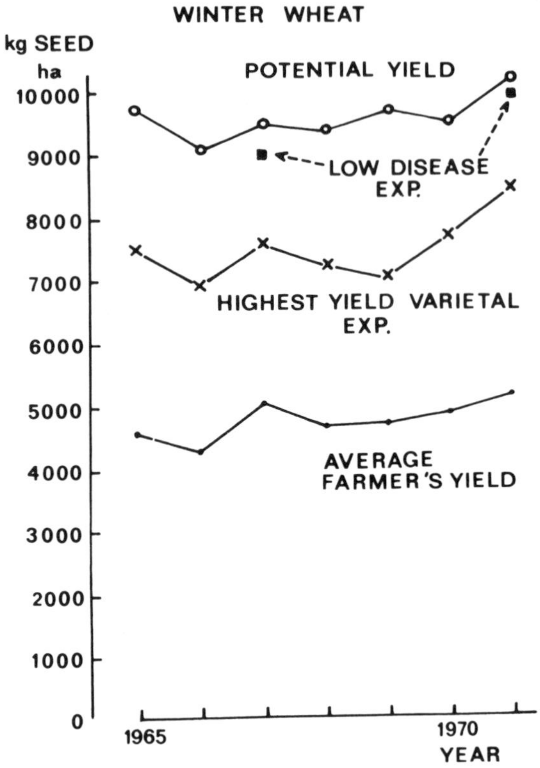

FIGURE 2. Calculated and obtained wheat yields in the Netherlands since 1965. (From de Vos, N. M., *Neth. J. Agric. Sci.*, in press. With permission.)

ha for rice, as shown in Table 5, was exceeded in several countries. In Australia, for instance, a yield of 12.4 tons per ha was achieved, in the Philippines 12.5, in India 12.6, in Ceylon 13.3, and in Senegal 14.0.[10,11] One rice crop was reported to be 16.4 tons per ha, but in this case the growth period was more than one year.[20]

Data of maximum yields, however, are rather scarce, particularly for crops other than cereals and potatoes. The highest yield found for yam was even obtained without fertilizer application.

As one person needs about 1 million kcal per year, it can easily be seen from Table 5 how many persons can be fed from 1 ha of the various crops if they reach the target yields. This ranges from 20 to nearly 100, with potentialities in the tropics about twice as high as in the temperate regions. Other calculations come to an average of 50 persons per ha.[34,37] This is about 12 times as much as the nearly 4 persons per ha who presently can be fed (see first section). However, one should consider that although some extension of farmed area is possible, on at least half of the current arable area, target yields cannot be realized mainly due to lack of water.

Future Potentials

The potential yields mentioned above are based on calculations and field experiments with the high yielding varieties of today. In the future, potential yields will undoubtedly be higher; how much higher depends mainly on two factors: research and price ratios.

Research will continously be directed toward improvement of varieties and of know-how about optimal conditions with regard to soil preparation, sowing (correct spacing), control of weeds, pests and diseases, irrigation and drainage, harvest and processing, etc. For instance, one particular aim in breeding rice and wheat, pulses, and root crops could be the selection, perhaps through mutation, of plants without photorespiration, or research could be directed toward developing chemical compounds which inhibit respiration; perhaps the results could increase potential yields substantially.[6,40]

Modern agricultural techniques cost money. Only if prices are remunerative will farmers increase their input and consequently their yield per hectare. If price ratios in the temperate zone would make it remunerative to increase temperature, CO_2 concentration, and light, food crops could be grown industrially, as is done already with vegetables, grapes, flowers, mushrooms, etc., and potential yields could increase considerably. In this case, potential food production per hectare per year in the temperate zone could increase 5 to 10 times since several crops per year would then be possible. This, however, is only possible on a large scale if per capita world income could rise substantially. Even without application of the above-mentioned techniques, industrialization of food crop growing based on the best known agricultural practices of today could increase average yields very fast.[34]

One should remember that in this chapter only the most important food crops could be dealt with. Many other crops take a big share in food production and food consumption in specific areas, such as chickpeas, dry broadbeans, pigeon peas, lentils and cowpeas, sugar cane and sugar beets, oil crops, bananas, and sago. Of these crops, particularly sugar cane as a photosynthetically efficient species has a very high yield potential in the tropics, while sugar beets have a remarkably high yield potential in temperate regions. Together they supply an ever increasing part of the calories in the human diet.

EXPECTED YIELD INCREASES

Which portion of the potential yields mentioned in the former section may be expected to be realized in the near future?

The main determining factors for each country are likely to be the yields of today, the increase in food demand of the increasing population, the input-output price ratios for the farmer, and the rate with which know-how, production means, credit facilities, and marketing facilities become available to the farmer. Most of these factors are highly dependent on the policy of the government concerned.

The FAO has made an extensive study, the Indicative World Plan (IWP), of the extent to which agriçultural production should be increased and of the measures which should be taken to make these increases possible.[23] Table 7 shows the targets set by the IWP for yield increases between 1962 and 1985 in percentages per year.

In developing countries, internal demand for cereals is expected to rise between 3.0 and 3.2%, for starchy roots between 2.7 and 4.1%, and for pulses between 3.1 and 3.9% per year. Part of the production increase is expected to be realized through an increase of the cultivated area, which part is different for each crop and each region.

According to the IWP, it is hoped that, in view of the nutritional value, the increase in root crop production for human consumption will go mainly to sweet potatoes and yam instead of to cassava.

The IWP does not give figures for Europe, North America, and Oceania. For Europe and North America, there seems to be no reason why yield increases in the near future should differ greatly from those realized in the past decade. The expected yield increases in these regions depend on food demand. If export demand from outside these regions does not change substantially, as was presupposed in the IWP, population increase within these regions will permit only an increase in production of crops such as wheat and rice directly for human consumption of about 1% per year. Income increase, in particular, will cause an increase in demand for animal products and hence a demand for fodder crops, such as corn, soybean, sorghum, millet, and cassava of several percent per

TABLE 7

Targets for Yield Increases in Percentage per Year Between 1962 and 1985*

	Asia	Near East	North Africa	Africa South of Sahara	South America
Rice	2.7	2.0	0.3	1.6	0.7
Wheat	4.3	2.8	3.2	2.2	1.5
Corn	3.8	–	4.7	1.6	1.3
Sorghum + millet	2.6	–	0.2	0.9	0.9
All cereals	3.0	2.4	3.3	1.3	1.7
Root crops	1.4	1.1	1.1	0.7	0.9
Groundnuts	3.3	–	–	1.2	0.2
Dry pulses	2.2	1.4	1.4	1.0	1.7

Figures for 1950 are 5-year averages (1948–52), figures for 1970 are 3-year averages (1969–71).

*(After reference 23.)

year. Demand for the first two crops is expected to go mainly to North America, demand for the last crop to tropical regions, while sorghum and millet could be supplied by both tropical countries and North America.

Because of the great dependence on weather, local production and hence availability of food crops may fluctuate greatly from year to year, requiring the maintenance of large buffer stocks and transportation facilities.

As noted in Table 3, there is a large difference in yields between countries, showing clearly the possibility for large yield increases in countries where average yields are still very low. The potential and target yields given in Table 5 show great possibilities even in countries with high average yields. But it should be repeated that the traditional ways to increase production, such as by enlarging the cultivated area and by increasing human labor per ha, are nearly exhausted in many densely populated areas. Large yield increases are possible, but the know-how and often also the means have to come from outside the rural community. This means that the realization of an adequate increase in food crop yields for several decades ahead is possible, but will depend largely on the policy of the government concerned, and on the concerted policy actions of governments on a world scale.

Acknowledgments

The author wishes to express his gratitude to Prof. Dr. C. T. de Wit for his critical remarks and to his colleagues Dr. T. A. El Baradi, Prof. Dr. G. Giesberger, Ir. J. P. Thijsse, and Dr. G. Verhaar at the Royal Tropical Institute for their assistance in preparing this chapter, to Miss J. M. van der Horst for making the drawings, and to Miss S. Kranenberg and her co-workers for typing the manuscript.

REFERENCES

1. **Alberda, Th., Brouwer, R., van Dobben, W. H., de Wit, C. T., and Wit, F.,** *De Groene Aarde (The Green Earth)*, Aula nr. 250, Het Spectrum, Utrecht, 1966.
2. **Alberda, Th.,** Actual and potential production of agricultural crops, *Neth. J. Agric. Sci.,* 10, 325, 1962.
3. **Ashbel, D.,** *New World Maps of Global Solar Radiation During I.G.Y.,* The Hebrew University, Jerusalem, 1961.
4. **Ashbel, D., Eviatar, A., Doron, E., and Ganor, E.,** *Solar Radiation in Different Latitudes,* The Hebrew University, Jerusalem, 1965.
5. **Aykroyd, W. R.,** The Nutritive Value of Indian Foods and the Planning of Satisfactory Diets, Special Report Series No. 42, Indian Council of Medical Research, New Delhi, 1966.
6. **Black, C. C., Chen, T. M., and Brown, R. H.,** Biochemical basis for plant competition, *Weed Sci.,* 17, 338, 1969.
7. **Bonner, J.,** The upper limit of crop yield, *Science,* 137 (3523), 11, 1962.
8. **Brougham, R. W.,** The relationship between the critical leaf area, total chlorophyll content, and maximum growth-rate of some pasture, and crop plants, *Ann. Bot. N. S.,* 24, 463, 1960.
9. **Bull, T. A.,** Photosynthetic efficiencies and photorespiration in Calvin cycle and C_4-dicarboxylic acid plants, *Crop Sci.,* 9, 726, 1969.

10. **Chandler, R. F.**, Maximum yield potentialities for rice, *Philipp. Agric.*, 46, 167, 1962.
11. **Cooke, G. W.**, *Fertilizing for Maximum Yields,* Crosby Lockwood, London, 1972.
12. **van Dobben, W. H.**, Influence of temperature and light conditions on dry-matter distribution, development rate and yield in arable crops, *Neth. J. Agric. Sci.,* 10, 377, 1962.
13. **Ferguson, T. U. and Haynes, P. H.**, The Chinese yam as a commercial proposition, *Farmer* (Jamaica), 75, 372, 1970.
14. **Gaastra, P.**, Photosynthesis of leaves and field crop, *Neth. J. Agric. Sci.,* 10, 311, 1962.
15. **Goldin, E. and Har-Tzook, A.**, Groundnut cultivation in Israel, *World Crops,* 18(2), 68, 1966.
16. **Hatch, M. D., Osmond, C. B., and Slatyer, R. O.**, Eds., *Photosynthesis and Photorespiration* (Proceedings of a conference), Canberra, November 23–December 5, 1970, John Wiley & Sons, New York, 1971.
17. **Idso, S. B.**, A holocoenotic analysis of environment plant relationships, Tech. Bull., 264, Agric. Exp. Stat., University of Minnesota, St. Paul, 1968.
18. **van Ittersum, A.**, A calculation of potential rice yields, *Neth. J. Agric. Sci.,* 20, 1, 1972.
19. **Loomis, R. S. and Williams, W. A.**, Maximum crop productivity: an estimate, *Crop Sci.,* 3, 67, 1963.
20. Mineral (the) nutrition of the rice plant, *Proceedings of a Symposium at the International Rice Research Institute,* February, 1964, Los Baños, Philippines, The Johns Hopkins Press, Baltimore, 1965.
21. **Monteith, J. G.**, Light and crop production, *Field Crop Abstr.,* 18, 213, 1965.
22. *Production Yearbook 1971,* FAO, Rome, 1972.
23. *Provisional Indicative World Plan for Agricultural Development,* Vol. 1, FAO, Rome, 1970.
24. Rapport du Secteur du Rwanda-Burundi pour les Exercices 1960, 1961 et 1962, Publication de l'Institut National pour l'Etude Agronomique du Congo (INEAC), 1963.
25. **Rijtema, P. E. and Endrödi, G.**, Calculation of production of potatoes, *Neth. J. Agric. Sci.,* 18, 26, 1970.
26. **Rostron, H.**, The growth and productivity of sugar-cane, *Proceedings 45th Annual Congress South African Sugar Technologists Association,* South African Sugar Technologists Association, Mount Edgecombe, Natal, 1971, 152.
27. **Sibma, L.**, Growth of closed green crop surfaces in the Netherlands, *Neth. J. Agric. Sci.,* 16, 211, 1968.
28. *Statistical Yearbook 1971,* United Nations, New York, 1972.
29. **Tanaka, A. and Kawano, K.**, Effect of mutual shading on dry-matter production in the tropical rice plant, *Plant Soil,* 24, 128, 1966.
30. **Tanaka, A.**, The relative importance of the source and the sink as the yield-limiting factors of rice, *Tech. Bull.* 6, A.S.P.A.C., Food and Fertilizer Technol. Centre, Hokkaido University, Japan, 1972.
31. **de Vos, N. M.**, Actual and potential yield of wheat, paper submitted for publication to *Neth. J. Agric. Sci.,* 1973.
32. **de Vries, C. A., Ferwerda, J., and Flach, M.**, Choice of food crops in relation to actual and potential production in the tropics, *Neth. J. Agric. Sci.,* 15, 241, 1967.
33. **Wallace, D. H. and Munger, H. M.**, Studies of the physiological basis for yield differences. II. Variations in dry-matter distribution among aerial organs for several dry bean varieties, *Crop Sci.,* 6, 503, 1966.
34. **Wassink, E. C.**, Plant physiology, and some aspects of future agriculture, *Neth. J. Agric. Sci.,* 18, 49, 1970.
35. **Watson, D. J.**, The physiological limitations of crop yield, and the possibilities of increasing it, *Landb. Tijdschrift,* 68, 590, 1956.
36. **de Wit, C. T.**, Photosynthesis of leaf canopies, *Agric. Res. Rep.,* 663, Pudoc, Wageningen, 1965.
37. **de Wit, C. T.**, Overbevolking zonder ondervoeding, in *De Groene Aarde (The Green Earth),* 425. Alberda, Th., Brouwer, R., van Dobben, W. H., de Wit, C. T., and Wit, F., Het Spectrum, Utrecht, 1966, 425.
38. **de Wit, C. T.**, Food production: past, present, and future, Stikstof (nitrogen), *Dtch. Nit. Fertil. Rev.,* 15, 68, 1972.
39. **Zaman, M. B. and Khan, A. A.**, Description and performance of some soya bean varieties at the Pakistan Forest Institute, Peshawar, *Pak. J. For.,* 19(1), 129, 1969.
40. **Zelitch, I.**, *Photosynthesis, Photorespiration, and Plant Productivity,* Academic Press, New York, 1971.
41. **van der Zijl, C. E.**, Improvement of Cassava Production Through Field Experiments, Ph.D. Thesis, Agricultural University, Wageningen, 1930.

INCREASING OUTPUT OF ANIMAL PRODUCTION: TECHNICAL MEASURES FOR INCREASING PRODUCTIVITY

K. L. Blaxter

TABLE OF CONTENTS

Introduction 127
  Human Food from Animals – the Present Situation 128
  Plants and Animals as Food Sources for Man 130

The Restraints on Animal Production 132
  Land and Water Resources 132
  Animal Disease 133
  The Limits Placed by Climate on Livestock Production 135
  Social, Religious, and Cultural Restraints 135

Methods of Augmenting Animal Production 136
  Disease Control – the Major Enzootic Diseases 137
  Disease Control – Local Disease and Parasitism 138
  The Provision of Feed for Livestock 139
    Nonpastoral Livestock 139
    Pastoral Farming 140
  Animal Breeding and Reproduction 141
  Environmental Control 143

Agricultural Policies and Production 144

References 146

INTRODUCTION

Domesticated livestock are kept for a variety of reasons. In almost all communities they are husbanded to provide protein-rich foods in the form of meat, milk, and eggs. They also provide hides, wool, and hair for the manufacture of clothing and textiles, while in sophisticated economies a series of biological products not readily synthesized chemically is prepared from their organs and tissues. In some areas of the world, animals are used extensively for transport and for draught, while in many developing countries possession of animals is indicative of the wealth of farmers and these animals then represent a reservoir of capital.

Any assessment of the contribution that livestock make to the life of a community and any consideration of increasing their productivity should take into account these varied products and uses of livestock. In this chapter, however, emphasis has been placed, virtually exclusively, on their value as sources of human food. The implications of such an emphasis should be realized. If the primary purpose of animals is to produce food, then it follows that a replacement of draught animals in developing countries by machines or an erosion of those social, religious, and economic customs that cause farmers to retain animals which contribute little to human food supplies necessarily augments productivity. Such a conclusion only follows the initial restricting assumption;

when different assumptions about the role of livestock in the cultures of different countries are made, then different conclusions and emphases necessarily emerge.

Human Food from Animals – the Present Situation

Productivity of livestock in the limited sense of their value as food producers can be estimated for different countries simply as the amount of protein produced from them per person in the population. Such a statistic measures production rather than consumption of animal products by the population and can be calculated from data compiled by F.A.O.[1] The statistic is not an exact one. Not only are the primary data on production of carcasses, milk, and eggs, and of human population subject to error, but certain assumptions have to be made in converting the data to a common basis of protein. Even so, and as shown in Table 1, the results show a very wide variation of productivity from region to region of the world. Oceania is clearly highly productive; the region includes Australia and New Zealand which have large export markets for livestock products. South America, a region which includes countries in which protein-energy malnutrition in man is rife and in which consumption statistics are well below these estimates of productivity, is also an exporting region. Europe, North America, and the U.S.S.R., regions in which exports and imports are on the average not major factors, however, produce much more protein from livestock than do Africa and Asian regions. These geographic regions are not synonymous with developed and developing countries; the fact that the range in livestock productivity in Table 1 is well over tenfold suggests, however, that differences between developed and developing countries are even greater.

The amount of food protein produced each day by the livestock industry of a country expressed per person in that country can be regarded as the product of the number of livestock kept per person and the average productivity of the individual animal. Such a separation is useful, for the overall provision of animal protein in a country can be increased either by increasing livestock populations or by increasing the yield of milk, meat, or eggs obtained from the average individual. Table 2 summarizes, by F.A.O. region, the numbers of farm livestock per 100 people. The

TABLE 1

The Mean Productivity of Farm Livestock in Different Regions of the World Expressed in Terms of the Daily Production of Protein per Person in the Population

	Daily production of protein g/day				
FAO region	From cattle and buffalo	From sheep and goats	From pigs	From total	From all classes
Europe	33.6	1.7	8.8	8.6	53
North America	45.1	0.5	10.4	23.0	79
South America	17.5	0.8	2.0	2.8	23
Near East	6.2	4.0	0.0	1.7	12
Far East	3.4	0.4	5.3	1.1	10
Africa	5.3	1.7	2.7	1.0	11
Oceania	93.8	30.4	4.0	7.6	136
U.S.S.R.	36.9	1.7	4.4	5.7	49
People's Republic of China	1.6	0.3	3.3	2.8	8
World	13.5	1.1	3.1	4.3	22

Calculated from data of F.A.O. for 1970-71.

TABLE 2

The Farm Animal Populations of the World

Region	Human population x 10^6	Cattle and buffalo	Horses, asses, and mules	Pigs	Sheep and goats	Poultry
		Number of animals/100 people				
Europe	462	27	2	30	30	273
North America	227	56	4	33	10	241
Latin America	284	88	15	36	60	242
Near East	171	27	6	0	120	98
Far East	1162	30	1	4	16	60
Africa	305	47	5	2	75	121
Oceania	19	175	3	18	1231	166
U.S.S.R.	243	41	3	28	59	247
People's Republic of China	850	11	2	26	15	138
World	3723	34	3	39	18	149

The numbers of agricultural animals/100 people estimated from F.A.O. statistics for 1970-71.

values are interesting for several reasons. First, in the world as a whole, the biomass of domesticated livestock is about five times that of the human population. Second, and with the exception of pigs, the populations of livestock in the Far East and Africa per person are in many instances greater than those in Europe. In Africa, for example, per person the population of cattle and buffalo is 174% of that in Europe, that of horses 209%, and of sheep and goats 250%. Latin America has more of each of the five livestock classes per head of the population than has North America, but reference to Table 1 indicates that food production from animals in Latin America is less than a third that in North America. The conclusion is inescapable that the productivity of individual animals varies widely from region to region of the world, and that this variation is, broadly speaking, greater than is that of livestock populations relative to human populations in the same regions. This has been illustrated for cattle, which account for about two thirds of the world's production of edible protein in Table 3. It is at once apparent that the mean annual output of protein as meat and milk from the 500 million cattle and buffalo in Africa and the Far East is less than one tenth that obtained from the average animal in Europe. Table 4 shows a similar comparison for pigs. The annual productivity of the average pig in the Far East and the People's Republic of China, two regions which together possess 40% of the world's domesticated pigs, is less than half that of the average European pig.

While the above approach, in which the output of animal industries is related to the human population, reveals these large differences in the productivity of livestock and thus suggests a considerable possibility for improvement of the food output from existing populations, it does not throw light on the potential of different countries in terms of livestock production. Land and feed resources for livestock are ignored. An alternative approach is to assess output per unit area, that is, meat and milk output per hectare or animal protein output per hectare per year. If this is to be done, questions arise with respect to whether the base of the calculation should be the agricultural area alone or the whole land area of the country other than urban land and forests, or whether desert and mountain areas should be excluded. These problems of land designation and classification make interregional comparisons difficult to interpret; indeed the only rational way in which to assess the potential for animal production in the

TABLE 3

Crude Productivity of Cattle and Buffalo by World Regions

Region	Cattle and buffalo population x 10^6	kg carcass/year per animal	kg milk/year per animal	kg protein/ /year/animal (carcass + milk)
Europe	123	70	1118	45.4
North America	127	87	487	29.4
South America	249	26	95	7.3
Near East	46	18	179	8.4
Far East	354	4	116	4.2
Africa	145	14	57	4.1
Oceania	34	45	397	19.6
U.S.S.R.	100	47	828	32.8
People's Republic of China	93	24	35	5.1

Calculated from F.A.O., 1972.

TABLE 4

Crude Productivity of Pigs by World Regions

Region	Pig population x 10^6	kg carcass /year/animal	kg protein /year/animal
Europe	139	89	10.7
North America	75	96	11.5
South America	103	17	2.0
Near East	<1	(–)	(–)
Far East	49	40	4.8
Africa	7	41	4.9
Oceania	3	68	8.2
U.S.S.R.	67	48	5.8
People's Republic of China	223	38	4.6

Calculated from data of F.A.O., 1972.

world is to examine the possibilities for livestock farming in each and every locality and then attempt a global summation. This has not been done, although many individual countries have obviously considered how best their land resources might be used and the part that livestock farming might play in their development. Even so, there is abundant evidence that the land resources of the world are not fully utilized in producing food for man, whether directly from plants or from animals.

Plants and Animals as Food Sources for Man

The above considerations of the present productivity of livestock populations show that in many regions of the world, as far as protein production is concerned, farm livestock do not contribute a major part of the protein needs of people, currently assessed as an optimum of 50 to 70 g protein/person/day. Much protein in all regions is derived from grains, pulses, and vegetables. Similar conclusions apply when livestock, as sources of edible fats, are considered. It could be argued that to increase the protein supply of people in areas where dietary protein is in short supply, emphasis should be given to an augmentation of primary crop production rather than to a secondary production of animal products. An extension of this argument is that since the human population is growing so rapidly, in the foreseeable future livestock populations will have to be curtailed since they compete directly with man for the primary produce of land. There are several fallacies in these arguments and, as with many similar generalizations, some elements of truth.

There is no doubt that an increase in the primary production of crops is usually an essential preliminary to the development of an agriculture which includes animals.[2] An increase in the productivity of a peasant farmer from an annual output of 300 to 400 kg grain/year allows him to keep an animal for draught purposes, thereby increasing his output still further. When his productivity exceeds 500 kg/year, milk and meat production emerge. On a larger scale, as countries move into cereal surplus, they then consider the development of highly intensive animal industries heavily dependent on grain, such as broiler poultry and intensive pig industries. In this sense, animal industries for food production emerge when human needs for crop products have been satisfied.

This, however, ignores the vast areas of the world, probably totaling more than 60% of the total agricultural area of the world, that are not readily cultivated, that is, the natural grazings and scrublands. These, because of topography, climate, accessibility, and, in some instances, poverty of soil, cannot be used to the advantage of man other than through meat and, to a lesser extent, milk obtained from grazing stock. In addition, the simple view that it is surplus grain that provides the basis of animal economies ignores the integral aspects of livestock and cropping systems in agriculture. Animals also utilize those parts of crop plants which are inedible by man, and the return to the soil of residues of these crops in dung and urine conserves plant nutrients and in some instances augments soil fertility. This occurs also in certain types of pastoral farming, as in Africa where stock are grazed on open pastures by day and herded in compounds at night, and excreta are used to support a small intensive agriculture. Crop residues are not necessarily those which remain on farms such as the straws of cereals and pulses and the leaves and crowns of root crops; they also include products of the industrial processing of the crops sold from farms. These comprise the outer coats of the cereal grains from wheat flour or rice polishing processes, bagasse and crude molasses from sugar production from cane, the residues of oilseeds remaining after the extraction of vegetable oils, citrus pulp from industries concerned with preparation of citrus juices or with canning, grape seeds or extracted barley which are the residues from industries concerned with the manufacture of alcoholic beverages, and many others. Included here are the by-products of the fishing industry in the form of fish meals, of waste mycelial felts from fermentation industries, and even waste cellulose from timber pulp. These industries are not dependent on agriculture at all. Even when agriculture is at subsistence level, household refuse and the by-products of crop production mean that the animal makes little demand on grain resources. Farm livestock are thus not obligatory competitors of man; rather they are commensals and their use leads to a more rational use of the primary production of land. The cropping of land for livestock through the cultivation of coarse grains, fodder crops, and of sown pasture species is an extension of this rationalization which has additional overtones emphasizing integral aspects. Most of these relate to the maintenance of soil fertility. Thus, rotation of crops and avoidance of monocultures have long been accepted as methods for the control of soil-borne diseases of primary food crops, while the introduction of fodder legumes results in an increase in the nitrogen available to subsequent crops through the symbiotic nitrogen fixation propensities of these plants. These integrative aspects of farming are not so apparent in highly developed countries where animal production methods have become industrialized. Ease and cheapness of transport of feed supplies in those countries entails spatial separation of primary production from the secondary production of livestock. The interdependence of cropping and stocking, however, is basically the same.

When livestock and crops are considered as alternative sources of human food their supplementary value is ignored. This applies not only to supplementary values as sources of nutrients, as exemplified by the value of milk protein, rich in lysine, as a supplement to the lysine-poor proteins of cereal grains, but also to supplementary values in the preparation of appetizing meals. This last aspect is often overlooked.[3] It appears that in societies that aspire to western-type food habits – and many communities in the Far East, notably Japan, are doing this – aspirations include a desire to consume some 600 g milk and 200 g carcass meat daily. These amounts of milk and meat, together with the protein obtained from other dietary components, certainly provide more than the minimal needs of protein calculated to maintain health. There is no reason to suppose that such amounts in excess of the minimum impair health; they are simply amounts which people wish to consume. On the basis of the present world population and its projected growth, to meet these aspirations would entail doubling world milk production by the year 2000 and quadrupling world meat production. Technically this is feasible. To do so, however, it is necessary to identify those factors which are responsible for the present low productivity and to plan the complex of socioeconomic agrarian policies inseparable from programs of agricultural improvement and to ensure that technical measures are fully and sensibly exploited.

THE RESTRAINTS ON ANIMAL PRODUCTION

There are innumerable factors operating to prevent the full realization of the potential of farm livestock in producing human food. They can conveniently be classified into those which relate to the provision of feed, those which prevent livestock from making best use of feed resources, notably disease and the vicissitudes of climate, and those which relate to the socioeconomic context in which livestock production takes place.

Land and Water Resources

The most productive animal industries of the world are largely concentrated in the cool temperature zone, that is, between latitudes 35° and 55° N.[4] Here temperature conditions provide an adequate growing season and precipitation is usually sufficient to allow plant growth or can be supplemented sufficiently by irrigation. Winter conditions are not so severe as to prevent the use of perennial crops. The least productive land areas in terms of livestock – neglecting the tundra and areas of permafrost – are those which may loosely be classed as the arid areas and the humid tropics.

The arid zones of the world account for some 35% of its land surface. A first division of the zone is to distinguish the extremely arid deserts, as exemplified by the Arabian desert, the Sahara, and the South American coastal desert. Here there is little or no immediate possibility for agriculture or animal husbandry on any major scale. The arid and semiarid areas, which account for some 24% and 5% of the world's land, respectively, support vegetation – the natural grasslands, the savannahs, veldt, and bush scrub. These areas include animal husbandries of various types ranging from nomadic pastoralism through transhumance to large-scale sedentary livestock farming in conjunction with crop and fodder production often supported by irrigation. Precipitation and the distribution of rain are all-important not only for crop and grassland production but equally in the long process of soil formation. Drought is common and because of ill-controlled grazing its effects on the land are exacerbated. Denudation of the surface leads to reduced penetration of rain when it falls, an accelerated run-off, and poor reestablishment of native grass species. Poor management of semiarid areas of Africa, as for example in Botswana, can lead to severe gully and sheet erosion with serious deterioration of the whole environment. Bush and scrub encroach following denudation of grassland and constitute an additional problem; for although bush plants provide some feed for emergencies, they represent a reduction in overall productivity in terms of feed. Even when scrub is used for emergency feeding, deaths of grazing livestock due to hunger and thirst are commonplace during drought and productivity of survivors is very poor. It is not unusual for cattle to calve only once every two or three years since feed supplies can be so poor that recovery from the nutritional strain of pregnancy and lactation is protracted. Water supplies from boreholes are often highly mineralized and not suitable for irrigation or for livestock. In more favored areas, and with irrigation, cropping is feasible; indeed drought-resistant grains can be grown in many years under dry farming conditions in more favored areas. The restraints imposed on animal production in these arid areas are mostly related to the effects of climate and water supplies on the soil, on plant growth, and indirectly on livestock.

The humid tropics account for about 12% of

the world's land resources. In the equatorial tropics rainfall is in excess of trans-evaporation, soils are heavily leached, and the climax is a rain forest with tropical vegetation. These areas which include the Congo Basin, the Guinea Coast, and the Amazon Basin are not major areas for livestock.[5] In the monsoon areas and those parts of the humid tropics in the trade winds, rainfall is seasonal; these are some of the most densely populated areas of the world and include parts of southeast Asia, India, and the Caribbean. Problems of feed provision are not overriding, although its conservation for the seasonal drought is necessary. In most of the humid tropics the potential for animal production has not been realized and the restraints are of other types entirely.

Any classification of world agriculture into a limited number of divisions is open to criticism, for it ignores the obviously wide variety of topography, soil type, climatic conditions, and the patterns of development that have led to types of husbandry in different countries. Even so, it is apparent that certain general statements can be made about the limitations placed by the climatic and soil environment on the development of livestock farming. Two are outstanding, namely, that of water supplies for crops and stock in about one third of the world, and present inabilities to utilize livestock to the fullest in the humid tropics, which account for a further tenth of the land area. There are many other limitations. Soil and hence plant deficiencies of phosphorus, first recognized on the grasslands of South Africa, are known to be of world importance and soil deficiencies of copper, cobalt, and selenium are known to be widespread. Shortages of these elements result in poor performance of grazing livestock, if not overt deficiency disease, and the full extent of such deficiencies has not been yet mapped on a global scale.[6] Their importance can be judged by the increases in productivity that have taken place in Australia and New Zealand as a result of the control of the cobalt deficiency diseases, "bush sickness," "coast disease" and "wasting disease"; control of the copper deficiency disease in cattle in southwest Australia, "falling disease"; and of the selenium responsive diseases in New Zealand, notably "white muscle disease" and "hoggett ill thrift."

Not only may mineral elements essential for the well-being of stock be deficient in soils, they may also be in excess. The best example is selenium. Selenium poisoning is enzootic in all types of livestock over considerable areas of the great plains of North America, notably in Dakota and Montana, and in more localized areas of Australia, Ireland, the Soviet Union, and Israel; it has recently been found in Iran. The accumulation of selenium in plants leads on their ingestion to "alkali disease" or "blind staggers." Again chronic endemic fluorine poisoning is enzootic in considerable areas of India and North Africa as a result of consumption by grazing stock of waters from boreholes heavily contaminated with fluorine from underlying strata. These toxicity problems place considerable restrictions on animal production and are less easily remedied than are deficiencies of nutrients.

Animal Disease

Even in countries with highly developed animal husbandries, communicable disease causes a considerable reduction in productivity through death of stock and through varying degrees of morbidity. Infections of the mammary gland result in diminished yield, while respiratory tract infections cause poor growth in young animals. Enteric disease is a further cause of loss in all species. Many of these diseases are associated with highly intensive types of animal production, where stock are kept in confinement in large numbers. Nor are some of these countries free from the major diseases of livestock. Foot-and-mouth disease in ruminants and pigs and Newcastle disease in poultry occur and result in serious economic loss.

In developing countries most attention is presently paid to the major enzootic and epizootic diseases and particularly to the zoonoses which are those animal diseases communicable to man. There is no reason to believe, however, that intensification of animal production in these countries will not result in the emergence of similar disease problems to those which diminish the output of animal production systems in highly developed countries. Indeed these diseases certainly occur, but are overshadowed by the depredations caused by the major ones. Some examples are given below.

Paralytic rabies in cattle transmitted by vampire bats, which are the natural host, has been estimated to cause the death of over half a million cattle annually in South and Central America.[7] The virus now appears to be transmitted to frugivorous and insectivorous bats in North

America, but since they do not suck blood they constitute but a minor hazard to animals and man. In Africa and Asia rabies in livestock is associated with virus transmitted from urban dogs and wild carnivores. The extent of losses in livestock has not been documented.

Perhaps one of the best documented accounts of the effects of an animal disease on the livestock industry is that relating to the rinderpest epidemic in Africa in the 1890's.[8] The disease was introduced from Asia, possibly into Egypt, spread into east Africa, and crossed the Zambesi into the Transvaal and the Cape. The losses in the Union of South Africa alone were 2½ million cattle and it has been estimated that between 80 and 90% of cattle, buffalo, eland, giraffe, wildebeest, kudu, and antelope died. The Masai of Kenya were reduced to starvation, their numbers and tribal supremacy fell, and their lands were subsequently colonized by settlers. Rinderpest is still a major disease of cattle. It is a major impediment to sustained economic development in Africa and the East, for the cost of control, using attenuated living virus vaccines, is high. Furthermore, sporadic outbreaks occur though not on the scale of the African one of 1890–1905. Happily Latin America is so far free of rinderpest.

Nagana, or animal trypanosomiasis, denies large areas of land to productive animal enterprises in Africa. The eradication of the tsetse flies that transmit the disease is a slow and costly process with existing technical knowledge. Control of the tsetse flies would, however, release 4½ million mi^2 of land in the Central African belt and allow the pasturage of 125 million cattle, an increase in Africa's population by one third.[9] The Arboviruses (an internationally agreed contracture for arthropod-borne virus diseases in which are included blue tongue of cattle, Nairobi sheep disease, and Rift Valley fever) also cause serious economic loss. African swine fever, originally a disease of wart hogs and bush pigs and now present in domestic pigs in West Africa with clear evidence of spread to the Mediterranean, is a further disease which can only be controlled by a stringent slaughter of infected animals.

Of all the major diseases of livestock, foot-and-mouth disease causes the greatest depredations. In terms of world economic importance, its effects exceed those of all the diseases hitherto mentioned combined. The North American continent, Australia, New Zealand, and the U.K. are free of the disease but as recently as 1966–67 half a million livestock were slaughtered in England to maintain this freedom. In other countries vaccination policies, some of dubious efficacy, are adopted in attempts to contain it. The disease is highly infectious, no respecter of national boundaries, and is airborne. Its effects can be catastrophic. In a major outbreak in Turkey in 1964, for example, out of 4 million cattle, buffalo, sheep, and goats in the infected provinces 1½ million were infected, many to die, and the remainder to suffer marked reductions in productivity. Figure 1 shows the world distribution of foot-and-mouth disease incidence. In South America where it is enzootic, all the major cattle raising areas are involved.

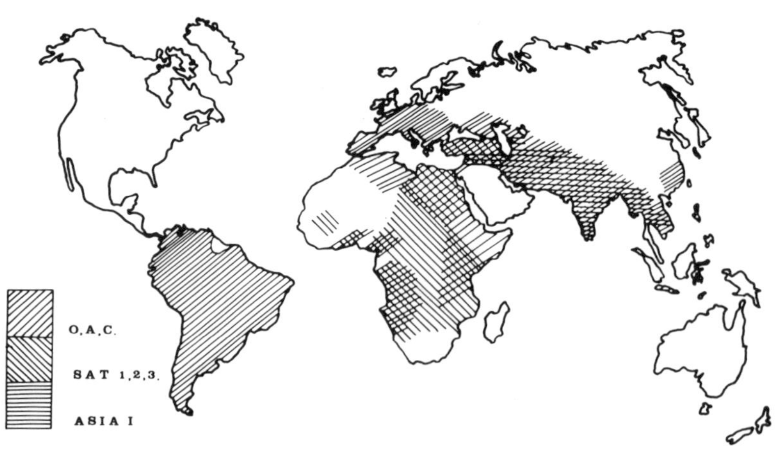

FIGURE 1. World distribution of foot-and-mouth disease classified according to type of virus.

To these restraints on production due to disease must be added those due to parasites – both internal and external. Perhaps the best measure of the restraints on production caused by disease is given by statistical information from Brazil. It was estimated in the mid-1960's that infectious and parasitic disease, coupled with disease caused by malnutrition, resulted in the annual loss of 3 million cattle, 10 million pigs, and 2 million sheep and goats. These losses do not include the diminution in productivity which results from parasitism and disease in survivors. Global estimates of death rates of domesticated livestock due to disease, parasitism, and malnutrition place them between 25 and 30% of the present populations per annum.

The Limits Placed by Climate on Livestock Production

The primary effect of climatic factors on animal production is the indirect one of reducing the food and water supply. In addition, climate has more direct effects, in that environmental temperature, air humidity and velocity, and solar radiation affect their productivity.[10] With all livestock the range of climatic conditions in which normal productivity is maintained is fairly wide but at extremes it is reduced. Milk yield in cattle, a particularly sensitive indicator, is reduced at temperatures below about $-5°C$ and above $30°$, depression at higher temperatures being particularly apparent if humidity is simultaneously high. In poultry, air temperatures in excess of $30°$ reduce growth, the number of eggs produced, and the weight and shell quality of individual eggs. There is, in addition, much evidence to show that high temperatures interfere with fertility, reducing it in particular in the male. The climatic environment is far from stable and with unhoused animals catastrophes leading to much loss of life occur from time to time due to severe weather. In western Canada and the northwest U.S., for example, a combination of severe winds and snow led to the losses of thousands of range cattle and sheep in the winter of 1966, and in the U.K. the winter of 1947 was so severe that about one third of the total sheep stocks perished. In Australia many thousands of sheep have died immediately following shearing when rain, cool conditions, and wind have occurred. Deprived of insulation and penned without feed before being returned to pasture, relatively mild weather constituted a severe stress to them. These catastrophes are rare but constitute a serious hazard. In hot climates weather catastrophes are usually those associated with lack of rain, drought, and failure of feed and water supplies, although overheating of day-old chicks during transport when insolation is high is a commonplace.

Much has been written about the deterioration of European-type cattle in tropical countries which is thought by many to be a direct result of heat stress to which these animals cannot accommodate. Equally there is doubt about the conclusion, for the physical environment is but one component of the tropical environment.

Weather affects parasites and disease vectors as well. Parasitic nematodes, for example, require high temperatures and moisture to hatch from eggs shed in feces to form infective larvae, and similar conditions are necessary for the hatching of the eggs of those Diptera which lay their eggs in the fleece of sheep to cause myiasis. Blue tongue transmission depends on conditions favorable for the *Culicoides* species which are vectors and there are seasonal variations in the incidence of tsetse fly. Indeed, the northward migration of the Fulani cattle herdsmen in west Africa corresponds with the high incidence of the tsetse fly in the lands they leave.

Social, Religious and Cultural Restraints

A distinction has to be made between the animal economies of the New World and the Old, which is central to any considerations of methods of augmenting production. The pastoral economies of the New World are recent and were established with commercial aims in mind; those in the Old World are the development of an ancient culture. In Brazil, for example, cattle rearing began quite recently simply to provide meat for workers in the sugar cane and coffee plantations. In the Old World pastoral life has remained unchanged for thousands of years from the times of the nomadic Semites. It is understandable that traditional and religious factors loom particularly large in the Old World for they are part of a cultural heritage.

A series of taboos on the consumption of animal products limits the expansion of certain types of animal production. Muslims and Jews, a population of 400 million, do not eat pig meat, and hence the production of pigs is anathema. The Hindus, population about 300 million, do not eat beef and because of doctrinal and legal restraints do not kill cattle. Meat from female pigs is regarded as unclean by some Melanesian peoples; eggs are not eaten by women of the Mashona tribe; Eskimos reject and ceremoniously bury the entrails of caribou as an act of atonement for killing them; and the Kazak of Turkestan dislike and rarely eat meat from cattle, but eat horse meat as a luxury item in their diet.

Religious beliefs can impede progress in other ways. For example, in the vaccination campaign for rinderpest control in Cambodia, a Buddhist country, difficulties ensued because of religious prohibition of any form of mutilation of animals. The branding, tattooing, or earmarking of vaccinated animals was thus not allowed and it was only after much discussion that the vaccinated animals could be marked with a red plastic eartag, red being a color of religious significance. Similarly, in the Near and Middle East it is traditional to eat meat from freshly killed animals at religious festivals so that thousands of animals are moved to consuming centers. These are moved on foot or by dhow within the region but in addition animals are brought in live by chartered vessels from Africa, Argentina, and eastern Europe. They cannot be quarantined in such numbers and constitute a serious hazard to the health of the native livestock, a hazard which could be overcome in large measure by an importation of carcasses.

In addition, ownership of animals is woven into the social structure. This can be an extremely complicated arrangement. The Mashona in South Africa, for example, have bride price paid in cattle, fines for adultery are similarly paid, and a beast can be given in payment for services of a herdsman. This cannot be used as bride price but its offspring can! A beast may be sold for millet but to have no cattle means that on marriage the man must work for his father-in-law.[11] Prestige is based on number, not on quality of animal, yet the Masai, for example, themselves value the lyre-horned cattle more than their productive short-horned brethren. In the New Hebrides tusked boars take in part – and with many differences – a similar role to that of cattle in pastoral Africa. It will be only too evident that to attempt to inject a highly commercialized animal economy into such situations is to destroy much which is of more subtle worth.

As important is the absence of a tradition of livestock husbandry particularly in tropical areas.[12] Management of animals is sometimes difficult to learn – even such matters as recognizing individual animals. The place of tradition here is considerable. The Lapp reindeer herders, for example, have some 50 names for coat color and distribution of markings, about the same number for antler conformation, and about a dozen to describe sex and age combination. A combination of these serves to describe an individual in a herd.

Pastoral peoples, particularly nomadic or partially nomadic ones, tend to be aggressive. Many tribal wars have been fought over grazing rights, these now being in part replaced by legal battles. In this regard, political instability and resultant modern war lead to effects of far-reaching significance on animal populations since, particularly with large animals, breeding stocks take long to replace. When war is associated with such insensate acts as widespread defoliation of forest and grazing lands, or blanket bombing, or the destruction of the whole social infrastructure, animal production takes many years to recover.

METHODS OF AUGMENTING ANIMAL PRODUCTION

The sheer variety and complexity of animal production systems throughout the world, their intricate interrelationships with other aspects of economic and social development, and their dependence on an infrastructure of marketing and distribution necessarily mean that the impact of single measures to increase productivity is often extremely difficult to ascertain. To be effective, measures to augment productivity must be part of an integrated whole. It is, for example, of little value to improve the genetic potential of stock if disease, malnutrition, and poor husbandry prevent its realization. Equally, to control an enzootic disease without consideration of consequences in terms of the marketing of the stock which have been so safeguarded is to create new and sometimes more intractable problems. Nevertheless, considerable advances have taken place in the last 30 years in animal production to show that the application of new knowledge, sometimes in a piecemeal fashion, has done much to improve the productivity of livestock. Mistakes have been made where countries have focused major attention on improvement of large animal stocks through importation of superior animals from temperate zones without simultaneously considering questions of disease and feed supplies and results have often proved disastrous. Generally it can be stated that in programs for increasing the output of human food from livestock, the first emphasis should be on the control of disease to be followed by attention to nutrition and husbandry and then by genetic improvement. It is in this order that methods of augmenting productivity are here discussed. Emphasis is given, through examples, to those practices which have proved successful, sometimes on a limited scale in contexts of developing countries, rather than to possibilities that emerge from experience gained in developed ones.

Disease Control – the Major Enzootic Diseases

In dealing with the major enzootic diseases of livestock there is no doubt that control must involve the central governments of states and intergovernment collaboration, sometimes on an international basis. Such control systems exist for many diseases and have been extremely effective. Not all can be dealt with; foot-and-mouth disease and rinderpest are given prominence.

Foot-and-mouth disease is caused by a virus of which there are seven known immunologically distinct types and more than 50 subtypes.[13] While the veterinary services of each country undertake their own measures for control, international agencies help in this task, notably the Office International des Epizooties, the Pan-American Foot and Mouth Disease Commission of F.A.O., and the Inter-African Bureau of Animal Health. In addition, the Animal Virus Research Institute in the U.K. is designated by F.A.O. as the World Reference Centre for typing and subtyping virus. These organizations monitor the incidence of the disease and coordinate control measures.

The methods used involve both compulsory slaughter of affected stock where an outbreak can be contained, or, where it assumes epizootic proportion, the vaccination of susceptible animals using an inactivated vaccine effective against the virus type concerned. Two general types of vaccination are employed. The first is the creation of a barrier by vaccination of all animals in a buffer zone to prevent spread of the disease. Thus, a barrier is maintained in Argentina to protect the provinces to the south of the Rio Negro and in eastern Europe Russia maintains a barrier of vaccinated stock – and indeed stock-free zones – to protect the susceptible animals in Czechoslovakia, Poland, and Rumania, this barrier being continued into Bulgaria. The spread of the South African foot-and-mouth virus from Turkey to Greece in 1962 was in fact contained by barrier vaccination. In May 1972, the same barrier methods were used to prevent the same virus subtype reentering from infections in Turkish Thrace. The second method, ring vaccination, is adopted where infection has occurred to prevent spread from an initial focus to a highly susceptible population and involves vaccination of all animals in a radius of 6 miles.

Vaccination thus plays an important role in the control of the disease and prevention of its spread. The main problem is that to maintain protection a continuing vaccination program is necessary. Where the disease is endemic, such a scheme need not cover the whole population at risk since a high proportion of vaccinated animals leads to a degree of national herd immunity which results in a diminution of the number of primary outbreaks if the disease does occur. Subsidiary measures relate to the presence of the disease in wild animals, the movements of which cannot be controlled. In South Africa this problem has been met by erection of enormous stretches of game-proof fencing to ensure that the game in the Kruger National Park and the Kalahari Gemsbok do not have contact with contiguous cattle stocks. Other measures relate to control of international trade in livestock and livestock products, for the virus can persist in bone marrow and other nonmuscular tissues for many months.

The control of foot-and-mouth disease continues to be a daunting undertaking. It is, however, one of the major successes in terms of international collaboration and if present technical measures continue to be employed, then considerable increases in animal production can be envisaged.

A similar situation applies to the control of rinderpest.[14] A massive campaign of vaccination in Southeast Asia has virtually eradicated the disease. The scale of operations was, and is, immense; 250 million cattle were vaccinated. Currently, the joint campaign against rinderpest in Africa is achieving a similar success, for incidence of rinderpest in the Sudan, Somalia, and Ethiopia is now declining rapidly. It would seem that the final stages of the campaign have now been reached and the problems that emerge are those of differential diagnosis of rinderpest in a disease environment which includes the mucosal disease complex and blue tongue. As with foot-and-mouth disease, international collaboration has achieved and is achieving control and eradication.

The elimination of the tsetse fly and the treatment and control of trypanosomiasis in both animals and man are tasks of an equally formidable magnitude in which success is not yet in sight.[9] The control of the *Glossina* species which are the vectors to break the cycle of the parasite can be achieved in several ways. Discriminatory clearing of bush, guided by a knowledge of the ecology of the *Glossina* species concerned, has made and continues to make a contribution, but often clearance schemes have not been associated with schemes for cultivation and resettlement and in many instances the areas have reverted to become tsetse habitats once more. The older practice of indiscriminate extermination of wildlife as a means of removing a reservoir of infection on which the tsetse fly can feed has largely been discontinued since all calculations show that the density of animals cannot be reduced rapidly enough to be below that which would prevent tsetse fly from feeding. The main control method is undoubtedly the use of organochlorine compounds, notably dieldrin and DDT. Blanket spraying by aircraft certainly covers large areas quickly but ground application, being selective, has great advantage, particularly in view of the environmental contamination and the destruction of natural ecosystems which would result from aerial spraying of an area of 4 million mi^2. Experimental studies of the possibilities of biological control through the use of genetically sterile males or through ecological steps made to encourage predators and parasites of *Glossina* populations are being made but so far they do not suggest rapid emergence of new and more acceptable measures of control.

As far as affected livestock are concerned, a series of drugs is used to effect cures and also as prophylactics. The latter include quinapyramine salts and phenanthridinium compounds. A disturbing feature is that the trypanosome can develop resistance to these compounds. Drug-resistant trypanosomes are then readily transmitted by the tsetse to retain their resistance on repeated passage through the flies and the mammalian hosts. Immunity to trypanosomes does occur and some breeds of cattle, for example, the N'dama in west Africa, can survive in situations in which it seems probable that they are inoculated by tsetse fly with infected trypanosomes virtually every day. Importation of these trypanosome-tolerant cattle has been successful in the Congo in increasing production. Attempts to adapt susceptible cattle to a trypanosome-infected environment coupled with judicious drug treatment have not, however, been very successful.

With African trypanosomiasis, even though many measures of control can be taken, it seems that scientific knowledge is not yet sufficient to enable a wholesale eradication program to commence. The reward that would accrue from finding an acceptable control system is immense, for it could open the way to a revolution in animal husbandry on that continent.

There are many other diseases of livestock which are enzootic in developing countries and which, on occasion, reach epizootic proportions. For many of these, control measures are available. For example, hemorrhagic septicemia, a pasteurellosis, is one of the more important diseases of livestock in Southeast Asia where it has a distinct relationship to weather conditions, outbreaks reaching a peak during the monsoon immediately following hot dry summers. It can be prevented by vaccination. Again the possibility is being considered of commencing an African campaign to eradicate contagious bovine pleuro-pneumonia since effective vaccines are available, and many African countries have instituted control measures independently.

Disease Control – Local Disease and Parasitism

Disease and parasitism are ubiquitous and emphasis on the major enzootic diseases implies neither that local problems are not equally important, nor that control and treatment measures are less effective. They differ in that they are problems of the individual herd or small area rather than of national magnitude. Considerable knowledge has been gained about treatment of these diseases and the efficacy of drugs, anthelmintic and antibiotic therapy in dealing with these conditions. The limitations in applying them are for the most part those related to the shortage of trained personnel to put methods of control into effect. An indication of the difficulties is given by the following statistics. In the United Kingdom there is 1 veterinary surgeon to every 2,000 cattle and in the U.S., 1 to every 4,700. In

Nigeria the ratio is 1:300,000 and in India 1:22,000. Among measures to increase productivity, the training and provision of adequate animal health services including veterinary staffs to provide day-to-day services must rank extremely high.

The Provision of Feed for Livestock

Study of the nutrient needs of farm livestock has been, and continues to be, a major research endeavor in developed countries, and much investigation is being, and has been, made of the value of different feeds and pastures in meeting these needs. The continuing effort in these complementary fields comes about from a realization that small changes in nutrient input and small differences in the substitution value of feeds have considerable effects on profitability and on output. Optimal nutrition is seen more and more to be best defined in economic terms, and recent changes in livestock production in developed countries reflect this. Thus, current trends in the livestock industries of developed countries are toward greater intensification, implying adoption of methods which result in greater outputs per unit time and per unit labor. Examples are the intensive poultry industry and to a lesser extent the intensive pig industry, while feed-lot fattening of cattle and some dairying industries are similar operations. They are characterized by their scale, by their high capital requirements, and by the fact that they depend heavily on grain. Some developments are taking place in the less advanced countries on much the same lines, but while they are suited to certain situations, they are not suited to the pastoral areas where different organizational problems have to be solved. The technical measures for increasing feed provision and ensuring nutritional adequacy are thus best dealt with in two sections, one dealing primarily with situations in which grain or by-products of human food production are available and the other with pastoral farming.

Nonpastoral Livestock

The effects of the new varieties of cereals on livestock farming are both direct and indirect. First, local surpluses of food grains can develop to provide feed and second, not only have yields of coarse grains – notably maize – also been increased, but it is being increasingly realized that it is necessary, to maintain fertility to crop with legumes or with fodder crops for livestock. An example is the use of berseem (*Trifolium alexandrinum*) in Egypt in rotations which include cereals and cotton. As yields and living standards rise so does the incidence of such multiple cropping, which usually means that livestock can profitably be kept.

There is every possibility that with new cereal varieties and with the new cropping and fertilizer technologies they indirectly encourage, cereal surpluses will occur more frequently than in the past. Admittedly these may be somewhat sporadic, for in areas of low rainfall variability of rainfall from year to year is of such magnitude that it can cause major changes in cereal yields. It is for this reason that poultry industries are the most favored ones to employ in these situations. Not only are poultry efficient converters of cereals to human food, but their populations can be expanded rapidly. The technology of so doing is relatively simple, particularly if development takes the form of the introduction of large-scale units. Furthermore, large units, particularly if encouraged to develop as contract-type enterprises in which individual farmers supply eggs or broilers to central packing stations or plants, can act as foci for dissemination of new knowledge. The poultry industry in Ghana commenced on the basis of imported feed and day-old birds and has led to growth of a number of similar smaller enterprises, though not so far to a major growth of coarse grain production to service it. Pigs are an alternative to poultry, although the pig is a more omnivorous animal and can grow satisfactorily on a wider range of feeds than can poultry, leading to a greater resilience in terms of use of resources.

The use of high-yielding cereal grains can lead to the development of similar intensive systems with cattle. Local surpluses of maize in Kenya, for example, have resulted in the development of a beef production system on feed-lot lines. Similar experiments are taking place in Malawi where considerable use is made of milling residues from maize. In all these intensive systems based on cereals, whether for ruminants or nonruminants, diets have to be adjusted to ensure that they are adequate sources of protein, minerals, and vitamins. In many instances local surpluses of by-products of the oilseed industry or the fishing industry ensure that this can be done. A primary measure to enable use to be made of surplus cereals by livestock is the provision of facilities for compounding rations and control of their nutritive adequacy.

Surpluses of by-products create different problems. In India, for example, until recently surpluses of feed were of oilseed residues rather than of cereals. Under such circumstances the problem is to make best use of the excess by ration formulation and feed processing. Citrus pulp again creates problems of a similar type. All these problems are capable of solution and can lead to profitable animal enterprises. Molasses derived from cane sugar production has been the subject of much investigation in Cuba, to lead to a new type of cattle feeding based on molasses supplemented with a small amount of roughage and urea (a source of nonprotein nitrogen which ruminants can use as a protein source by virtue of microbial synthesis in their rumens). This new technology is currently exciting much interest in countries producing sugar cane, for it converts a relatively low-value by-product, molasses, to a high-value one, meat.

The measures necessary to increase productivity in these types of economy are primarily those related to augmentation of crop yield and the technical efficiency of secondary processing of crops to yield by-products for stock of high value and of low variability. In addition, however, are those agricultural practices which are concerned with the integration of fodder crop production with cash cropping, and with the techniques of feed formulation and forward planning of feed supplies.

Pastoral Farming

There are wide variations in the patterns of pastoral farming in different areas of the world, and the extent of their dependence on cultivation. In any system of pastoralism the main problem is to match the productivity of grazings with the number of stock carried, bearing in mind the probability of drought and seasonal declines in the availability of herbage. Several measures can be taken to deal with this, depending on land and climate. In favored environments, control of grazing, a development which usually entails fencing, ensures adequate recovery of grazed lands and the accumulation of reserves of feed to meet seasonal scarcities. The conservation of seasonal surpluses to meet seasonal dearths and the adoption of a wide range of techniques in hay and silage making are included here. In addition, pasture improvement by the introduction of improved species or varieties of pasture grass or legume increases production. Other phases of development include separation of stock classes and the control of pasture supplies of feed to ensure that young animals or milking animals receive better treatment than do dry or nonproductive stock. Combinations of approaches such as these have led to considerable advances in, for example, cattle production in Queensland and the older sheep production in Victoria. In the latter, wheat production and sheep husbandry on sown pastures alternate and the systems include strategic reserves of feed for drought feeding.

As lands become more arid, pasture improvement by reseeding becomes more difficult, and the vegetation becomes less and less suitable or sufficient for conservation. The management of the semiarid lands for cattle and sheep grazing is a hazardous business for rainfall, and even in minimal amounts, cannot be relied on every year. The greatest danger is in overgrazing, particularly when this is exacerbated by continued drought. Marginally, and particularly in areas where there is a seasonal rainfall, improvement can be made using drought-resistant species of legumes and grasses, and techniques of range management and improvement can be applied. Important here are the widespread deficiencies in the soil of many of these areas of phosphorus and of traces of mineral elements which, when remedied, increase productivity. In arid areas, nomadism and consequent overgrazing are commonplace; their replacement by ranching systems, in which the young stock are taken off for finishing in better environments and stocking is suited to the feed resources available, is a clear way of making better use of an enormous resource.

In semiarid areas or areas in which rainfall is highly seasonal, pasture herbage during the summer months becomes very fibrous and its protein content falls to 2% or below. The nutritive value of this material can be improved markedly by the addition of nonprotein nitrogen (NPN) usually in the form of urea or biuret.[14] In addition, inclusion of phosphate and sodium chloride makes up for these deficiencies in the dried herbage. Methods are now available whereby NPN can be made available under these circumstances, notably by pasture spraying – a method incurring an element of risk if a shower of rain does occur to wash the NPN from herbage – and by the provision of blocks containing a mixture of 40% urea and over 40% salt together with molasses which animals can lick at will.[15] There is much evidence to show that these devices result in better survival and better productivity of stock grazing poor mature herbage during drought conditions. Their productivity is, however, still low by normal standards; the gains achieved by these measures are to be interpreted relative to the poverty of productivity otherwise achieved.

In the tropics, where moisture is adequate for large parts of the year, the potential growth of pasture species is enormous, but many of the native species rapidly become of low nutritive value per unit weight as they mature. Establishment of new pastures based on Townsville lucerne or Townsville stylo has considerable potential in many situations and its use has already transformed animal production in subtropical Queensland.

Wherever livestock feed is kept over from one harvest or season to meet subsequent shortages, it is essential that such supplies are not subject to depredations. The losses of human food of vegetable origin as a result of insect infestation of grain, rodent damage, and fungal spoilage have often been emphasized.[16] A much quoted figure of 10% losses due to spoilage for all the cereals, pulses, and oilseeds produced in the world is exceeded grossly by the statistics emanating from surveys particularly in Africa and India. In Kenya, for example, storage of maize cobs in cribs has been shown to lead to losses of 23% due to insect damage. These losses apply equally to feed destined for stock. Admittedly some food so spoiled can be used as feed for livestock but these marginal gains are overshadowed by the continued losses. The measures for control range from the simple prevention of rodent access to stored crops to the complex fumigation of bulk grain. Their efficiency varies and even in highly developed countries losses of feed in these ways are not always small.

Each and every climate region of the world presents different problems and indeed a variety of solutions when it comes to considering methods for augmenting feed supplies. Technical knowledge is available about many of these problems and numerous examples could be given of their successful application. Economic factors and the context of farming systems, however, have to be considered in such applications. It will be evident that what may be feasible for a government to apply in terms of land and crop improvement on government lands with a view to increasing animal output is very different from that which can be adopted by an individual farmer with limited resource. It can be anticipated that for this reason alone, overall improvement of livestock production will tend to lag behind growth of knowledge and clear demonstration of its effective application.

Animal Breeding and Reproduction

The wide variety of types of livestock in different parts of the world no doubt reflect a continuous process of natural and artificial selection which has resulted in the survival of animals well adapted to climate and other environmental factors. The prevalence of haired sheep in desert areas, and of fat-tailed sheep in arid zones are examples, so too are the prevalence of *Bos indicus* (Zebu) types in tropical areas and *Bos taurus* types in temperate ones.[7] Such adaptations relate to survival of the stock; they do not necessarily entail maximal productivity of food for man. European cattle usually have much higher yields of milk and propensities for rapid growth than have the breeds native to Africa or India. Understandably there have been many attempts to introduce European improved livestock into countries in which the productivity of native stock is poor, either to maintain herds of pure bred stock or, by crossing them with native stock, to attempt to improve the latter's productivity while retaining those attributes which are of importance in conferring resistance to environmental stress. The vast herds of Hereford cattle in both North and South America are examples of the pure breeding of European type cattle in new environments, and others could be cited. In addition, there have been many highly successful crossbreeding enterprises with cattle which have led to the emergence of new breeds. Examples here are the Santa Gertrudis breed which includes both *Bos indicus* and *Bos taurus* blood and the Bonsmara of South Africa. The South African developments are illustrated in Table 5. The new breed calved for the first time before the indigenous one, the calving percentage for the new breed was higher than that for both the indigenous and exotic breed, calf mortality was much lower than in imported stock, and mature size and growth rate higher. Again the long-term projects at the

TABLE 5

The Productivity of Beef Cattle in South Africa Showing Superiority of a New Breed Including Indigenous and Exotic Blood

	Africander Indigenous stock	Imported Hereford stock	Synthesis – the "Bonsmara" Breed
Birth weight, kg	32	35	34
Weaning weight, kg	179	177	207
Mature weight, kg	477	495	547
Age at first calf (months)	43	38	35
Calving %	81	88	92
Mortality of calves %	7.7	25.8	11.5

Allahabad Agricultural Institute, India, in which native Red Sindhi cattle were crossed with imported Jersey and later Brown Swiss cattle have shown an earlier calving and a higher milk yield of the crosses than the Red Sindhi. Over several decades improvement of lifetime production has been as much as 2.7-fold through crossbreeding.[18]

Breeding studies in Africa, North Australia, India, and in America have shown that Zebu cattle have certain merits in crossbreeding programs. *Bos indicus* types vary widely, including the Sahiwal from India, the Boran from East Africa, the Brahman, and Africander. Many of these have an innate heat tolerance higher than that of European cattle and, in addition, a resistance to ticks (*Boophilus* sp.) and other arthropods. Tick infestation reduces feed intake and gain so that the latter is less than half that of uninfested stock. Zebus, however, are not good milk producers nor do they respond as well as *Bos taurus* cattle to higher nutritional inputs.[10]

There are many problems in breed replacement and a large number of experimental introductions of new breeds have not been successful. Tropical Africa provides an example. Because of disease problems, poor resistance to high temperatures, and poverty of feed supplies, many of the attempts made by former colonial powers to improve the output of native stock by replacing them with European breeds failed. Breed replacement or a simple crossbreeding system might seem a simple panacea for low productivity, but unless associated with special provision for the imported stock and a simultaneous improvement of the nutritional, parasitological, disease and husbandry environment for the crossbreds, it is not likely to succeed.

In temperate countries the genetic improvement of dairy herds and to a lesser extent beef herds has come about through the widespread use of artificial insemination, whereby sires of proven worth have been used very widely to lead to thousands of progeny from particularly superior animals. Developing countries have followed this example and a number of artificial insemination schemes have been promoted, notably in Thailand, Kenya, and India. In hot countries this might seem to have advantage since high temperatures reduce semen production and a few bulls could well be kept under conditions which mitigate this environmental stress. The use of coconut milk as a semen diluent and the introduction of liquid nitrogen for low-temperature storage and transport of semen have helped to attain reasonable levels of fertility in inseminated cows in such areas. Even so, all the evidence suggests that the improvements in production that have come about as a result of artificial insemination are small, and that many artificial insemination schemes have elements of prestige rather than improvement as their basis.[19] Any improvement that has occurred appears in many instances to be accounted for less by genetic gain than by the presence on farms of the operators who can advise on simple nutritional and husbandry operations. The inseminators in Kenya, for example, make decisions about which animals to inseminate on the basis of the probability of calf survival and the likelihood that surplus bulls according to need will be castrated and used for meat. In making their decision they necessarily give advice. The overriding difficulties are obvious: those of transport and of creating orderliness of a service in some native communities. Despite these difficulties, artificial insemination does provide the means of systematically improving the productivity of livestock. It results in an economy in the use of males kept on farms solely to sire calves. It also provides the means of introducing new genetic material into environments in which imported stock might not survive. For example, imported Jersey cattle in Ghana did not survive very long; they mostly succumbed to snake bite – presumably native cattle were more aware of the hazard and treated snakes with due respect.

With poultry and particularly with large-scale intensive developments in which birds are well housed, distribution of genetically superior breeds developed in Europe and America leads to an immediate harvest in terms of increased productivity. The same is true of other types of animal enterprise in which a special environment is created for the exotic stock. Indeed several feed-lot systems have developed near new population centers based on importation by air of young calves from overseas and their subsequent fattening for meat. Again, provided exotic cattle can be protected from disease and heat and feed supplies are assured, small dairy industries can be created using housed animals and local feed. Such enterprises may be economically viable when there is a large demand for fresh animal produce in a large urban area nearby, but are unlikely to result in widespread improvements in overall productivity for their scale may well be too small, relative to the native stocks and husbandry systems.

Environmental Control

Livestock industries have developed in many inhospitable and apparently unsuitable environments. The severe winters of Northern Europe are such that livestock need considerable protection to survive. In cold northern climates most cattle are housed for months of the year, while in extreme conditions such as those in Norway and Iceland sheep are also kept indoors during the winter. Thus housing constitutes environmental control, though there are aspects of these practices more concerned with facilitation of hand feeding of stock than they are with protection of animals against the effects of weather. The cost of housing is high and there are the alternatives of transfer of stock from regions of high weather risk to those where they can survive. The movement of the reindeer herds of Lapland, the valley wintering of beef herds in British Colombia, and the restriction of the use of alpen pasture land to the summer are examples, and so are some other types of transhumance in Africa. In many instances the provision of winter shelter for stock does enable the resources of feed of cold climates to be used more effectively, for in those situations the limit on stock numbers is placed not by the availability of summer feed but by winter stock carrying capacity.

In hot environments, shelter is equally important, for solar radiation can produce heat stresses in animals which result in diminution of their productivity. In hot sunshine grazing stock seek shade, some breeds more so than others. The amount of feed consumed is reduced, with consequent lowering of growth rate, milk yield, and reproductive performance. With dairy cattle the provision of shelter during the heat of the day as roofed buildings with roof coverings of materials such as aluminum sheeting to reflect solar radiation, if combined with adequate ventilation, can be integrated with grazing management practices to increase productivity. Spraying of cattle and provision of water in which buffalo can wallow are additional methods. Problems arise, however, particularly in humid climates, for such shelters soon become mudholes and heavy sources of parasitism and infection. Provision of simple shade and the gearing of management practices to the diurnal variation in the heat load imposed on stock are about the limits to which any degree of environmental control can be used to augment the productivity of beef cattle and sheep which are usually kept under more extensive conditions than are milking buffalo cows.[20] With more intensive modes of livestock production, a greater degree of environmental control is possible. Poultry housing in particular has been studied and design features that enable birds to be kept at high productivity are known.[21] Traditionally in hot arid areas, housing for man and animals has made use of the heat capacity of thick walls to absorb heat by day and release it by night, while in hot humid areas housing has, through experience, been kept very light and designed to provide maximal air movement. Economic considerations and ventilation needs preclude the use of traditional thick walled houses in arid areas and the use of new heat-reflecting materials and, where water is available, evaporative coolers for the whole building become an alternative. In Malaya and

Singapore the combination of local materials with newer products has resulted in houses in which production can be sustained at high levels provided that the houses are erected to make use of all those factors that modify air movement.

AGRICULTURAL POLICIES AND PRODUCTION

The difference between the highly productive animal industries of developed countries and those of the less well-developed ones is not simply a matter of difference in the extent to which modern techniques of animal husbandry, genetics, nutrition, and disease control are employed. It also includes a series of aspects of the social and economic organization of the countries concerned. To increase productivity entails undertaking measures not usually regarded as technical ones, notably those which relate to farmer incentives, agrarian structure, and the whole institutional framework in which animal production takes place. Furthermore, just as the various technical and scientific measures interact in leading to advancement, so too do those same measures interact with, and require modification to accord with, the economic and social climate in which the livestock producer lives and works. Livestock production does not occur in an agricultural vacuum; it is an integral part of the economic life of the community.

Decisions about the measures to be taken to provide optimal conditions in which technical advance can be made are beset by several difficulties.[22] First, animal production operates over much longer time periods than does primary crop production with the sole exception of tree crops and forestry. The time scale of improvement is equally long, which contributes to the conservatism of livestock farmers and their resistance to change. Second, livestock products are perishable, a fact that creates difficulties if markets are not local ones, difficulties which reach major magnitude if overseas markets are envisaged. Third, modern livestock farming depends on industrial inputs. Some of these are direct-feed supplements, veterinary pharmaceuticals, sera and vaccines, fencing wire, and dairy equipment. Others are indirect, that is, are concerned with increasing crop and pasture production on which livestock depend – fertilizer, seed and machinery.

These difficulties imply that in planning for improvement in the livestock sector, governments have to consider very carefully the nature of price or other incentive for the farmer and the fiscal policies and credit facilities required to put them into effect. They must consider too the provision of marketing facilities, including adequate transport and roads, abattoirs, dairies, refrigerated storage, dehydration, canning and freezing plants, and the opportunities of markets overseas together with any restraints on their entry to these markets. Furthermore, planning cannot neglect the provision of feed plants and fertilizer plants together with other more sophisticated inputs, some of which may imply foreign exchange commitment. In addition, they must consider that in their country livestock farming may well be a separate entity from crop production and that no stratification within their livestock industry exists. To integrate crop and stock production and to arrive at new agrarian structures entail a further consideration of incentive, market and trading facilities, and other provisions.

Specific measures involve political as well as economic judgments. For example, in dealing with questions of incentive, problems arise with respect to the pattern of land tenure and of inheritance in the countries concerned and social antagonisms between nomadic livestock farmers and settlers. These modify appreciably an individual farmer's willingness to invest and innovate. As in Moslem countries, customs of inheritance lead to land subdivision which mitigates against livestock development. This type of problem is particularly apparent in Malaysia and Indonesia where peasants own the land they cultivate. If, as in parts of Africa, the lands are tribal, cultivation is shifting and livestock husbandry involves transhumance and incentive policies for improvement must involve community relations. Many farmers in Nigeria travel miles on foot or bicycle to their farms from the villages where they live. This sort of existence is possible when farming involves crops alone; it is hardly a possible social structure in which livestock farming can develop. This mode of existence in west Africa is very different from that in the east of Africa where the farmers live on their holdings. This pattern has emerged as a result of the partial and continuing replacement of tribal ownership by private freehold ownership of land, and latterly by the replacement of expatriate occupiers by natives, following the achievement of independence from colonial powers. The land tenure situation in native America derives from Spanish settlement and the ideas of feudal Spain. Solutions which are central to modern development range from the cooperatives of Cuba to the revival of Indian tribal systems of tenure as in the Mexican ejido, and clearly have considerable political implications. Changes in systems of land tenure in many instances thus seem prerequisites for large-scale improvement of livestock production. Some resilience must be maintained. The effects of the political factor involved in land tenure are well illustrated by the fall in agricultural output which took place when Dutch-owned estates in Indonesia, many of which were well integrated under agency control, were placed under a central state control, in which restrictions on ownership were imposed. The long-term implications of political decisions involving land tenure can well be realized as exemplified by the lessons of Polish collectivization.

Again, while the emphasis in agricultural advance in developed countries has been to judge successive steps by economic criteria, a process which has inevitably led to increase of scale and an economy of labor, it can be questioned whether measures to promote improvement in developing countries should emulate this pattern. Rural unemployment, with consequent rural drift to urban centers where employment opportunities are equally poor, occurs as agricultural production increases under western influence in many developing countries, for example, Mexico. In Mexico City, unemployment due to the influx of rural populations is a major problem. Obviously, to avoid unemployment, advance in the livestock industries in developing countries can only be toward the form of that in the developed ones if industrialization proceeds at a very rapid pace. The pace of industrial development in its turn may depend on the presence of other natural resources, notably power supplies and mineral reserves in a country. It can be argued that there is much merit in many areas of the world in retaining intensive labor systems of livestock husbandry. Certainly such policies would preserve the close link between domesticated animals and man which is a part of the culture of the peoples concerned. Replacement of animals as sources of motive power by machines that are imported is an illustration of a process which, while it might lead to greater food production, does not necessarily result in maintenance even of existing levels of employment. The measures that may be taken by governments to provide the climate in which farmers would increase their livestock production are relatively simple, but they have complex overtones and political implications.

The provision of market opportunities, including overseas markets for animal products, involves considerable capital investment in terms of abattoirs, milk processing, and other plants. They are essential to progress, but may equally conflict with policies relating to industrialization in the urban sector. Clearly the decisions to be made on overall priorities in developing countries are far more difficult to make than are those relating to modifications of modern technological processes to enable them to improve productivity.

Whatever technical processes are to be employed, whether at the farm, in marketing, processing, or provision of essential inputs, their adoption and continuance requires skilled people, educational programs, and major investment in extension services. This is well recognized and the measures necessary have been and are being taken in most developing countries. There may well be a tendency in some to concentrate on higher education and to be concerned with prestige aspects of university education to the neglect of the further education and rudimentary training of those who care for animals or provide essential services. Equally there are differences of view about the extent to which the state should take direct responsibility for such training. Even so, it is without question that to enable the livestock industries of many countries to expand, considerable numbers of able men and women with skills that can be taught and then expanded through experience are required. It is only in this way that the vast store of knowledge about the means of improving the production of food from livestock can be put to practical use, to be adjusted on the basis of local test to create new and productive industries. Technically there are few limits to increasing livestock production and there is no reason why growth in the provision of food of animal origin should not match and exceed growth of the human population. The main limitations are those associated with the political, institutional, social, and economic factors which determine whether this technology is in fact applied.

REFERENCES

1. F.A.O., *The State of Food and Agriculture*, 1970, F.A.O., Rome, 1970.
2. **Clark, C. and Haswell, M.,** *The Economics of Subsistence Agriculture,* Macmillan, London, 1967.
3. **Blaxter, K. L.,** Domesticated ruminants as sources of human food, *Pure Nutr. Soc.,* 29, 244, 1970.
4. **Duckham, A. N. and Masefield, G. B.,** *Farming Systems of the World,* Chatto & Windus, London, 1970.
5. **Perpillou, A. V.,** *Human Geography,* Longmans, London, 1966.
6. **Underwood, E. J.,** *The Mineral Nutrition of Livestock,* C.A.B. and F.A.O., Rome and Aberdeen, 1966.
7. **Chalmers, A. W. and Scott, G. R.,** The ecology of rabies, *Trop. Anim. Health Prod.,* 1, 33, 1969.
8. **Mack, R.,** The great cattle plague epidemic of the 1890's, *Trop. Anim. Health Prod.,* 2, 210, 1970.
9. F.A.O./W.H.O., African Trypanosamiasis, Report of a Joint F.A.O./W.H.O. Expert Committee, F.A.O. Agricultural Studies No. 81, 1969.
10. **Hafez, E. S. E.,** *Adaptation of Domestic Animals,* Lea & Febiger, Philadelphia, 1968.
11. **Gelland, M.,** *Diet and Tradition in African Culture,* E. & S. Livingstone, Edinburgh, 1971.
12. **Ucko, P. J. and Dimbleby, G. W.,** *The Domestication and Exploitation of Plants and Animals,* Duckworth & Co., London, 1969.
13. Committee of Enquiry on Foot and Mouth Disease, 1968, Part I, H.M.S.O., London, 1969.
14. **Briggs, M. H.,** *Urea as a Protein Supplement,* Pergamon Press, Oxford, 1967.
15. **Alexander, G. I.,** Non protein nitrogen supplements for grazing animals in Australia, *World Anim. Rev.,* 4, 11, 1972.
16. President's Scientific Advisory Committee, *The World Food Problem,* Vol. 2, Report of the Panel on the World Food Supply, The White House, Washington, D. C., 1967.
17. **Temple, R. S.,** Temperate and indigenous beef cattle breeds in the tropics, *World Rev. Anim. Prod.,* 8, 39, 1972.
18. **Mahadevana, P.,** *Breeding for Milk Production in Tropical Cattle,* C.A.B. Farnham Royal, England, 1966.
19. **Rollinson, D.H.L.,** Further developments of artificial insemination in tropical areas, *Anim. Breed. Abstr.,* 39, 407, 1971.
20. **Rendel, J. M.,** Breeding cattle for the Australian north, *World Rev. Anim. Prod.,* 8, 48, 1972.
21. **Ferguson, W.,** Poultry housing in the tropics – applying the principles of thermal exchange, *Trop. Anim. Health Prod.,* 2, 44, 1970.
22. **Bunting, A. H.,** *Change in Agriculture,* Duckworth & Co., London, 1970.

INCREASING OUTPUT OF ANIMAL PRODUCTION RELATIVE POTENTIAL OF SPECIFIC MEAT-PRODUCING ANIMALS

R. W. Phillips

TABLE OF CONTENTS

Introduction 147

Animal Products in Man's Food Supply 148

Some Reasons for Variations in Supplies of Animal Products 151
- General Considerations 151
- Numbers vs. Productivity 152
- Genetic Levels of Productivity 152
- Relation of Economic Levels to Demands for Animal Products 153

Potentials for Increasing Animal Production 154
- Potential of Various Types of Animals 154
  - Farm Animals 154
  - Wildlife 155
  - Fisheries 156
- Potentials for Increases in Different Regions 157
  - Europe 157
  - North America 158
  - Oceania 158
  - Latin America 158
  - The Far East 159
  - The Near East 159
  - Africa 159
- General Observations on Potentials for Future Increases in Production 161

References 162

INTRODUCTION

Animals contribute a great deal to man's food supply and to the nutritional quality of his diet. Yet, for a number of reasons, there are wide variations in the levels of those contributions in different countries and regions of the world. Thus, in some countries the supplies of animal products are generous, in others they are modest or low, while in some they are scant indeed.

If man's present and future needs for animal products are to be met, great increases in production will be necessary. There are substantial possibilities for achieving such increases, but there are also limitations. The factors that impose limitations upon increases in production are geographic, climatic, biological, economic, and social in nature.

The object of this chapter is, therefore, threefold: to provide background information on present supplies of food of animal origin; to discuss the reasons for the variations in levels of supplies; and to consider the potentials for increases in the output of animal products. Within these contexts, the meat-producing animals are interpreted as including those which also produce milk or eggs. In addition, some attention is given to game animals and to fish.

ANIMAL PRODUCTS IN MAN'S FOOD SUPPLY

Countries vary a great deal in the amounts of food they have available for their peoples. These variations are most easily expressed in terms of calories, total protein, and animal protein available per person per day. The variations are greatest for animal protein, an indication that countries vary considerably more in the quality than in the quantity of the diets of their peoples. The variations in supplies of animal protein also reflect substantial differences in levels of animal production and/or in economic capacities to import animal products.

Data assembled by FAO[1] on these three yardsticks of the quantity and quality of man's diet in 90 countries are reproduced in graphic form in Figure 1. The countries are arranged in descending order of calorie supplies and the range is from 3,450 cal per person per day in Ireland to 1,770 cal. in Somalia; thus, the best-fed country in this respect has nearly twice as many calories as the poorest fed. For total protein, the range is from 111.7 g per person per day in Uruguay (No. 13 in the chart) to 41.4 g in Indonesia (No. 87), i.e., Uruguay has nearly 2¾ times as much total protein per person as Indonesia. For animal protein the range is much greater. Uruguay, which ranks first in this respect also, has 77.4 g per person per day, or over 21 times that available in the country with the lowest level, i.e., Rwanda (No. 86), which has only 3.6 g.

To show the variations in total protein supplies more clearly, the data set out in graphic form in Figure 1 (minus those for calories) have been rearranged in Figure 2 in descending order of total protein supplies. Even a casual examination of this chart reveals that among the 30 best-fed countries in terms of total protein, roughly half the protein is from animal sources and half from plant sources on the average. In the remaining 60 countries, much more of the protein is obtained from plants than from animals. However, it may be noted that among the 30 countries having the greatest

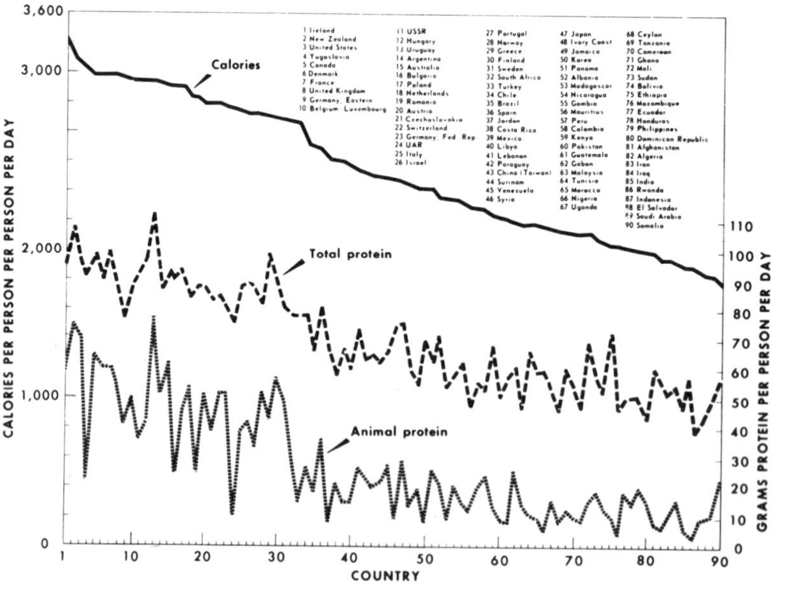

FIGURE 1. Amounts of calories, total protein, and animal protein in national food supplies of 90 countries, arranged from left to right in descending order of amounts of calories. (From Phillips, R. W., in *Animal Agriculture,* Cole, H. H. and Ronning, M., Eds., W. H. Freeman and Company, San Francisco. Copyright © 1973. With permission.)

supplies of total protein, there are a number that depend more on plants than animals, most notably Yugoslavia (No. 8 in the chart), Bulgaria (No. 13), and Romania (No. 22).

The data on animal protein supplies that are included in Figures 1 and 2 are reassembled separately in Figure 3 to distinguish even more sharply the extremely wide variations among

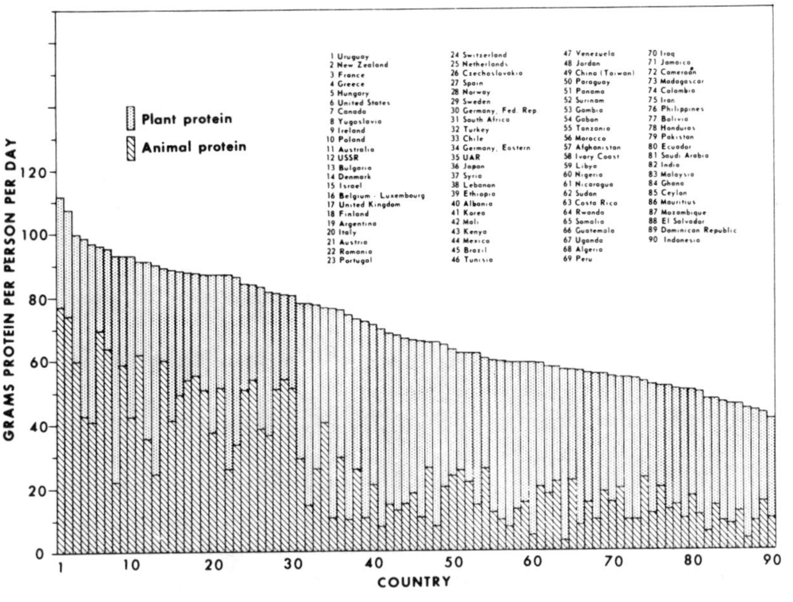

FIGURE 2. Amounts of total protein and proportions of animal and plant protein in food supplies of 90 countries, arranged from left to right in descending order of amounts of total protein. (From Phillips, R. W., in *Animal Agriculture,* Cole, H. H. and Ronning, M., Eds., W. H. Freeman and Company, San Francisco. Copyright © 1973. With permission.)

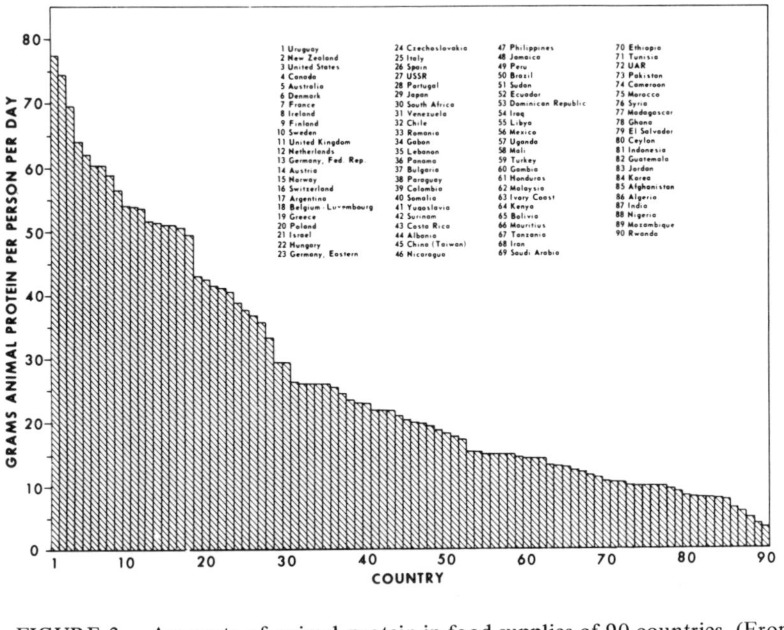

FIGURE 3. Amounts of animal protein in food supplies of 90 countries. (From Phillips, R. W., in *Animal Agriculture,* Cole, H. H. and Ronning, M., Eds., W. H. Freeman and Company, San Francisco. Copyright © 1973. With permission.)

countries in such supplies. Among the 90 countries, some like Uruguay, New Zealand, the U.S., Canada, and Australia have generous supplies of 77.4, 74.3, 69.6, 64.1, and 62 g, respectively. But 62 of the countries have less than 30 g, and of these 17 have 10 g or less per person. Since these are average amounts in national food supplies, not amounts actually consumed, it is evident that many of the world's people consume very little animal protein.

For the most part, animal protein comes from four major products: milk, meat, eggs, and fish. Since this chapter is concerned with potentials for increased output of such products, it is also worthwhile to examine the variations among countries in the present output of these products. Data, assembled by FAO[2] for the same 90 countries that are included in Figures 1 to 3 and arranged in the same sequence as in Figure 3, i.e., according to level of animal protein supplies, are arranged in Figure 4.

Finland (No. 9 in the chart) ranks first in milk production per person per day, with 899 g. Indonesia (No. 81) and Korea (No. 84) are at the other extreme, with only 2 g. Uruguay (No. 1) ranks first in meat produced per person, or 310 g, compared with only 4 g in India (No. 87). For eggs, the range is from 58 g in Israel (No. 21) to an amount too small to record in Rwanda (90), while ten other countries are shown as having only 1 g per person per day. Japan (No. 29) has the most fish per person, 89 g, while at the low end of the scale there are five countries, Bolivia (No. 65), Iran (No. 68), Syria (No. 76), Afghanistan (No. 85), and Rwanda (No. 90), with no recorded quantities. It is noteworthy that while fish are important nutritionally and are of special importance because a large share of the supply is taken from international waters, the amount in food supplies corresponds closely with the amount of eggs.

An overall examination of Figure 4 suggests something of the potential that exists for increasing the output of animal products. If, for example, the production levels in countries No. 21 through 90 in the chart could be raised to levels corresponding generally with those in countries No. 1 through 20, there would indeed be a remarkable change in the overall level of nutrition of the world's people.

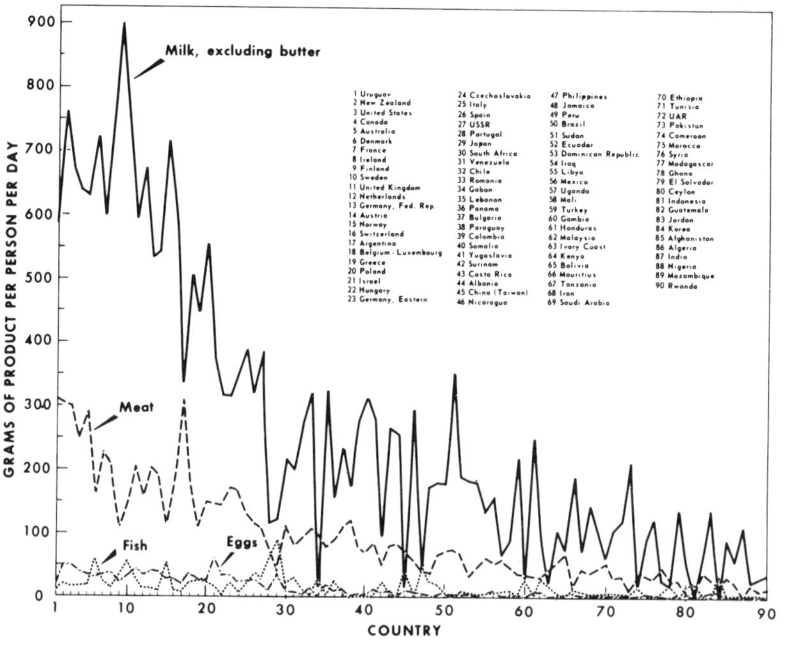

FIGURE 4. Amounts of milk, meat, eggs, and fish in the food supplies of 90 countries. The countries are arranged from left to right in descending order of animal protein supplies, i.e., in the same order as in Figure 3. (From Phillips, R. W., in *Animal Agriculture,* Cole, H. H. and Ronning, M., Eds., W. H. Freeman and Company, San Francisco. Copyright © 1973. With permission.)

SOME REASONS FOR VARIATIONS IN SUPPLIES OF ANIMAL PRODUCTS

General Considerations

Some rough estimates have been published by FAO[3] that indicate the wide differences which exist in levels of productivity in different major regions of the world. These estimates are shown in Table 1. These differences among geographic regions also suggest some of the basic causes of the wide variations between regions and countries and between areas within countries.

Agriculture is on the whole a more intensive enterprise in Europe than in North America. Moreover, North America has large range areas where cattle can be grown and subsequently fattened on feeds produced in intensive farming areas such as the Corn Belt. Consequently, North America has both specialized beef and dairy industries. In Europe, however, the dual-purpose animal prevails and a much larger proportion of the total cattle population is used for milk production. As a result of these interrelated factors, Europe has a larger production of milk per head in the total cattle population, while North America has a larger output of beef.

Compared with either North America or Europe, Asia has very low levels of production of both meat and milk. In much of Asia, human population densities are great, farms are small and are intensively cultivated to produce human food, little land can be devoted to the production of animal feed, and cattle are used primarily for draft purposes, while milk production, and in particular beef production, are secondary roles. Furthermore, in one major country – India – religious beliefs prevent most of the population from consuming beef. Also, the low level of per capita incomes throughout most of Asia means that the average person cannot afford the luxury of many animal products but must rely primarily upon foods of plant origin.

TABLE 1

Production of Meat and Milk per Head of Cattle Population in Major Regions 1966/67, in kilograms per head per year

Region	Beef	Milk
North America	87	520
Europe*	59	1,016
Oceania	47	512
Latin America	27	89
Africa	14	76
Asia**	11	80

*Including U.S.S.R.
**Including Mainland China

Africa, which also has quite low levels of productivity compared with North America and Europe, is faced with some of the same difficulties but it also has some different problems. Much of the continent is not densely populated, so is unlike Asia in this respect. But income levels are low, so the stimulus to production that comes from a high level of demand is not present. Also, large sections of Africa are either arid or covered by tropical jungle, and thus not adapted to intensive animal production. Tsetse fly infestation is also a factor limiting cattle production in substantial portions of the continent. Customs among some tribes lead to emphasis upon numbers rather than productivity in terms of meat and milk. Thus, ownership of large numbers of animals is a prestige matter and their productivity or marketable offtake is a secondary matter. Cattle are also a form of currency, for example, for the purchase of brides among some tribal groups. In other circumstances, the emphasis is upon numbers as a matter of survival. The Masai, who live in a hot, dry area of East Africa, normally bleed their cattle and consume the blood, thus keeping the animals alive as a continuing source of food. In many areas where increases in productivity should be possible, epizootic diseases such as rinderpest and foot-and-mouth disease are still a threat, thus limiting the possibilities for exporting live animals or carcasses. For these and other reasons, neither specialized beef nor dairy production has been developed to any marked degree in most parts of Africa.

In Latin America the regional average production of beef is somewhat higher than in Asia and Africa, owing to the considerable attention to beef production in a few countries, particularly Argentina and Uruguay. However, for much of the region there are limitations imposed by low incomes of the people, such as wet tropical, high mountain, and semiarid areas unfavorable to cattle production, lack of feed for fattening cattle, presence of parasites and diseases, inadequate marketing and processing facilities, and other factors. Since Latin America is a highly diverse region, the particular combination of factors limiting production varies a great deal in different subregions and countries.

Much more could be said about the reasons for variations among regions in productivity of cattle, as portrayed in Table 1. Also, similar analyses and conclusions could be made for sheep, goats, swine, and poultry, although the limiting factors vary somewhat with differences in species. For example, the dense populations and small farms of Southeast Asia place less of a limitation upon the development of swine and poultry production than upon production by ruminants, which requires extensive grazing areas or other sources of roughage. As a further example, a special limitation is placed upon swine production in those areas of Asia and Africa where the Moslem religion prevails.

The foregoing should be sufficient to indicate the broad range of factors that place limitations on animal production. However, a few of the limiting factors are of such importance in all the regions where animal products are now in scarce supply that they are worthy of more detailed examination, i.e., numbers vs. productivity, genetic levels of productivity, and the relation of economic levels to demands for animal products.

Numbers vs. Productivity

Reference has already been made to the concern with numbers of animals, rather than with productivity, in parts of Africa. But the problem of low productivity in relation to numbers is much more widespread. It exists for a variety of reasons throughout most of the developing countries.

There is a common misconception that the densely populated, heavily tilled areas of the world, and Asia in particular, have relatively few farm animals. On the contrary, the numbers in most such areas are substantial. For example, Phillips[4] has pointed out that Asia had 30.8 % of the world's cattle, 39.5 % of the pigs, 22 % of the sheep, 50 % of the goats, 96.9 % of the water buffaloes, and approximately 30 % of the poultry. Yet the productivity of these animals in terms of meat, milk, and eggs is quite low.

Thus, as Phillips[4] has shown, there are 11 countries in Asia that have more cattle and water buffaloes per 1,000 hectares of arable land than does the U.S. Yet, leaving aside one anomaly in the available statistics, the U.S. outranks all except Israel in terms of beef and veal produced per 1,000 animals, is outranked only by Israel and Japan in milk produced per 1,000 animals, and is first in terms of the amounts of milk and of beef and veal produced for each 1,000 persons. To pursue this point one step further, the U.S. is outranked by 13 Asian nations in numbers of poultry per 1,000 hectares of arable land, yet in terms of poultry meat, and eggs produced per 1,000 birds, the U.S. outranks all the Asian countries, most of them by a very wide margin.

These low levels of production in the developing countries result from a number of causes. Much of the draft power on farms is provided by cattle and water buffaloes, emphasizing the capacity to work rather than meat or milk production. Neither the art nor the science of animal production is well developed in most of these countries and leaders as well as institutions devoted to animal science are few. Neither is the thinking of farmers tuned to specialized animal production nor do most of them have the capital to undertake such enterprises. Consequently, as has been pointed out by Phillips,[5] efficient systems of animal production have not been evolved and integrated into the overall pattern of farming. Furthermore, the development of improved, productive strains through breeding has not taken place to a degree that is at all comparable with that which has occurred in the temperate zones.

Genetic Levels of Productivity

Although various geographic, climatic, economic, and biological factors related to feeding and to diseases and parasites place serious limitations upon animal production in many countries, the restriction placed upon such production by low genetic capacities is one of the most important, not only of itself but because it limits the beneficial effects that might otherwise result from improvements on other fronts, particularly improved feeding and management.

Some impressive types and breeds of animals have evolved under the relatively poor conditions of production existing in the poorer countries, where supplies of livestock products are small, as has been pointed out by Phillips,[6] Joshi and Phillips,[7] and Joshi, McLaughlin and Phillips.[8] Also, some types, which of themselves are not very efficient producers, have traits that might be utilized in developing more productive strains. One example of such a trait is the apparently high level of fertility in some types of Chinese swine, as described by Phillips, Johnson, and Moyer[9] and

Phillips and Hsu.[10] However, many of the types and breeds found throughout the tropics and subtropics, in high mountain areas, and other difficult environments do not have the high levels of genetic capacity for meat, milk, and egg production found in many breeds and types in the Temperate Zones, where conditions are generally favorable to animal production and where much attention has been given to improvement through breeding, while at the same time providing improved feeding and management.

This point can perhaps best be illustrated with chickens, where eggs laid provide a precise measure of productivity. Although accurate statistics on production are difficult to obtain in many developing areas of the world, such figures as are available indicate that the native types of hens lay about 40 to 60 small eggs per year on the average. Production as high as 100 eggs per year is exceptional. By contrast, U.S.D.A.[11] data indicate that the average laying hen in the U.S. produces approximately 220 eggs per year. This difference in genetic capacity to respond to adequate feeding is of importance, both because of the increased output obtained from superior strains and because of the increased efficiency associated with high levels of production. Regarding efficiency, a hen that lays only 40 normal-sized eggs per year may need up to 850 g of dry feed to produce 1 egg. If, however, production is increased to 120 eggs, the feed requirement drops to about 300 g per egg, while at a level of 240 eggs per year, the feed requirement drops to about 180 g per egg, according to FAO.[12]

The point may also be illustrated with cattle, using milk production as the measure of performance. India, which has more cattle than any other country, is also a country which lays great store on its cattle, both for religious reasons and because in the words of Lord Linlithgow, a former viceroy of pre-partition India, "The cow and the working bullock bear on their patient backs the whole structure of Indian agriculture." As this quotation indicates, most of the cattle are used primarily for draft purposes and the cows produce only enough milk to nurse their calves, or if milked at all, they yield only limited amounts of milk – about 500 to 2,000 lb per lactation – beyond that taken by the calf. However, some milking breeds, such as the Sahiwal, Red Sindhi, and Gir, have evolved. But the cows of such breeds yield amounts only in the 3,000 to 6,000 lb per lactation range under conditions of good feeding and management; only an occasional exceptional animal exceeds these levels according to the data assembled by Joshi, McLaughlin, and Phillips.[8] By contrast, the average yield of milk cows in the U.S. is over 9,000 lb per lactation; 9,166 lb in 1969 and 9,388 lb in 1970, exclusive of milk sucked by calves, according to the USDA.[13]

Relation of Economic Levels to Demands for Animal Products

Data presented in graphic form earlier in Figures 1, 2, and 3 indicate that the poor countries are generally the poorly fed countries, both in terms of calories and in terms of dietary quality as measured by amounts of protein, and particularly animal protein, in the diets of their peoples.

The calorie level in national food supplies tends to rise rapidly as annual incomes per person increase from around $60 up to $300, after which there is less response to increases in income; beyond annual incomes of about $1,000 per person there appears to be little increase in energy supplies as incomes increase further.[14] The level of total protein also increases rather rapidly until incomes reach about $300, and more gradually thereafter.

Animal protein supplies bear an even closer relationship to level of income, as may be seen from Figure 5. This chart, compiled by Brown,[14] shows this close relationship among 30 countries. The one marked exception to the general trend is Argentina which, although not a rich country, has a long tradition of livestock production and a high level of meat consumption.

Since somewhat over half the world's people live in countries where the average annual income per person ranges from well under $100 up to around $700, most of them simply do not command the purchasing power necessary to permit the consumption of sizeable amounts of animal products.

For example, Schertz[15] points out that in India, where the annual income was about $63 per person, $36 or about 10 cents a day was being spent for food, which included an allowance for home-produced food. Compared with this level of expenditure for food, a day's ration of protein of say 30 g from one of the plant sources could be purchased for about 1/3 to 1 2/3 cents, or from skim milk powder for about 2 cents. However, if that amount of protein was obtained from a source such as beef, cheese, or eggs, the cost would range from 7.4 to 13.6 cents.

Thus, under circumstances of low incomes the effective demand for most animal products is quite low and the stimulus to production which results from an active demand is largely absent.

It follows that such countries do not have the purchasing power to import substantial quantities of food supplies of animal origin from countries that have developed the capacity to produce such products surplus to their own needs. Hence, much of the international trade in animal products is among the developed, relatively affluent countries, where both the market demands and the capacities to produce, process, and market exist.

POTENTIALS FOR INCREASING ANIMAL PRODUCTION

Against the foregoing background of factors that affect levels of animal production and in which problems that impose limitations on animal production have been emphasized, a background that is by no means exhaustive, what are the potentials for increasing the output of animal products? These potentials vary among species, among production areas, and of course among countries or areas with different economic levels.

Potentials of Various Types of Animals

Farm Animals

Data summarized earlier in this chapter indicated that there is a wide gap between protein needs and protein supplies in many countries. FAO,[16] in its *Provisional Indicative World Plan for Agricultural Development,* gave considerable attention to this problem. It was recognized that, although animal products are important, much of the world's protein supply comes from plants. For example, in Latin America about two thirds of all the protein is of plant origin, while in other developing regions about 80% comes from plants. Therefore, needed increases in protein must come in part through breeding of cereals for higher protein content, through the development of higher yielding pulses, and through more attention to increased ouput of protein-rich oil seeds and the higher-protein varieties of root crops. However, these increases would leave a substantial share of the protein gap to be filled from animal sources.

If this portion from the animal side is to be filled, it must be provided to a substantial degree by the two rapidly reproducing, more efficient converters, pigs and poultry. Taking the developing region as a whole, it was estimated that with an 11% increase per annum in poultry and 5% in pork, or alternatively 10% in poultry and 5.8% in pork, it would be possible to close the protein gap by 1985. Such increases, while technically feasible, would require the production of 110 million tons

INCOME AND SUPPLY OF ANIMAL PROTEIN PER PERSON

Selected Countries

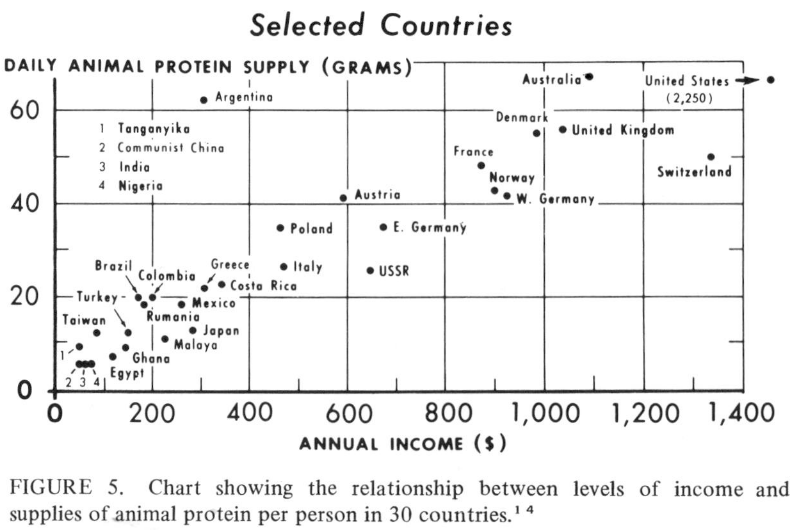

FIGURE 5. Chart showing the relationship between levels of income and supplies of animal protein per person in 30 countries.[14]

of concentrates by 1985, compared with only 31 million tons in 1962. Thus, there would have to be a satisfactory ratio between feed grain and livestock product prices and a breakthrough in cereal production to ensure an even flow of grain for animal feeding. Also, a change would have to come about in consumption patterns, since such a shift would mean that 47% of all meat consumed in developing countries by 1985 would be pig and poultry meat, compared with 24% in 1962. Even so, around 50% of all meat supplies in the world would still be beef and veal and the constraints imposed by a long reproductive cycle will limit the possibilities of keeping beef and veal production adequate to meet the needs of a rapidly expanding human population.

Other factors also limit the expansion of production by ruminants, particularly cattle. The techniques for large-scale industrialized production of pigs and poultry are fairly readily transferable from developed to developing countries. But transfers of the improved technology for ruminant production are beset by a number of nontechnical problems including social customs, usage, and institutions; bringing about an increase in productivity often means the creation of a new market-oriented institutional and social structure. Such changes are not readily accepted by farmers, nor is the need for them always understood by agricultural leaders in developing countries.

FAO[17] also points to some other reasons why maintenance of adequate ruminant production of meat will be difficult. There appears to be little doubt that demands for beef in developed countries will be well in excess of those countries' production potential. In the developing countries, production of beef and mutton apparently kept pace with domestic demands until the 1950's through herd enlargements and production in new areas, but scope for this type of expansion has diminished in many countries. However, domestic demand has continued to increase and the availability of local beef and mutton per person has tended to decline in a number of developing countries. Increases in production and especially of exports are also constrained by animal disease problems, and the livestock industry is being forced increasingly onto land of marginal productive capacity.

Increasing the offtakes, particularly in African countries with large cattle populations, where numbers rather than productivity have been emphasized, offers considerable potential for increasing the availability of beef. Moreover, once unproductive animals are removed, their feed can be utilized for productive purposes, and the structure of the herd may also be shifted to include more breeding cows. However, once these avenues of increase are utilized, other means of improving productivity must be sought.

All these considerations point rather clearly to the conclusion that among the farm animals, increasing emphasis must be placed upon pigs and poultry if man's requirements for animal protein are to be met.

Wildlife

Various types of wildlife have received increasing attention in recent years as sources of food, particularly in Africa where substantial resources still exist in the form of large game animals.

There is a basic conflict of interest between the development of cropland and the continuing use of adjacent areas for grazing by wild animals. Also, there is a conflict of interest between those wishing to develop range livestock production and those who prefer to see such lands used for the maintenance of wild herds. Moreover, the question of which type of production is the more efficient and beneficial to a country is by no means resolved.

However, a substantial body of opinion is accumulating in support of the view that particularly on arid bush savanna lands, a sensible and economically sound solution rests in the development of game management for sustained meat production as a legitimate form of agricultural land utilization. Among the arguments cited by Roth[18] for this approach are that such land use: (a) is a substitute for cattle production where cattle cannot be kept; (b) supplements cattle ranching in marginal areas to such an extent that low stocking rates in conjunction with game utilization became economical; (c) permits a reduction of wild animals which are detrimental to agriculture, in favor of meat-productive species; (d) materially justifies the existence of game animals and thus contributes to their conservation; (e) helps to maintain the ecological equilibrium and ensures that marginal areas remain productive; (f) limits poaching and thus reduces illegal traffic in game products and the associated danger of disease dissemination; and (g) provides conditions under which authorities can investigate disease problems, reduce the danger of disease outbreaks, control the spread of diseases, and reduce public health hazards in respect to wildlife products.

Apart from the management and harvesting of meat of game animals maintained in the wild state, a case is developing for game farming or ranching, wherein the animals are maintained in semidomesticated and perhaps eventually domesticated circumstances. Kyle[19] points out some of the advantages of wild species, compared with cattle, and discusses the possibilities of using various species in game ranching.

Cattle are completely excluded from about 37% of the total land mass of Africa, owing to the transmittal of trypanosomiasis by the tsetse fly. Although the zebu is better able to cope without good supplies of water than the European cattle, even its ability in this respect falls far short of most game animals. The rate of reproduction in African cattle is generally low, as is also their rate of growth. Even improved breeds, such as the Boran, fall well short of the East African antelopes in these respects, according to Kyle.[19]

Among the antelopes, the common eland is one of the most promising. It is relatively easy to domesticate, yields a lean carcass of high quality, and is able to thrive even when no drinking water is available. Since its main diet consists of bushes which draw on a relatively deep water table, it does not destroy the shallow-rooted grasses in times of drought. Also, it is quite mobile in its grazing habits, so does not overgraze limited localities. Its combined abilities to resist disease, drought, and heat stress enable the eland to thrive in arid conditions in Africa which are marginal or submarginal for cattle.

There are some 80 major species of antelope in Africa and many of them are reported to be more capable than cattle of producing high quality meat under arid conditions. Among those mentioned by Kyle[19] are Thomson's Gazelle, Impala, Springbok, Grant's Gazelle, Topi, Kongoni, and Wildebeest. The African Buffalo also offers possibilities in the wild state, but efforts at domestication have not been successful. Other species that have been cropped to some extent are the giraffe, elephant, and hippopotamus, the latter two particularly under park conditions where, with protection, their numbers regularly become excessive. The growth rates of the elephant and hippopotamus are such that their meat production capacity is about the same as the conventional meat producers, or about 1 1/3 lb/day. Kyle[19] reports that while the meat of the elephant is somewhat coarse, that of the hippopotamus is very pleasant and not unlike pork.

Approaches to management of wildlife for meat production and to game ranching are still essentially experimental in nature, and a great deal of study and experience is yet needed before their real places in the scheme of things in Africa become clear. However, they seem to offer enough promise, particularly when coupled with their economic value in relation to tourism, to justify further exploration.

A main expense in such cropping schemes results from the fact that slaughtering must usually be done in the field. Thus, as Kyle[19] points out, trucks are needed to bring animals from the bush to processing stations for dressing, inspection, and freezing. If the bush areas to be cropped are quite extensive, mobile processing units may be necessary. In either event, cold storage trucks are needed to carry the meat to warehouses in population centers. However, under ranching conditions, where animals are accustomed to handling, it should be possible to transport animals to market points in the same way as cattle.

Most of the ranching schemes developed thus far have been of a small, private nature, too small to arouse serious commercial interest. Only as larger-scale trials are carried out will it be possible to arrive at sound assessments of the practical possibilities.

Fisheries

The output of the world's fisheries increased steadily following the reconstruction of fishing fleets after World War II through 1968. The estimated average annual world catch of fish, crustacea, and mollusks during the 1948–52 period was 20,790,000 metric tons. By 1968, according to FAO,[20] it had risen to 57,410,000 metric tons. There was a moderate decline in 1969, but the level rose again to 62,090,000 metric tons in 1970. Preliminary estimates for the first half of 1971 again indicated a reduction, with fish meal output more than a quarter lower than a year earlier in the six most important producing countries, while there were also poorer catches of some important food-fish species in North America and Europe.

A number of factors combine to indicate that fish production is not apt to increase as fast in the near future as it did during the 1960's. Some important stocks are already under heavy fishing pressure and cannot be expected to yield much more. There are relatively few sizeable under-developed resources; since these have not yet attracted investment, they will remain largely untouched until plans for raising the capital for their exploitation and utilization are made and put into effect. Rapid technical obsolescence of fishing equipment, debt burdens, rising labor costs, and lack of skilled skippers are among the factors impairing efficiency in many countries. Marine pollution is also having adverse effects, including the actual withdrawal of some fish, considered potentially dangerous, from markets.

Therefore, although efforts are being intensified on many fronts to conserve and develop fishery resources and to increase efficiency and lower costs, overall increases in world supplies of fish are apt to be modest.

Potentials for Increases in Different Regions

Any attempt to estimate the potentials for increases in animal production is beset with many difficulties, not only because many factors affect the potential within any particular region, but also because possibilities of importation and exportation between regions have a direct bearing on the possibilities in many instances. Also, it is hardly possible to undertake a really comprehensive review of such a complex set of problems in the space available here. However, drawing upon the studies made by FAO[20,21] in respect to livestock fisheries and other sources, the prospective situation in each region is set out below in capsule form.

Europe

The consumption of beef and veal rose 70% in Southern Europe, 24% in the six Common Market (EEC) countries, and 6% in other Northwestern European countries between 1960–61 and 1968. Consumption increased more rapidly than production in all except the latter group of countries. Owing to an increase of 9% in the cattle herd in the EEC, large dairy surpluses developed. Steps are being taken by the EEC countries to reduce dairy output and, over the longer term, to bring about some increase in beef production. The demand for beef and veal is expected to continue to grow faster in Southern Europe than elsewhere in the region, reflecting a rapid increase in incomes and the initial low level of consumption.

The net deficit of production compared with consumption is expected to increase over the next decade or more, so imports are apt to rise rapidly in Southern Europe, and to a less marked degree in the Federal Republic of Germany and the United Kingdom.

The consumption of pork increased by 27% for Western Europe as a whole between 1960–61 and 1968, or somewhat faster than beef. Production approximately kept pace with consumption. The demand is expected to continue to rise more rapidly than for beef and veal and production will probably keep pace with demand. Policies are not yet clear as to how the extra feed supplies will be obtained, but there are some indications that stimulation of domestic production may be given priority over imports.

Although there was a period of stagnation in mutton and lamb consumption in the early 1960's, there was an overall rise of 8% in Western Europe between 1960–61 and 1968. The increase was greatest in EEC, 22%; but it was also substantial in Southern Europe where the demand rose 13%. However, production lagged well behind consumption, rising only 4% for Western Europe as a whole. The overall deficit in production is expected to grow, particularly in Southern Europe and the EEC. In addition to the United Kingdom, a traditionally large importer, France, Greece, and Yugoslavia appear likely to be major importers.

In Eastern Europe and the U.S.S.R. higher incomes resulted in a shift in demand from staples to higher-cost animal products. The steady rise in consumption witnessed during the 1960's has been difficult to maintain owing to difficulties encountered in getting the livestock sector of the economy on a more efficient long-term basis. There has been a falling off in numbers, particularly of beef cattle in countries such as Hungary and Czechoslovakia. In some countries, exports of meat were reduced and larger purchases have been made outside the region.

Increasing production of meat, milk, and eggs appears to be a primary policy target of most of the Eastern European countries and the U.S.S.R. Emphasis is apparently being placed on both large-scale specialized production units and on the increase of production on small family plots. Indicative of the emphasis being placed upon improving supplies of feed is the large-scale agreement made recently by the U.S.S.R. with the U.S.

for the import of substantial amount of feed grains over a three-year period.

For fisheries, the amount of catch taken by Western European countries has increased somewhat over the last decade, 10,960,000 metric tons in 1970 compared with 7,720,000 in 1960; but this region's share of the world's catch has gradually declined. On the other hand, the U.S.S.R. and most other centrally planned countries have plans for expansion of fisheries and are apt to be responsible for a considerable portion of increases in the world catch over the coming years. As a group, these centrally planned countries increased their catch from 3,400,000 to 8,210,000 metric tons between 1960 and 1970.

North America

As the population grew and per capita incomes rose, the consumption of meat, particularly beef and veal, increased markedly in North America during the 1950's and 1960's. Per capita consumption of red meat (beef, veal, mutton, lamb, pork) rose from 64.3 kilos in 1948–52 to 79.1 kilos in 1967. Meat prices also rose sharply, indicating that the level of consumption may in fact have been restrained somewhat by lack of supplies.

In this connection, it should be noted that consumption increased more rapidly than did domestic production during the 1950's, and the aggregate foreign trade in fresh, chilled, and frozen meat shifted from a small net export to a net import of more than 250,000 metric tons. Beef and veal accounted for most of this increase, although the proportionate increase in mutton and lamb was much greater, while the region continued to be a small net exporter of pork.

Within the U.S., the rising level of imports led to enactment of legislation under which imports could be limited. Following this, a number of supplying countries exercised "voluntary restraints." The effect of this action upon the region as a whole resulted in a sharp drop in imports between 1963 and 1965. However, demand remained high and although imports increased gradually during the remainder of the 1960's, supplies were not adequate to meet the demand, and prices for meat and meat animals rose sharply, especially during 1969. The trend continued into the 1970's and led, in mid-1972, to steps to encourage imports into the U.S., rather than to limit them.

The continuing rise in population and in individual incomes is expected to result in a continuing rise in demand for meat in the region. By 1985 it is expected to exceed the 1961–63 annual level by more than 50%. The region has the land and potential feed supplies as well as the technical possibilities to achieve production increases of this magnitude. However, it is not at all clear that the domestic livestock industry will be able to command the capital and labor required to maintain even the present level of self-sufficiency.

Although the catch of U.S. fisheries has increased somewhat over the last decade, i.e., from 3,750,000 metric tons in 1960 to 4,090,000 metric tons in 1970, its share of the world catch has been gradually declining, a trend that appears likely to continue.

Oceania

This region has long been known, not only for a high level of domestic consumption of meat, but also for its meat exports. These exports consist almost entirely of beef, veal, mutton, and lamb. Owing to a strong export demand, the exports rose from 445,000 metric tons per year in 1948–52 to 932,000 metric tons in 1968.

Cost-price relationships in meat production promise to remain internationally competitive in Australia and New Zealand. Assuming reasonable access to markets overseas, a further expansion of livestock production, as a part of overall diversification of agriculture, appears likely. Pork production in the region, which has been limited, offers possibilities for increase, particularly if incomes and import demands rise in those Far Eastern countries where pork is traditionally a favored article of the diet.

Oceania's take of fish has been quite limited and has increased from 110,000 metric tons in 1960 to 150,000 metric tons in 1970. Some modest growth is anticipated in the years ahead, but appears apt to remain small in relation to this region's output of meat.

Latin America

In this region, livestock contribute in a major way to the economies of Argentina, Brazil, Mexico, Paraguay, and Uruguay, while in the remainder of the region they are of less importance. Meat accounts for about 65% of the value of animal products; milk and dairy products 20%;

and eggs, wool, hides, and skins for the remaining 15%. Cattle account for about 70% of the meat production and nearly all the milk. Pigs contribute 17% of the meat, while sheep and poultry contribute only about 6% each.

Argentina and Brazil, which had 51 million and 90 million head of cattle, respectively, in 1968, account for about 70% of the region's beef production, while Colombia, Mexico, and Uruguay account for about 5% each.

Most pigs are managed in an extensive manner, and particularly in Central America they often scavenge for their feed. Scarcity of feed grains is an obstacle to pig production and, although pig numbers increased at an annual rate of about 2.4% over the 1960 decade, there is little evidence that production methods are changing. Although there is a substantial potential for increased pork production, there appears little likelihood of its being realized so long as emphasis is given to such a great extent to beef production.

As noted above, attention to sheep and poultry production is limited. There appears little likelihood for any major increase in the output of mutton and lamb. However, as modern techniques for the production of broilers and eggs are introduced, the contribution of poultry to the total animal production of the region is growing. The potential for expansion of modern poultry production is still quite large, however, since most of the birds in the region are still found in small flocks maintained under traditional subsistence production conditions.

The largest increase in fishery production during the 1960's occurred in Latin America, for use in the making of fish meal. Although Peru is the leading country, others in the region and particularly those on the East Coast have participated in the growth and are expected to contribute to further growth in the overall world fisheries catch.

The Far East

Livestock play an important part in the agriculture of this region, although their contribution to the GNP is estimated at only 4%, or 12% of the agricultural component of the GNP. These statistics do not take account of the fact that more than half the total energy used in farming in the region is supplied by draft cattle and water buffaloes. The farm animals are also the source of manure, which continues to play an important part in maintaining soil fertility. It also seems probable that much of the domestic production for family subsistence and village use is never recorded. However, recent trade trends indicate that progress in animal production is lagging behind the region's requirements.

Imports of pork by countries in the region, excluding Japan and Mainland China, rose from 5,340 tons in 1963 to over 24,000 tons in 1968, while poultry imports increased by 225% to 27,695 tons. More moderate increases occurred for other meats. These amounts are marginal, compared to the overall production and consumption of meat in the region. Also, much of the imported meat went to Singapore and Hong Kong. However, imports of dairy products, which also increased steadily, were more evenly spread among the countries of the region. Japan has not only stepped up its production of beef, milk, pork, and poultry meat, but has also increased its imports of meat, particularly pork, as well as its imports of feed grains. Also, although Japan has maintained its position as the world's second largest producer of fish, some 10% of the domestic consumption is now from imports. Although information on Mainland China is limited, there is some indication that pig production has been increased on both collective and limited private holdings.

In its *Indicative World Plan,* FAO estimated an annual excess in demand for meat products over prospective production in the region by 1985 of approximately 3,300,000 metric tons and a deficit in milk of 26,200,000 metric tons. The lack of land and capital, as well as the rather long reproductive cycles, places heavy restraints on increasing beef, veal, mutton, and lamb production in much of the region. Hence, insofar as needs for meat can be met from domestic production, the supplies will have to come largely from pigs and poultry, and in fact outputs of pork and poultry products rose much faster than beef and mutton during the period from 1963 to 1969.

Japan is the leading fishing nation in the region, but other countries catch substantial amounts. The total catch for the region, exclusive of Japan, increased from 4,740,000 metric tons in 1960 to 9,440,000 metric tons in 1970. It appears likely that this region will share in further increases in world fisheries output.

The Near East

Livestock contribute in an important way to the agricultural sector of the national economies of most of the countries of the region. Also, for many people, animal husbandry is a way of life. For example, in Afghanistan about 80% of the people are nomads or seminomads, while in Somali at least two thirds of the people raise livestock in the traditional migratory pattern. A transition from this subsistence pattern to a market economy has not yet been achieved. Even so, there has been some growth in animal production outputs in response to increases in population and levels of income. However, production has not kept pace with consumption; imports of livestock products into the region rose from $150 million per year in 1964–66 to $195 million in 1968.

The demand for livestock products has been projected by FAO[16] to rise between 1962 and 1985 at an annual rate of 4.7% for meat, 4.9% for eggs, and 4.4% for milk. In view of the low rate of increase in the past, it seems impossible to meet growing demand from domestic production, while imports to meet the full deficit would impose an excessive strain on the balance of payments of most countries. Consequently, consumption targets upon which the above projections were based were set below the real demand projections, except for the oil-rich countries. Even so, at constant prices, the import bill for this region would rise from about $100 annually in 1961–63 to around $545 in 1985.

The real obstacle to increased production in this predominantly dry region is how to provide more and better feed. Extension of cultivation to marginal lands is carried out in most countries at the expense of grazing. In turn, range land is overgrazed and forest areas are encroached upon, since in most countries of the region controlled grazing and pasture improvement are practically nonexistent. Improvement of range lands and changes in nomadic patterns of life are by their nature long-range problems. Thus, in the short run, hope for improvement in domestic production lies primarily in the expansion of intensive feeding and fattening with concentrated feeds, and increasing feed and fodder production from irrigated lands.

Poultry production has proved to be one of the quickest and most economic ways of producing the needed animal protein, but so far only Lebanon has undertaken intensive, rapid development. However, efforts are being made to introduce modern production methods in Iraq, Jordan, Kuwait, Saudi Arabia, and Egypt. Among the constraints are inadequacy of feed (although some is being imported), incentives for investment, poultry technicians, knowledge of housing and management requirements, and health and disease problems.

In spite of the difficulties imposed by the region's climate and other factors, countries of the region are devoting increasing attention to livestock problems. However, the problems are of such magnitude that rapid progress cannot be anticipated.

Likewise, prospects for progress in fisheries are not great, except for those countries having access to the Indian Ocean where some increases appear likely.

Africa

This region has a considerable potential for livestock development. However, there are also substantial restraints which limit the speed of expansion, particularly of beef and dairy production. These restraints include the pastoral system of husbandry, inadequate marketing methods and facilities, and the basic problem of animal disease, especially trypanosomiasis. Also, fluctuations in grazing conditions and in availability of water in many areas result in variations in numbers and potential output from year to year and season to season. Moreover, the development of more intensive production methods, not only for beef and dairy cattle but also for pig and poultry production, is generally limited by inadequate feed supplies. Crop residues and processing by-products, such as those from oilseed pressing, are often wasted or not fully utilized. Therefore, expansion of the output of the cattle industry is essentially a long-term process. However, a number of countries are taking steps to increase the output of animal products.

A breakthrough in tsetse fly eradication would have a marked effect on cattle production in the large portion of Africa where this insect exists. Several countries are undertaking pilot activities to make infested areas safe for cattle production, but with existing technology eradication of the tsetse fly will be very expensive. However, the potential benefits are sufficient to justify a high priority for continuing research on this problem.

In East Africa some attention is being given to improved range management and to stratification of the cattle by taking feeder cattle from the more extensive, less productive areas to areas where more intensive feeding is practicable. By development of improved ranching systems, particularly in Ethiopia, Kenya, Madagascar, Tanzania, Uganda, and Zambia, increases are being brought about in the beef supply and conditions are being created under which nomads will be encouraged to settle.

One of the results of use of high-yielding varieties in Kenya has been a surplus of corn, which has led to the carrying out of pilot cattle-fattening trials. The growth of agricultural processing industries such as pressing of peanuts and other oilseeds and the milling of cereals is making feed available for fattening of animals. Slaughterhouses and cold storage facilities are also being developed. For example, in West African countries like Ghana and the Ivory Coast, such facilities are being built in the main consuming areas to process animals driven from the North. Also, some meat canning facilities for meat to be exported are being developed, as in Kenya, since sanitary regulations of importing countries prevent the export of fresh meat. Schemes to expand milk, poultry meat, and egg production are also being undertaken in a number of African countries.

Also, as pointed out earlier in this chapter, the value of wildlife as a source of meat as well as a tourist attraction and the desirability of conservation are being realized and steps are being taken to protect and utilize this resource. Attention to both marine and inland fisheries is also increasing, and some modest growth may be expected in this sector.

General Observations on Potentials for Future Increases in Production

Granting that economic conditions remain generally favorable, strong demands for meat and most other animal products seem likely to continue in both the developed and the developing countries. Population pressures will certainly continue to rise and incomes are also expected to increase. Prices for animal products, especially beef, are high, reflecting the strong demand, so production will be encouraged. In the cattle industry there is a considerable time lag between price increases and expansion of production. Also, as FAO[22] has pointed out, rapid production increases following World War II, which were achieved to a large extent by better utilization of calf reserves for beef and veal production, may not be possible to match in the longer run because calf reserves are extremely low in many countries and a strong demand for veal frequently raises calf prices to where holding them for beef production is no longer profitable. Thus, although increases in the output of beef and veal are forecast for 1972 and 1973 and continuing increases may be expected, more rapid increases seem likely to occur in pork and poultry production, since they reproduce more rapidly and convert feed more efficiently than the meat-producing ruminants.

There are substantial resources that can be devoted to increased outputs of animal products to meet the increasing demands. These are to be found in widely varying circumstances: in the highly productive agricultural areas of the Temperate Zones where much of the intensive animal production is now practiced; in the range areas of the Temperate Zones, where many of the world's feeder cattle and sheep are now produced; in the densely populated, intensively tilled areas – for example, in Japan, Southeast Asia, the Nile Delta – where, with high-yielding varieties and improved crop production practices, grains surplus to human needs may become available for livestock and poultry feeding; in mountain areas where marginal lands may be turned more to animal production and less to subsistence farming; in the wet, humid tropics where practical techniques for the utilization of the high plant growth potential in such climates are receiving attention; and in the tropical and subtropical savannas and other dry areas where, with more efficient management, range livestock and perhaps game animals or a combination of range animals and game can yield greater outputs. There are also possibilities for the closer integration of range land resources with those of feed-producing areas where the offtake of range lands can be finished for marketing.

Whatever the circumstance under which animals are produced, it appears certain that the world must move toward more intensive approaches to animal production if the needs for animal products are to be met. That intensification will find expression in a variety of ways, as Phillips[23] has pointed out. More productive, better adapted types of animals will be sought or developed from existing types for use in many circumstances. More effective disease and parasite control programs will be developed, especially in those parts of the world where lack of such programs now imposes serious limitations on production. New approaches to efficient feeding will be found. In highly intensive agricultural areas, systems of integrating animal production with crop production will be developed, along the lines already being used to some extent in Japan. In areas where animals move from range lands to feedlots, more intensive management of those feedlots may be anticipated; one man can feed upwards of 5,000 cattle in a modern feedlot. More intensive approaches to broiler production may also be expected; with modern feeding systems one man can now care for 60,000 to 70,000 birds. More effective management of range lands may be foreseen. Even under the most extensive conditions of production, where only game animals are harvested or where game and range animals share the use of the land, more intensive handling of the resource may be expected.

Thus, while it is unlikely that all man's needs for animal protein or even for some animal by-products such as leather can be met over the decades ahead, there are potential resources – both in animals and in land and feed supplies – which can and no doubt will be devoted to efforts to meet a considerable portion of those needs.

REFERENCES

1. FAO, *The State of Food and Agriculture 1970,* Food and Agriculture Organization of the United Nations, Rome, 1970, 210.
2. FAO, *The State of Food and Agriculture 1970,* Food and Agriculture Organization of the United Nations, Rome, 1970, 209.
3. FAO, *The State of Food and Agriculture 1970,* Food and Agriculture Organization of the United Nations, Rome, 1970, 170.
4. **Phillips, R. W.,** Animal agriculture in Asia – present and future, in *The Role of Animal Agriculture in Meeting World Food Needs,* Proc. 15th Ann. Meeting, Agr. Research Institute, National Academy of Sciences/National Research Council, Washington, D.C., 1966, 147.
5. **Phillips, R. W.,** Animal agriculture in the emerging nations, in *Agricultural Sciences for the Developing Nations,* Pub. No. 76, American Assoc. for the Advancement of Science, Washington, D. C., 1964, 15.
6. **Phillips, R. W.,** Untapped sources of animal germ plasm, in *Germ Plasm Resources,* Pub. No. 66, American Assoc. for the Advancement of Science, Washington, D.C., 1961, 43.
7. **Joshi, N. R. and Phillips, R. W.,** *Zebu Cattle of India and Pakistan,* Agr. Study No. 19, Food and Agriculture Organization of the United Nations, Rome, 1953.
8. **Joshi, N. R., McLaughlin, E. A., and Phillips, R. W.,** *Types and Breeds of African Cattle,* Agr. Study No. 37, Food and Agriculture Organization of the United Nations, Rome, 1957.
9. **Phillips, R. W., Johnson, R. G., and Moyer, R. T.,** *The Livestock of China,* Pub. No. 2249, U. S. Department of State, Washington, D.C., 1945, 117.
10. **Phillips, R. W. and Hsu, T. Y.,** Chinese swine and their performance compared with modern and crosses between Chinese and modern breeds, *J. Hered.* 35, 365, 1944.
11. U.S.D.A., *Agricultural Statistics 1971,* United States Department of Agriculture, Washington, D.C., 1971, 430.
12. FAO, *Report of the Third FAO Meeting on Livestock Production in the Americas,* Food and Agriculture Organization of the United Nations, Rome, 1955, 109.
13. U.S.D.A., *Agricultural Statistics 1971,* United States Department of Agriculture, Washington, D.C., 1971, 382.
14. **Brown, L. R.,** *Man, Land and Food,* Foreign Agr. Econ. Rept. No. 11, United States Department of Agriculture, Washington, D.C., 1963.
15. **Schertz, L. P.,** Food Supplies and Economic Growth in Developing Countries – the 1970's, presented at Annual Meeting, Western Agr. Econ. Assoc., Oregon State University, Corvallis, 1969.
16. FAO, *Provisional Indicative World Plan for Agricultural Development: Summary and Main Conclusions,* Food and Agriculture Organization of the United Nations, Rome, 1970.
17. FAO, *The State of Food and Agriculture 1970,* Food and Agriculture Organization of the United Nations, Rome, 1970, 170.
18. **Roth H. H.,** The conflict between beef production and the use of wild animals for food in Africa (in German), *D. Fleischwirtschaft,* 46, 114, 1966.
19. **Kyle, R.,** *Meat Production in Africa – The Case for New Domestic Species,* Bristol Veterinary School, Bristol, 1972.
20. FAO, *The State of Food and Agriculture 1971,* Food and Agriculture Organization of the United Nations, Rome, 1971, 8.
21. FAO, *The State of Food and Agriculture 1970,* Food and Agriculture Organization of the United Nations, Rome, 1970, 46.
22. FAO, Report of Second Session, FAO Inter-Governmental Group on Meat, Food and Agriculture Organization of the United Nations, Rome, 1972.
23. **Phillips, R. W.,** Toward an Intensified Animal Agriculture, Proc. VIIth Internatl. Zootechny Symposium, Milan, Italy, in press.

REDUCING CROP LOSSES

L. Chiarappa

TABLE OF CONTENTS

A Short Historical Review 163

Identifying, Quantifying, and Expressing Crop Losses 165

Some Selected Examples of Actual and Potential Crop Losses 166
The Pingalap Disease of Breadfruit in the Pacific Islands 166
The "Unknown Diseases" of Coconut 167
The Bayoud Disease of the Date Palm in the Sahara 167
The Moko Disease or Bacterial Wilt of Bananas 168
New Wheats and Old Pathogens: The Risks of the "Green Revolution" 169

Strategies for Effective Control 169
The "Hungry Locust" 170
The Post-war Experience in Japan 172

The Promise of the Future 174

References 176

A SHORT HISTORICAL REVIEW

There is every indication that insects, fungi, and other biologic crop adversities preceded man on earth. Fossil fungi have been discovered in pre-Cambrian cherts, while fragments of small arthropods have been recovered from Devonian cherts.[1,2] Also, there can be little doubt that soon after man started to engage in primitive forms of agriculture, pests and diseases began taking their toll from his crops. Written accounts of the damage caused by locusts, mildews, and blights on cultivated plants are present in the Old Testament, while weeds are graphically represented as problems in growing crops in a Sumerian Tablet from Nippur in Iraq dated 1700 B.C.[3] However, it was only with the Greek and Latin authors that descriptive accounts are given of pests and diseases and of some of the losses they caused. For example, Theophrastus of Eresus (370 to 286 B.C.), in dealing with diseases of cereals and pulses, wrote: "As to diseases of seeds – some are common to all, as rust, some are peculiar to certain kinds; thus chick-pea is alone subject to rot and to being eaten by caterpillars and by spiders; and some seeds are eaten by other small creatures. Some again are liable to canker and mildew as cummin. But creatures which do not come from the plant itself, but from without, do not do so much harm; thus, the Kantharis is a visitor among wheat, the phalangion in vetches, and other pests in other crops."[4]

The observed phenomena were so little understood that they encouraged philosophers and writers to speculate on their possible causes. Pests and diseases were believed to arise spontaneously from within or without the plant (a concept retained for many centuries afterwards) and to occur at special times because of sin and acts of divinity. The Romans were in fact so concerned about the appearance of rust diseases on cereal crops that they had special rites in the spring, called "Robigalia," to propitiate the goddess Robigo, today identified as the disease itself, and then recognized as the *maxima segetum pestis* (worst crop pest). Similarly in Japan a mythical legend describes Otoshino-Kami, the Goddess of Farming becoming angry with farmers after being told that they had engaged in planting rice against her will, and punishing them by releasing pests into rice fields and destroying their crops.[5]

Knowledge of losses caused by pests and diseases in ancient times is extremely meager and nothing is actually known of their social or economic impact. In the western world, with the decline of the Roman empire and the advent of the Dark Ages – a period roughly extending from 400 to 1200 A.D. – this situation worsened. Many of the previous advances made by the Greek and Roman naturalists were lost or came to a halt; agricultural lands were either abandoned or overrun by foreign armies, the economies stagnated, and diseases of men and crops did the rest in either reducing populations or in rendering their life extremely difficult. Under such conditions it is no wonder that interest in agriculture and natural history was replaced by a paralysis of intellectual activities, blinding dogmas, and hopeless ignorance. Meteorological factors such as persistent rains, frosts, droughts, etc. were more readily understood than any biologic cause of loss. For example, early British records show that between 500 and 1500 A.D. there were 124 crop failures resulting in great famine, mostly indicated to be due to adverse climatic conditions.[6] Similar crop calamities occurred in other parts of the world as shown by records of medieval China or by recent studies of the Aztec civilization in Central America.[7]

It took many centuries before man could free himself from the belief that all these failures were due to celestial-meteorological agents or otherwise supernatural causes.

A complete intellectual change was required to break the bonds of scholasticism and dogma, and to liberate man's imagination and interest in a rational exploration of natural phenomena. This change came gradually, starting with the Renaissance in Europe and then progressing more rapidly after the Church Reformation. However, the study of insects and plant diseases could only receive greater attention after the development in the 17th century of optical apparatus. While the foundations were then laid for modern botany, entomology, and microbiology, the real causation of many plant diseases was not yet readily understood. This was most evident during the severe potato blight epidemic of 1845 – 46 in Ireland which virtually destroyed the potato crops and resulted in a great famine causing hundreds of thousands of people either to die from malnutrition or to emigrate. Although close association of the fungus (*Phytophthora infestans*) with blight of the potato foliage or rotting of the tubers was accepted by all who studied the disease in Ireland, the general conclusion was that the fungus was the result rather than the cause of the disorder. Several years had to elapse before experimental evidence of fungus pathogenicity could be obtained, thus opening the way to the recognition of the real causes of such crop losses. This knowledge proved essential for the development of more effective forms of control. In fact, the beginning of man's effort to reduce or prevent crop losses with the use of chemicals dates from the year 1860, when arsenicals were first used to control the Colorado beetle in the U.S., and 1884, when Bordeaux mixture was found to be an effective fungicide in France. Soon afterwards other forms of control were developed including the breeding of resistant varieties and the use of plant quarantines and sanitation measures. There is no question that some very remarkable successes in pest and disease control were obtained during the following century, but surprisingly enough, the vulnerability of man's crops to losses has remained high during all this time and has possibly increased in recent years. This has been mainly due to two factors:

the great flexibility of man's competitors (insects, fungi, viruses, etc.), which permits them to easily adapt to new conditions, and the introduction of certain practices of intensive farming (such as the use of fertilizers, sprinkler irrigation, crop uniformity over large areas, etc.). An example of this increased crop vulnerability is clearly underlined by the 1970 epidemic of Southern Corn Leaf Blight in the U.S. when approximately 90% of U.S. corn (consisting of 70,000,000 acres) was planted to maize varieties sharing a common source of cytoplasm. As a result of the sudden appearance of a new race of the causal organism (race T of *Helminthosporium maydis*), the maize crop was very severely damaged.

A third factor which has probably slowed man's progress in effectively controlling pests and diseases has been the lack of a full appreciation of the amount of loss they actually cause and the resulting socioeconomic implications.

It is evident from this brief historical review that man has experienced losses in his crops from the very beginning of agriculture. During the course of the centuries, he has advanced from a period in which he was ignorant of the true causes of loss to the time when he learned about causation but not about remedies. This was followed by our modern era, when both causes and remedies were known, but crops still remain vulnerable to pests and diseases. Ignorance still persists about the entity and economics of losses. The implications of this situation will be briefly examined.

IDENTIFYING, QUANTIFYING, AND EXPRESSING CROP LOSSES

Some plant pests and diseases are quite spectacular; they kill, stunt, wilt, and ostensibly reduce the quantity and/or the quality of crops. But many other pests and diseases are not so evident; they subtly destroy great fractions of yield, but can only be detected after some form of control is developed and an accurate measurement of the resulting increases in yield can be made. For example, potato latent mosaic virus has been present for at least 20 years in practically every potato grown in the U.S. The measured amount of loss caused by the disease (as established by independent research in England, Australia, and America) is equivalent to 13% of a healthy crop. Applied to American production over the same 20 year-period, this figure reveals a loss of 1.1 billion bushels of potatoes.[8] The insidious, invisible but steady decline of production caused by certain plant parasitic nematodes in crops is another example. There is no question that these plant parasites have been feeding on crops since man's early history. But only in 1943, following the report by Carter of the nematocide action of D-D, was it possible to have a clear definition of the yield-depressing effect of nematodes.[9] Today, 30 years after this first demonstration, yearly losses caused by plant parasitic nematodes are estimated to be about 1.6 billion dollars in the U.S. alone.[10]

These examples clearly indicate the need of identifying losses for a fuller evaluation of the problem and for the proper development and use of economically effective control measures.

There are various types of losses that must be considered. At the farm level, losses may consist of one or more of the following elements:

Reduction in quality or quantity of produce
Extra costs for harvesting and/or grading
Costs for extra fertilizers, irrigation water, etc.
Cost of replanting and of delay in production and harvest
Cost of early crop abandonment;
Cost of growing substitute crops and of adopting certain rotations
Cost of chemical control.

Outside the farm, crop losses are of different types, depending on where they occur and which segments of the social matrix they affect. For example, when growers suffer from losses as a group in a market-oriented agriculture the whole economic life of the depending community is affected. A good example is the recent appearance of the pear decline disease on the west coast of the U.S., where the disease killed or took out of production more than one million pear trees.[11] The total value of the California pear crop prior to the outbreak was more than $66 million. Of this, only 41% was the gross return to the growers and 59% was the return to nongrowers such as agrochemical industries, packers, trucking companies, etc, who suffered equally from the disease.[12]

When losses occur within the context of subsistence farming, their consequences go far beyond the economy of a given farm or dependent community. Large strata of populations including those living in big cities are affected with starvation and famine. This is more common and especially severe where nutritional requirements are normally met with difficulty and where the accidental loss of 5 to 10% of the normal crop can cause critical food shortages. The famine of Bengal of 1942–43 is an example.[13]

Directly or indirectly, crop losses have also an important effect on state finances. This includes reductions in tax paid by loss-affected farmers, state subsidies given to them, and extra expenses paid by the state to finance plant quarantine and inspection services (including destruction of pest-infested shipments), plant protection work (including support to research institutes and advisory services), and, more recently, to resolve pollution problems derived from agrochemicals.

It is evident that in the final analysis in a free-market economy, the consumer is the one most directly affected by crop losses. He must pay higher taxes to maintain the state subsidies and activities mentioned above, but also, because of the increased market price of a given commodity, he must pay for losses incurred in the field, during storage, transport, wholesale, and retail sales.

In spite of the importance of crop losses due to pests and diseases, very little reliable information on their magnitude is available. This is due partly to the intrinsic difficulties of defining what "loss" really is, and partly to the difficulty of assessing losses.

For example, the reduction in yield of a given crop, resulting from pest and disease attack, need not automatically reduce income to the individual farmer. On the contrary, the farmer may be compensated by a higher market price resulting from a crop shortage. In this case, it is evident that there is not an economic loss but possibly a financial gain at the farm level. This same fact prompted the farmers of Enterprise, Ala. to put up a monument to the boll weevil because it made cotton growing difficult and kept the price for this crop high.[14]

Although this situation is exceptional, it illustrates some of the difficulties involved. If we consider loss solely in terms of reduction of quantity or quality of crops, there is a tremendous annual tax on human labor, land, and natural resources in order to "feed" insects and nematodes, to grow weeds, or to perpetuate plant diseases on cultivated crops. This tax is paid by the community as a whole. To quantify this tax we must depend on the availability of reliable field methods of crop loss measurement. It was this philosophy which prevailed at the FAO Symposium on Crop Losses.[15] This has prompted many scientists in the field of entomology, nematology, plant pathology, and weed science to unite their forces in an international collaborative effort to develop better methods for the assessment of crop losses.[16] The need, value, and use of such a program has been recently reviewed.[17]

SOME SELECTED EXAMPLES OF ACTUAL AND POTENTIAL CROP LOSSES

The influence that insects, plant diseases, and other biological adversities can exert on man's food supply and his environment is probably best illustrated by a few examples of recent outbreaks or epidemics purposely selected for the particular socioeconomic settings in which they have occurred. Some additional examples are also given for a number of particularly dangerous situations now existing in the world and constituting a most serious hazard to man's food availability.

The Pingalap Disease of Breadfruit in the Pacific Islands

The breadfruit (*Artocarpus communis* L.) is a vigorous, rapidly growing tree particularly well adapted to the ecological conditions of the Pacific Islands. It is known to withstand severe windstorm damage and to rapidly regenerate adventitious stems when blown down during typhoons. From ancient times the breadfruit has provided a major source of carbohydrate food and utilities such as timber for boats and construction, latex, foliage, etc. to the islanders.

Starting in 1957, a disease attacking breadfruit trees of bearing age made its first appearance in the Pingalap Atoll in the Eastern Carolinas.[18] The disease soon assumed epidemic proportions, causing the death of trees within one to six months from the onset of symptoms. It soon spread to other Eastern Carolina islands, to the Gilbert and Ellice Islands, to Guam and Saipan of the Marianas, and to American Samoa. The extent of losses varied from as little as 2 to 3% to as many as 80% of the trees killed. In Guam the disease was particularly severe, leaving whole sections of land as if ravaged by fire. The repercussions of Pingalap disease to the economy and well-being of the islanders can be easily understood if one considers that the replacement value of breadfruit as a food crop to the peoples in the Pacific basin, Indonesia, and Southern India could well be in terms of billions of dollars annually. Although many attempts have been made to identify the causes of the disease, these have been so far unsuccessful.

The "Unknown Diseases" of Coconut

The coconut palm (*Cocos nucifera* L.) is called in the tropics the "tree of heaven" for its unique capacity to provide food, drink, oil, shelter, timber, etc. No other tree can offer so many and varied uses for so many years. In fact, palms grown in good soils can maintain production for as many as 80 years. While the cultivation of this crop in India and East Asia is at least 1,000 years old, in the Philippines it is said that the first plantings were established following an edict of the Spanish government in 1768 compelling each Philippine farmer to plant an area of at least 200 ft^2. Today, the Philippines is the largest coconut-growing country in the world both with regard to area under the crop (above 1 million hectares) and production of nuts (about 5,000 million). Coconut is also important on the west coast of Africa and in the Caribbean area (Cuba, Jamaica, etc.).

World coconut production is seriously threatened by two major diseases: one confined to the Philippines, and locally called "cadang-cadang," and another common in many countries of the Caribbean area and called "lethal yellowing." A third killing disease, likely to be the same as lethal yellowing, occurs in West Africa where it is variously called Kaincopé (in Togo) or Cape St. Paul Wilt (in Ghana). Because agents of these diseases are still unidentified, they have been improperly grouped under the name of "unknown diseases."

In the Philippines, cadang-cadang was first described in 1937 after it had been observed in the San Miguel Island in 1931.[19] The disease spread at first southeastward and by 1962 only 80 healthy palms remained out of a population of 250,000. Later the disease was found in the four provinces of the Bicol peninsula, Catanduanes, Masbate, and the northern shores of Samar, and recently all the way from Infanta, Quezon (east-northeast of Manila) to the southeastern tip of Samar. Accurate loss estimates are not available. However, conservative appraisals of the toll paid so far to cadang-cadang are 10 million dead palms. Affected trees first cease to bear female flowers and thus become useless for nut production. They later die, usually within three to ten years from the onset of symptoms. The final result is that only crownless trunks are left to indicate where flourishing plantations had given abundant harvests in earlier years. The threat posed by cadang-cadang to other provinces still free from the disease cannot be overemphasized. It is estimated that some 8 million people, more than one third of the entire population, could be seriously affected if the disease should ever become generally established in the Philippines.

Lethal yellowing is probably just as devastating in the Caribbean and West Africa. For example, in Key West, Fla. the disease has been responsible for the total disappearance of tall coconut palms, once an essential part of the landscape and tourist attraction. Likewise, the disease is responsible for the "new look" of the coconut industry in Jamaica where the susceptible "Jamaica Tall" has been killed at the rate of 60,000 to 100,000 palms a year (Figure 1) and where the resistant "Malayan Dwarfs" have been replanted to save the island's oil production. An important development in lethal yellowing research, which may remove this problem from the list of "unknown" diseases, has been the recent discovery that it might be due to a mycoplasma.[20]

The Bayoud Disease of the Date Palm in the Sahara

The date palm (*Phoenix dactylifera* L.) is a unique monocotyledonous plant particularly well suited to desert conditions due to its innate ability to withstand arid weather, extreme climatic variation, and high soil and water salinity. It is an irreplaceable part of the flora of the oases of the Sahara and Arabian Deserts where, in addition to producing food, it provides much needed shade for the growing of other crops as well as timber for local construction, fuel, etc. Dates are an indispensable part of the diet of nomadic populations as well as of the few sedentary farmers living in the oases. For some of these populations, living exclusively on a diet of dates and semolina or of dates and camel's milk, consumptions of 500 to 700 g of dates per day are not uncommon. A poor date crop can easily mean starvation to such people. Dates are also important as a medium of

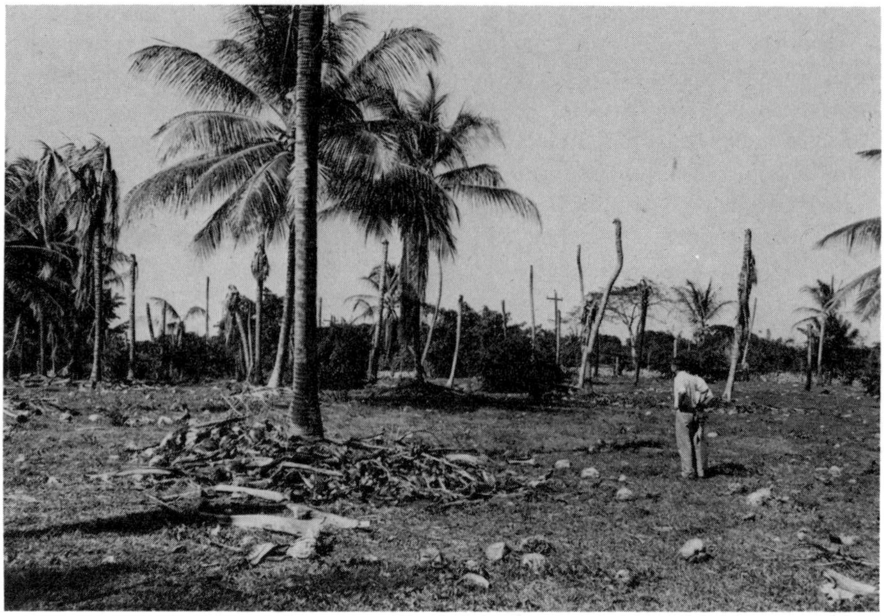

FIGURE 1. Devastating effect of lethal yellowing disease on tall coconut palms in Jamaica.

exchange, such as for bartering against sheep or camels with the Tuaregs, or as a source of cash income when the crop is sold for export south of the Sahara or to European markets.

At the beginning of this century, a lethal disease of the date palm was first observed in the Draa Valley of Morocco. The disease, called "el bayoud" (meaning in Arabic "the whiteness"), appeared as a sudden drying of one or more of the palm fronds, followed by total wilting. Once established in any one area, the disease was seen to spread through the soil from palm to palm. The soil remains contaminated and unsuitable for replanting with date palms. From the original focus of infection in the Draa Valley, the bayoud disease has moved to nearly all oases of the western and central Sahara, leaving behind a trail of death and destruction. For example, of the 15 million palms in Morocco 70 years ago, only 4 1/2 million now remain. This country is now importing considerable quantities of dates where it used to be a large exporter.[21]

The major concern for bayoud at present is in Algeria where the disease is gradually moving in the direction of the highly valuable groves of Deglet-Nour palms in the eastern region, in the area where the government is making a special effort to raise living conditions of nearly a half-million people. In this area, dates ensure the highest annual revenue from agriculture (estimated around $12 million a year) and it would be disastrous to the socioeconomic structure of the local "wilaya" if bayoud disease should become established. The disease is spread over thousands of kilometers by nomads who cannot understand its infectious nature. The government's efforts to prevent movement from oasis to oasis of plant material infected with the causal organism (*Fusarium oxysporum* f.s. *albedinis*) has so far proved unsuccessful. If no early solution can be found to this serious problem, man himself will be responsible for creating with his own hands the "desert within the desert."

The Moko Disease or Bacterial Wilt of Bananas

More than 40 species of *Musa* are loosely included under the common name of "banana." Of these only a very few are currently cultivated throughout the tropics: the bananas of international commerce (used for fruit or dessert consumption) and the more starchy plantains (used for cooking).

Most of the cultivated varieties have evolved from wild *Musa* species originating in Ceylon, India, Burma, and Malaysia. Likewise, most of the insect pests and diseases of bananas also originated in these areas. An exception to this is the Moko disease, an extremely important wilt caused by *Pseudomonas solanacearum.* This bacterium is soil-borne and currently known to occur only in certain zones of the American continent. Several strains of the bacterium have been identified and some have proved to be extremely important. For example, the so-called SFR strain oozes out of male floret scars and is spread to other bananas by visiting insects. This insect dissemination is responsible for the seriousness of epidemics in Honduras, Guatemala, El Salvador, and Nicaragua. In a few years, thousands of square miles of staple food plantains of the susceptible Bluggoe banana have been destroyed.[22]

As already indicated, the bacterium causing Moko disease is limited geographically to the Americas where it is a native parasite of indigenous species of Musaceae which have high levels of resistance to it. However, no cultivated bananas which originated in southeast Asia appear to possess resistance. Any of the strains of Moko attacking banana (especially those insect-transmitted) could reach the African continent or the banana-growing areas of Southeastern Asia and the western Pacific. The consequences can easily be visualized, especially where large populations still depend on plantains as a major part of sustenance.

New Wheats and Old Pathogens: The Risks of the "Green Revolution"

Anyone who has recently visited India, Pakistan, or the Near East and North Africa must have been impressed by the rapid progress in wheat production which has occurred in these countries over the last ten years. Yields per unit area have increased greatly (doubling over local varieties in many instances) as a result of what is popularly referred to as the "green revolution." The main factors in this revolution have been the new Mexican varieties of wheat which share two major characteristics: semidwarfness and stiffer straw (which makes them better suited to fertilizer usage) and nonsensitivity to day length (which makes them adaptable to different growing conditions). These varieties have now been used in no less than 25 countries and over an area that has expanded from 9,300 hectares in 1966 to 12 million hectares in 1970–71.[23] It is said that the farmer in India or Pakistan who has adopted the new Mexican varieties has increased his average net income from 37 to as much as 162 U.S. dollars.[24] This is indeed a tremendous achievement and an effective demonstration of what could be done to raise the standard of living of many countries, to increase world food availability, and to forestall famine. However, plant protection specialists are fully aware of the implications of such rapid progress and of the dangers that the green revolution may also pose.

In fact, from a strict epidemiological point of view, it is extremely dangerous to grow crop varieties over large areas, especially when they all share a common and narrow genetic background. The recent experience in the U.S. with Southern Corn Leaf Blight disease is a good example. An analysis of Mexican varieties made in 1969 revealed that they share many parents in common and that some of these have been used as much as 12 times or more.[25] Furthermore, resistance in Mexican varieties to such an important disease as stem rust (*Puccinia graminis* f. sp. *tritici*) has been derived only from two or three parent lines.[26] This type of resistance is of the "vertical," gene-specific type which is known to be short-lived and to 'break down,' especially under conditions favoring development of new races of the pathogen (genetic uniformity and monoculture of the host). The story of plant pathology is full of failures of new wheat varieties due to loss of resistance and particularly full of severe crop losses following wheat rust epidemics.[27] But such losses have a very different significance in countries which are just emerging from traditional types of agriculture and where rapid economic progress could be lost and the future jeopardized.

STRATEGIES FOR EFFECTIVE CONTROL

With enemies as subtle as insects, fungi, viruses, nematodes, etc. it is not easy to develop a strategy conducive to effective and long lasting control. Furthermore, difficulties often arise when such strategies must be translated into field tactics requiring much organization and the smooth interplay of technical, political, legal, financial, and administrative factors. However, two examples, can be given of crop losses that have been substantially reduced thanks to the development and application of an overall international or national strategy.

The "Hungry Locust"

With this appropriate title, Huskell has described the serious losses caused to agriculture by the swarming locusts.[28] A large swarm of the African Migratory Locust (*Locusta migratoria migratorioides*) in West Africa or the Desert Locust (*Schistocerca gregaria*) (Figures 2 and 3) in northern and eastern Africa and the Near East can contain from 35 to 70 million locusts per square kilometer, with swarms covering 1,000 km^2 and

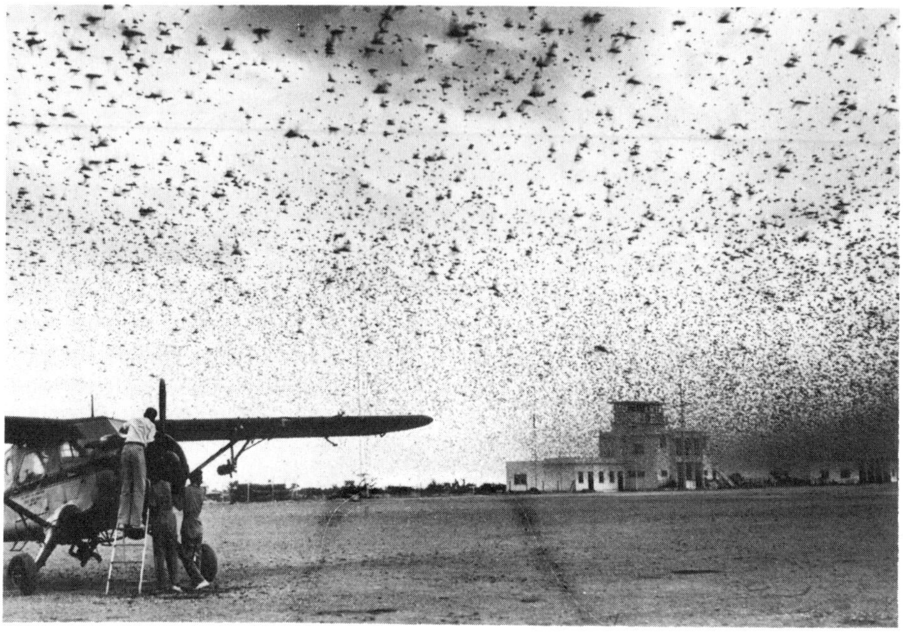

FIGURE 2. A swarm of desert locusts invading an airport in Somalia.

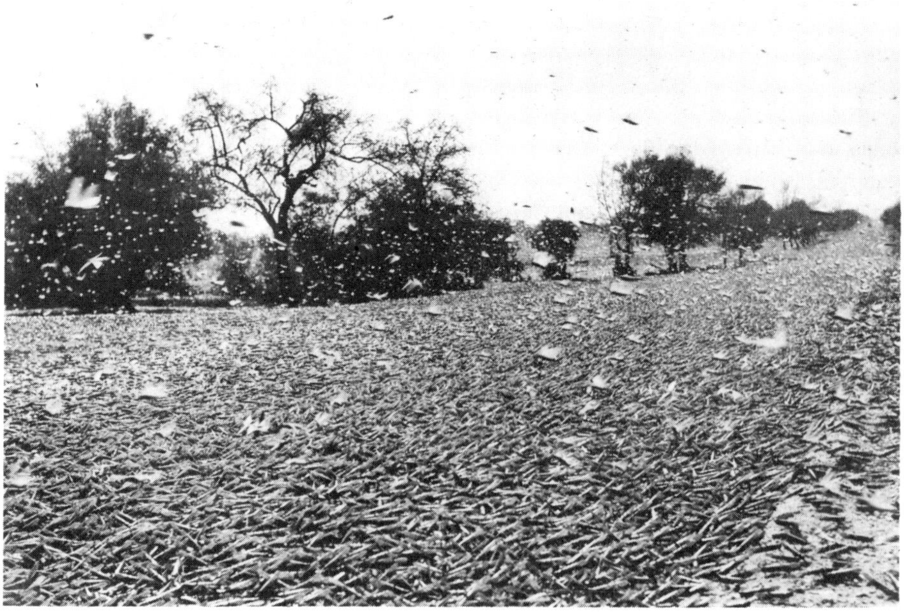

FIGURE 3. A solid carpet of locusts feeding on grasses during an invasion in Morocco.

total populations as high as 40,000. Each adult locust, weighing about 2 g, is capable of eating its own weight in food each day. This means that a large swarm can eat as much as 80,000 tons of plants in a single day. There are estimates of human food lost following locust plagues in some African countries. For example, in Sudan there were 55,000 tons of grain lost in 1954, while in Ethiopia 167,000 tons of grain were lost in 1958 due to the desert locust. This food was sufficient to feed one million people for one year.

One of the intrinsic problems with locusts is that the origin of any outbreak is usually limited and relatively small. From this confined place the locust produces migrant, gregarious forms which congregate into larger swarms and which then fly out to the so-called "invasion areas." Here, if the conditions are favorable, new swarms are produced which in turn fly further afield, invading increasingly large territories. This means that "outbreak areas" are usually confined to only small places within a given country where low density locust populations, well below damaging levels, are not always detected or controlled (Figure 4). Once, however, the swarms have expanded to the "invasion areas," damage occurs at once to many countries and control becomes increasingly more difficult and costly. With several locust species,

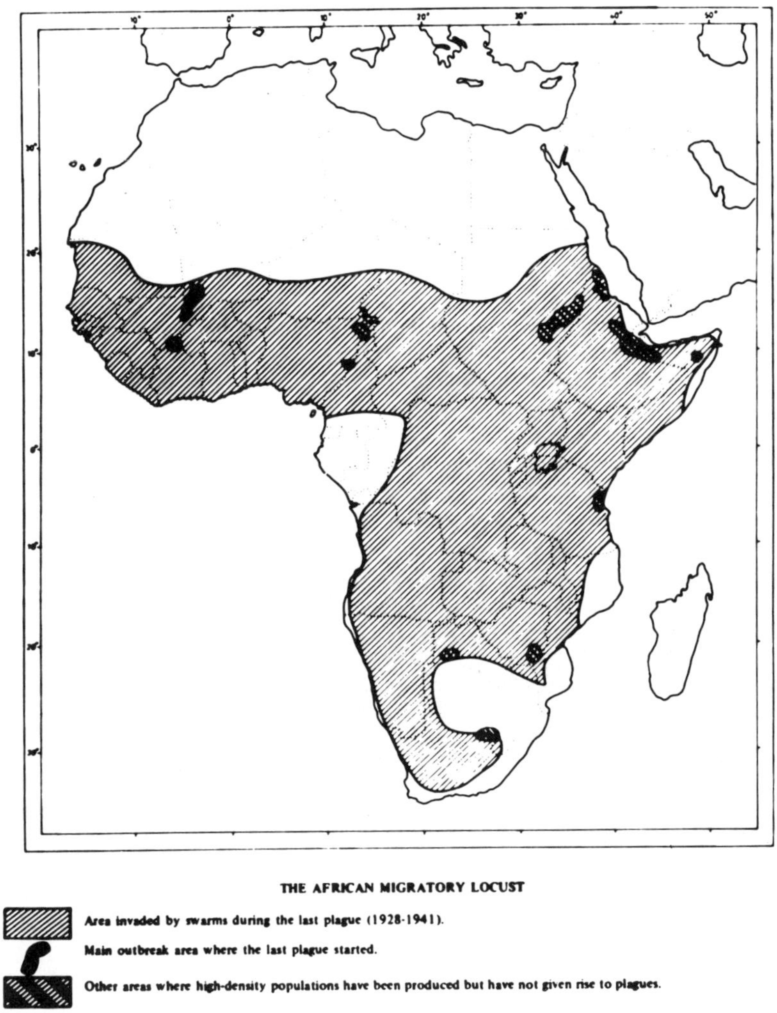

FIGURE 4. Outbreak and invasion areas of the African migratory locust. (From *The Locust Handbook,* The Anti-Locust Research Centre, London, 1966, 1.2.1.)

such as the desert locust, there are no "fixed" outbreak areas and identification of these breeding areas requires intensive reconnaissance work in very inhospitable, desertic regions and over huge territories, often involving as many as 40 countries (Figure 5).

It is clear that such a problem cannot be solved by any one individual country. Control of the "hungry locust" and of the severe crop losses it causes must depend on an overall stragegy developed in very close international collaboration. It is for this reason that in 1952 FAO (Food and Agriculture Organization of the United Nations) initiated a coordinated program involving training, research, surveying, communication, and reporting, as well as international control campaigns embracing all the affected countries from Afghanistan and India to Morocco. Thanks to this collaboration and to the large-scale project financed in 1960 by the United Nations Development Program, much has been achieved in controlling locusts. In fact, it can be said with full confidence that as long as such international collaboration can be maintained there will be no danger of the "hungry locust" again threatening man's food supplies over vast areas of the world.

The Post-war Experience in Japan

Japan is probably one of the few countries where a nationwide, comprehensive strategy on the intensive use of plant protection measures was developed under the pressure of post-war need and where the effect of controlling pests and diseases on the production of certain crops can be best evaluated thanks to the richness and accuracy of available records.

A tradition of inducing farmers to engage in pest and disease control has existed in Japan for many years.[29] In fact, as early as 1896 the Insect Pest Control and Prevention Law was enacted to give authority to prefectural governors to issue ordinances under which farmers were requested to control certain pests and diseases considered of "national" importance. These ordinances, however, fell short of expectation and it was not until the post-war years 1945–1950, when an acute food shortage crippled the country, that an entirely new strategy was developed and a new approach was launched. This was based on the assumption that one of the quickest and surest ways of increasing food availability was that of preventing crop losses in major staple food crops such as rice, wheat, barley, and soybean and that this had to be achieved by an integrated program involving demonstrations to farmers, incentives, and, of course, legislation. A new Plant Protection Law was thus enacted in 1950 to establish the necessary plant protection infrastructures (including a Plant Protection Section in the Ministry of Agriculture and Forestry) as well as to improve actual field control of pests and diseases. This law ensured that control operations were to

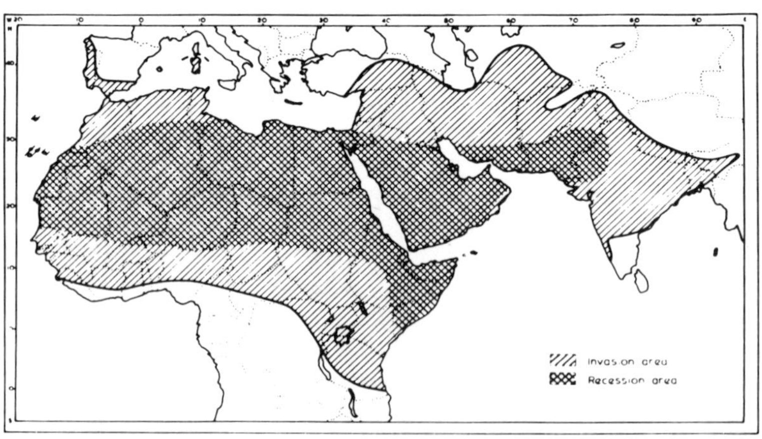

The distribution of the Desert Locust. Map showing the maximum area liable to invasion during plagues and the smaller area where locusts have been found during recessions.

FIGURE 5. Distribution of the desert locust and spread of its invasion area. (From *The Locust Handbook,* The Anti-Locust Research Centre, London, 1966, 1.2.)

be based on recommendations derived from field research, that the forecasting system for pests and disease outbreaks was to be applied nationally, that appropriate reserves of pesticides were to be established to meet peak demand during the growing season, that spraying and dusting equipment for the timely application of pesticides was to be leased out to the farmers, and, finally, that government subsidies for the purchase of chemicals or of applicators were to be channeled to the growers.

A special effort was also directed to the use of helicopters for controlling rice pests and diseases and of herbicides in order to save human labor. The use of helicopters rose from approximately 1,000 hectares of rice in 1958 to 833,000 hectares in 1965. The increase in herbicide use is shown in Figure 6 and the resulting reduction of human labor is illustrated in Figure 7.

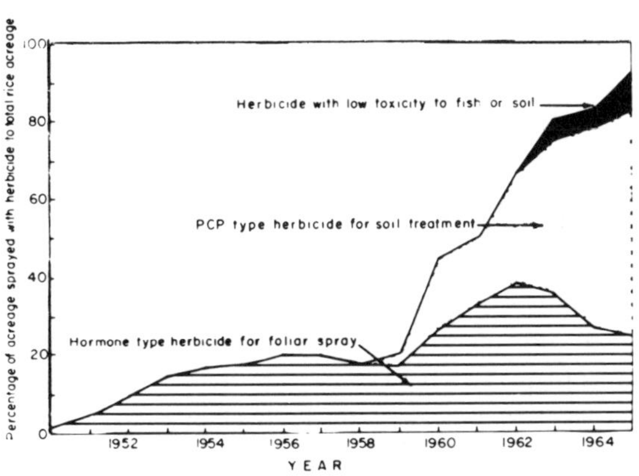

FIGURE 6. Trend in herbicide use in rice growing in Japan. (From Hori, M. and Hishikura, H., Eds., *Plant Protection in Japan. Agriculture, Asia,* Association of Agricultural Relations in Asia, Tokyo, 1967, 81.)

The results are best illustrated by the effects on rice production. Until 1950, production and availability of this commodity had been characterized in Japan by great fluctuations in yield due to the effect of pests and diseases, occasionally coupled with adverse weather conditions.[5] The post-war development of new and more effective pesticides, combined with the knowledge accumulated by the Forecast and Early Detection Service System, and the measures already described both effectively controlled rice pests and diseases and stabilized rice production by eliminating serious fluctuations. These two events are graphically expressed in Figure 8 where the occurrence of rice pests and diseases, weather adversities, and yearly production of brown rice are plotted against the period 1926–1966. After 1955, when the country-wide strategy came into full operation, minimum rice production (in year 1956) was higher than any yield experienced during the previous 31 years. There was also a remarkable yield stabilization. These outstanding results were obtained mainly through the reduction of losses by pests and diseases, as shown in Figure 9.[30] However, there were also indirect increases because certain new agronomic practices which were not previously possible, due to the adverse effect of pests and diseases, could be introduced. These included early planting, which

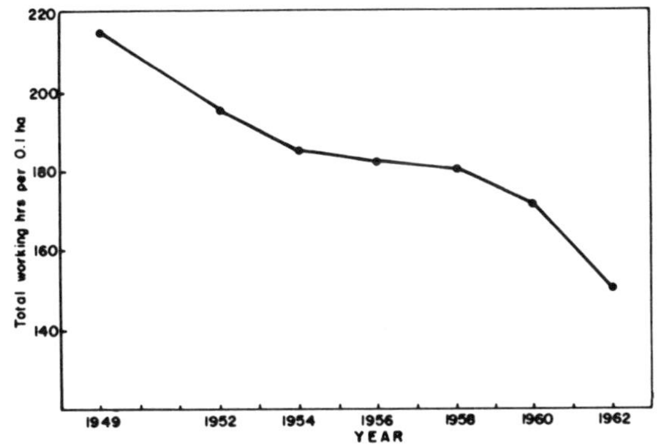

FIGURE 7. Yearly reduction in man's working hours in rice fields resulting from mechanization and herbicide use. (From Hori, M. and Hishikura, H., Eds., *Plant Protection in Japan. Agriculture, Asia,* Association of Agricultural Relations in Asia, Tokyo, 1967, 82.)

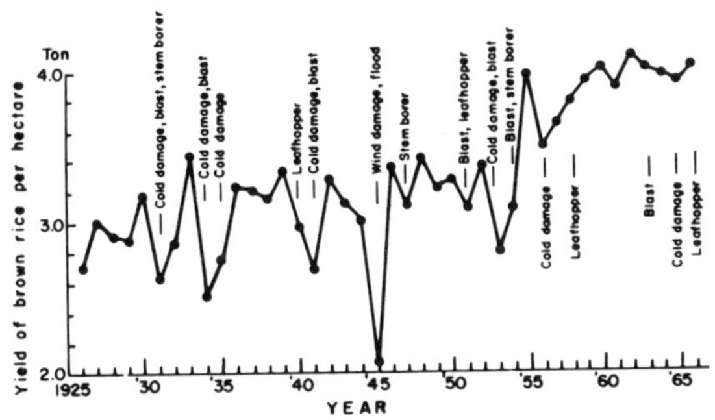

FIGURE 8. Average rice production in Japan and major causes of yield reduction over a 40-year period. (From Hori, M. and Hishikura, H., Eds., *Plant Protection in Japan. Agriculture, Asia,* Association of Agricultural Relations in Asia, Tokyo, 1967, 30.)

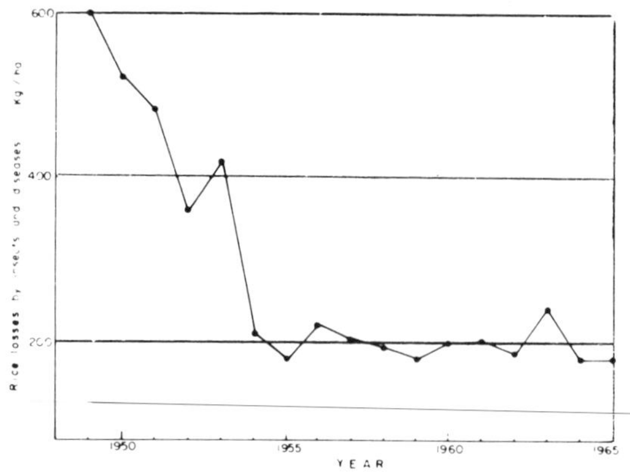

FIGURE 9. Average crop losses caused by pests and diseases in rice over the period 1949-1965. (From Hori, M. and Hishikura, H., Eds., *Plant Protection in Japan. Agriculture, Asia,* Association of Agricultural Relations in Asia, Tokyo, 1967, 109.)

enabled crops to escape typhoon damage, denser spacings, and, most important, increased rates of fertilizers.

Ishikura estimated that an average of 300 kg of rice per hectare was saved. This is an estimated 1.05 million tons of brown rice in the 3.5 million hectares grown in Japan, valued at approximately 109 billion yen. The total expenditure on control of pests and diseases is estimated at only 40 billion yen.[5]

If the situation in Japan is closely analyzed, one can easily see that the "boom" in plant protection and the remarkable results achieved in reducing crop losses are the result of several concurrent factors. Among these the following can be easily singled out: available technical know-how on intensive farming, perfection in organization (including an efficient extension service), a stable price support policy for the commodities to be "protected," and clear, convincing evidence to the grower of the economic advantage of his plant protection activities. All these factors have been backed by a strong agrochemical industry and by an aggressive group of manufacturers of agricultural machinery (including aircraft) which have cheaply and efficiently provided the necessary inputs.

This kind of situation does not exist in most countries of the world, where one or more of such factors are lacking. This is particularly true in the countries of the developing world where farming is still primitive and where many other factors of crop production must be improved before pests and diseases can be efficiently and economically controlled. Pest control activities must also be accommodated within the overall framework of a given society, keeping in mind the reality of local pricing and marketing systems, the educational level of farmers, their habits and traditions, land tenure, etc.

THE PROMISE OF THE FUTURE

Before concluding this rapid review on preharvest losses and on their effect on man's food availability, it may be useful to look briefly into the future of plant protection. This would help in understanding some of the still unsolved problems and in focusing on some of the responsibilities and new activities that plant protection scientists face in the future.

There is little doubt that the "green revolution" will continue to expand in most areas of the developing world involving a broader spectrum of crops and growing conditions. Likewise, there will be a greater intensification of agriculture in the industrialized countries to produce more, better, and "healthier" crops per unit of land. All this will undoubtedly call for greater investments in the form of technical inputs at the farm level (machinery, fertilizers, pesticides, virus-free propagating material, etc.) as well as at the level of collateral activities (food processing plants, cold storage, etc.). Concern over the safeguard of the environment on the one hand and on the side effect of agrochemicals on the other hand will continue to grow and to create public anxiety. Consequently, different approaches in the control of crop pests and diseases will have to be sought. In this situation, the plant protection scientist will find himself in the very front line of agricultural progress. He will be responsible to society for overcoming the risks of the expanded "green revolution," safeguarding the greater investments in agriculture, and eliminating or reducing the hazards of a contaminated environment.

Can plant protection scientists meet all of these challenges and fulfill these obligations? Based on recent experience, the answer is "yes." In fact, already new approaches to control pests and diseases in a more stable form and in a "cleaner" and "safer" agriculture are under way and give promise of achieving these goals. Two deserve mention: the integrated control approach and breeding for "horizontal" resistance.

Integrated control has developed in recent years mainly to free economic entomology from its overdependence on chemical pesticides in favor of a sounder and broader ecological basis. Following the discovery and exploitation of synthetic pesticides in the 1940's and their excessive use in the 1950's, many undesirable phenomena appeared, such as insect resistance, rapid resurgence of pest populations following treatments, increased costs to growers, toxicological hazards to man and wildlife, outbreaks of secondary pests, etc. To overcome these problems, the integrated approach has tried to make better use of ecological, managerial, and biological factors of control in combination, where necessary, with the minimum usage of chemicals which are less injurious to nontarget insect species, to man, and wildlife.[31] Although such an approach is complex (requiring knowledge of insect biology and seasonal fluctuation, biotic factors and biological control agents, damaging population levels, host plants and alternate crops, etc.), there is no doubt that it will give rewarding results in the future.

"Horizontal" resistance instead defines a completely different approach to control plant disease through breeding. Most of the breeding work conducted over the past 50 years has been on so-called specific or "vertical" resistance. This type of resistance is oligogenically inherited and thus easily handled in a plant breeding program. However, vertical resistance is usually short-lived. Therefore, new crop varieties, particularly of cereals such as wheat and barley, have been obtained and released just as rapidly as new pathogenic races of their disease agent have developed. In Kenya, for example, nearly four varieties of wheat were released each year to replace "lost" varieties during the period 1960–68.[32] "Horizontal" resistance is polygenically inherited. It is certainly more difficult to handle, but has the great advantage of being stable. Inbreeding crops, such as wheat and barley, present great difficulties for breeding for horizontal resistance, although very recently plans have been put foward to overcome this limitation.[33] If they should prove feasible, man will have acquired a powerful new tool to combat plant diseases and to stabilize his green revolution.

In conclusion, we have seen how insects, fungi, and other biologic adversities have posed a great and continuous challenge to man's food supply from the very beginning of history. During all this time man has accepted losses of crops, first as an inescapable act of extraterrestrial forces, then, soon after recognition of their nature, he has tried to control them with increasing and varying degrees of success. Lately, man has also made serious attempts to obtain a clear view of their entity through reliable appraisal.

Today many loss-causing agents still remain unknown and uncontrolled while several dreadful disease agents are confined to certain parts of the world, posing new serious threats to man's food supplies and requiring constant attention and vigilance. Serious situations of crop vulnerability exist due to the green revolution and of the same requirements for crop uniformity over vast areas dictated by modern agriculture.

Many control measures have proved difficult or of short duration while comforting examples exist of successful reduction of crop losses at the national and international levels. There is no doubt that agriculture will continue to move rapidly ahead in the future at an acceleration that will be nearly exponential. In many countries of the developing world the critical transition period for "take-off into sustained growth" has been achieved thanks to the green revolution. But to make sure that this will remain as "green" as we like to see it and to ensure that "two blades of grass will grow where only one grew before," plant protection scientists will have to develop considerable new knowledge and use it with great imagination and dedication in the years to come. This will require a great deal of hard work. But as Plato said, "Hard is the good" and a poet much before Plato had also recognized that:

> "Before the gates of Excellence the high gods have placed sweat.
> Long is the road thereto and steep and rough at the first,
> But when the height is won, then is there ease."

REFERENCES

1. **Tyler, S. A. and Barghoorn, E. S.,** Occurrence of structurally preserved plants in pre-Cambrian rocks of the Canadian Shield, *Science,* 119, 606, 1954.
2. **Carpenter, F. M.,** Fossil insects, in *Insects – The Yearbook of Agriculture,* USDA, 1952, 14.
3. **Kramer, S. N.,** *From the Tablets of Sumer,* Falcon's Wing Press, Indian Hills, Colorado, 1956.
4. **Theophrastus,** *Enquiry into Plants and Minor Works on Odours and Weather Signs,* 2 Vols. (Engl. transl. Sir Arthur Hort), W. Heinemann, London and G. P. Putnam's Sons, New York, 1916.
5. **Ishikura, H.,** Present situation of disease and insect pest control for important crops. A. Rice, *Agric. Asia* (spec. issue), 5, 29, 1967.
6. **Orlob, G. B.** History of plant pathology in the Middle Ages, *Ann. Rev. Phytopathol.,* 9, 7, 1971.
7. **Schultze, L.,** *Wahrsagerei, Himmelskunde und Kalender der Alten Azeteken,* Kohlhammer, 64 Stuttgart, 1950.
8. **Starr Chester, K.,** Plant disease losses: their appraisal and interpretation, *Plant Dis. Rep.* (suppl.), 193, 190, 1950.
9. ~~**Carter, W.,** A promising new soil amendment and disinfectant, *Science,* 97, 383, 1943.~~
10. Anon., Estimated crop losses due to plant-parasitic nematodes in the United States, Soc. Nematol., Spec. Publ. No. 1, 1971.
11. **Stout, G. L.,** *Annu. Rep. Bull.,* 43rd Bureau of Plant Pathology, Calif. Dept. Agr., 52, 109, 1963.
12. **Reed, A. D.,** Ramifications of the pear decline disease in the general economy, *Calif. Agric.,* 15, 2, 1961.
13. **Padwick, G. W.,** *Losses Caused by Plant Diseases in the Colonies,* Phytopathol. Paper No. 1, Commonwealth Mycological Institute, Kew, England, 1956.
14. **Howard, L. O.,** *The Insect Menace,* Century Co., New York and London, 1931.
15. Report of the FAO Symposium on Crop Losses, FAO Report PL/M/6, Rome, 1967.
16. **Chiarappa, L.,** FAO international collaborative programme for the development of reproducible methods for the assessment of crop losses, *FAO Plant Prot. Bull.,* 18, 29, 1970.
17. **Chiarappa, L., Chiang, H. C., and Smith, R. F.,** Plant pests and diseases: assessment of crop losses, *Science,* 176, 769, 1972.
18. **Morwood, R. B.,** Report on plant disease investigations in the Trust Territories of the Pacific Islands, Office of the High Commissioner, T.T.P.I., Saipan, 1958.
19. **Ocfemia, G. O.,** The probable nature of "cadang-cadang" disease of coconut, *Philipp. Agric.,* 26, 338, 1937.
20. **Plavšić-Banjac, B., Hunt, P., and Maramorosch, K.,** Mycoplasmalike bodies associated with lethal yellowing disease, *Phytopathology,* 62, 298, 1972.
21. **Toutain, G.,** Note sur l'épidémiologie du Bayoud en Afrique du nord, *Al Awamia,* 15, 37, 1965.
22. **Buddenhagen, I. W.,** Banana diseases in the Pacific area, *FAO Plant Prot. Bull.,* 16(2), 17, 1968.
23. **Hafiz, A.,** Present status of wheat research and production programmes in Near East region, CIMMYT Wheat Workshop, El Batan, Mexico, Sept. 22-29, 1971.
24. **Smith, R. F.,** The impact of the green revolution on plant protection in tropical and subtropical areas, *Bull. Entomol. Soc. Am.,* 18, 7, 1971.
25. **Poulsen, K. K.,** Parents used in the development of Mexican wheat varieties, *Inf. Bull. Near East Wheat Barley Improve. Prod. Proj.,* 6(2), 33, 1969.
26. **Stewart, D. M., Hafiz, A., and Abdel Hak, T.,** Disease epiphytotic threats to high-yielding and local wheats in the Near East, *FAO Plant Prot. Bull.,* 20, 50, 1972.
27. **Vallega, J. and Chiarappa, L.,** Plant disease losses as they occur worldwide, *Phytopathology,* 54(11), 1305, 1964.
28. **Haskell, P. T.,** The hungry locust, *Sci. J.,* January, 1970, 61.
29. **Hori, M.,** The development of recent plant protection in Japan, *Agric. Asia* (spec. issue), 5, 1, 1967.
30. **Fukunaga, K.,** Recent development of agricultural chemicals. A. Use and development of agricultural pesticides, *Agric. Asia* (spec. issue), 5, 107, 1967.
31. **Smith, R. F. and Reynolds, H. T.,** Principles, Definition and Scope of Integrated Pest Control, Vol. 1, Proc. FAO Symposium on Integrated Pest Control, Rome, Italy, 1971, 11.
32. **Pinto, F. F. and Hurd, E. A.,** Seventy years with wheat in Kenya, *East Afr. Agric. For. J.* (spec. issue), 36, 1, 1970.
33. **Robinson, R. A.,** Horizontal resistance, *Rev. Plant Pathol.,* in press.

REDUCING FOOD SPOILAGE AND DETERIORATION

J. C. Ayres

TABLE OF CONTENTS

Introduction 177

Time 177

Temperature 178

pH 179

Water Activity (a_W) 181

Oxygen Tension 184

Nutrients 185

Inhibitory Substances 186

Pests 187

References 188

INTRODUCTION

When a plant or animal dies, it begins to decompose. Such decomposition is recognized in many ways. The appearance of the product changes: meat surfaces become sticky, slimy, or even putrid; vegetables wilt or become flabby; milk products develop disagreeable odors and tastes; and fruits display soft areas or rot. There are many factors responsible for food spoilage, but microbial proliferation in and on the product is probably the most important. Insects, mites, and vermin also are responsible for enormous wastages of food. Continued enzymatic activity within the tissues results in overmaturity, discoloration, excessive oxidation, bitterness, and/or off-odor. Other chemical reactions bring about changes in color, flavor, and appearance, e.g., nonenzymatic browning, rancidity, and darkening. In a similar manner, physical changes caused by excessive heat or cold, dehydration, and pressure also cause the food to become undesirable.

The likelihood that a food will spoil depends upon many factors including time, temperature, pH, water activity, oxygen tension, nutrients, inhibitory substances, and pests.

TIME

Very few completely stable foods exist but there are several, such as salt, sugar, flour, and rice, that do not spoil even after long storage periods unless they become wet or are subjected to insect or rodent infestations. On the other hand, some foods such as meats, poultry, fish, shellfish, eggs, dairy products, and many fruits and vegetables are highly perishable. A third or intermediate category would comprise commodities such as apples, onions, potatoes, nutmeats, and dried fruits that slowly deteriorate even when properly handled.

TEMPERATURE

The ultimate storage life of foods is generally a function of loss of water content due to storage temperature fluctuations, particle size, lipid content, volatile flavor and colors, and enzymatic activity. Many foods can be held in the frozen state for months, but it is considered practically impossible to sterilize foods by freezing. Meats, fish, poultry, eggs, milk, butter, fruits, and vegetables should be kept as cool as possible, but above the point of freezing. Some of these foods, such as bananas, berries, cucumbers, eggs, lemons, lettuce, peaches, peppers, potatoes, sweet potatoes, and tomatoes, are severely injured by freezing, while others such as beets, cabbage, parsnips, rutabagas, and turnips are damaged little. Most foods other than nuts freeze at temperatures between 0 and -4°C (Table 1). When held at room temperature or higher, fresh foods discolor and develop disagreeable putrefactive odors. The whites and yolks of eggs become thin and fragile and break easily; also, the air cell of the egg enlarges. Milk sours, curdles, and often undergoes a "stormy" fermentation; butter becomes oily, deepens in color, and becomes rancid; cheese softens, "oils-off," and develops off-odor. Many vegetables ripen and soften rapidly and fruits become mealy or soon lose much of their characteristic flavor. Lutz and Hardenburg indicated that sweet corn loses 60% of its sweetness in 1 day at 30°C but only 6% when refrigerated at 0°C, and that as much ripening takes place in apples held at 20°C for 1 day as in 10 days at -1°C.[1] Delaying picking or holding apples in a warm sacking shed may shorten their storage life by as much as 30 days even if the apples are later stored at -1°C. Pears are unusually sensitive to temperature. Porritt reported that the storage life of Anjou and Bartlett pears is 35 to 40% longer at -1.1° than at 0°C.[2]

TABLE 1

Approximate Freezing Point of Selected Foods

°C	Commodity
0.0	Water
	Cucumbers, lettuce
-0.5	Cabbage, turnips
	Celery, tomatoes
-1.0	Spinach, peas, beans, berries
	Carrots, parsnips
-1.5	Broccoli, peaches, pears
	Limes, poultry
-2.0	Beef, veal, lamb, fish, lemons
	Pears, American grapes, oranges, eggs
-2.5	Pork
	Avocados, beets, cranberries
-3.0	Brazil nuts
-3.5	Bacon
	Peanuts, bananas
-4.0	Emperor grapes
	Coconut
-5.0	
-6.0	American walnuts
-7.0	Persian walnuts
	Pecans

Data on fruits and vegetables adapted from *U.S.D.A. Handbook 66* (viz. Ayres[7]).

When foods are frozen slowly, ice crystals grow to large size, puncturing tissue cells so that when the product is thawed, structural damage results and there is leakage of cellular fluid. Fluctuating temperature during storage also permits ice crystal growth and damages protoplasmic content. Furthermore, since water freezes out of such solutions, the increased concentration of electrolytes in the unfrozen residue causes permanent colloidal changes such as may be evidenced by the curdling of cream sauces or the coagulation of milk protein.

The loss of moisture vapor by sublimation from the surface of frozen foods causes a serious dehydrated condition called "freezer burn." In foods displaying freezer burn, the appearance, texture, palatability, and even the nutritive value are irreversibly changed. Ice-glazing, spray- or dip-coatings, or impermeable packaging films are used to avoid freezer burn.

Cutting, chipping, slicing, dicing, and grinding foods greatly increase the surface area exposed to microbial action and oxidation. In addition, the mixing associated with these processes spreads the surface flora throughout the food mass. Discoloration is produced by enzymes activated by atmospheric oxygen in direct relation to their time-temperature exposure.

Oxidative deterioration takes place during frozen storage of foods containing significant amounts of fats or oils. Animal tissues are more susceptible than plant tissues to the development of rancidity. It is generally agreed that the order of reactivity of fats in flesh foods is fatty fish > turkey > chicken > pork > mutton > beef.

Care must be taken to avoid cross transfer of odors in storing various food commodities. Apples, pears, and citrus fruits should not be in the same cold storage quarters as cabbage, carrots, celery, dairy products, eggs, fish, meats, onions, or potatoes. Milk, butter, eggs, and meats readily absorb odors from apples, pears, and citrus fruit, and these fruits, in turn, acquire an unpleasant earthy odor and taste when stored with potatoes.

All fleshy fruits and in particular apples, bananas, melons, peaches, pears, and tomatoes produce ethylene during ripening. This gas stimulates the ripening of many fruits and vegetables, but has an adverse effect on the color of acorn squash, cucumbers, leafy vegetables, and peppers; ethylene causes bitterness in carrots.[3]

Enzyme activity is temperature dependent, but is also enhanced by pH and substrate concentration. While some of the peroxidases, such as those in pickles, are fairly heat resistant, heating to 80°C is sufficient to inactivate most enzymes. On the other hand, enzymes continue to function, although at a slow rate, far below the freezing point.

The total temperature range for the growth of bacteria, yeasts, and molds extends from approximately -7°C to 80°C. It is well known that bacterial growth can occur on frozen meat at -3°C and that yeasts and molds have been found to grow at as low as -7°C. Bacterial growth has been recorded at -7°C on supercooled media.[4] The minimal temperature for microbial development is set by the point at which their substrate freezes and nutrients in the organism's microenvironment become unavailable. There is an inverse relationship between the rate of freezing and the loss of microbial viability. Bacteria die more rapidly at -1° to -5°C than at lower temperatures. Haines attributed this phenomenon to more pronounced protein flocculation at temperatures slightly below the freezing point than at lower temperature.[5] With quick freezing, heat is rapidly removed so that the temperature of the product passes through the zone of maximum crystal formation in 30 min or less.

When foods remain unfrozen, storage life usually decreases as the temperature increases. The type of microbial flora responsible for spoilage varies with the temperature. Some microorganisms prefer low temperatures and others very high temperatures. Organisms generally are separated into psychrophilic, mesophilic, and thermophilic groups on the basis of their preferred temperature for growth. While few true psychrophiles (cold-loving) bacteria grow on refrigerated foods, a large variety of species of *Pseudomonas, Achromobacter, Flavobacterium,* and *Alcaligenes* can tolerate a temperature of 5°C or less. These organisms quickly adjust to low temperatures and are often associated with the production of off-odor and slime on meats, fish, and poultry.

Many fermentative bacteria (*Streptococcus lactis, Leuconostoc,* and *Lactobacilli*), molds, and yeasts grow well at room temperature and persist for long periods at somewhat lower temperatures, but fail to survive above 40 to 45°C. However, coliforms and enteric pathogens find 35 to 45°C much to their liking. *Lactobacillus thermophilus, Bacillus thermoacidurans,* and *B. stearothermophilus* grow well at still higher temperatures, i.e., 55 to 60°C and cause spoilage in underprocessed canned foods (Figure 1).

pH

Foods can be placed in different classes according to their free hydrogen ion content [H] or pH ($\log \frac{1}{[H]}$). Very few foods are basic (alkaline); egg white, soda crackers, lye hominy, and lutefish are almost the only examples.

Most bacteria prefer substrates that are almost neutral, i.e., only slightly acid (pH 6.0 to 7.0). When foods become more acid or alkaline, microbial growth generally is retarded. Those foods lowest in effective acidity (pH > 4.5) include meat-, fish- and shellfish-, poultry-, and milk-products, and most vegetables. Many mesophilic and thermophilic spore-forming bacteria as well as a large number of molds, yeasts, and nonspore-forming microorganisms grow well on these substrates. Since low acidity is necessary for growth of food poisoning organisms and, particularly, staphylococci, salmonellas, *Clostridium perfringens,* and *C. botulinum,* these foods present the greatest hazards to health. Fairly severe heat treatments are used when canning these items to assure that they are safe.

High acid foods (pH < 4.5), such as fruits and fruit juices and fermented vegetables , may be further subdivided on the basis of their acidity. Those foods with the greatest acidity (lowest pH)

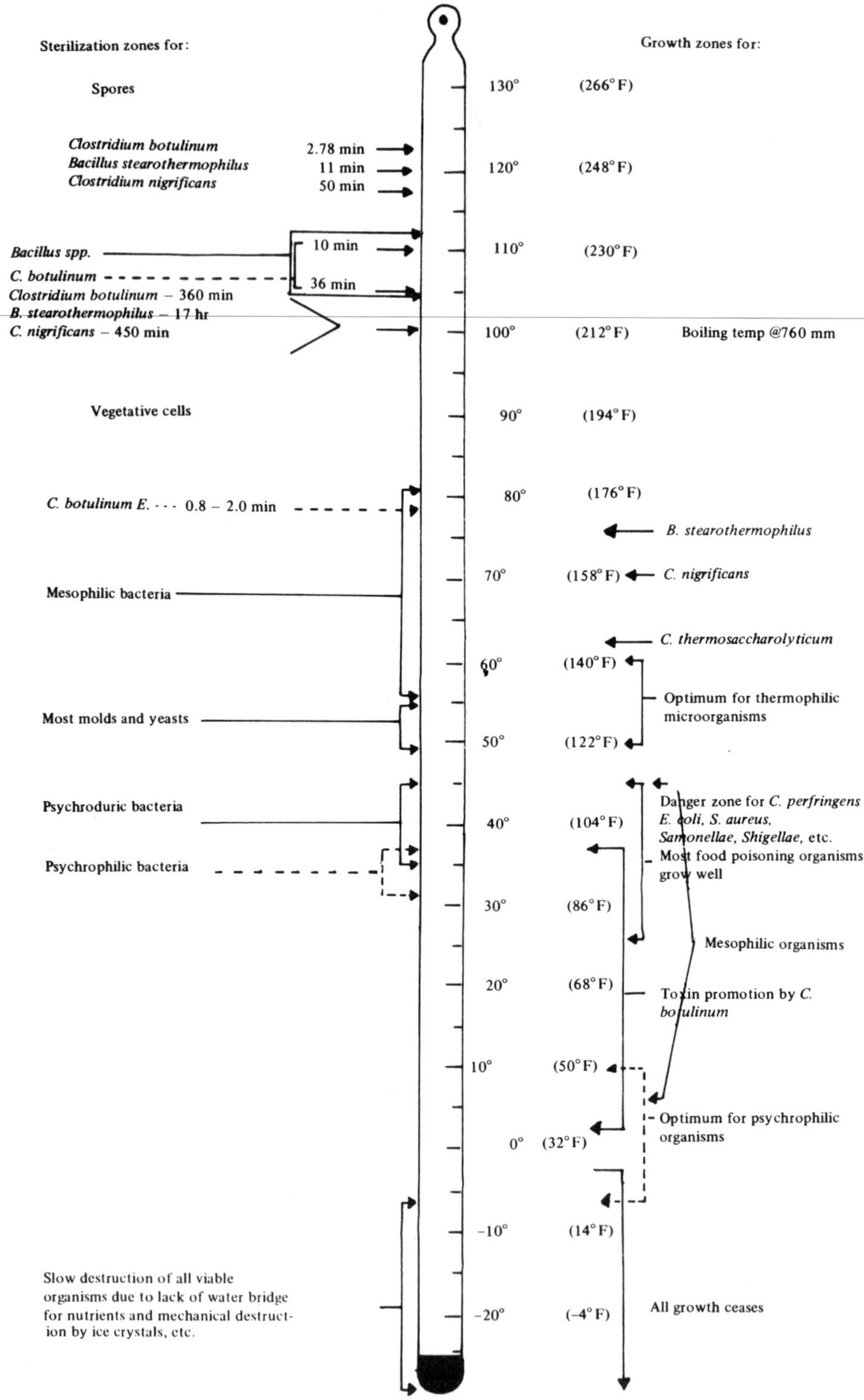

FIGURE 1. Temperature relations for growth and survival of microorganisms.

include citrus fruits, most stone fruits, grapes, apples, berries, pickles, sauerkraut, etc. (see Figure 2). Spoilage of this group is effected by yeasts and molds and a few nonspore-forming bacteria. Heating for a few minutes at 77°C is sufficient to destroy any of these organisms in canned foods. Within the high acid foods the subgroup having higher pH (lower acidity), such as tomatoes, figs, pears, some apricot varieties, ripe pineapple, etc., is subject to spoilage not only by yeasts, molds, and nonspore-forming bacteria, but also by a group of heat resistant, spore-forming anaerobes. This latter group grows well at pH 4.5 and slowly down at about pH 3.7. They produce considerable amounts of gas and butyric acid in canned foods.

High acid-high solid foods include items such as jams, jellies, preserves, purées, and catsup. Molds and yeasts are able to grow in high concentrations of acid and sugar or solids and so are primarily responsible for spoilage of these foods. Vegetative cells and spores of both of these forms of life are sensitive to heat and are quickly destroyed at 70°C.

WATER ACTIVITY (a_w)

The chemical potential of the water relative to that of pure water at the same temperature and pressure is called water activity or a_w. By definition $a_w = \frac{P}{P_o}$ where P represents the water vapor pressure of the solution and P_o that of pure water. A large proportion of the cellular content of plant and animal tissues consists of water. For example, the value for fresh meat is $a_w = .99$ (see Figure 3). When the surrounding atmosphere is drier than this, the surface of the meat begins to dry and the meat loses its desirable moist, glistening appearance or "bloom." Prolonged storage in an atmosphere having a low relative humidity causes the meat to dehydrate to such an extent that the surface becomes so dried that it is almost impervious to further loss of water, i.e., "case hardened." With cured meats, a_w values needed to assure a desirable product vary with the fat content, degree of microbial action to which the product is subjected, amount of smoke it receives, and its salt content.

Many fruits and some vegetables (cucumber, egg plant, peppers, tomatoes) have a cuticle that prevents rapid loss of moisture from the surface. However, other fruits wrinkle and lose weight, and vegetables such as beets, cabbage, celery, chard,

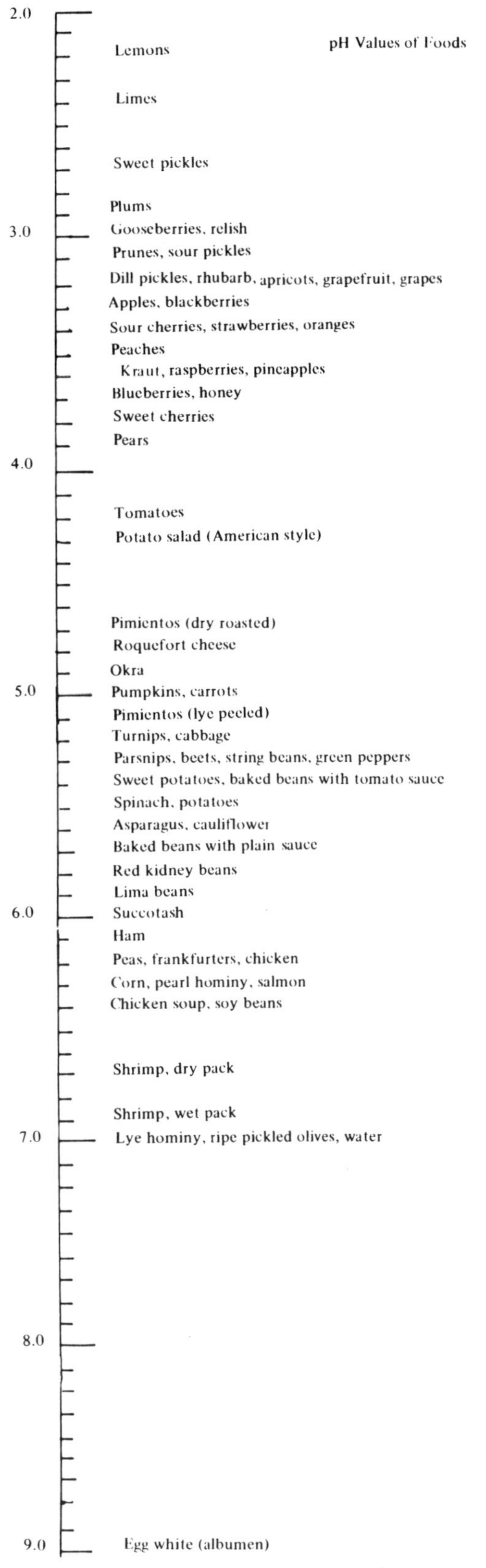

FIGURE 2. pH values of foods.[8]

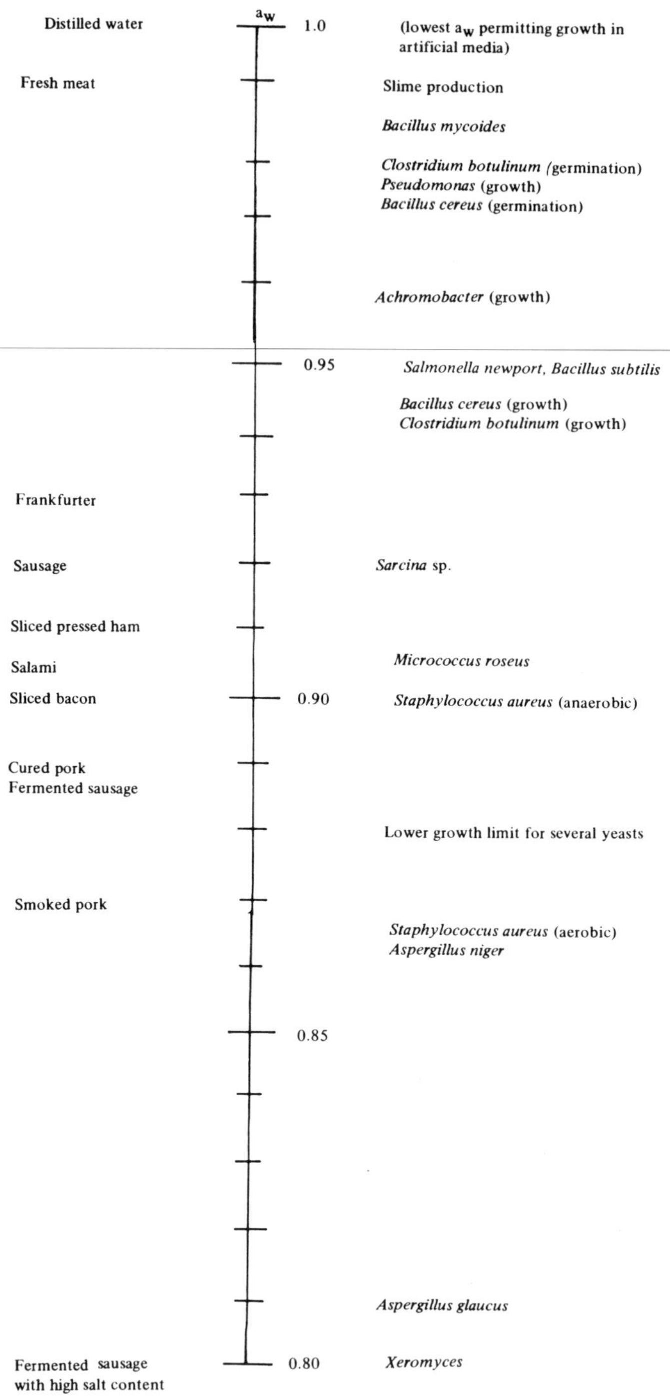

FIGURE 3. Comparison of water activity values for various meats with those limiting the germination or growth of microorganisms.[9,10]

green beans, lettuce, peas, spinach, etc. wilt and become inedible if exposed to dry atmospheric conditions for a prolonged period of time. Celery and rhubarb have the ability to rehydrate when saturated with moisture, but most of the leafy vegetables do not possess this characteristic. When foods are held at refrigeration temperatures, it is essential that the air be nearly saturated with moisture (Table 2). Since microbial growth is favored at high relative humidity, the processor attempts to hold food products under conditions that minimize shrinkage and do not promote spoilage. Sudden pronounced changes in humidity may cause "sweating" or moisture condensation on the cool surface of the food commodity. Sweating promotes the spoilage of eggs and the decay of fruits and vegetables.

The amount of moisture that is available to various microorganisms determines if they will grow or not. Generally speaking, molds require less available moisture than yeasts and they, in turn, are less demanding than bacteria. If the water is bound by solutes such as salt or sugar dissolved in the water, these solutes create an osmotic pressure that draws water from the cells when the concentration of dissolved materials in that unit is greater outside of the cell than inside. Slime-producing bacteria such as the pseudo-

TABLE 2

Optimal Storage Temperatures and Relative Humidities of Commodities Susceptible to Cold Injury When Improperly Stored[1]

	Lowest safe storage temperature	R.H.	Symptoms of injury when stored below safe temperature
Apples	2-3	85-90	Internal browning, brown core, soggy breakdown
Bananas	12-13	90-95	Dull color when ripened
Beans (snap)	7	90-95	Pitting, russeting on removal
Lettuce	0	90-95	Discoloration, water soaked areas, decay
Oranges, Florida and Texas	0	85-90	Rind pitting, rot
Oranges, Arizona	3-9	85-90	Rind disorders
Lemons	11-13	85-90	Internal discoloration, pitting
Limes	8-10	85-90	Pitting, brown blemishes
Watermelons	4-5	85-90	Pitting, objectionable flavor, decay
Squash, Winter	10-12	70-75	Keep relatively well
Sweet potatoes	12-16	85-90	Require curing at 30°C and r.h. of 85 to 90% for 4 to 7 days to prevent chilling injury, pitting, and decay
Tomatoes, ripe	7-10	85-90	Softening and decay
Tomatoes mature green	12-13	85-90	Poor color when ripe, rot
Nuts	0-2	65-75	No damage if moisture content is low
Shell eggs	0	90-95	Cracking, watery consistency, tendency to spoil quickly
Carcass beef[2]	−2	90-95	Rupture of cells, increase in drip loss

[1] Data on fruits and vegetables adapted from *U.S.D.A. Handbook 66* (viz. Lutz and Hardenburg[1]).

[2] Beef, pork, lamb, poultry, fish, and shellfish keep satisfactorily in the frozen state.

monads growing on the surfaces of cut meats, fish, and poultry require a very "wet" substrate. The lowest a_w at which these organisms grow is 0.97. The limiting a_w value for *E. coli* and *C. botulinum* is 0.95 but that of *Staphylococcus aureus* is 0.86 (see chart). The lower a_w limit for a beer yeast is 0.94, while that of baker's yeast is 0.91. However, osmophilic yeasts have been reported to grow in syrups with a_w values as low as 0.62 to 0.65. A minimal a_w value of less than 0.62 is necessary to stop all mold growth, but most food spoilage molds are inhibited at a_w values less than 0.70.

If given sufficient time, molds will grow in a saturated solution of sugar and it is known that their enzymes remain functional in almost saturated salt solutions. During the production of soy sauce, a heavily overgrown cooked soybean-roasted wheat mixture is suspended in a 24% salt solution for several months during which time the mold (and yeast) enzymes slowly convert the protein to glutamic acid.

On jams and jellies the presence of a thin film surface moisture provides a site with reduced solids content upon which the mold may proliferate and secrete enzymes that hydrolyze the substrate and convert it to alcohols, acids, and other decomposition products. The same phenomenon is considered responsible for the spoilage of honey by osmophilic yeasts. A moisture content of 20% is considered critical. When the amount of water in honey exceeds that level, the surface of honey is diluted due to its hygroscopic property and contaminative yeasts quickly adapt and bring about spoilage.

OXYGEN TENSION

Oxidation and reduction reactions are electrical in nature and involve the ability to transfer electrons. During oxidation electrons are lost, while during reduction there is a gain of electrons and the O-R potential, or E_h, is a measure, in volts, of the electrons that are exchanged. The iron in blood and muscle pigments is readily oxidized from the ferrous (Fe^{++}) to the ferric (Fe^{+++}) state so that in raw meats the native reduced purple-red myoglobin is converted to a brownish discolored metmyoglobin. Similarly, with nitrate ($NaNO_3$ or KNO_3), the exposure of cured meats to air and/or heat results in profound pigment changes. The actual curing agent was found to be the nitrite produced by the bacterial reduction of the nitrate salt and a legal limit of 200 ppm of $NaNO_2$ is permitted in meat. The nitrite serves as a source of nitric oxide which reacts with myoglobin and the nitrosomyoglobin, in turn, is converted to a nitrosohemochromogen, the pink-red cured meat pigment. If there is further oxidation, pigments are produced that cause the meat to become brown, gray, or even greenish in color. High nitrite content causes the pigment of cut lean surfaces to oxidize, while insufficient nitrite in the cure results in fading. Some bacteria, in the presence of acid such as in vinegar-pickled cured meats, cause excessive nitrite reduction, "nitrite burn," or greening.

A vast array of enzymes occurs in plant and animal tissues that catalyze the oxidation of a variety of compounds. An example is the enzyme peroxidase in fruits which causes them to darken quickly in the presence of air. Autoxidation in lipids results in the development of rancidity in meat fats and other fats and oils. This form of spoilage can be prevented by the use of antioxidants such as butylated hydroxyanisole (BHA) and butylated hydroxytoluene (BHT) or delayed by adding a synergistic agent such as ascorbic acid.

In general, animal fats are poorly poised and while their O-R potential would predict the type of change that takes place, the poising effect and the oxygen tension of the microenvironment are important in determining the extent of change. The addition of ascorbic acid serves to poise the fat at a reduced O-R level for longer time. It behaves similarly to prevent the enzymatic browning of fruits and vegetables.

The type of microbial growth that takes place in foods is related to its oxygen-reduction potential. Aerobic bacteria require strongly positive E_h conditions for respiration and cease to grow when free oxygen has been depleted. The respiration of anaerobes is inhibited when the oxygen (Figure 4) available to them is not combined with a substrate nutrient. Facultative organisms respire under either aerobic or anaerobic conditions, while microaerophiles require free oxygen but at reduced tension. The latter type of microbial proliferation prevails in sausage emulsions when the thermal process is insufficient to kill greening bacteria in the core area of the sausage. These organisms cause considerable spoilage when wieners are underprocessed and a viable fairly heat resistant residual population

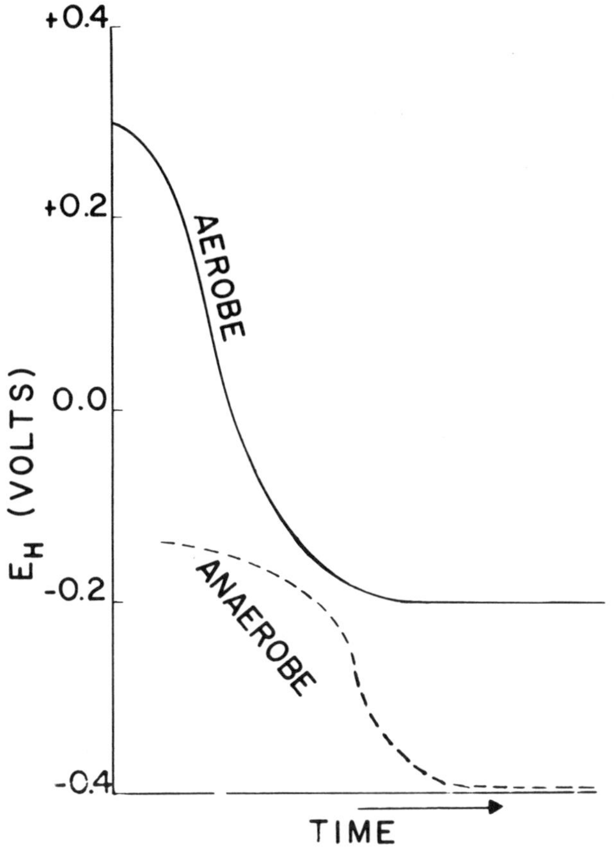

FIGURE 4. E_h conditions for an aerobe and an anaerobe.[11]

quickly proliferates, causing the core areas to turn green when the temperature is appropriate.

NUTRIENTS

Most foods contain proteins, lipids, carbohydrates, vitamins, minerals, and other accessory food substances and water. Many plant tissues are excellent sources of carbohydrates, whereas animal tissues are often considered the preferred sources of proteins. Yet the content of these several components varies widely among the several foods that comprise man's dietary. Cane and beet sugar are almost entirely carbohydrate; protein and water are the main constituents of egg white. Only a trace of fat and less than 1% carbohydrate are present. In an earlier section, it was pointed out that food spoilage is dependent upon many factors; thus, the complement of nutrients that a food possesses does not necessarily predict its storage life. Substrate concentration is of great importance. The unavailability of moisture in sugar, starch, flour, and cereal products prevents these products from spoiling. Anatomical features also greatly contribute to the storage life of foods. For example, oranges, eggs, carrots, and milk have approximately the same moisture content. Yet the spoilage that these four foods undergo varies greatly. With oranges, eggs, and carrots the presence of a protective rind, shell, or skin serves as a partial barrier to microbial invasion. The proteins that comprise the shell membranes of the egg are difficult for many microorganisms to penetrate and attack. On the other hand, molds experience little difficulty in penetrating the membranes that separate the several sections of the orange. Carrots and oranges have roughly similar carbohydrate compositions. The cuticle of carrot and its higher ash content prevent rapid microbial penetration. Since the available acidity of the orange is much greater than for the other three foods, it is more susceptible to mold and yeast growth, while the carrot is often subject to bacterial attack. Structural features of these two commodities contribute greatly to differences in their storage life. Since milk is fluid, motile bacteria readily migrate to all portions of the container with ease. Also, with changes in temperature, nonmotile microorganisms are transported by convection.

Skin surfaces and viscera of meat animals, poultry, and fish are heavily contaminated with microorganisms. It is impossible to completely avoid exposing the edible flesh to some of this contamination when hides, feathers, scales, and viscera are removed. Juices seeping from the severed flesh or from pieces of fat or meat cut from the carcass provide an excellent source of nutrients for bacteria. Equipment, cutting block, saws, knives, and other utensils are often vehicles for spreading microorganisms from one place to another, as are the hands and clothing of workers and the water used for rinsing working surfaces. Insanitary, inadequate, or poorly controlled processing procedures result in products that have high initial microbial loads. As Figure 5 shows, the storage life of ground or sliced beef directly reflects the precautions taken to control contamination during processing. When high numbers of organisms are present, these bacteria cause meats to develop off-odor at refrigeration temperature (4.4°C or 40°F) in two days, and by four days the counts reach such a large number that the

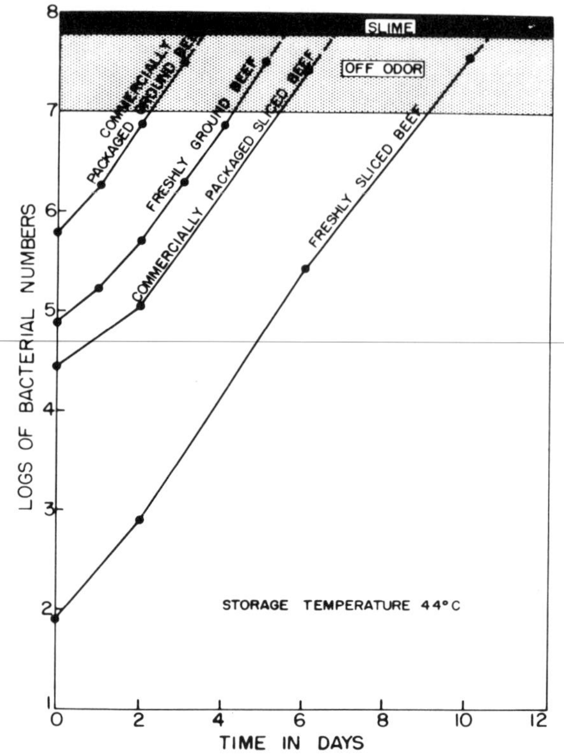

FIGURE 5. Effect of initial bacterial populations on storage life of sliced and ground beef.

coalescing cells produce a malodorous surface slime. While freshly ground meat has a large number of bacteria, the load is only about one tenth that of comminuted meat made from the bits and pieces that are generally prepared into hamburger. Also, the storage life of carefully prepared ground beef is about double that of a poorly handled product.

A similar but even more dramatic contrast pertains to sliced meats. When clean knives and sanitary slicing tables are used, meats with counts of less than 100 bacteria/cm^2 and a storage life of nine days are possible. More typically, surfaces of sliced beef have 20 to 30,000 microorganisms/cm^2 and keep for only five days.

INHIBITORY SUBSTANCES

Acids such as ascorbic, benzoic, citric, lactic, malic, oxalic, salicylic, and tartaric are initially present in various plant tissues. Ascorbic acid is found in most fresh fruits and vegetables. In addition to its use as a vitamin, ascorbic acid is often employed to retard browning; but since it is readily destroyed by oxidation, its protective effect is only temporary. Benzoic acid occurs naturally in cranberries and serves as an effective yeast inhibitor. Almost all plant materials contain citric acid or citrate, but much of the acid utilized commercially for the production of beverages and foods is prepared by mold fermentation rather than from fruit juices. Lactic acid exists in nature in certain plant juices and in the muscles and blood of animals. This acid is commonly produced from the carbohydrate present in cabbage, cacao, coffee, cucumber, olive plums, milk, and tea and, under controlled conditions, yields desired end products. Under other circumstances, lactic acid production may result in deterioration of wine, beer, and cheese.

Fruits vary in their content of malic and tartaric acids. In some fruits, e.g., apples, peaches, and pears, malic is the predominant acid; in grapes and currants, tartaric acid occurs in considerable quantity. Malic acid does not give the tartness of citric acid, while tartaric acid has a more bitter taste; however, both acids have better buffering action than citric acid.

Spinach and rhubarb have higher oxalate contents than most other foods and, supposedly, sporadic poisonings have occurred from the ingestion of rhubarb leaves. Small amounts of salicylic acid occur in most fruits. By decreasing the pH in foods, organic acids exert antiseptic effect and the undissociated acid controls microbial growth. When used in too large an amount, any of the fatty acids damage cell membranes. Benzoic, oxalic, and salicylic acids also interfere with enzymatic processes.

Formaldehyde and several phenolic and cresylic compounds occur as minor components of hardwood smoked meat, fish, poultry, and cheese. These agents combine with proteins in cells to form protoplasmic poisons and insoluble proteinates. While their desired function is to contribute flavor and retard microbial growth, gastric carcinoma has been attributed to the consumption of very heavily smoked fish and mutton over extended periods.

The alcohol content of beer, ale, and unfortified wine is sufficient to limit microbial growth but does not prevent the eventual spoilage of these products. Lactic acid bacteria, called tourne bacilli, form acid from the sugars in wine and produce a sour, "mousy," discolored wine.

Many raw foods contain antivitamins. Cereals and liver have been shown to be rachitogenic; fish oils destroy vitamin E; the lipoxidase of raw soybeans oxidizes and destroys carotene; raw fish flesh contains the enzyme thiaminase that destroys thiamin; and raw egg white has a battery of inhibitory substances including the protein avidin that binds biotin.

Among inhibitors, the antienzymatic substance solanine, associated with "green" potatoes, sometimes presents a real health hazard. This alkaloid is a powerful cholinesterase inhibitor; since cholinesterases control nerve impulses, solanine may block the normal functions of nerve activity.

There are many trypsin inhibitors among plant species and several antitrypsins of animal origin. These agents result in excessive losses of essential amino acids.

Almost all raw legumes contain proteins that are able to agglutinate red blood cells. When hemagglutinin levels exceed 0.5% for kidney beans or 1.0% for black beans, growth of experimental animals is probably inhibited due to failure of nutrients to be absorbed through the intestinal wall.

PESTS

Flies, roaches, rats, mice, cats, dogs, and flying birds are the usual vectors for transmitting disease and filth via foods. Flies, being the most common of the pests, often are tolerated to a certain extent. Yet their habits are the most despicable. They breed in manure, garbage, and decaying or fermenting matter. In addition to depositing microorganisms by walking over the food, they excrete fly specks on food materials, utensils, and equipment. They are particularly fond of sugar-containing foods and often solubilize these products by secreting saliva and using their sponge-like labella to draw up the moisturized product through their tubular proboscis.

There are several kinds of cockroaches with which the food processor must contend. These disgusting nocturnal insects inhabit sewers, basement areas, and other damp and/or dark places and, alternately, feed, breed, and reside on food surfaces. These insects soil far more food than they consume and unless commodities to which they have access are thoroughly washed or cleaned, molted roach parts, egg cases, eggs, nymphs, and even adult roaches may become a part of the processed product.

Aphids, fruit flies, and gnats are more discriminating than flies and roaches in habitat and their presence in foods carries less public health implication. Aphids and plant lice are sucking insects that are associated particularly with leafy vegetables, broccoli, brussel sprouts, cabbage, and cauliflower since the juices of these plants are their preferred nutrients. These insects are most difficult to remove or wash free. Usually fruit flies and gnats are associated with fermenting fruit and vegetable products. Great care must be taken to avoid having fragments of these insects in products prepared from apples, apricots, bananas, beans, berries, cabbage (family), corn, cucumbers, dates, figs, olives, peaches, pears, peas, plums, potatoes, sweet potatoes, and tomatoes. The cheese skipper, the larva of a fly which gets its name from its jumping habit, bores into cheese and cured meat, causing meats to become slimy and, in the case of cured meats, to rot these infested products.

Scores of other insects are injurious to raw food commodities and to stored and finished products. The larval stage of the Indian-meal-, the Mediterranean flour-, and the Angoumois grain-moths and of the yellow meal worm, is destructive in cereal products. The first two cause webbing together of products, while the larval stage of the Angoumois grain-moth eats round holes in grain and meal worm larvae eat cereal products, meal, bran, meat scraps, and even feathers. The confused flour beetle and many other beetles and weevils also chew holes in all kinds of grain, flour, starchy materials, beans, peas, baking powder, fruits, nuts, and chocolate. After other insects have damaged grain products, dried fruits, nuts, yeast, sugar, candy, or any dried plant food intended for human consumption, the saw-toothed grain beetle may eat or damage these products. The cadelle not only attacks all stored grain and seeds but also cuts holes in sacks and bores holes in wooden grain bins.

Adult ham beetles and larder beetle larvae feed on or slightly below the surface of cured meats and many other foods; ham beetle larvae bore through the meat and cause it to rot. Several species of mites also attack meats, feeding on the surface and giving the affected parts a powdery appearance. These tiny arachnids (1/32 in.) may be carried into storage areas or deposited on foods by flies, ants, or other insects.

Rodents damage foods in many ways other than by ingestion. Rodent hairs, droppings, urine, nests, foreign matter, dead animals, and filth are distributed in portions of foods not consumed. Rats and mice cannot exist where either food or shelter is lacking and while mice can live without water for long periods, rats will not remain where water is unavailable. The U.S. Fish and Wildlife Service estimates the population of mice in this country to exceed 1 billion and indicates that a single pair of mice may consume 4 lb of food during the fall and winter months. Also, each mouse eliminates about 48 droppings per day and voids about 1/2 ml of urine. Similarly, a pair of rats consumes about 27 lb of food during the fall and winter and voids 25,000 droppings and 1 1/2 gal of urine.[6] Occasionally, cats and dogs are employed to reduce rodent populations. This practice should be discouraged since cat or dog hair may be responsible for adulterating the food.

Bird contamination is a problem only where windows, doors, ventilators, or other openings afford access to feeds and foods and nesting places. English sparrows and pigeons are the most troublesome, but on occasion other species may cause damage as well. Stored seeds and grains are the products that are generally consumed and/or fouled. Occasionally these species also spread salmonellosis and ornithosis.

REFERENCES

1. **Lutz, J. M. and Hardenburg, R. E.,** *The Commercial Storage of Fruits, Vegetables, and Florist and Nursery Stocks,* Agriculture Handbook No. 66, United States Department of Agriculture, Washington, D.C., 1968, 6.
2. **Porritt, S. W.,** The effect of temperature on post-harvest physiology and storage life of pears, *Can. J. Plant Sci.,* 44, 568, 1964.
3. **Carlton, B. C., Peterson, C. E., and Tolbert, N. E.,** Effect of ethylene and oxygen on production of a bitter compound by carrot roots, *Plant Physiol.,* 36, 550, 1961.
4. **Haines, R. B.,** Microbiology in the Preservation of Animal Tissues, Gr. Brit. Dept. Sci. Ind. Research Food Invest., Special Report 45, 1937.
5. **Haines, R. B.,** The effect of freezing on bacteria, *Proc. Roy. Soc. B.,* 124, 451, 1938.
6. **Dykstra, W. A.,** Rodent filth in food, *Pest Contr.,* 22(7), 9, 1954.
7. **Ayres, J. C.,** Temperature and moisture requirements, in *Proceedings Low Temperature Microbiology Symposium,* Campbell Soup Co., Camden, N.J., 1962.
8. **Bigelow, W. D. and Cathcart, P. H.,** Relations of processing to the acidity of canned foods, Nat'l. Canner's Assoc., Bull., 17-L, 1921.
9. **Hansen, N. W. and Riemann, H.,** Mikrobiologische Beschaffenheit von vorverpacktem Fleisch und vorverpackten Fleischwaren, *Die Fleischwirtschaft,* 14, 861, 1962.
10. **Scott, W. J.,** Water relations of food spoilage microorganisms, *Adv. Food Res.,* 7, 83, 1957.
11. **Hewitt, L. F.,** *Oxidation-Reduction Potentials in Bacteriology and Biochemistry,* 4th ed., London County Council, London, 1936; read in **Porter, J. R.,** *Bacterial Chemistry and Physiology,* John Wiley & Sons, New York, 1946, 57.

PRODUCTION AND USE OF UNCONVENTIONAL SOURCES OF FOOD

N. W. Pirie

TABLE OF CONTENTS

Introduction 189

For Whom Should the Unconventional Foods Be Made? 190

The Need for Unconventional Foodstuffs 191

The Possible Sources of Food Proteins 192
- Edible Plants or Parts of Plants 193
  - Vegetables 193
  - Seeds 193
  - Underground Parts 195
- Plant Products That Need Some Form of Processing 195
  - Mechanical Fractionation 195
  - Conversion by Animals 196
    - On Land 196
    - In Water 197
- Unconventional Photosynthetic Plants 198
- Microbial Conversions 199
- Synthesis 200

The Nutritional Value of Unconventional Foods 200

Conventionalizing the Unconventional 201

References 202

INTRODUCTION

"So long as freedom from hunger is only half achieved, so long as two thirds of the nations have food deficits, no citizen, no nation, can afford to be satisfied. We have the ability, as members of the human race. We have the means, we have the capacity to eliminate hunger from the face of the earth in our lifetime. We need only the will."

That statement by the late President Kennedy, opening the World Food Congress in 1963, is more effectively phrased than many others made during the past 20 years. Every year, however, some government committee or committee set up by the International Agency says much the same thing in language appropriate to the group that is being addressed. Unofficial organizations are equally vocal; an early example was a collection of essays[1] presented to Lord Boyd Orr, the first Director General of the Food and Agriculture Organisation, on his 70th birthday in 1950. The contributors argued that existing scientific knowledge, if energetically used, could make it possible to feed everyone in the world adequately. The population has increased since then – but so has skill, knowledge, and the ability to use both. If we had the will, today's job could be done; the future is more problematic.

The potentialities of conventional methods of agriculture have been assessed in earlier chapters of this book. It is obvious that when fully exploited, they will improve the food supply enormously. Even without an increase in the area farmed or the distribution of improved varieties, merely by bringing the standards of the less efficient up to the level reached by the more efficient farmers in a neighborhood, the present food deficit could probably be abolished. To accomplish that, a radical change in outlook is needed. Farming tends to be a despised occupation in those regions most in need of food. Instead of trying to improve conditions in villages, the more enterprising people try to leave them and get jobs in town. This is understandable. The policy in nearly every country is to pay agricultural workers less than industrial workers because it is thought that industrialization is the key to progress. It is possible that this policy will work, but there is no historical precedent for it. Those countries that are now well fed are industrialized, but their industrialization was preceded by a period of efficient, progressive, and often prosperous farming. Even when unconventional foodstuffs are being discussed, it would be prudent to assume that production will depend to a large extent on skilled farmers satisfied with the esteem accorded to them by the community.

FOR WHOM SHOULD THE UNCONVENTIONAL FOODS BE MADE?

Many unconventional foods are already being eaten. Dried skim milk and corn-soy-milk mixture are outstanding examples. Communities suffering from various types of misfortune have been given more than 3 million tons of dried skim milk during the past 15 years and the school lunch program in India is dependent on donated corn-soy-milk to a large extent. Although these nearly tasteless powders were not the conventional foods of any community, they, or similar products, will probably soon lose their unconventional status, for infant feeding at any rate. So far they have been used by poor and often starving people. "Texturized" foods, usually based on soy, come at the other extreme. Either as novelties, because they are acceptable to vegetarians or because they are cheaper than meat, they are now winning acceptance in relatively affluent communities. Even in affluent countries there are extremely poor people. A survey organized by the U.S. Public Health Service[2] suggested that one sixth of the population of the U.S. was malnourished. The American Medical Association[3] found the position particularly bad in the Southeast, along the Appalachians, and in Indian reservations. Surveys in Britain have given similar results. It may be argued, therefore, that cheaper and possibly unconventional food is needed in all countries whether poor or affluent, developing or industrialized.

The reasons for the existence of malnutrition in different countries differ. The U.S. produces an overabundance of food; at the moment, Britain can buy whatever food is needed. Malnutrition in these countries could, therefore, be prevented by changes in the economic structure. The desirability of different types of change is obviously a matter of opinion. This author's opinion is that the basic foods should be supplied free. It seems anomalous that countries that do not find their political stability shaken by free education or a free health service should shudder at the thought of free food. Be that as it may, it will be agreed that the problem in affluent countries could be solved by means other than changes in the technique of farming or in the character of the foods produced.

However, in most of the world this is not so. At the moment there is so little food in some nations that one result of an increase in the wage rates of those who are now worst paid would be the disappearance of food from the shops. The cause of individual malnutrition is poverty, but the relief of individual poverty would cause a general food shortage. The greatest need for improved food supplies, and possibly for unconventional sources of food, is therefore in the developing countries.

This conclusion is sometimes disputed. It is said that if these countries bought food with all the money they now spend on armaments, they could eat well. Though preferable, that arrangement would still leave them dependent on overseas aid for much of their food; this can hardly be looked on as a desirable permanent state of affairs. Small countries, such as Britain, can rely on exports and overdrafts; large ones cannot. It is said that the people in developing countries are lazy, feckless, and apathetic. If this is any truer of them than of people in industrialized countries, it is probably a consequence of malnutrition; few of us would retain our energy and enterprise after several years on the usual diet in Central America or India. It is well to remember that Cicero advised Atticus not to get British slaves because they were too stupid and uneducable to be used in a Roman household. Racial comparisons should be postponed until such time that the groups that are being compared are living on comparable diets and have done so from infancy. One of the more striking results in an experiment in Britain in 1924[4] was the greater liveliness of boys getting an extra pint of milk a day; this was shown by their being more often in trouble for minor offenses against order than the control group.

Conventional foods can, or could, meet the needs of the industrialized countries and it is likely that they will continue to do so in spite of some increase in population. It is possible that these foods will meet the needs of the industrialized parts of developing countries. But it is a pure assumption that they will also meet the needs of those living in relatively primitive conditions far from towns; the assumption is especially improbable in the wet tropics. Rural inhabitants of the wet tropics are presently the worst fed group in the world; there are about 1000 million of them and it is unlikely that there will be fewer by the end of the century. It is this group, therefore, that greatly needs unconventional food; the foods that will be of most use to them are those that can be made from local produce by simple methods. The methods already used by many primitive people, e.g., grating, washing and fermenting cassava, brewing, and improving various beans by fermentation, show that sophisticated processes can be managed without elaborate equipment. It would be better to try to build up new technologies from the existing basis, rather than to try to introduce a completely alien type of technology. A village industry of the type that is now titled "Intermediate Technology," in which the most up-to-date scientific knowledge is applied to technically simple processes, is the type of innovation that is most likely to be useful.

THE NEED FOR UNCONVENTIONAL FOODSTUFFS

Unconventionality may involve no more than a change in quantity and place. It is, for example, unconventional almost everywhere except in the Far East to eat an amount of green vegetables supplying more than 1 or 2 g of protein per day or to eat fermented soy products.

The minerals and vitamins that we need are distributed so widely in conventional foods that there is little need to look for new sources of them unless they have been removed or destroyed by modern techniques of food handling, a form of unconventionality to which we have now become accustomed. The need can, therefore, often be met by returning to more primitive methods of food handling. In parts of the world where soil or water is deficient in elements such as calcium, fluorine, or iodine, the need for supplementation is well known. An ill-balanced diet, even if not subjected to sophisticated treatments, may be vitamin deficient. Unless ideology forbids it, the deficiency can be corrected with conventional foods. There is, for example, no need for vitamin A deficiency where green vegetables will grow or for vitamin C deficiency where potatoes or fruit will grow. The vitamin B group raises greater difficulties, but there is no basic unconventionality in supplying them by fermentation. Beer, especially if the yeast is still present, supplies several of them. Vegetarians often get a scanty supply of vitamin B_{12}. It is made by several molds so that it could be supplied by the minor unconventionality of "seeding" a cheese, yogurt, or fermented bean mixture with one of these effective molds as well as with the organisms usually relied on. Thus, the only unconventionality needed to satisfy the world's mineral and vitamin requirements is that we should think rationally about nutrition.

Plants synthesize fats and carbohydrates so efficiently that ensuring an adequate supply of them is more an administrative than a scientific problem. If the agricultural policies outlined in earlier chapters are implemented effectively, there is no physical reason preventing human energy requirements from being adequately met. Of course, it will not be easy to overcome the nonphysical obstacles; however, we should question the wisdom of proposals to make fats or carbohydrates by total synthesis in factories when they could be made as cheaply and abundantly by intelligently managed agriculture. The position with proteins is radically different: proteins differ in quality, methods for producing adequate amounts in all regions of the world are not known, and we are bedeviled by arguments about the amount needed. Purely biochemical and physiological considerations should specify how much protein each person needs. Communities or individuals who apparently eat as little as 40 g of protein a day may show no blatant signs of malnutrition, whereas those that apparently eat 100 g may show no signs of plethora. Energy intake varies much less. The question is: would the first communities fare better on more protein or the second on less? A naive approach is to measure how much protein an individual needs to be in nitrogen balance. Obviously, someone not in balance is getting too little protein and will go on being depleted until an equilibrium is established at which metabolism is depressed so much that it matches intake. But it is unwarrantable to assume that as soon as the balance is struck, say at about 40 g protein per person per day, nutrition is adequate. Furthermore, if the average protein consumption in a community is 40 g a day, half get less than this. Communities vary in the extent to which food is evenly distributed. But there are few communities in which those most in need of protein, children and pregnant or lactating women, get preferential treatment. Foods rich in protein are usually the most highly esteemed parts of the diet and, through custom and selfishness, men tend to get more than their share of them. It will be necessary to supply much more than the minimum amount of protein to ensure that everyone gets that minimum.

The ideal is easily stated: a person whose energy intake is adequate is not getting enough protein when well-being is increased by eating more protein. The ideal is easy to state but less easy to define or measure. With domestic animals we know what we want – rapid growth, a certain bodily conformation, a large milk yield, or abundant eggs. Although children grow much more slowly than domestic animals, their growth rate is a good index of the amount of protein in the diet. There is no evidence that rapid growth is desirable; some experiments on animals even suggest that it shortens the ultimate expectation of life. Life tables, however, do not suggest that the nonobese members of well-fed communities have suffered.

No one would wish casually to increase the difficulties of countries with a food shortage by urging on them inflated nutritional standards; they should not, on the other hand, be encouraged to live in a 'fool's paradise,' and much of the money they now spend goes on prestige projects of more debatable value than improved nutrition. When we consider the diets actually eaten by the more productive members of the community, including members of official committees that give niggardly trophological advice to others, it seems reasonable to think that lack of protein makes many members of apparently well-fed communities less healthy and responsive than they could be. It is possible that the average amount of protein eaten should be as great at 100 g a day. This opinion is shared by those who organize the U.S. space program; astronauts, the most up-to-date elite group, get 120 g. Most countries offer their Olympic athletes even more.

In countries with an overall food shortage, the primary need is for more food and, for as long as the daily energy intake is inadequate, it would be extravagant folly to advocate any great emphasis on the protein content of the food. Until energy needs are satisfied, the expensive protein would simply be used by the body as fuel. That has been obvious for half a century; it recently seems to have come as a blinding revelation to many officials. Organizations that, for a decade or more, have stressed the need for more protein and have suggested means for getting it, now issue statements suggesting that protein and energy are, in a sense, alternatives. This is absurd. Both are needed, but methods for increasing the supply of the protein-deficient foods are already known. That is why the United Nations set up a Protein Advisory Group, but has not seen any need for a Carbohydrate Advisory Group or a Fat Advisory Group.

Therefore, this author's conclusion is that it is reasonable to restrict discussion about unconventional sources of food to protein concentrates that could be produced by simple techniques from resources that are or could be made available in the wet tropics. The greatest need is at present in the wet tropics, and any work done to improve the food supply there will automatically be applicable in other parts of the world. By contrast, improvements in the techniques used in industrialized countries will probably not be useful soon in the wet tropics. Work planned for the benefit of the industrialized countries will not necessarily have the same breadth of application.

THE POSSIBLE SOURCES OF FOOD PROTEINS

All proteins contain between 15 and 20% of nitrogen and the amount of protein that is present in a food is usually calculated from its nitrogen content. For a few years, agriculture can depend on the supply of nitrogen in soil and nitrogen slowly becomes available as igneous rock weathers; continuous farming depends on biological or industrial fixation of atmospheric nitrogen which is abundant. There is more variety in the sources from which carbon comes, which are shown to the left of Table 1. It is interesting to note that the most abundant source, the carbonate rocks which contain 1 to 2 kg of carbon per cm^2 of the earth's surface, contributes little to the food supply; the products of past photosynthesis, coal, oil, and gas which contain several g of carbon per cm^2, are just beginning to be used; and carbon dioxide, with only 80 mg of carbon per cm^2, is the source of almost all our food. Small as this source may seem to be, it is constantly replenished by respiration and rotting in spite of the annual removal of about 100,000 million tons of carbon by land and sea plants. Clearly, this is likely to remain our primary carbon source; unconventionality will be mainly directed at our method of exploiting it.

Edible Plants or Parts of Plants

Vegetables

Leaves, immature flowers, seeds, tubers, and other underground parts of plants are traditional foods almost everywhere. The species selected for use are not always the most productive or those with the most valuable balance of nutrients; they are those that are relatively free from fiber and harmful or strongly flavored components, and permit convenient peeling, podding, or threshing. Varieties with these qualities have been deliberately selected from among the wild plants for several thousand years. Unconventionality, therefore, will not be involved if this process continues and if it is extended to species with which Europeans were not, until recently, familiar. There are many groups of tropical leafy plants, e.g., Amaranthus and Basella, that have already had about as much selection as the Crucifers had had by 1700. They could probably be greatly improved by modern methods of selection and induced mutation. If the International Vegetable Research Institute, proposed by FAO,[5] is established, this should be part of its program. The use of new species of vegetable is an obvious unconventionality; there are others. Very few communities eat as much leafy material as is desirable, bearing in mind that leaves contain 20 to 30% of protein and are rich sources of carotene (pro-vitamin A). In many parts of the tropics where they grow readily and where vitamin A deficiency is common, leafy vegetables are eaten to a much smaller extent than they are in Europe and U.S. The popularization of vegetable eating would be a valuable innovation. A first step toward this, and possibly an easier one, would be to persuade those concerned with vegetable production to publish such complete records that the yields of edible protein per hectare and year could be calculated. The figures would probably be so impressive that interest in leafy vegetables would increase greatly.

Seeds

Although the cereal seeds supply more than half the protein eaten in well-nourished countries and a still greater proportion in malnourished countries, the seeds of conventional strains contain little protein. Furthermore, the mixture of proteins they contain is not as favorable nutritionally as protein from most animal sources. The recent increase in interest in the amount and quality of the protein in food quickly led to the recognition that some strains of maize, which had been unesteemed for 35 years, were better sources of lysine than conventional strains. Many institutes are now searching for cereal strains with all the merits – large yield, good quality protein, large percentage of protein, and disease resistance. The results are encouraging. There are sorghums with 3 to 4% of nitrogen in the grain, wheats with up to 3.8%, barley with 3.1%, and oats with 4.8%. Experience with other cereal seeds suggests that almost all the nitrogen will be contained in proteins; it is too early to tell how well these strains satisfy the other requirements.

Little need be said about legume seeds; their use is traditional throughout the subtropics and those parts of the tropics where rainfall is so distributed that they can ripen. The only unconventionality envisaged, with those that can be eaten with no more pretreatment than cooking, is in such aspects of husbandry as adequate use of manures, protection from disease and predation, and encouragement of those insects, ants, etc. that are necessary for fertilization. The yields commonly attained are probably much smaller than those that are possible. Groundnuts (*Arachis* or *Voandzeia*) can yield 500 kg of protein per hectare in four months. The more productive

TABLE 1

- Sources of carbon for human food
  - Atmospheric carbon dioxide used by photosynthesis
    - Edible plants or parts of plants
    - Plants or parts of plants that need processing
      - Extraction
        - (with Edible plants or parts of plants:) Only the size of the edible units distinguishes these two types of plant protein concentrate
      - Conversion by animals
        - Fish
          - From the sea and other large bodies of water
          - Supplied with food in ponds
        - Birds and single-stomached mammals
        - Ruminants, stall-fed or grazing on potentially arable land
          - (Supplied with food in ponds; Birds and single-stomached mammals; Ruminants, stall-fed or grazing on potentially arable land:) Except when wastes are used these compete directly with people
        - Ruminants, domestic or wild, maintained on nonarable land or agricultural by-products
      - Microbial conversion
        - (with the Microbial conversion below:) The "biomass" may need extraction or conversion by an animal
  - Reduced forms of carbon, e.g., coal, oil, gas
  - Carbonates after chemical reduction
    - (Reduced forms of carbon; Carbonates after chemical reduction:)
      - Microbial conversion
      - Purely chemical transformation
        - Amino acids
        - Carbohydrates
        - Fats

strains of *Phaseolus* can, in ideal conditions, yield as much as that; yields from *Cajanus, Vigna, Cicer,* and *Pisum* are smaller. Obviously, two or even three crops can be grown in a year in some climates. A hectare devoted to growing legume seeds could, therefore, supply about 1 ton of protein per year as a concentrate containing 25 to 30% protein. The Indian Agricultural Research Institute has published two valuable surveys of recent research on seed proteins.[6]

It is now unconventional to eat seeds from plants other than cereals and legumes, although there is evidence that *Chenopodium* seeds were at one time a staple in Europe, and nuts are eaten on a small scale. Quinoa, a member of the *Chenopodium* family, is eaten in the highlands of South America. Although it has not been subjected to any up-to-date selection and is probably suboptimally fertilized, it yields up to 3 tons of seed per hectare. The seed contains 15% protein. It seems to be a crop much more worthy of attention than buckwheat (*Fagopyrum*), which contains only 10% protein.

Underground Parts

Except for groundnuts, which are legume seeds that bury themselves as they develop, the underground parts of plants seem to be protein deficient. Some of the yams contain 2.5% nitrogen. If this is mainly protein nitrogen, it might be worthwhile trying to breed strains that are still richer in protein, because some yams are well adapted to wet tropical regions where seeds do not ripen readily. However, the use of cassava, potatoes, yams, etc. is so widespread that the use of improved strains hardly amounts to an unconventionality.

Plant Products That Need Some Form of Processing

Many plants, or parts of plants, contain good quality protein that is not useable as human food because it is accompanied by other materials that are indigestible, unpalatable, or harmful. The other materials may be useful sources of energy, but become troublesome diluents when a protein concentrate is being sought. To get a protein concentrate, all that is necessary is fractionation. This procedure must be sharply distinguished from conversion in an animal and from the use of a protein-deficient material, fortified with a cheap source of nitrogen, such as ammonium phosphate, so as to enable microorganisms to grow. One or the other of these processes is sometimes unavoidable if the material is not to be wasted. But conversion is a successful method for making a protein concentrate only because the animal excretes (wastes from our egocentric standpoint) even more of the carbon than the nitrogen in its fodder, thus accumulating protein.

Mechanical Fractionation

The method of fractionation that can be used most effectively with a seed or nut depends on the manner in which protein is distributed within it. In rice, protein is concentrated in a layer immediately under the bran; it can be separated from the main body of the endosperm by suitably contrived abrasion; equipment for doing this is in use in various parts of the world. Starting with rice containing only 8 or 9% protein, fractions containing up to 21% protein can be separated. It is claimed that by combining abrasion with solvent extraction the yield of the protein-rich fraction can be increased. This process also concentrates the thiamine and riboflavin; these products are already being used commercially in baby foods. In a somewhat similar manner, coarse wheat flour is separated in an airstream into protein-rich and protein-depleted fractions. This is more convenient than the traditional wet process, developed in China hundreds of years ago when gluten (*mien chin*) was separated, and introduced to Europe by Beccari in 1728. Fractions containing 30% protein can be made.

The problems raised by cottonseed differ from those raised by cereal seeds. It is already a concentrate which, after defatting, contains 50 to 60% protein, but contaminated with various brown pigments and with gossypol, a phenolic aldehyde that combines with lysine and makes it unavailable. There are strains of cotton free from these substances, but they are more subject to insect attack than normal cotton. These harmful substances are contained in discrete glands which can be separated from judiciously milled cottonseed by flotation or classification in an airstream. The exploitation of these methods has elevated cottonseed from being a source of oil and cattle fodder to the status of a human food which is gaining acceptance in Central America largely through the enterprise of INCAP in Guatemala.

Recognition of the potentialities of coconut protein has come much more slowly. Dry copra contains 20 to 25% protein and so it could be regarded as a protein concentrate, but the presence of 12 to 16% fiber limits the amount that can be eaten. Early attempts to separate protein and fiber were partly frustrated by the use of dried copra, expeller residue, or autoclaved coconuts. All of these pretreatments, to varying extents, coagulate the protein and so impede separation. Technologists in Mysore, the Philippines, and elsewhere have now stopped trying to be original and have reverted to the method that is traditional in the Pacific Islands: they disintegrate coconut meat with water warm enough to liquefy the fat but not to coagulate the protein. The resulting emulsion is "broken" and the protein coagulated from the aqueous layer. The concentrate contains 74% protein and the oil made in this way is of better quality than oil made by the usual procedure of drying and screw expulsion. There seems to be no serious obstacle to the widespread adoption of this wet-processing method; it would make 0.7 million tons of protein available for human nutrition that are presently either wasted or used as animal feed.

Seed residues left after expressing oil contain more than 30 million tons of protein (Table 2). Less than 1% of this is now used as human food and presently only about five times as much measures up to the quality standards that would make it acceptable as a food source. This very large potential protein source will not become useful until the producers realize the value of the residue and handle the crop, at all stages from harvest to processing, carefully and cleanly.

In arid regions or regions with seasonal rainfall, seed crops may yield better than leaf crops. In regions such as Britain, with well-distributed rain, leaf crops yield better than seed crops, and in regions where it rains nearly every day, seed crops tend to rot rather than ripen. In Britain, therefore, leaves are more productive than any other crop; in still wetter tropical regions leaves and coconuts are probably the only source from which protein concentrates can be made reliably.

TABLE 2

World Production of Seeds Yielding a Protein-rich Residue

	million tons/year	
Soy	46	Total protein content about 30 million tons
Cotton	22	
Groundnut	18	
Sunflower	10	
Rape	6.5	
Linseed	4	
Coconut	3	
Sesame	2	
Castor	1	

When the juice expressed from pulped fresh leaves is coagulated and the coagulum is filtered off, three products, protein coagulum, material soluble in water, and leaf fiber containing some unextracted protein, are made (Table 3). Each product must be used both for economy and to prevent local pollution. At different times and places, each has indeed been regarded as the main product with the others as by-products. At Rothamsted we attach most importance to the extracted protein and have designed equipment both for extracting crops on the 1 to 3 ton (wet weight) an hour scale and for making precise agronomic measurements on a laboratory scale. These pieces of equipment and the equipment used commercially in Hungary and the U.S. are described in Handbook 20 of the International Biological Program.[7] That handbook also describes the separation and purification of the protein and gives information about its composition, nutritional value, and presentation on the table.

By using a succession of crops on the same land, the yield of dry extracted protein can, in a favorable year, exceed 2 tons per hectare; five cuts of cocksfoot yielded 1.67 tons in a less favorable year. The actual yield in any year depends greatly on the weather, especially on rainfall in late spring and early summer. With increasing skill and the use of irrigation water when necessary, we think it should be possible to get 3 tons in Britain regularly. In parts of India where cold weather does not stop growth, 3 tons have already been reached and 5 tons should be possible. In suitable regions, leaf protein production gives a greater yield of edible protein than any other method of land use. Furthermore, the crops used are harvested regularly or when young and so are less at risk to many pests, predators, and diseases than other crops.

Conversion by Animals

On Land

There is nothing unconventional about feeding an animal vegetable matter and then eating the animal, its milk, or its eggs. However, it seems to be unconventional to think carefully about the merits of different types of animal and about the optimal use of different types of resource. Land that is too rough or steep to plow or that is kept unplowed as an amenity either maintains ruminants or it produces no human food. The only question of principle raised is "Are the most productive types of animal used to graze and browse on it?" What evidence there is suggests that a mixed fauna makes better use of the land than a single species for the very simple reason that it can crop the vegetation at more levels, thus wasting less of it. The point seems to be geometrically inescapable but it requires rigorous experimental verification. If land were used extensively in this way, some of the meat produced would have an unfamiliar texture because meat from wild herbivores tends to contain less fat than meat from domestic animals. It is said that the "gamey" flavor often associated with the meat of wild animals is not intrinsic, but develops because of the way in which the meat is handled.

In many countries it would be very unconventional to eat invertebrates. Locusts are an important food in East Africa, insect eggs in Mexico, and the giant snail (*Achatina*) in West Africa and parts of the Pacific. It may not be worthwhile cultivating these animals in place of larger and more familiar animals. Even that is not certain; an acre of water is said to yield 4 to 5 tons (dry matter) of midge larvae in a year! But if the invertebrates are there and if it is the local custom to eat them, visiting "experts" should not disparage the custom merely because they find it unconventional.

There is more disagreement over the use of arable land. It can produce either animal food or human food along with some wastes and by-products that can be given to animals. Animals return between 5 and 20% of the protein they eat as edible protein. The use of potentially arable land primarily to produce animal fodder is, therefore, a pleasant extravagance that wealthy countries can indulge; it is astounding to find FAO[5] urging similar extravagance on protein-deficient countries. Wastes and by-products that are inedible because they contain too much fiber should be supplemented with urea or some similar source of nitrogen and used as ruminant feed instead of being burned or allowed to rot as they often are now. Domestic wastes that we prefer not to eat are potential feed for nonruminants such as pigs and chickens. But the maintenance of more animals than can be fed on by-products or on nonarable land is misguided in a country that is deficient in protein.

In Water

Unconventional ways of using fish are widely advocated because perishability complicates distribution. This advocacy may be questioned; it may be an attempt to find a technological solution for a problem that it would be better to solve by social or economic changes. In many countries, fish-marketing and fish preservation by smoking or drying are still in a medieval state. Improvements in the distribution of marine fish, so that they could move quickly a few more miles inland, and the application of the principles of Intermediate Technology to fish preservation, would do as much to increase fish consumption as the industrial production of tasteless, odorless, and structureless fish powders will do. However, when the productive fishing grounds are far from land, the fish must either be frozen or processed at sea. The course preferred depends on costs and the value to be placed on the common preference for fish that still tastes of fish.

The ocean yields potential foods besides fish. FAO[5] estimates the potential cephalopod harvest as 9 million tons (wet weight) of which less than 1 million tons are now caught. A major culinary revolution will be needed before this resource is fully exploited. Antarctic krill are even more abundant. The potential is thought to be 50 million tons (wet weight) a year. The dried material, after solvent extraction, contains more than 70% protein; the 6% of chitin that it also contains is probably useless in human nutrition, but there is no reason to think it harmful. The policy at present seems to be to exterminate whales and then catch what had been their food for use as pig and chicken feed; to an outsider it would seem more sensible to let the whales do the fishing and exploit them optimally. Where ocean currents bring in a regular supply of new food-laden water, mussels can be very productive if they are supplied with points of attachment and protected from predators. Ropes hung from rafts perform both duties and the yield of protein (dry weight) can then exceed 2 tons per hectare a year. This yield, though impressive, is obviously not strictly comparable to a photosynthetic yield because most of the mussel's food grows elsewhere and is merely eaten at the site where measurements are made. Nevertheless, there are many

TABLE 3

The Three Products Made by Fractionating a Fresh Leafy Crop

Juice, which gives after coagulation	coagulum containing	proteins fats starch	Food for man and other nonruminants
	fluid containing	amino acids amides sugars salts, etc.	Medium for the growth of microorganisms
Fibrous residue containing	most of the	cellulose hemicelluloses lignins pectin	Still a fodder for ruminants and a substrate for microbial fermentation
	some of the	proteins fats starch	

suitable unused sites and an estimated 1.5 million tons of potential food are suspended in the oceans. There seems to be a case for the popularization of clam chowder.

The point made in the last paragraph applies with equal force to freshwater fish farming. Many claims made for it are unrealistic because the fish are maintained on food grown elsewhere and do not differ in principle from pigs in a pen. Herbivorous fish, living on vegetation growing in and around a pond or canal, are rapidly gaining recognition as a means of controlling water weeds. The Chinese grass carp (*Ctenopharyngodon*) is particularly favored because of its prodigious appetite – it eats its own weight in weeds daily. Although the idea of using fish to keep waterways clear may be unconventional, there is nothing unusual about the flesh of the fish. The manatee, a wholly aquatic herbivorous mammal, can also be used to keep waterways clear. Its meat has a characteristic flavor and texture; it could not, therefore, be disguised as the meat of a land mammal, but it is so acceptable as a food that difficulty is foreseen in discouraging poachers.

Unconventional Photosynthetic Plants

The assumption underlying this discussion so far is that the plants on which future food supplies will depend will be of familiar types or, if unfamiliar, will be those that grow wild. The photosynthetic yield of these plants in normal conditions is considerably less than that attainable in theory. Possibly, the yields would be greater if unconventional plants were used, which might be advantageous in spite of the unfamiliarity of the material produced. During the past 30 years, most attention has been given to single-celled green algae, such as *Chlorella,* which, when cultivated in carefully controlled laboratory conditions, outyielded ordinary agriculture. But in comparable conditions there is no evidence that they are any more efficient than familiar plants; nothing would be gained by digging ponds in arable land so as to cultivate algae in them. There are, however, circumstances in which algal cultivation is sensible. In sunny regions they grow well in sewage, purify the water, and, at the same time, produce a mixed mass of algae and bacteria; this can be used as chicken feed but probably not as human food. Because they are submerged and do not transpire, they do not need as much water as higher plants and so could be useful in deserts. Some, notably the multicellular blue-green alga *Spirulina,* flourish in alkaline lakes and are a traditional human food in North Africa and Mexico. Because of this ability, *Spirulina* is now being grown commercially as human food.

Most Temperate Zone crops use light less efficiently as it gets stronger. Many tropical plants, notably maize and sugar cane, have a different photosynthetic mechanism and work efficiently even in full sunlight. Some desert plants hold the record for rate of photosynthesis per unit of leaf area. Unfortunately, desert plants are sparse so that the yield per hectare is small, and most of the material synthesized is not edible. Now that the possibility of achieving rates of photosynthesis greater than those to which we are accustomed is realized, it will be the job of the agronomist to see whether a potentiality can be turned into agricultural reality and the job of biochemical engineers to see what use can be made of the products.

Microbial Conversions

Logical classification is always difficult and sometimes impossible. The feature unifying previous discussion is that the methods discussed depend on atmospheric carbon dioxide and photosynthesis, regardless of the size of the plant photosynthesizing. The microorganisms considered in this section do not photosynthesize, but depend on carbon supplied by other plants, either present or past, and on the photochemically produced oxygen of the atmosphere. The prefix micro is, by convention, not used rigidly; fungi large enough to be handled are included in the category. Conversion by animals has been discussed separately, although the process does not differ in any essential respect from conversion by microorganisms.

Microorganisms have two roles in food production. Without multiplying to such an extent that they become a major component of the final product, they can alter the texture of an inedible raw material, digest a component in it to which human digestion is unadapted, destroy a harmful or unpleasant component, and contribute a desired flavor. Alternatively, they can grow so extensively that they consume the greater part of the raw material, so that what is finally harvested consists almost exclusively of microbial material, commonly called "biomass."

Soy is traditionally made more digestible and palatable in the Far East by fermentation with various microorganisms; one third of the protein eaten in Indonesia comes from fermented soy and groundnut. These methods could usefully be applied to other inedible or unattractive beans. They are well adapted to use on a small scale for local production, unlike more thoroughly investigated methods which depend on extracting the protein or destroying harmful substances by controlled heat treatment. The idea of using the many microorganisms that make enzymes that are able to convert the cellulose in fibrous materials into smaller molecules that are metabolizable by nonruminants, including man, is attractive, but it has not proved practical so far. The isolated enzymes are eaten in Japan in the hope that they will carry out the digestion within the consumer, but there is no definite evidence of success.

Part of the carbohydrate in protein-deficient foodstuffs can be converted to protein by using them, with an inorganic nitrogen source, as substrates for microbial growth. This method has been used to double the percentage of protein in the final products from barley, rice, and wheat for animal feed and it is being studied as a means of increasing the percentage of protein in foods based on cassava.

In principle, it makes little difference whether microorganisms are grown on a substrate produced by agriculture, a substrate such as coal, gas, or oil in which the carbon is already reduced, or limestone in which the carbon is oxidized. In practice, it makes an immense difference. Beer and wine making is so nearly universal that it is obvious that no community would have difficulty in managing a fermentation system using molasses, where this is abundant, and other fluids elsewhere. In the Philippines 1 million tons of coconut water are wasted annually and 0.3 million tons of whey solids are wasted annually in U.S.; the quantity of sugar-rich effluent increases yearly as more vegetables and potatoes are processed industrially. A small potato-processing factory sends out as much clean organic matter as is contained in the sewage from a town with 100,000 inhabitants and there will be much useful effluent when leaf protein production begins on an industrial scale. With present arrangements, most of this valuable material goes to increase the pollution problem and cause eutrophication in rivers and lakes.

Solid agricultural wastes are less tractable and the simple solution of feeding them to ruminants may be the best. Town refuse, even when screened, is unsuitable for animals because of the risk that it will contain broken glass and other noxious material. Fermentation with the help of cellulose-digesting organisms could be applied to it also; the resulting fluid would then be used as the substrate for growing another useful microorganism. That would solve the problem of noxious solids in the waste but such a system would be a risk to soluble poisons. It might be better to make use of the fact that the larger fungi grow upward and so automatically free themselves from the material on which they grow. What is envisaged is the seeding of pulped waste with fungus, incubating the mass until cap formation is imminent, and then spreading out the mass in thin layers for the brief period of rapid growth. The whole process could be mechanized in countries not suffering from unemployment.

Fermentation is a form of combustion; part of the substrate is oxidized to carbon dioxide, which is the process that produces energy for growth. As in all such systems, energy transfer is incomplete and some appears as heat. When carbohydrates are the substrate, heating is a trivial problem. It is formidable with gas or oil; the heat generated is about half what would have been generated had the gas or oil been burned and it has to be removed at a temperature low enough to permit microbial growth. This difficulty can be partly resolved by preliminary partial oxidation of the substrate, e.g., by turning CH_4 into CH_3OH, which could yield heat at a useful high temperature rather than at an embarrassing low one.

This point is not raised captiously, but to dispel the illusion spread by the popular media that an area the size of Manhattan could satisfy the world's protein needs from oil. The fermentation tanks might be fitted onto Manhattan, but the Hudson River would not suffice to cool them. Microorganisms grown on the products of past photosynthesis are most likely to contribute to the nutrition of those who now need food by supplying pig and chicken food for affluent countries. This will minimize the consumption in affluent countries of protein concentrates (such as fish meal and groundnuts) produced by malnourished communities that should be using these concentrates at home. However, this should cause no distress. Annual production of oil is less than 2,000 million tons, of which a tenth is the straight-chain paraffin fraction that the oil companies wish to dispose of to food manufacturers; photosynthesis supplies 100,000 million tons of carbon a year, mostly without human help. Still more will be brought into circulation when agriculture is more efficiently organized.

Synthesis

Bearing in mind the initial argument that the most important types of unconventional food are those that could be made from local products for local consumption by people without great technical capacity, synthetic foods are not likely to be important. However, few communities will prosper unless they engage in some trade with industrialized countries; some synthesizable components of an adequate diet are needed in small amounts only. The vitamins are one example, but, as already pointed out, foods rich in them can be produced by conventional means. Some of the amino acids are now synthesized and put into animal feeding stuffs; in this way a cheap but incomplete protein can be given the nutritional value of a better but more expensive one. It may be worthwhile adding amino acids to human foods also. This will be discussed in the next section.

The entirely false idea has been spread by popular writers that eating could degenerate into swallowing a few synthetic pills every day. Regardless of the sources from which our food comes or the form we choose to give it, the weight (dry matter) eaten each day by an average adult will remain 400 to 500 g because the necessary amount of metabolizable energy cannot be packed into less. That would make a formidable pile of pills.

THE NUTRITIONAL VALUE OF UNCONVENTIONAL FOODS

The production of adequate amounts of carbohydrate and fat raises no serious scientific problems and their merits are easy to assess. People cannot metabolize every type of fat and carbohydrate, but those that are metabolized are of equal value. Fortunately, most plants that grow vigorously make starch or sucrose. The amino acids in proteins are the essentials in food; eight are particularly important because people cannot synthesize them or use others to substitute for them. But there is no need for all eight to be present in the correct ratio in any single protein. It is the amino acids in the diet as a whole that matter. The merits of a protein source, therefore, cannot be judged without knowing what other proteins are being eaten along with it. Two proteins completely devoid of different essential amino acids, so that neither could be the sole protein source in an adequate diet, could be the protein component of an adequate diet if eaten together. Unfortunately, two or three of the amino acids are scarce in almost all proteins except those in milk and eggs. There are, therefore, limits to the upgrading that is possible by judiciously mixing the dietary proteins. Proteins rich in those amino acids that are usually scarce are now being looked for in many different plant species and varieties. There have been a few successes, but no good plant source of the sulfur-containing amino acid, methionine, has been found. Fortunately, this could be added as it can be synthesized. Addition of a synthetic amino acid is not necessary unless a protein is nearly free from that amino acid; a mere deficiency can be compensated for by eating more of the protein.

Judgments on the nutritional merits of different proteins, based on chemical analysis, must be confirmed by tests on animals with digestive systems similar to our own because the protein may not be digestible and some of the amino acids in it may be linked to other substances in a manner that makes them unavailable. Interpretation of the results is not always easy because it may take weeks for the digestive system of an animal to adapt to a new type of food, and the tests should be prolonged lest another component in the potential food should be harmful.

CONVENTIONALIZING THE UNCONVENTIONAL

Most articles on the world's food supply assert that it is difficult to change food habits and suggest that the attempt may be scarcely worth making. The conclusion is quite unfounded. Any middle-aged person in an affluent country can look back on many changes in local food habits. The readiness with which people in poor countries spend money on imported novel foods of doubtful value distresses all those working on child welfare in those countries. The present author has given[7,8] many examples of changes, both for the better and worse. Strictures on commercial concerns that claim to be selling nutrition, when all they are actually selling is convenience, appear regularly in such journals as *Cajanus,* the newsletter of the Caribbean Food and Nutrition Institute.

Attempts to change food habits must be made with intelligence and sympathy. Many months of expert work in the kitchen are needed to determine how to present the unconventional food acceptably and in a manner adapted to the cooking facilities and eating habits of the recipients. Those who are advocating change must be convinced that the change would benefit the recipients; they must be regular and obvious users of the food themselves and must not expect immediate success. If possible, the food should be given prestige by being accepted by a few prestigious local people; it may be used in clinics so long as it is served as a food and not a medicine, but it should not be introduced first in such places as refugee camps, orphanages, and prisons. A stigma is hard to rub off.

A few valuable unconventional foods have achieved economic success; notably the cottonseed-based product, Incaparina, in Central America and fish sausage in Japan. However, the probability of early commercial success is small. Beneficial changes are not likely to be made without support from a government, foundation, or international agency. This point has been made repeatedly by groups of varied political commitment, e.g., the World Health Organization,[9] the Harvard Business School,[10] the U.S. President's Science Advisory Committee,[11] and the U.N. Economic and Social Council which advocates a "protein development tax" on various luxury items.[12] Nevertheless, many economists still consider the food supply in old-fashioned economic terms.

When the job of ensuring that the world is properly fed is taken seriously, some reallocation of the effort put into different forms of research and development will be needed. It seems anomalous that the senior staff of the International Rice Research Institute in the Philippines numbers 17, whereas that of the Rubber Research Institute of Malaya numbers more than 100. Within food research there are anomalies arising from history, commercial interest, and unawareness of potentialities. More effort is devoted to soy than to all the other legume seeds together, and a thousand times more to microbial conversion of oil than to leaf protein, although the latter is potentially the most abundant of the protein sources and is particularly well adapted to the wet tropics. In Britain, 2% of the value of the fish landed is spent on research and development, whereas the average for the food industry is considerably less than 1%. The more adequately financed directions of research and development are well worth the money spent on them; there is every reason to think that more effort devoted to the more unconventional lines discussed in this paper would be equally rewarding.

REFERENCES

1. **Le Gros Clark, F. and Pirie, N. W.,** *Four Thousand Million Mouths,* Oxford University Press, London 1951.
2. **Schaefer, A. E.,** quoted from *Time,* January 31, 1969.
3. Malnutrition and hunger in the United States, *J.A.M.A.,* 213, 1, 1970.
4. **Corry Mann, H. C.,** Diets for boys during the school age, *Med. Res. Council Special Report* 105, H.M.S.O. 1926 (reprinted 1930).
5. *Provisional Indicative World Plan for Agricultural Development,* Vol. 1, FAO, Rome, 1969.
6. Recent Research on the Improvement of Protein and Nutritive Properties of Food and Feed Plants, I.A.R.I. Research Bulletin (New Series No. 6) New Delhi, 1971; New Vistas in Pulse Production, Indian Agricultural Research Institute, New Delhi, 1971.
7. **Pirie, N. W.,** *Food Resources: Conventional and Novel,* Penguin Books, Harmondsworth, Middlesex, 1969.
8. **Pirie, N. W.,** The direction of beneficial nutritional change, in *Ecology of Food and Nutrition,,* 1279-294, 1972.
9. World Health Organization, Review of expansion of production and consumption of protein-rich foods prepared by industrial processing, Report to UNCTAD, 1966.
10. Harvard Business School, *The Protein Paradox: Malnutrition, Protein-rich Foods, and the Role of Business,* Management Reports, Boston, Mass., 1966.
11. President's Science Advisory Committee. *The World Food Problem,* Vol. 1, Report of the panel on the world food supply, Washington, D. C., 1967.
12. U.N. Department of Economic and Social Affairs, Strategy statement on action to avert the protein crisis in the developing countries, United Nations, New York, 1971.

IMPROVING NUTRIENT COMPOSITION OF PLANTS THROUGH GENETICS AND AGRONOMIC PRACTICES

H. T. Hopkins

TABLE OF CONTENTS

Introduction 203

Element Composition and Nutritional Status of Plants 203

Soil and Other Site Factors in Relation to Nutrient Composition of Plants 205

Nutritional Quality of Foods and Feeds of Plant Origin 207

Improving Nutritional Quality of Plants Through Genetic and Agronomic Measures 209
- Proteins, Vitamins, Hormones, and Other Substances 209
- Inorganic Elements 211
- Effect of Herbicides in Improving the Protein Content of Plants 212

Conclusions 212
- Acknowledgments 212

References 213

INTRODUCTION

The purpose of this chapter is to examine various practices, primarily genetic and agronomic, for improving the nutritional quality of foods of plant origin. Due to the scattered nature of information relative to this question, an exhaustive analysis of pertinent literature was not attempted. Rather, an effort has been made to be selective and to identify certain ideas, principles, and institutional positions relating to this question.

ELEMENT COMPOSITION AND NUTRITIONAL STATUS OF PLANTS

Investigators in plant nutrition have generally striven to identify soil conditions, amounts and sources of inorganic elements, plant hormones, light, water, temperature, and other factors determinant to the optimal growth and yield of field crops. Element composition of plant tissue, in theory at least, reflects the nutritional status of higher plants. Concentrations of certain inorganic elements in leaves and other plant tissues can be related to crop performance.[1,2]

Sixty-eight years ago Hall[3] advanced the notion, accepted by almost all later workers, that the element composition of plants reflects the amount of the element available to plant roots as measured by crop yield. Macy[4] pointed out, however, that this view embodied the concept of the *sufficiency* of one nutrient relative to all other factors influencing yield response rather than the absolute nutrient supply. For example, in data reported by Hall[3] and further extended by Gilbert,[5] season had a greater effect on the nitrogen composition of wheat than the addition of extra soil nitrogen, but the response data showed that when the nitrogen supply was high, it was definitely more sufficient because grain yield was increased 57% in the "poor" season and 230% in the "good" season. As the yield increased in the "good" crop year, the nitrogen concentration of grain decreased irrespective of the addition of extra nitrogen. These data illustrate the well-known inverse relation between yield and protein content of grain and reflect a competitive relation between straw and grain for factors which ultimately limit yield. Schlehuber and Tucker[6] discussed certain misinterpretations of this inverse relation appearing during the first decade of the 20th century, as follows: With a constant and suboptimal soil nitrogen supply, increased crop yields dilute the protein content of the grain. Recent work by Warner et al.[7] indicates that nitrate reductase activity level in corn plants is related directly to corn yields. Interestingly, the F_1 hybrid resulting from crossing two inbred lines of *Zea Mays L.* had a higher heterotic level of nitrate reductase than either parent.[7]

Macy[4] grew alpha barley plants in triplicate on two different soils using six levels of nitrogen applied as sodium nitrate. Results indicated the existence of a threshold optimum nitrogen level (the so-called critical percentage) in the grain above which there was luxury consumption and below which there was poverty adjustment. Below the latter there was the minimum percentage of nitrogen. The threshold optimum for nitrogen content was considered an inherited trait.[4] Environmental factors other than nitrogen supply could change the nutrient composition, but they did not change the relation between the minimum percentage, poverty adjustment, and luxury consumption. Threshold optimum nitrogen content was considered to be connected intimately to the relation between vegetative and reproductive phases during the growth cycle. Poverty adjustment was defined as a partially limiting factor. In essence, this suggests a form of homeostasis, or an internal nutrient element balance.[8]

Existence in rose clover (*Trifolium hirtum*) of a four-step relation between yield and magnesium concentration (all other essential nutrients not limiting) was reported by Specht[9] as follows: minimum percentage, poverty adjustment, luxury consumption, and toxic level. Using solution culture techniques and 17 levels of magnesium replicated ten times, data were obtained supporting the view that plants possess a mechanism which controls degrees of variability of element content in their tissues. Underlying this hypothesis were three concepts, as follows: (1) degree of variability in concentration of a given element may be related to the level of its concentration in plant tissue; (2) action of a variation control mechanism during the growth cycle may produce element-variability patterns defining optimum growth ranges for nutrients; and (3) the magnitude of element interaction phenomena may be subject to the action of a variation control mechanism in the plant. Pertinent to these concepts, Specht[9] cited the need for having a backlog of compositional data on specific plant tissue that can serve as a reference base, homogeneity of sample materials relative to physiological factors, and standardization of analysis and interpretation of plant composition. These concepts and principles could be used in the assessment of the status of any substance in plants relative to environmental factors.[9] Magnesium content of clover forage could be increased almost tenfold over the range of external supply from acute deficiency to luxury consumption. As the supply of magnesium was increased further, the yield remained unchanged or decreased, but the magnesium concentration continued to increase up to the toxicity level. Thus, the action of the variation-control mechanism was keyed to the internal concentration of a given nutrient.[9]

In a somewhat similar study, Bould[10] noted that the fruiting stage in strawberry plants was the most sensitive for diagnosis of nutrient status of the leaves. In the absence of non-nutritional limiting factors, fertilizer responses were obtained if the levels of nitrogen, phosphorus, potassium, or magnesium were lower than those in the so-called deficient class. No fertilizer response was seen if leaf values were higher than those classed as sufficient.[10]

Field crop engineering was reported by Clements[11] on the industrial crop sugar cane (*Saccharum officinarum L.*). Sixteen crops were grown at two locations in the Hawaiian Islands. Weight, moisture content, dry matter, total sugar, hydrolyzable carbohydrate, total nitrogen, phosphorus, potassium, calcium, and magnesium were determined on each of four different tissues collected at about 35-day intervals. After evaluating more than 100,000 bits of data by partial regression, it was found that the leaf sheath of young mature leaves (i.e., leaves three, four, five, and six from the top leaf) was best for monitoring the "well-being" of sugar cane during its growth cycle. This procedure was referred to as the crop log.[11] Under these conditions, sugar cane yield was judged more dependent upon the energy level of light and solar heat than upon soil factors. Maximum yields, however, can be obtained only by maintaining high tissue moisture levels.[12] Actual levels of sheath tissue moisture, nitrogen, potassium, and total sugars of the sheaths are found within 48 to 72 hr after sampling, whereupon they are plotted on the log and compared with "normal" levels and the necessary corrective action can be taken. At times the crop log data are backed with root and soil pH data covering the potentially toxic trace elements, manganese, zinc, and copper. Imposition of a mild moisture stress can prevent blossoming of sugar cane.[12]

These four studies suggest that leaf, organ, or total plant analyses done several times during the growth cycle permit one to define levels of specific mineral elements, soil management practices, or other factors required for the near optimal growth and yield of specific crops. When this strategy was used on sugar cane, both the yield and the quality of the sugar cane were improved.[12] Additional information on crop yields relative to the nutrient supply in soils is given by Steenbjerg and Jakobsen.[13]

For mineral elements not mobile in the phloem, leaves may not be the tissue of choice for monitoring the nutrient status of plants.[14] What is important here is that *tissue* analysis, when done on specific plants for specific nutrients at specific times, can provide a useful guide to plant breeders, biochemists, plant physiologists, and others as they work together toward improving the nutritional quality of foods of plant origin.

According to Wallace et al.,[15] the entity of crop yield is made up of multiple characters. Expression of yield depends on the functioning and interaction of many physiological components within the plant itself. Certain limiting physiological components within the plant tend to vary between plant varieties. Genetic control of yield occurs *indirectly* through control of physiological components which interact to produce an economic yield. Plant growth and grain yield of corn are the end result of a series of biochemical reactions each of which is catalyzed by one or more specific enzymes.[16] Functional effectiveness of enzymes may vary, both within and between cells and tissues during seed germination, growth, maturation, and fruiting.[16]

Vegetative and reproductive growth patterns differ among plants. Vegetative growth is determinant to both the potential number of seeds and the photosynthetic (leaf) capacity to sustain growth and maturation of the seed.[15] During ontogeny, one would expect to find many critical nutrient interactions, competitive and otherwise. More rapid and predictable yield improvement may be expected from planning crosses so as to maximize the segregation of genotypes possessing the physiological complementation and balance of biochemical and physiological processes.[15] For example, excessive activity of one enzymatic component may limit another to a level below the optimum.[17]

Judging from these various observations, it is apparent that higher plants contain heritable physiological components, primarily enzymatic, which may or may not respond to fertilizers or other manipulations at certain times during their growth cycle. Apparently, one desirable stratagem for further improvement of the mineral and trace element quality of foods of plant origin would be to maximize the segregation of genotypes having a greater competence to respond to specific inorganic nutrients under a wide range of moisture, temperature, and light regimes.

SOIL AND OTHER SITE FACTORS IN RELATION TO THE NUTRIENT COMPOSITION OF PLANTS

Evaluation of soil and other site factors relative

to nutrient composition of plants growing in the temperate and humid tropic zones may be categorized as follows: (1) soil inventory and (2) soil management systems.[18] Soil inventories are based on the detailed mapping of soils presently used for areas of intensive cropping and irrigation schemes, as well as those areas having relatively infertile soils but with good potential for future use. In the humid tropics, the latter areas refer, in part, to the microvariability associated with termite mounds and the microrelief.[18] Topographic and other features included in soil survey maps and reports are essential in hilly terrain where slope exposure can be rather decisive for crop yields if experience in the temperate zone can be used as a guide. Recently, in experiments reported from West Virginia on the effect of slope orientation on the yield of bluegrass (*Poa pratensis L.*), yield responses during a three-year period were two- to sixfold greater when growing on north slopes than on south slopes, each of which received nitrogen applications ranging from 112 to 448 kg/hectare.[19] Interestingly enough, the average percentage of nitrogen in bluegrass leaves was essentially the same on either the north or south slopes, irrespective of the level of nitrogen applied. This suggests an important area for improvement of bluegrass yields, particularly with reference to the likelihood that nitrate reductase activity in bluegrass leaves was inhibited by temperature and moisture stresses.

Current soil management practices in tropical areas are usually subject to improvement generally within the socioeconomic conditions of that area.[18] Fertilizers need not be the only component of the soil management system. For example, manipulation of physical and chemical properties of soils as a means of controlling accelerated erosion, improving water infiltration rates, subsurface drainage, and improving the biological properties of soils can be practiced more widely.[18] Use of natural fallows should be continued and improved wherever feasible in the humid tropics. Practices such as the no-tillage systems used with corn culture in the U.S. could be explored for use in all areas.[20]

In the heavily cropped and leached soils of the temperate and tropical zones, soil nitrogen is the nutrient most often limiting crop growth and animal performance.[18,21]

Methodology for assessing the nitrogen-supplying capacities of temperate and humid tropical soils should be evaluated.[18] For example, movement and leaching patterns of nitrogen and trace elements need more detailed study to develop more efficient approaches to the application of these nutrients to soils.[18,22,23] Especially needed are more critical evaluations in tropical soils of biological nitrogen fixation such as the inoculation and management of leguminous crops and the evaluation of nonsymbiotic nitrogen fixation.[18]

Transfer of liming procedures as used in soils of the temperate zone to tropical zones appears to have done more harm than good. Many tropical soils not only have a high percentage of exchangeable aluminum saturation at soil pH values below 5.0, but also contain (as for certain temperate zone soils) low exchangeable calcium and magnesium.[18] Aluminum tolerant crops should be identified and new varieties developed having high resistance not only to aluminum, but also to sodium, zinc, copper, and manganese.[14,24]

Feed and food plants may grow normally, yet still not meet the dietary requirements of some animals.[21,24] Conversely, plants may grow normally, yet still contain levels of trace elements such as selenium, cadmium, and molybdenum that can trigger either direct toxicity or metabolic imbalances in animals.[24] Furthermore, plant growth will cease or be slowed when grown in soils containing high levels of arsenic, iodine, beryllium, fluorine, nickel, and zinc before these elements will be absorbed and accumulated at dangerous levels in plant tissue. To a degree, the soil-root-shoot system exerts a buffering action on the environmental cycling of trace elements.[24]

Particularly intriguing is the configuration of the root system in relation to nutrient uptake.[25] Resistance of soils to the transfer of mobile ions from widely spaced roots can actually lower the rate of ion uptake by plant roots when convection is minimal in the soil solution. High root densities can overcome resistance to ion transfer from the soil solution to root surfaces, except for the most immobile elements. Lack of knowledge of functional differences between roots of different age and form puts severe limits on present ability to interpret inorganic element uptakes.[25]

Inherent differences among hybrids with respect to depth of rooting was thought by Baker et al.[26] to influence the relative concentrations of elements accumulated in ear leaves of corn hybrids selected for low and high phosphorus accumulation by roots. These workers concluded that the concentration of phosphorus in corn seedlings can be used to predict the availability of soil phosphorus. On the basis of previous work, certain corn hybrids exhibited partial genetic control for the accumulation of phosphorus, potassium, calcium, magnesium, strontium, and zinc.[27-29]

In a discussion of soil dynamics, Nikiforoff[30] has warned that future replacement of wild vegetation and low yielding plants by plants designed to yield more protein, starch, and other nutrients for animals and man can be considered a rather drastic meddling with the driving force of short geochemical cycles. Conceivably, this might lead to disastrous results for man if this effort should be undertaken without a thorough understanding of soil genesis and dynamics. He concluded by saying that the order of the day should be a critical review of these concepts in the light of geochemistry and geophysics.[30]

Worldwide agricultural research should have as its primary goal the achievement of a continuous rise in the economic yield of crops per unit area per unit time, while maintaining the long-term productivity of the soil base.[31] Hybrid strains should be developed with the capability of giving an economic response both under dry land and controlled irrigation and fertilization practices.[31,32] Aside from efforts to increase crop and protein yields by fertilizer use, additional effort is needed to increase the nutritive quality of tuber crops, food grains, legumes, fruits, and vegetables to improve the nutrition of economically handicapped sections of the world population.[31]

Several years ago, Maynard[33,34] advanced a number of generalizations relative to the relationship between soil factors and the nutritive content of plants, as follows: (1) Addition of commercial fertilizers to the soil is an important step toward betterment of human health because it serves to increase the level of certain mineral elements in the soil, and leads to an increased yield or total amount of foods of plant and animal origin on a per hectare basis. (2) Addition of commercial fertilizers to the soil results in an improvement of the nutritive value of foods because it permits the production of vegetables and fruits having an inherently high nutritional quality. (3) Addition of fertilizers to the soil or other means of increasing the supply of mineral elements in the soil does not contribute importantly to variations in nutrient content or to variations in nutritional quality of foods. (4) Genetic and climatic factors are more important in governing variations in nutrient content of a specific harvested crop than are soil factors. (5) The relation purported to exist between the content of an element in a food crop and ultimate nutritive value of animal tissue, thereby implicating soil factors, is untenable. (6) Endemic goiter is the only established example of a direct relationship between a soil deficiency (iodine) and a human disease.

With respect to Maynard's first and second generalizations, let it be said that fertilizer effects should always be given in terms of specific crops, nutrients, and soils.[35] Irrespective of the effect of fertilizer additions to the soil on the concentration or variation of specific nutrients in a given crop, the overall effect usually observed is an increase in the total amount of a crop as well as the total amount of nutrients obtained from each hectare of land. Thus, the plane of nutrition with respect to specific nutrients in those foods making up the overall diet, in theory at least, should be increased.

Concerning the third and fourth generalizations set forth by Maynard,[33,34] it can be said that the chemical composition and, at times, the nutritional quality of plants can be affected by soil factors.[35] Soil factors such as structure and nutrient status interact with the genetic make-up of a plant within a closely interrelated mesh of climatic factors. Furthermore, there is other evidence from studies in which genetic and soil factors are eliminated as variables to show that the amount of solar radiation incident upon plant leaves can set ultimate limits to crop yields.[36] Also, in terms of ontogeny, it is essential to recognize that specific tissues of the plant interact concomitantly with soil and climatic factors.[11,16] Genetic factors in and of themselves, however, operate significantly in the plant kingdom with respect to different capacities to accumulate alkali cations.[37]

NUTRITIONAL QUALITY OF FOODS AND FEEDS OF PLANT ORIGIN

Practical steps to meet basic or optimal human requirements for mineral and trace elements can be meaningful only if the differing "availabilities" of these nutrients from various foods are measured on animals and man within well-defined confidence limits.[38] For example, the availabilities of iron, zinc, selenium, and chromium in foods can vary from 0 to nearly 100% of an optimal reference compound.[38]

In the evaluation of protein quality in foods, microbiological and chromatographic analyses are used to measure individual amino acids.[39] Available amino acids are estimated by chemical, microbiological, and biological assay methods. In the latter methods, at least five different evaluations can be made. These include animal growth and protein efficiency ratio (PER), net protein retention (NPR), net protein utilization (NPU), the nitrogen balance index, and the net dietary protein calories percent (ND_pCal %). Most of these methods cannot be applied to man without various modifications.[39]

Principal clinical methods useful in protein evaluation in infants and man are growth measurements and nitrogen balance.[39] Important considerations in the evaluation of protein quality in man relate to the effects of individual stressors on protein metabolism, such as infection, injury, undernutrition, climatic stress, severe exertion, psychological stress, and physiological state.[39]

Clinical methods for the evaluation of mineral and trace elements have not reached the same level of sophistication as for protein. With respect to all of these nutrients, the problem of adequate sampling is still bothersome.[38-40]

In commenting on the research effort to improve the composition of the plant from the nutritional viewpoint up to that time (1946), Beeson[41] observed that workers have not generally given clear definition to their objectives, and that too few experiments dealing with human foods have been reported. After the passage of nearly three decades, these views still apply very much.

According to Mangelsdorf,[42] during his history man has used fewer and fewer plant species as food. Today about 13 plant species feed the majority of the world's people, as follows:

three cereal crops (rice, wheat, and corn)
two sugar crops (sugar cane and sugar beet)
three root crops (white potato, sweet potato, and casava)
two legumes (common bean and soybean)
two tree crops (coconut and banana)
one peanut crop

Fundamentally, a real need exists for the discovery of new sources of plant germ plasm useful for human food. For example, of about 250,000 species known to man, about 250, or 0.1%, have been used to produce the world's supply of food and fiber.[43]

Recently, Kaldy[44] made an evaluation of the protein value of various food crops based on their biological value of protein per hectare. White potato was found second only to soybean with reference to the biological value of the protein produced per hectare, outranking such foods as corn, beans, peas, and spring wheat.

In 1955 Beeson[45] reported on experiments to test the effect of the addition of phosphate fertilizer to a North Carolina soil, deficient in available phosphate, on the yield and nutritional quality of soybean forage. Experiments began in 1945 and continued for several years. Accordingly, the first year after application of phosphate fertilizer, both the yield of the soybean forage and the phosphate concentration in the forage were increased. This response would be expected since the soil had been analyzed and found deficient in available phosphate.

When this forage was fed to sheep, those receiving forages from soils treated with the phosphate fertilizer gained the most weight. Supplementary feeding tests[46] showed that the superiority of the fertilized forage was due to the extra phosphate it had accumulated from the treated soil. Rabbits placed under a similar dietary regimen confirmed and extended the data obtained on sheep.[46] Following additional study, it was found that the soybean hay grown on soils fertilized with phosphorus contained qualities other than increased phosphate or protein which enhanced rabbit growth.[46]

In other experiments it was determined that application of lime to the soil increased the calcium and phosphorus concentrations of lespedeza hay.[45] Animals fed this hay grown on soils treated with the highest lime rates showed significantly better growth despite the fact that the calcium content of lespedeza hay from unlimed soils already contained sufficient calcium for optimal growth of rabbits. Implications of these data are impressive from the standpoint of global nutrition of animals and man.

Certain problems inherent to studies of this

type are selection of the test animal, choice of diet components that develop sufficient stress in the animal so as to emphasize differences in nutritional quality of plants from different environments and agronomic practices, preparation of lots of feed (or food) that represent each specific soil or site condition, and the design of experiments so that the experimental error includes both the site and animal variations.[45] Enough reports are available on the increases induced in the nutritional value of crops by addition of certain fertilizers to the soil to make exciting the possibility of producing crops of high nutritive value on most soils.[45]

In 1956 Maynard[34] discussed data from a ten-year experiment on ruminants which he considered as supporting his contention that application of fertilizers to soils affects only the yield and not the nutritional quality of a crop. Other aspects of this problem have been discussed elsewhere.[47] Detailed examination of this experiment is justified because of apparent misconceptions concerning its objectives.[34,48,49] First, the work was described as dealing largely with ruminant nutrition in which the nutritive value of a secondary product, milk, was determined by feeding it to nonruminants (i.e., the rat).[21] The test soil was described as a fine sandy loam of "fair" inherent productivity. In the course of 100 years of farming no lime or commercial fertilizer had ever been added to this soil. Apparently no crop had been grown on the farm for 25 years prior to the study. The soil was analyzed and judged highly deficient in nitrogen, phosphorus, and potassium, but sufficient with respect to trace elements essential for plant growth. Control and treated soils received the same levels of nitrogen fertilizer (from 20 to 60 lb/acre depending on the crop) and the same forms of nitrogen (NH_4NO_3 or urea) to induce sufficient plant growth to allow machine harvesting. Significantly, the so-called depleted soils were treated with the same levels of nitrogen fertilizer as the other soils which received additional phosphorus and potassium fertilizers.[21] This experiment does not meet the rigorous criteria required in the evaluation of soil factors in relation to the nutritive value of plants because only one level of phosphorus and potassium was involved. Nevertheless, the experiment was useful in showing notable reproductive failures among the dairy herd due to the failure of all soils to supply enough cobalt to the forage.[50]

IMPROVING NUTRITIONAL QUALITY OF PLANTS THROUGH GENETIC AND AGRONOMIC MEASURES

Proteins, Vitamins, Hormones, and Other Substances

Judging from past experience, nutritionally improved crops will be adopted by growers provided they give good yields and they all have an acceptable texture, flavor, color, and other esthetic qualities.[51] Pricing policy is also important. For example, premium prices might be paid to growers for producing high quality protein in grains and legumes.[52] One important obstacle to the realization of this practice for cereal grains is the frequently observed (but resolvable[53]) inverse relation between grain yield and grain protein.[3,53] Also, broad classes of wheat quality have emerged throughout the world based on the end use to which wheat products are put.[53]

Until very recently, the quantity and nutritional quality of cereal protein had received little attention from plant breeders, largely because of a lack of rapid and accurate methods for measuring amino acid profiles in foods.[54] Apparently, significant increases in protein content of wheat can be achieved through breeding without sacrificing wheat yield. Nature has provided the genetic variability needed for nutritional improvement of cereals, including rice.[53,54]

Serious lowering of protein content and the concomitant alteration of the favorable balance of amino acids may be avoided if both parents possess genes for above average protein content.[53] The recent report by Eilrich and Hageman[55] showed, for example, that the application of different rates of nitrogen fertilizer [$Ca(NO_3)_2$] to soils supporting certain wheat varieties resistant to lodging prevented the depression of the percentage grain protein when grain yields were increased. High nitrogen application rates during the reproductive phase maintained a high nitrate reductase activity. Also, seasonal nitrate reductase activity was significantly and positively correlated with yield of wheat grain.[55]

All cereal grains except the high lysine corns, opaque-2, and floury-2[56] lack the balance of essential amino acids needed for animals and man.[53,54] Lysine in cereals is the most limiting amino acid. Therefore, the improvement of protein quality in cereals should begin with lysine.[57] Carpenter[51] maintains, however, that although lysine is the first limiting amino acid in cereals when eaten alone, in all examples of average national total diets it has been found that methionine and other sulfur containing amino acids are usually the first to become limiting to humans.

Reports of heterogeneity in the methionine content of different fractions of soybean storage proteins suggest that progress in the improvement of these legumes is also feasible.[56] Development of strains lacking or low in toxic compounds (e.g., estrogens, coumarins, and goitrogens) would provide another means of increasing the quality of readily available plant proteins.[56]

Variations in soil and microclimatic factors exerted a greater effect on the bread-making quality of seven different wheat cultivars than genetic factors.[59] That is, all seven wheat cultivars responded alike to comparable environments during a seven-year test at eight different locations. Similarly, the average protein content of grain differed more significantly with location than with the cultivars. Statistical correlations made between protein content and location strongly suggested that available soil nitrate played a major role in these effects. In all seven cultivars, grain protein was negatively correlated with grain yield.[59]

Nutritive value of pearl millet (*Pennisetum typhoides*) has received little detailed study.[60] This cereal crop is unusually tolerant of drought and heat and produces grain for human consumption in areas of the world considered too hot and dry for other cereals. Yet, pearl millet contains more iron than wheat, sorghum, or rice. As with other cereals, however, its amino acid profile is deficient in lysine. Limited genotype assessment suggests that protein and lysine content can be improved. Pearl millet oil contains more palmitic, stearic, and linolenic acids and less oleic and linoleic fatty acids than corn oil.[60]

Protein content of certain rice varieties is significantly influenced by nitrogen fertilization, crop season, planting date, and environment.[61]

Provitamin A (beta carotene) content of tomatoes (Rutgers var.) was increased from 5 μg/g fresh weight to about 80 μg/g fresh weight by the introduction of one gene. Fruit color was changed to orange-red (from red) when gene B was introduced.[62]

Plant cytokinins as well as other hormones may participate in regulating the size of barley grain perhaps by influencing the accumulation of metabolites during the grain "filling" period.[63] Evidence was also obtained indicating that cytokinins are synthesized in barley roots, as judged by the lowering of the cytokinin content of grain when the oxygen supplying power of the soil was decreased by saturating the root zone with water, especially in the earlier stages of growth. Size of barley grain appears to be regulated by the relative vigor of the root system. As with corn, the activity of cytokinin per kernel decreased sharply during the maturation phase.[63]

Workers at the Indian Agricultural Research Institute (Swaminathan et al.[64]) have shown that fertilizer treatments that increase protein levels in wheat by 10 to 15% increase lysine and tryptophan levels and yield a protein with balanced amino acid composition. Therefore, genetic improvement of wheat offers great scope for evolving new varieties responsive to nitrogen fertilizers in which additional protein that is synthesized will be of better quality. An increase in protein content per se by regular breeding techniques appears to be the most rapid method for enhancing the nutritive quality of bread, wheat, and rice.[64] In rice, considerable scope exists for the redistribution of protein in rice grains in a manner that will prevent the reduction of protein content during milling.[61,64]

In unripe cereal grains, lysine and tryptophan are present in large amounts, but they are incorporated during ripening into the endosperm storage proteins whose main function is to supply amino nitrogen to the growing embryo at germination.[64] The so-called nonessential amino acids of cereal grains, glutamic acid, aspartic acid, and alanine, account for more than half of the total nitrogen. Thus, nutritional imbalances of cereal grain protein result from the physiological function for which they are synthesized in the seed. Embryo proteins, on the other hand, have a more balanced amino acid content. New knowledge at the molecular level is needed to find ways of modifying patterns of protein synthesis during grain maturation and ripening.[64] Reduction in the prolamine fraction in maize, sorghum, and several millets leads to an increase in the lysine content of the grain. *Panicum miliaceum,* among minor millets, is rich in lysine.[64]

Reduction of the fibrous envelope in seeds of *Paspalum* sp., *Setaria* sp., and *Eleucine* sp. can improve the digestibility of these grains. Protein quality in cereals may also be improved by selecting grains with large embryos.[64]

Addition of nitrogen fertilizer to soil supporting pearl millet enhanced the prolamine content by about 40%, thereby decreasing the lysine content and enhancing tryptophan levels. Breeding research aimed at improving protein quality in pearl millets should take these factors into account.[64]

Good cultivars of *Cicer arietinum* and *Cajanus cajan* have been treated with physical and chemical mutagens to develop a greater variability (now lacking) in the protein content of these crops. Also, mutation breeding appears feasible on *Lathyrus sativus* to remove neurotoxic components from seeds.[64]

Genetic upgrading of the protein quality of cereals, pulses, and other food and feed crops requires the use of rapid, nondestructive screening techniques.[65] The nondestructive micro-dye-binding capacity (DBC) developed originally for rice (*Oryza sativa*) has been found equally reliable on maize (*Zea Mays L.*), wheat (*Triticum aestivum*), mung bean (*Phaseolus aureus*), red gram (*Cajanus cajan*), sorghum (*Sorghum vulgare*), and millet (*Pennisetum typhoides*). Similar improvements are being sought in histological techniques by use of protein specific radioactive dyes. Radioactivity is measured in uniformly cut cross sections using a conventional liquid scintillation counter. With these methods the mean frequency distribution of 321 wheat strains in the F_5 generation has been shifted toward superior protein quality, suggesting that further scope for selection is still possible.[65]

Inorganic Elements

Ample evidence is at hand indicating that the absorption, translocation, and utilization of inorganic elements are under genetic control.[14] Genetic effects operating in the nitrogen nutrition of corn were examined in detail 33 years ago by Burkholder and McVeigh.[66] Plant breeders have been successful in obtaining resistance to toxic levels of manganese and aluminum in the grasses *Lolium* sp. and *Agropyron* sp. On a global basis, the most deleterious element in soils appears to be salt.[14]

Cell walls of higher plants may constitute part of an internal chelating mechanism for bestowing tolerance to high levels of zinc and copper in *Agrostis* sp.[67] The pectate fraction of cell walls of zinc tolerant *Agrostis tenuis* contained five to six times as much zinc as the nontolerant plants growing on the same site. However, the tolerance mechanism for zinc in *Agrostis stolonifera* was located mostly in the soluble RNA fraction.[67] Tolerance to high external concentrations of heavy metals appears determined not by single genes but by multiple genes.

According to Wallace et al.,[15] the minimum and simplest estimate of gene number controlling crop yield is based on the assumption that each physiological component is controlled by a single gene. On the other hand, maximum estimate of gene number is based on the assumption that all genes of a plant affect the yield. The latter estimate may be the closest to reality.[15]

Using chromosomal translocations in corn (*Zea Mays L.*), Barber and Thomas[68] postulated a minimum of six genetic loci affecting relative phosphate accumulation by the ear leaves of corn.

Agronomic control points relative to trace element problems in the U.S. have been discussed by Allaway[24] in relation to soil selection, addition of trace elements to soils or as foliar sprays, soil management, crop selection, and crop management practices.

Feed grain production has been shifted inadvertently from the selenium deficient soils of the Great Plains states to the northeastern U.S. where soils are not deficient in selenium. Peat and muck soils in some parts of the U.S. lack one or more trace elements for all crops grown on these soils. Eighteen states have reported zinc deficiency in corn, apparently due to the influence of higher corn yields.[69]

Selenium concentrations in certain plants can be increased at least tenfold by applications of selenium to the soil without visibly changing plant growth.[24] The practice of adding trace elements to soils or plants is confined primarily to the elements zinc, copper, iron, boron, molybdenum, and manganese.

Addition of lime to acid soils usually leads to an increased uptake by plants of trace elements that enter as anions (e.g., boron).[24] Heavy applications of phosphate fertilizers usually reduce the uptake of metallic trace elements which enter plants as cations. Addition of lime usually decreases the uptake of manganese, aluminum, and potassium. Use of irrigation to increase available soil moisture sometimes leads to an increased uptake of cobalt and molybdenum in certain plants grown on certain soils. When sulfate is added to soils containing high levels of selenium (assuming low native sulfate levels), the uptake of selenium by plants can be reduced.[24]

Effect of Herbicides in Improving the Protein Content of Plants

When certain auxin-like chemicals are applied to the soil or to plant leaves at sublethal levels, protein synthesis can be increased.[70,71] Application of herbicidal levels of 2,4-dichlorophenoxyacetic acid (2,4-D) to the leaves of cucurbits produced an inhibition of nitrate reductase in the leaves and decreased the synthesis of protein. In corn seedlings, however, nitrate reductase activity was enhanced by the application of 2,4-D, accompanied with increased levels of protein in the grain.[70]

In comparable studies using the triazine Simazine [2-chloro-4,6, bis(ethylamino)-*s*-triazine], Singh et al.[71] reported that this material generally stimulated the activities of nitrate reductase, glutamic-pyruvic transaminase, alpha amylase, starch phosphorylase and ATPase of bush bean leaves. Addition of Simazine to field soils at Logan, Utah at a rate of ½ or ¼ lb/acre significantly increased the percentage of total nitrogen and the soluble protein in pea seeds. In treated plants the total concentration of amino acids (including protein and free amino acids) was greater than in untreated controls. These gains were observed not to produce any qualitative differences in the amino acid patterns of the seeds of treated and untreated plants.[71]

One interesting aspect of these data is that auxin-like chemicals may, in combination with other soil treatments such as nitrogen fertilization, lessen the pressure for massive applications of nitrogen to increase the protein quality of food and feed plants. Caution is advisable in the use of these chemicals, however, until safe levels have been established for food consumed by humans.

CONCLUSIONS

Chemical methods are available for the determination in plants of practically any of the nutrients known to be essential to the growth of higher plants, animals, and man. Questions arise, however, with reference to the tissue to be sampled, chemical or biochemical entities that are critical for plant growth and economic yield, the frequency of sampling, the time of sampling, number and homogeneity of samples, compositional data reference base, standardization of analyses and interpretations, and cost factors, among others.

Field engineering or crop "logging" studies have been successfully used for many years to improve the yield and quality of sugar cane. This approach, or modifications thereof, could be used by plant breeders and others to "fine tune" their short- and long-range efforts to develop and select plants having improved protein, vitamins, trace elements, and other qualities, provided the plant breeder receives the correct information from plant and animal nutritionists and other knowledgeable groups of workers. Much yet remains to be done in the effort to improve the nutrition of economically handicapped sections of the world.

Precautions have been issued as to the effect of the wholesale replacement of world vegetation and low yielding plants by plants tailored to yield more protein and other nutrients, with reference to the impact of these measures on the driving forces of short geochemical cycles. Clearly, an assessment of the possible effects of these measures on world soils should be made in the light of geochemical and geophysical knowledge.

Soil and crop management practices should be used that are optimal for specific crops grown on specific soils, if a continuous rise in economic yield is to occur while at the same time maintaining long-term productivity of the soil base. Strains of plants useful as food for man should be developed and selected having the capacity to respond to fertilizers (primarily nitrogen) both under dry land and controlled irrigation systems. The technological breakthroughs achieved at the International Rice Research Institute will in due course be transferred to other food crops.

Acknowledgments

The author expresses his thanks to Dr. Miloslav Rechcigl, AID, for his interest and encouragement, and to all other persons who provided assistance during the preparation of this report.

REFERENCES

1. **Goodall, D. W. and Gregory, F. G.,** *Chemical Composition of Plants as an Index of their Nutritional Status,* Tech. Commun. Imp. Bur. Hortic. No. 7, Imp. Agric. Bur., Penglais, Aberystwyth, Wales, 1947.
2. Reuther, W., Ed., *Plant Analysis and Fertilizer Problems,* Publ. No. 8, American Institute of Biological Sciences, Washington, D.C., 1961.
3. **Hall, A. D.,** The analysis of the soil by means of the plant, *J. Agric. Sci.,* 1, 65, 1905.
4. **Macy, P. F.,** The critical nutrient composition of plants, *Plant Physiol.,* 11, 749, 1935.
5. **Gilbert, J. H.,** Agricultural investigations at Rothamsted, England, U.S. Department of Agric. Offic. Exp. Stat. Bull., Govt. Print. Off., Washington, D.C., 1895, 146.
6. **Schlehuber, A. M. and Tucker, B. B.,** Culture of wheat, in *Wheat and Wheat Improvement,* Quisenberry, K. S. and Reitz, L. P., Eds., Am. Soc. Agron. Monograph No. 13, Madison, 1967, 134.
7. **Warner, R. L., Hageman, R. H., Dudley, J. W., and Lambert, R. J.,** Inheritance of nitrate reductase activity, in *Zea Mays L., Proc. Natl. Acad. Sci.,* 62, 785, 1969.
8. **Shear, C. B., Crane, H. L., and Myers, A. T.,** Nutrient element balance: a fundamental concept in plant nutrition, *Proc. Am. Soc. Hortic. Sci.,* 47, 239, 1946.
9. **Specht, A. W.,** Evidence for and some implications of a variation-control mechanism in plant composition, *Soil Sci.,* 89, 83, 1960.
10. **Bould, C.,** Soil and plant nutrient content in relation to crop yield, *Proc. Nutr. Soc.,* 24, 21, 1965.
11. **Clements, H. F.,** Environmental influences on the growth of sugar cane, in *Mineral Nutrition of Plants,* Truog, E., Ed., University of Wisconsin Press, Madison, 1961, 451.
12. **Eastin, J. D.,** Chairman, *Symposium on Physiological Aspects of Crop Yield,* American Society of Agronomy and Crop Science Society of America, Madison, Wisc., 1969, 339.
13. **Steenbjerg, F. and Jakobsen, S. T.,** Plant nutrition and yield curves, *Soil Sci.,* 95, 69, 1963.
14. **Epstein, E.,** *Mineral Nutrition of Plants: Principles and Perspectives,* John Wiley & Sons, New York, 1972, Chap. 12.
15. **Wallace, D. H., Ozbun, J. L., and Munger, H. M.,** Physiological genetics of crop yield, *Adv. Agron.,* 24, 97, 1972.
16. **Hageman, R. H., Leng, E. R., and Dudley, J. W.,** A biochemical approach to corn breeding, *Adv. Agron.,* 19, 45, 1967.
17. **Duffield, R. D., Croy, L. I., and Smith, E. L.,** Inheritance of nitrate reductase activity, grain protein, and straw protein in a hard red winter wheat cross, *Agron. J.,* 64, 249, 1972.
18. Committee on Tropical Soils, Agric. Board, National Research Council, *Soils of the Humid Tropics,* National Academy of Sciences, Washington, D.C., 1972.
19. **Bennett, O. L., Mathias, E. L., and Henderlong, P. R.,** Effects of north- and south-facing slopes on yield of Kentucky blue-grass (*Poa pratensis, L.*) with variable rate and time of nitrogen application, *Agron. J.,* 64, 630, 1972.
20. **Duncan, W. G.,** Cultural manipulation for higher yields, in *Physiological Aspects of Crop Yield,* Eastin, J. D., Chairman, American Society of Agronomy and Crop Science Society of America, Madison, Wisc., 1969.
21. **Dexter, S. T.,** Nutritive values of crops and cow's milk as affected by soil fertility, *Symposium on Nutrition of Plants, Animals, and Man,* Michigan State University Centennial, East Lansing, 1955, 9.
22. **Viets, F. G., Jr.,** Chemistry and availability of micronutrients in soils, *J. Agric. Food Chem.,* 10, 174, 1962.
23. **Hodgson, J. F.,** Chemistry of micronutrient elements in soils, *Adv. Agron.,* 15, 119, 1963.
24. **Allaway, W. H.,** Agronomic controls over the environmental cycling of trace elements, *Adv. Agron.,* 20, 235, 1968.
25. **Barley, K. P.,** The configuration of the root system in relation to nutrient uptake, *Adv. Agron.,* 22, 159, 1970.
26. **Baker, D. E., Jarrell, A., Marshall, L. E., and Thomas, W. I.,** Phosphorus uptake from soils by corn hybrids selected for high and low phosphorus accumulation, *Agron. J.,* 62, 103, 1970.
27. **Gorsline, G. W. and Baker, D. E.,** Inheritance of P, K, Mg, Cu, B, Zn, Al, and Fe concentrations in corn (*Zea Mays, L.*) leaves and grain, *Crop Sci.,* 4, 207, 1964.
28. **Gorsline, G. W. and Baker, D. E.,** Relationship of strontium-calcium within corn, *Crop. Sci.,* 4, 154, 1964.
29. **Baker, D. E., Gorsline, G. W., Smith, C. B., Thomas, W. I., Grube, W. E., and Ragland, J. L.,** Technique for rapid analysis of corn leaves for eleven elements, *Agron. J.,* 56, 133, 1964.
30. **Nikiforoff, C. C.,** Reappraisal of the soil, *Science,* 129, 186, 1959.
31. World Food Congress Commission I, Report of subcommittee on "the strategy of high-yielding varieties," *Plant Foods Hum. Nutr.,* 2, 106, 1972.
32. **Parker, F. W. and Nelson, L. B.,** More fertilizers for more food, in *Symposium Prospects of the World Food Supply,* National Academy of Sciences, Washington, D.C., 1966, 78.
33. **Maynard, L. A.,** Soils and health, *J.A.M.A.,* 143, 807, 1950.
34. **Maynard, L. A.,** Effect of fertilizers on the nutritional value of foods, *J.A.M.A.,* 161, 1478, 1956.
35. United States Department of Agriculture, The effect of soils and fertilizers on the nutritional quality of plants, Agric. Res. Ser., Agriculture Information Bull. No. 299, Govt. Print. Off., Washington, D.C., 1965.
36. **Black, J. N.,** The ultimate limits of crop production, *Proc. Nutr. Soc.,* 24, 2, 1965.
37. **Collander, R.,** Selective absorption of cations by higher plants, *Plant Physiol.,* 16, 691, 1941.
38. **Mertz, W.,** Human requirements: basic and optimal, *Ann. N.Y. Acad. Sci.,* 199, 191, 1972.
39. Committee on Protein Malnutrition, Food and Nutrition Board, National Research Council Publ. No. 1100, Evaluation of Protein Quality, National Academy of Sciences, Washington, D.C., 1963.

40. **Cannon, H. L., Papp, C. S. E., and Anderson, B. M.,** Problems of sampling and analysis in trace element investigations of vegetation, *Ann. N.Y. Acad. Sci.,* 199, 124, 1972.
41. **Beeson, K. C.,** The effect of mineral supply on the mineral concentration and nutritional quality of plants, *Bot. Rev.,* 12, 424, 1946.
42. **Mangelsdorf, P. C.,** Genetic potentials for increasing yields of food crops and animals, *Symposium Prospects of the World Food Supply,* National Academy of Sciences, Washington, D.C., 1966, 66.
43. American Association for the Advancement of Science, *Symposium on Germ Plasm Resources,* Hodgson, R. E., Ed., *AAAS,* Washington, D.C., 1961, 308.
44. **Kaldy, M. S.,** Protein yield of various crops as related to protein value, *Econ. Bot.,* 26, 142, 1972.
45. **Beeson, K. C.,** The effect of fertilizers on the nutritional quality of crops, *Symposium on Nutrition of Plants, Animals, and Man,* Michigan State University Centennial, East Lansing, 1955, 45.
46. **Matrone, G., Weldon, V., Smart, W. W. G., Jr., Sherwood, F. W., Smith, F. H., and Wise, G. H.,** Effects of phosphate fertilization and dietary mineral supplementation on the nutritive value of soybean forage, *J. Nutr.,* 52, 127, 1954.
47. **Hopkins, H. T., Stevenson, E. H., and Harris, P. L.,** Soil factors and food composition, *Am. J. Clin. Nutr.,* 18, 390, 1966.
48. **Harris, R. S. and Von Losecke, H.,** *Nutritional Evaluation of Food Processing,* John Wiley & Sons, New York, 1971, Chap. 1.
49. **Hollingsworth, D. and Martin, P. E.,** Some aspects of the effects of different methods of production and of processing on the nutritive value of food, *World Rev. Nutr. Diet.,* 15, 1, 1972.
50. **Ward, G. M., Weaver, E., Ely, R. E., and Dunn, K. M.,** Effect of fertilizer practices on nutritive value of feed for four successive generations of dairy cows, *Symposium on Nutrition of Plants, Animals, and Man,* Michigan State University Centennial, East Lansing, 1955, 52.
51. **Carpenter, K. J.,** Nutritional considerations in attempts to change the chemical composition of crops, *Proc. Nutr. Soc.,* 29, 3, 1970.
52. **Swaminathan, M. S.,** Report on the world food congress, *Plant Foods Hum. Nutr.,* 2, 105, 1972.
53. **Johnson, V. A. and Schmidt, J. W.,** Hybrid wheat, *Adv. Agron.,* 20, 199, 1968.
54. **Johnson, V. A., Schmidt, J. W., and Mattern, P. J.,** Cereal breeding for better protein impact, *Econ. Bot.,* 22, 29, 1968.
55. **Eilrich, G. L. and Hageman, R. H.,** Nitrate reductase activity and its relationship to accumulation of vegetative and grain nitrogen in wheat *(Triticum aestivum, L.), Crop Sci.,* 13, 59, 1973.
56. **Nelson, O. E.,** Genetic modification of protein quality in plants, *Adv. Agron.,* 21, 171, 1969.
57. **Johnson, V. A., Mattern, P.J., and Schmidt, J. W.,** The breeding of wheat and maize with improved nutritional value, *Proc. Nutr. Soc.,* 29, 20, 1970.
58. **Liener, I. E.,** Toxic constituents of plant foodstuffs, *Proc. Nutr. Soc.,* 29, 56, 1970.
59. **Johnson, J. A., Khan, M. N. A., and Sanchez, C. R. S.,** Wheat cultivars, environment, and bread-baking quality, *Cereal Sci. Today,* 17(10), 323, 1972.
60. **Burton, G. W., Wallace, A. T., and Rachie, K. O.,** Chemical composition and nutritive value of pearl millet [*Pennisetum typhoides* (Burm.) Stapf and E. C. Hubbard] grain, *Crop Sci.,* 12, 187, 1972.
61. **Houston, D. F. and Kohler, G. O.,** *Nutritional Properties of Rice,* National Academy of Sciences, Food and Nutrition Board, Washington, D. C., 1970.
62. **Tomes, M. L.,** Improving color and pro-vitamin A content in the tomato, *Proc. Sixth Int. Congr. of Nutrition,* Livingstone, Edinburgh, 1964, 631.
63. **Michael, G. and Seiler-Kelbitsch, H.,** Cytokinin content and kernel size of barley grain as affected by environmental and genetic factors, *Crop Sci.,* 12, 162, 1972.
64. **Swaminathan, M. S., Naik, M. S., Kaul, A. K., and Austin, A.,** The choice of strategy for the genetic upgrading of protein properties in cereals, millets, and pulses, *Plant Foods Hum. Nutr.,* 2, 119, 1972.
65. **Kaul, A. K., Dhar, R. D., and Swaminathan, M. S.,** Microscopic and other dye binding techniques of screening for proteins in cereals, *Plant Foods Hum. Nutr.,* 2, 113, 1972.
66. **Burkholder, P. R. and McVeigh, I.,** Growth and differentiation of maize in relation to nitrogen supply, *Am. J. Bot.,* 27, 414, 1940.
67. **Antonovics, J., Bradshaw, A. D., and Turner, R. G.,** Heavy metal tolerance in plants, *Adv. Ecol. Res.,* 7, 1, 1971.
68. **Barber, W. D. and Thomas, W. I.,** Evaluation of the genetics of relative phosphorus accumulation by corn (*Zea Mays, L.*) using chromosomal translocations, *Crop Sci.,* 12, 755, 1972.
69. American Chemical Society, Micronutrient shortage widespread, *Chem. Eng. News,* 39(38), 52, 1961.
70. **Beevers, L. and Hageman, R. H.,** Nitrate reduction in higher plants, *Ann. Rev. Plant Physiol.,* 20, 495, 1969.
71. **Singh, B., Wu, M. T., and Salunkhe, D. K.,** The use of chemicals to increase leaf and seed proteins of certain crops, *Plant Foods Hum. Nutr.,* 2, 171, 1972.

IMPROVING THE NUTRIENT COMPOSITION OF MEAT-PRODUCING ANIMALS

G. A. Lodge

TABLE OF CONTENTS

Introduction 215
The Patterns of Normal Growth 216
Species Differences in Body Composition 217
Breed Differences in Body Composition 218
Sex Differences in Body Composition 220
Nutritional Influences on Body Composition 221
Nutritive Value of Carcass Components 224
Protein Quality 224
Fat Composition 224
Conclusions 225
References 226

INTRODUCTION

Nowadays meat animals are kept primarily as sources of high-quality protein and so it is in these terms that possible means of improving their composition must be considered. Such was not always the case, however, for prior to the present widespread production and use of vegetable and mineral oils for dietary, domestic, and industrial purposes, muscle, as a protein source, was almost a by-product. The early livestock improvers, who originated the bases of many of our present-day breeds in the late 18th and early 19th centuries, selected their animals primarily for their ability to mature rapidly and deposit appreciable fat at an early age and light weight. Such breeds were suited to the husbandry methods of the day, based on bulk feeds of relatively low nutritive value, and provided animals which, when slaughtered at the mature weights characteristic of the time, produced carcasses with the considerable fat cover which appears then to have been the consumer preference.

The pig, in particular, was prized for its ability to convert carbohydrate into fat; the main task of the present-day breeder is to reverse the work of the early 'improvers' by reducing the ready ability of the pig to deposit fat without reverting to the original wild boar (*Sus scrofa*) with its slow growth rate and low reproductive capacity. A similar problem, but to a lesser degree, confronts breeders of beef cattle and sheep, with the increasing trend toward intensive feeding systems and the more rapid rates of growth which then ensue.

The evident success of the early livestock breeders in developing the type of animal they required from seemingly unpromising indigenous material indicates the variation which does exist among animals in the rates at which specific body tissues develop, for either genetic or environmental reasons, and consequently the scope which exists for influencing these at least in quantitative, if not qualitative, terms.

Unfortunately, however, fat deposition is a much more variable characteristic than is muscle growth or, even more so, protein synthesis. It cannot be expected, therefore, that improvements in rates of protein production by meat animals can be changed as readily as can rates of fat production. Clearly, an inverse relationship exists between proportions of fat and lean tissue in a carcass, but if restriction of fat deposition merely limits weight gain without enhancing muscle growth, there will be no real improvement in overall production of nutrients.

It is perhaps desirable at this stage to distinguish between consumer acceptability and nutritive value. It may be relatively simple to manipulate the normal growth patterns of the organs and tissues of meat-producing animals to increase the proportion of the most acceptable tissue, i.e., muscle, and reduce those of those less acceptable, i.e., bone, fat, and most of the internal organs. This, however, may have relatively little influence on the overall protein content or the basic composition of the fat, and so the true nutritive value may not be materially changed. In the sense, however, that people consume only what is acceptable to them unless under the duress of starvation, modification of growth to increase proportions of those relatively limited parts commonly deemed acceptable may be regarded as improving the overall nutrient composition.

This subject may best be approached by considering the pattern of what might be regarded as 'normal' growth and then, using the well-documented pig as the basis, the variations from this which can occur for genetic or environmental reasons.

THE PATTERNS OF NORMAL GROWTH

The classical work of Hammond and his colleagues at Cambridge clearly established the anatomical changes which occur in animals with increase in age. There are several excellent detailed reviews of this complex subject[1-3] from which the points of most relevance to the nutritive value of the ultimate carcass are that as the animal grows, its head, legs, and viscera decrease relative to the total body and the percentage of water also decreases, prenatally because of increases in the contents of protein and ash, but postnatally almost entirely because of increased deposition of fat. These trends are well illustrated in the pig (Tables 1 and 2).

At birth, the body composition of the pig, relative to total weight, is about 1.5 to 2.5% fat, 10 to 12% protein, and 3 to 5% ash.[4-7] This low fat percentage in the pig at birth, in contrast to about 9% for the seal, 10% for the guinea pig, and 16% for the human,[8] is common to the mammalian farm species.

In the pig, early postnatal growth is characterized by a rapid increase in fat deposition, from the value of about 2% at birth to about 10% at 7 days, and 14 to 15% by two weeks.[4-6] Calves and lambs appear to follow a similar trend, but to a much lesser degree.[9-12]

Following this initial, very rapid increase in body fat content, its proportion in the pig increases more slowly but consistently and may reach as high as 60% by a liveweight of 150 kg, or approximately 9 months of age,[13] although in some studies only 33% fat was reached by 120 kg, or approximately 7 months of age,[14] indicating the influence of genetic and/or environmental effects on rate of fat deposition.

Over the weight range 10 to 150 kg represented by Clausen's data,[13] the protein percent decreased from 16.7 to 10.2, ash from 3.4 to 2.0, and water from 67.3 to 28.4. In Hornicke's study,[14] the respective reductions over the weight range of 15 to 120 kg were 16.0 to 14.1% for protein, 3.7 to 2.7% for ash, and 70.4 to 50.4% for water. These data illustrate the relative constancy of protein and ash as proportions of body weight compared

TABLE 1

Chemical Composition of the Pig at Successive Stages of Prenatal Life†[7]

Age from conception (days)	Weight (g)	Body composition: Water (%)	Lipids (%)	Protein* (%)	Ash (%)
30	5	94.7	0.5	3.6	0.9
45	117	90.1	0.7	6.7	1.6
60	119	89.6	0.9	6.2	2.0
79	422	88.5	1.0	7.2	2.6
100	778	85.3	1.3	8.6	3.0
107	1137	83.6	1.4	9.7	3.2

*N x 6.25
†Derived from one litter of pigs at each age

TABLE 2

Chemical Composition of the Pig at Successive Stages of Postnatal Life[13]

Live bodyweight (kg)	Body composition			
	Water (%)	Lipid (%)	Protein* (%)	Ash (%)
<10	67.3	12.5	16.7	3.4
10–30	57.3	23.2	16.6	2.9
30–50	49.4	33.1	15.1	2.6
50–70	43.7	40.2	13.9	2.4
70–90	39.1	45.8	12.9	2.2
90–110	35.2	50.8	12.0	2.1
110–130	31.6	55.2	11.1	2.1
130–150	28.4	59.3	10.2	2.0

*N x 6.25

to the considerable changes which occur in fat and water, and support the contention that improving nutritive value of the carcass in protein terms is only within fairly strict limitations. This fact is also well illustrated by data on the body composition of Holstein steers following different feeding regimes and slaughtered over a wide range of weights, from 91 to 590 kg.[15] Over the full period from birth to 590 kg, carcass protein ranged only from a maximum of 18.5% at 227 kg to a minimum of 14.5% at 590 kg, whereas ether extract increased from 4.3% at birth to 35.1% at 590 kg at the expense of water, which declined over the same period from 75.6 to 49.2%. Energy intake of the steers influenced the relative proportions of the tissues at each weight, but the growth patterns were essentially unaltered. This relative constancy of protein content in cattle is equally evident in data on bulls slaughtered over a range of weights from 41 to 362 kg empty body weight,[16] in which ether extract content increased from 4.8 to 14.4%, while protein remained around 19% over the whole weight range. It is noteworthy, however, that in this experiment the proportion of protein in the *edible* parts of the carcass increased from 39 to 48%, mainly through decreasing proportions in head, hide, feet, viscera, and blood; to that extent, the nutritive value improved with increase in age of animal.

The factors which may be manipulated to effect changes in carcass value, in addition to age at slaughter, include species, breed, sex, nutrition, and other environmental parameters. Frequently it is difficult to interpret the relative effects of these factors from the published data because of interactions between them. In particular, species are difficult to compare at a common stage of development and age interacts with environmental restrictions.

SPECIES DIFFERENCES IN BODY COMPOSITION

As indicated above, the mammalian farm species are similar in body composition at birth but diverge postnatally to follow somewhat different courses to maturity. The most comprehensive study of interspecies differences in body composition is that of Reid and co-workers at Cornell University.[17] From a reevaluation of previously published data on considerable numbers of cattle and pigs, together with original experiments with sheep, involving several breeds, ages, sexes, and nutritional regimens, it was indicated that the interrelationship between body fat and body water was very consistent within species but differed between them; the rate of increase in fat percent per unit change in water percent was greatest in sheep and least in cattle. On a fat-free body basis, pigs had the least protein and ash (19.2 and 3.9%, respectively) and cattle had the most (21.6 and 5.3%, respectively), with sheep intermediate (20.4 and 4.8%, respectively). On a dry matter basis, however, pigs had the highest protein percent (83.4) and the lowest ash (17.0), while cattle had the lowest protein percent (80.2) and highest ash (19.7), with sheep again intermediate (81.1% protein and 18.9% ash).

A striking feature of the above data was the extremely wide range of values for all species (Table 3), indicating that the other influences previously mentioned are of greater significance than species in determining nutrient content of meat animals. However, it does appear that the pig has greater potential for fat production than either of the ruminant species and all have a similar limitation on protein content at about 20% of empty body weight.

Body composition in poultry, as influenced by age and growth rate, was studied in detail by Wilson,[18] who found that the proportions of bone, muscle, and fat were much more consistent than reported for sheep and pigs[19-22] because of the much lower content of the most variable component, body fat. At 24 weeks of age, cockerels following a high plane of nutrition had only 1.7% fat in the total body, in contrast to values of 25 to 33% reported for pigs and sheep of similar age. However, although there is this considerable difference in the proportions of body tissues between poultry and the mammalian species, in terms of protein all are comparable. Chickens at various weights and ages, following various dietary regimes, show a body protein content consistently around 19%, the apparent discrepancy between muscle data and protein data being accountable for by differences in moisture content.[23,24] The evidence for turkeys indicates that they also have body protein contents which remain in the 16 to 20% range, even though fat content may be doubled by dietary manipulation.[25,26]

In species evaluation, however, the relative proportions of the body tissues are of perhaps less significance than the efficiency with which meat protein is produced. Several such evaluations have been presented, varying with the values used for input and output and method of calculation,[27-32] an example of which, illustrating only the meat producing processes, is shown in Table 4.

As the production of protein for human consumption, not energy, is the main purpose of animal production, evaluation is given only in those terms but relative to inputs of both protein and energy. In efficiency of conversion in both respects poultry are preeminent, with pigs superior to the ruminants. It should be stressed, however, that nutritional and economic efficiency do not always coincide and that a production system which may be very inefficient biologically, e.g., beef from range cattle, may be quite acceptable economically because no more efficient system is possible within the environmental limitations. Also to be considered is the ability of ruminants to utilize nonprotein nitrogen sources in the diet, so that a poorer conversion of dietary protein to meat protein may be more than counterbalanced by the saving in true protein in the animal's feed.

BREED DIFFERENCES IN BODY COMPOSITION

Within species there are marked differences between genotypes in the rates at which the body tissues develop, hence the broad designations of early and late maturing, and possibly in ultimate mature composition. It might be anticipated that such differences would be greatest when a species is kept for two or more distinct purposes, as in cattle for either milk or beef, in sheep for wool or mutton, and in poultry for eggs or meat. Less difference might be expected between breeds of swine, for all of which the sole purpose is production of lean meat, although at one time in Europe some distinction was made between pork and bacon.

At either a common age or a common weight,

TABLE 3

Range in Body Composition* of Cattle, Sheep, and Pigs[17]

	Percentage composition			
Species	Water	Fat	Protein	Ash
Cattle (n = 256)	39.8–77.6	1.8–44.6	12.4–20.6	3.0–6.1
Sheep (n = 221)	39.6–73.8	4.9–46.6	10.7–19.5	1.7–5.8
Pigs (n = 714)	30.7–80.8	1.1–61.5	8.3–19.6	1.3–5.6

*On the basis of empty body weight

TABLE 4

Overall* Efficiencies of Protein Production from Farm Meat-Producing Species[31]

Species	Protein efficiency %†	g/mcal ME‡	g/mcal GE§
Beef herd	6	2.6	1.5
Sheep flock	3	1.3	0.8
Pig herd	12	6	4.0
Broiler flock	20	11	7.7

*Calculations include overheads of maintaining the breeding population
†(Edible protein x 100) ÷ (total food protein consumed)
‡ (Edible protein (g)) ÷ (total metabolizable energy consumed (mcal))
§(Edible protein (g)) ÷ (total gross energy consumed (mcal))

cattle do indeed show wide differences in body composition between breeds. Animals of the relatively large, late maturing 'dairy' breeds, e.g., Holstein or British Friesian, grow some 20% faster and have a higher muscle percentage than do those of the relatively small, early maturing 'beef' breeds at similar weight[33-35] or similar age.[9]

In general, the traditional beef breeds have a higher ratio of muscle:bone but a lower ratio of muscle:fat at normal slaughter weights than do animals of the dairy breeds.[36-38] There is an interaction in this respect with age, however, so that Herefords had more muscle and less bone than Friesians in early life but less muscle and more fat than Friesians at 6 months of age.[9]

The so-called 'exotic' beef breeds, i.e., those of more recent importation from Europe, typified by the Charolais, the Limousin, and the Chianina, are characteristically bigger animals than the traditional beef breeds of British origin (Hereford, Shorthorn, and Aberdeen Angus). Berg[39] found that Charolais crosses were between the British beef-breed crosses and the Holstein dairy breed in muscle:bone ratio and tended to have the least fat even though they were heavier than both in carcass weight. In a study involving numerous breeds and crosses, Mukhoty and Berg[40] found that differences between breeds in muscle:bone ratio were established early in life and thereafter the tissues grew at relatively constant rates; rates of fat deposition, however, differed widely between breeds.

These differences are generally attributed to differences between the breeds in physiological age at the time of slaughter, but in a comparison between Hereford, Shorthorn, and Aberdeen Angus steers grown under the same conditions and to similar ages and weights, Tulloh[41] found significantly less muscle and more fat in Shorthorns than in either of the other two breeds.

The distribution of muscles, as well as total muscle weight, could influence not only the commercial value of the carcass but also its nutritional value, since some muscles have higher protein content than others.[42,43] However, in extensive studies on this subject, Butterfield and co-workers[44-48] found negligible differences between cattle of widely divergent types in the weights of individual muscles as proportions of total muscle weight. This relationship may be modified, however, in the case of 'double-muscling,' i.e., muscle hypertrophy which occurs as a genetic abnormality in some breeds of cattle. The disproportionate development of a 'double-muscled' heifer of the Aberdeen Angus breed was not uniformly distributed but was greater in the femoral and humeroscapular muscles than in those more distally located.[49]

Difference has been reported[50] between beef-type and dairy-type breeds (Hereford vs. Holstein) in efficiency of energy conversion to body tissues, but the two were almost identical in their efficiency of protein production.

The breeds of sheep vary as widely in mature size as do those of cattle, but all appear to reach mature weight at a common age of about two years.[51] This would suggest that at a given slaughter age the muscle proportion of carcasses would be similar, but daily muscle growth to slaughter age would be greater for the larger breeds.

At a given body weight, however, the larger breeds would be less mature and so would be expected to have less muscle relative to bone and less fat than the smaller breeds. That such differences at a common weight do exist is indicated by the data of Reid et al.,[17] comparing body compositions of several breeds and crosses at common weights (Table 5). Breed comparisons on limited numbers of each must be treated with reservation, because of within-breed variation, but clearly, appreciable differences exist between genotypes in their protein yield at given weights; Suffolks contained more water and protein and less fat than

TABLE 5

Breed Differences in Body Composition of Sheep* at Successive Slaughter Weights[17]

Breed	Body composition according to EBW† (kg)								
	20			40			60		
	Water (%)	Fat (%)	Protein (%)	Water (%)	Fat (%)	Protein (%)	Water (%)	Fat (%)	Protein (%)
Suffolk	67.5	10.0	18.0	57.5	22.8	16.0	52.5	29.5	14.8
Hampshire	67.0	10.5	17.5	55.3	25.8	15.3	49.3	33.7	14.2
Corriedale	62.0	17.0	17.5	51.0	32.8	13.5	45.7	40.0	11.7
Shropshire	62.0	17.5	16.5	51.5	31.3	14.0	46.2	38.5	13.0

*All sheep were castrated males
†EBW = ingesta-free, wool-free body weight

the other breeds studied, while Corriedales and Shropshires showed the reverse.

Differences between breeds of pig in the proportions of body tissues appear to be less evident. In a comparison between purebred Yorkshires, Hampshire x Yorkshire, and Duroc x Yorkshire,[52] there were no significant differences in the tissue proportions at a common slaughter weight, but there were breed differences in rates of tissue gain.

Among the breeds of pig, the Belgian Pietrain is distinctive in being markedly different from others in its content of lean meat, being some 8% higher in this respect than the generally lean Landrace.[53-55] This advantage is offset, however, by the Pietrain's slower rate of gain[54,56] and higher water content in the muscle.[57]

It is evident from the foregoing discussion that considerable genotypic differences do exist in relative rates of development of the major determinants of carcass value and, therefore, substitution of breeds is one possible approach to improving the nutritive value of meat-producing animals. Another is to utilize the considerable differences which exist between sexes in rates of tissue growth.

SEX DIFFERENCES IN BODY COMPOSITION

Sex differences in rates of development of the body tissues are extensively documented and appear to be associated with differences between sexes in rates of maturity, such that the female at any given age or weight is relatively more mature than the entire male and, therefore, has more fat relative to muscle and bone.

The effects of castration on growth and carcass characteristics have been well reviewed by Turton[58] and by Field,[59] but recent Canadian studies[40,60-62] appear to be the only ones with cattle involving males, females, and castrates, thereby providing the direct comparison between the female and the entire male. Although exact interpretation of sex effects is prevented by differences in age at slaughter, it is clear that within genotypes, bulls are considerably leaner than steers or heifers, while the latter tend to be fatter than steers. Comparisons between castrates and females[63-65] and between castrates and bulls[34,66-70] support this conclusion that at a given weight the entire male is leaner than the castrate which, in turn, is leaner than the female. Since the bull also has the fastest weight gain,[34,71] it is evident that the entire male has an appreciably faster rate of muscle growth than the female and, therefore, is capable of producing a greater amount of edible meat in a given period of time. The disadvantages of bulls for meat production are largely managerial, but with increasing intensification of production methods, which allow attainment of desirable slaughter weights at relatively early ages, bulls are finding increasing use where intensive beef production systems are feasible.

Sex effects on body composition are well documented for sheep, as direct comparisons have been made between both intact and gonadectomized males and females.[72-74] Males are heavier at birth and grow muscle at a faster rate than females; intact animals of either sex grow muscle faster than do those gonadectomized. These differences exist even in early life, but the entire ram is appreciably the leanest, the ovariectomized female the fattest, and the castrate and the entire female similar and intermediate in this respect (Table 6).

In the pig, sex comparisons relevant to muscle growth have been confined mainly to intact females and castrated males. Here a species difference appears to exist, since in cattle the tendency is for the female to be fatter than the castrated male, whereas in the pig the reverse is the case.[52,66,75-85] The issue is confused, however, by the influences of age and nutrition. Thus, Lodge and Day[86] found in pigs fed ad lib and slaughtered at 60 kg, no difference in carcass lean content between intact males and females, both of which were superior to the castrates. In a later experiment[87] with pigs fed on restricted scales, there were no differences in carcass composition between castrates and females, again slaughtered at 60 kg. With restricted feeding Blair and coworkers[88] found that females and castrates had similar carcass lean content at 45 kg, but that the females were significantly leaner at 68 kg. In the sheep, on the other hand, entire females and castrated males interchanged in relative fatness between 8 and 28 weeks of age, at both of which ages they were virtually the same.[72,73]

The point which is abundantly clear, however, is that the entire male of all the species gives the highest output of lean meat in the shortest time, except in early life when commercial slaughter does not generally occur. Efficiency of meat production could be improved appreciably, therefore, merely by abandoning castration. This would present no problems in sheep production, or in cattle in confined systems where growth is rapid and the presence of bulls would not cause managerial problems. Only in the pig, and possibly the goat, where male sexual maturity is characterized by the presence in the tissues of odorous androstenone,[89] may castration be regarded as necessary except when slaughter is to be at an unusually early age.[90]

The use of exogenous sex hormones and related compounds to influence growth rate and carcass characteristics of meat animals has been widely practiced over the past decade. In general, the effects tend to parallel those observed between the sexes, but there are some anomalies. Estrogen treatment, which increases carcass fatness in entire lambs and bulls,[91,92] as might be expected, also increases bone and muscle growth in castrated animals, which is contrary to expectations from comparisons between castrates and entire females. Animals appear to be more responsive to exogenous hormones with approach of puberty,[74] so little benefit is likely to result in animals slaughtered at early ages.

As found by Everitt and Jury[72,73] in sheep of the different sexes, exogenous hormones also influence water content of muscle, in that increased leanness resulting from estrogen administration is accompanied by an increase in the proportion of water to protein in the muscle.[93-96]

NUTRITIONAL INFLUENCES ON BODY COMPOSITION

What might be regarded as the 'normal' pattern of tissue growth, as outlined earlier, may be considerably modified by a plane of nutrition. The relationship between overall rate of growth, as influenced by plane of feeding, and relative rates of development was studied intensively by the

TABLE 6

Sex Effects on Chemical Composition of Carcass Weight Change in Lambs[73]

	Stage of growth							
	0 to 12 weeks				12 to 24 weeks			
Sex	Water (%)	Fat (%)	Protein (%)	Ash (%)	Water (%)	Fat (%)	Protein (%)	Ash (%)
Entire male	45	36	15	4	43	42	11	5
Castrated male	41	41	14	4	15	80	3	4
Entire female	39	44	13	4	24	66	7	3
Ovariectomized female	36	48	12	4	22	74	0	4

students of Hammond in the 1930's[19–22,97] and has formed the subject of several subsequent studies. The conclusions reached by the Cambridge group were that undernutrition penalized body components differentially in reserve order of their maturity and affected primarily those undergoing most active development at the time of the restriction. As those tissues of major significance in determining carcass quality developed essentially in the order bone, muscle, and fat, the final composition of the carcass could be considerably modified by imposing feed restriction at the appropriate time to limit development of the least desirable tissue. Thus, as exemplified in the pig by McMeekan,[19–21] feed restriction in early life limited skeletal and, to a lesser degree, muscle development, and when such animals were later fed to a high level, they became excessively fat. Conversely, high plane feeding in early life followed by later restriction ultimately resulted in a carcass with a high proportion of lean to fat.

The interpretation of these results, that bone, muscle, and fat are all influenced differentially, has been subsequently questioned, first by Wallace[98] and later by Wilson[18,99] and Elsley et al.[100] The counterargument, further expounded by Fowler,[3,101] considers the true interpretation of the original data to be that restriction in total growth affects all tissues more or less equally with the exception of fat, the quantity of which was largely independent of the size of the rest of the body. The implication of this interpretation is that muscle:bone ratio is relatively constant, in contrast to fat:bone or fat:muscle ratios which will vary widely with plane of nutrition. McMeekan's data[21] indicate that this indeed is the case, showing overall variations between the extremes of 9% in muscle:bone, 105% in fat:bone, and 137% in fat:muscle. Elsley et al.[100] stress, however, that muscle:bone ratio is not constant over all possible feeding regimes and some differential curtailment of development occurs at extreme levels of restriction. In cattle, moderate degrees of feed and growth restriction failed to influence the muscle: bone ratio,[36,102] whereas severe restriction resulting in weight loss depleted both muscle and fat but had little effect on bone, thus narrowing the muscle:bone ratio.[45] In this latter experiment, rehabilitation of the cattle resulted in relatively rapid return to near-normal muscle:bone ratio, but fat required a prolonged period of recovery to return to the level found in animals with uninterrupted growth. In an experiment with calves up to 82 kg liveweight, Butterfield et al.[103] found that doubling the growth rate by high plane feeding had only minor influence on body components, but tended to increase both muscle and fat percents at the expense of bone.

It is evident that poultry also maintain a relatively constant muscle:bone ratio over a wide range of dietary variation, with protein remaining relatively constant and changes in fat occurring at the expense of moisture.[104–106]

Evidence on tissue response to plane of nutrition differing from both the above hypotheses has been presented in Australia[41] and the U.S.,[17] suggesting that body composition is weight dependent and largely uninfluenced by age or nutritional regime. Tulloh[41] reached this conclusion from a reevaluation of published data on carcass components of cattle, sheep, and pigs which showed linear relationships between empty body weight and weights of bone, muscle, and fat. However, the slopes of the regressions for the three tissues were different and the variations from the regression were greatest for fat and least for muscle. This indicated that as empty body weight increased, bone formed an ever decreasing portion of the total, fat an ever increasing portion, while the proportion of muscle remained almost constant, and that both bone and fat, but especially the latter, were more readily influenced than was muscle by factors other than body weight.

In a further report by Tulloh[107] of an experiment involving cattle slaughtered at similar ages but a variety of weights, growth coefficients for the individual tissues relative to increase in empty body weight were 1.0 for muscle, 0.7 to 0.8 for bone, and 1.5 for fat, thus confirming the earlier observations of Watson[108] and Callow[109] that skeletal muscle remained almost constant throughout life, at about one third of body weight.

The same conclusion was reached by Reid et al.[17] from an experiment in which chemical components of sheep carcass were determined following different dietary regimes and slaughter at either a common age or a common weight (Table 7). The body composition of animals of similar weight was approximately the same, even at ages as widely different as 374 and 613 days. The heavier animals had proportionally more fat and less water, and a tendency toward less protein.

This close relationship between body weight and body composition appeared to hold true over

TABLE 7

Relative Effects of Age and Weight on Body Composition of Sheep[17]

Animal	Feed intake (high or low)	Age (days)	EBW* (kg)	Body composition Water (%)	Fat (%)	Protein (%)	Ash (%)
1	H	270	28.2	57.4	24.4	15.0	2.9
2	L	270	19.9	61.5	18.5	15.6	3.9
3	L	349	28.7	56.6	23.9	15.8	4.0
4	H	381	49.6	46.1	38.1	13.1	2.6
5	L	381	27.7	54.5	27.7	14.3	2.8
6	L	583	47.5	46.1	38.5	12.6	2.7
7	H	374	58.3	46.2	38.4	12.8	2.4
8	L	374	31.8	56.3	24.1	15.8	3.3
9	L	613	56.0	46.0	38.5	12.7	2.8

*Ingesta-free, wool-free body weight

a wide range of growth rates, provided the animals were in a continuous positive energy balance; but partial fasting followed by refeeding resulted in a little more protein, considerably more water, and much less fat at a given body weight than occurred with a continuous body energy gain.

Although these different hypotheses on relationships between growth rate and body composition show points of disagreement, ranging from the very pliable association indicated by the Cambridge school, by which body composition at a given weight can be greatly modified by nutritional plane and growth rate, to the relatively rigid association expounded by Tulloh and the Cornell group, whereby body composition is a direct function of body weight regardless of age, there are aspects of unanimity. Of particular significance when considering ways to improve nutritive value of meat animals is the general finding that protein, or muscle where results are expressed in physical terms, is the least variable of the carcass constituents (see also Lohman[110]). In terms of individual muscle growth, Suess et al.[111] found that the relative growth of only the L. dorsi was influenced by moderate differences in plane of nutrition and that the rate of intramuscular fat deposition could be regulated by dietary means without altering rate of muscle growth. If fat was the main determinant of the nutritive value of meat it would be a simple matter to propose procedures for its enhancement, but it is evident that little can be done to increase protein content, apart from increasing total weight of animal. Taking animals to greater weights at slaughter clearly results in greater protein production, but at the expense of as much, or even more, carcass fat. There may be species differences, however, in the degree to which body composition is dependent on body weight. Reid et al.[17] noted a much less definite relationship in rats than in sheep, and work with pigs indicates that at least the proportions of 'fat' and 'lean' are quite susceptible to dietary manipulation.

In a study with pigs, designed to establish optimal energy and protein intakes for maximal muscle growth without incurring excess fat deposition,[112–115] growth and body composition responses to dietary energy increment were essentially linear, whereas responses to protein showed various curvilinear relationships (Table 8).

As the energy value of the diet was increased, daily weight gain and the percent of fat in the sample joint increased, the percent of lean decreased, while bone and skin were not significantly affected. Increase in protein content of the diet gave maximum growth rate on 18 or 21%, followed by a decrease on 24% dietary protein; maximum lean and minimum fat percents, however, were obtained on the highest protein level, 24%. These data show the conflict of interests which arises when establishing optimal performance in meat animals; carcasses of highest

TABLE 8

Composition of the Middle Section* of Pigs Slaughtered at 59 kg/liveweight Following Different Energy and Protein Intakes (from Cooke et al.[114])

Body component	Dietary energy level (Mcal/kg)				Dietary protein level (%)			
	2.8	3.1	3.4	3.6	15	18	21	24
Lean %	49.3	47.6	46.7	44.7	43.3	47.7	47.8	49.3
Fat %	27.8	31.0	33.9	34.9	34.2	31.7	31.6	30.1
Bone %	5.5	5.7	5.5	5.3	5.3	5.6	5.4	5.5
Skin %	5.7	5.6	5.6	5.4	5.3	5.5	5.8	5.7

*Half carcass less shoulder, ham, and belly

lean content, and therefore, perhaps, of highest nutritional acceptability, were obtained on the lowest energy and highest protein diet, but highest rate of muscle growth, which is the factor of perhaps greatest practical significance in a production system, was obtained with intermediate levels of both energy and protein. In evaluating possible means of improving nutrient output of meat-producing animals, it is necessary to think beyond the composition of the individual animal and consider the efficiency and rate of production of the complete system.

NUTRITIVE VALUE OF CARCASS COMPONENTS

Indicated above has been the degree to which proportions of muscle and adipose tissue, or protein and lipid, in a carcass may be modified by appropriate choice of genotype, sex, slaughter age, and diet. Consideration must also be given, however, to differences which may occur in the chemical composition, and therefore nutritive value, of the proteins and fats themselves.

Protein Quality

The fact that meats of different species differ so considerably in appearance suggests that differences in nutritive value might also occur. The low content of myoglobin in the skeletal muscles of pigs and breast muscles of poultry, relative to the general musculature of cattle and sheep, does influence the resulting meat quality but primarily through differences in postmortem change.

The paler muscles show a rapid decline in pH postmortem, which tends to denature the proteins. Generally, pork has a lower total nitrogen content than beef,[116,117] while chicken and turkey muscle have higher nitrogen contents than the red meats.[118]

In the avian species there are marked differences in composition between the light and dark meats, with the latter having 2 to 4% units more fat at the expense of protein.[119-121] The amino acid composition of the protein, however, is similar for all the meats, but the protein of turkey muscle appears to have a higher proportion and that of chicken a lower proportion of lysine than does beef or pork.[122,123] Evidence on the degree to which amino acid content may be modified within a species appears to be lacking.

Acceptability of meat, and therefore indirectly its nutritive value, is largely determined by its toughness. A major factor in this respect is the content of connective tisssue; although pork has considerably more collagen than corresponding beef muscle,[43,124] this does not appear to be associated with increased toughness or tenderness. Therefore, it can be concluded that the connective tissue of pork is of a different form to that of beef and mutton.[125]

Flavor is another aspect of acceptability, if not of nutritive value, and there is evidence that the flavor of meat from sheep may be influenced by the plant species which they graze upon prior to slaughter; generally, it would appear that leguminous plants impart a stronger flavor to the meat than do grass swards[126,127] and that grazing may impart more flavor than indoor concentrate feeding, even at very similar weights and ages.[128]

Fat Composition

Carcass fat composition differs quite markedly between the ruminant and nonruminant species, as a result of microbial hydrogenation of unsaturated dietary fats[129] in the former. As pointed out by Hilditch and Williams,[130] most land animals deposit fat in the proportions of one third C_{16} acids (mainly palmitic) and two thirds C_{18} acids. The relative proportions within the latter group determine the overall degree of saturation and the general tendency is for adult ruminants to have higher levels of the saturated stearic and lower levels of the unsaturates; oleic, linoleic, and linolenic.

Of major significance is the degree to which the depot fats can be influenced by the diet. In general, the proportion of unsaturates in adipose tissue of pigs and poultry can be increased appreciably by feeding unsaturated oils[131-136] or by substituting corn for barley as the basic cereal.[137] Administration of corn oil, either in the diet or directly into the abomasum, increased the proportion of unsaturated acids in body fat of lambs,[138] and the depot fats of cattle have also been increased in their content of total unsaturates by substituting an all-concentrate (primarily cereal grain) for an all-forage (pelleted alfalfa)[139] diet. Lambs fed barley-rich diets had unusually soft subcutaneous fat, which was related not to a higher proportion of unsaturates than in grass-fed sheep, but to considerably higher proportions of branched-chained acids and *n*-acids with an odd number of carbon atoms, which in turn was related to propionate production from the high-cereal diet.[140,141]

In ruminants, the dietary effect on fatty acid composition of adipose tissue appears to be essentially an indirect one, through an influence on the intraruminal microbial population,[142,143] rather than a direct effect of the fatty acid composition of the diet per se.

The question of dietary effects on body fat composition of ruminants is further complicated by the evidence of changes which occur with increase in age or weight. It is to be expected that the saturation of depot fat will increase in the young animal as rumen function develops, but there is evidence also to suggest that a peak is reached in cattle at around one year of age, followed by increases in proportions of unsaturated fats with advancing maturity.[144-146] This contrasts with evidence from sheep, either that saturation of adipose tissue increases with increased fat deposition,[147] or that over the common range of market weights neither rate of gain nor stage of development influenced the fatty acid content of depot fat.[148,149]

It cannot be assumed, however, that a real species difference exists in this respect, as other influential factors may confound the issue. Thus, stage of development is closely interrelated with diet, especially in comparisons between high-forage and high-concentrate feeds. There appear to be sex differences in the proportion of saturated acids in depot fats; in sheep, castrates were found to have a higher percent of saturates than rams,[148,149] while cattle have shown varying results between castrates and females.[150-152] Seasonal differences in cattle, uninfluenced by any dietary change, have also been reported.[145] Location of the fat within the body is clearly a major contributing factor to differences obtained in fatty acid composition of sample tissues; there are marked differences in this respect between different sites in the same animal both in ruminants[144,150,151,153] and in pigs.[136,154,155] Also, differences have been reported between adipose depots in poultry in their susceptibility to dietary change; abdominal fat was least resistant and liver fat most resistant to the influence of dietary fat.[156] There also appear to be differences between strains of poultry in the degree to which adipose tissue reflects the fatty acid and composition of the diet.[157]

CONCLUSIONS

It is evident from the data reviewed on variation in body composition of farm livestock, either in physical or chemical terms, that the musculature is not readily deviated from its normal pattern of growth, and the overall protein content is even less pliant. Adipose tissue is by far the major variable accounting for differences in weight, composition, and conformation of the meat-producing species and, therefore, any major improvements which can be effected in the nutrient composition of carcasses are essentially in terms of the quantity and quality of fat which accompanies the muscle or protein. The major area for improvement in meat production would seem to be in the efficiency with which protein is produced, by limiting energy expenditure on excess fat deposition, improving dietary protein utilization and the rate of body protein synthesis, minimizing the dietary cost of maintaining the animal, and improving reproductive performance so as to minimize the overhead costs of the breeding population. Prospects for increasing the protein content of the animal, other than by increasing overall weight, do not seem hopeful.

REFERENCES

1. **Hammond, J.,** *Growth and Development of Mutton Qualities in Sheep,* Oliver and Boyd, Edinburgh, 1932.
2. **Palsson, H.,** Conformation and body composition, in *Progress in the Physiology of Farm Animals,* Hammond, J., Ed., Butterworths, London, 1955, Chap. 10.
3. **Fowler, V. R.,** Body development and some problems of its evaluation, in *Growth and Development of Mammals,* Lodge, G. A. and Lamming, G. E., Eds., Butterworths, London, 1968, 195.
4. **Elsley, F. W. H.,** The physiological development of the young pig, *Ann. Zootechnol.,* 13, 75, 1964.
5. **Brooks, C. C., Fontenot, J. P., Vipperman, P. E., Thomas, H. R., and Graham, P. P.,** Chemical composition of the young pig carcass, *J. Anim. Sci.,* 23, 1022, 1964.
6. **Wood, A. J. and Groves, T. D. D.,** Body composition studies on the suckling pig. I. Moisture, chemical fat, total protein and total ash in relation to age and body weight, *Can. J. Anim. Sci.,* 45, 8, 1965.
7. **Salmon-Legagneur, E.,** Quelques aspects des relations nutritionelles entre la gestation et la lactation chez la truie, *Ann. Zootechnol.,* 14, 1, 1965.
8. **Blaxter, K. L.,** Lactation and the growth of the young, in *Milk: The Mammary Gland and its Secretion,* Vol. 2, Kon, S. K. and Cowie, A. T., Eds., Academic Press, New York, 1961, 305.
9. Anonymous, *Rept. of Major Beef Research Project,* The Royal Smithfield Club, London, 1966.
10. **Wallace, L. R.,** Factors influencing the efficiency of feed conversion by sheep, *Proc. Nutr. Soc.,* 14, 7, 1955.
11. **Barton, R. A. and Kirton, A. H.,** A comparison of whole milk with buttermilk in the rearing of calves for veal. 2. Slaughter and carcass composition data, *Anim. Prod.,* 3, 41, 1961.
12. **Butterfield, R. M., Johnson, E. R., and Pryor, W. J.,** A study of growth in calves. 1. Carcass tissues, *J. Agric. Sci. Camb.,* 76, 453, 1971.
13. **Clausen, H.,** George Scott Watson Memorial Lecture, Queens University, Belfast, 1953.
14. **Hornicke, H.,** Methods of estimating body composition of living animals with special reference to pigs. 5. Body composition of normally fed pigs during growth, *Z. Tierphysiol. Tierernahr. Futtermittelk,* 17, 28, 1962.
15. **Waldman, R. C., Tyler, W. J., and Brungardt, V. H.,** Changes in the carcass composition of Holstein steers associated with ration energy levels and growth, *J. Anim. Sci.,* 32, 611, 1971.
16. **Osinska, Z. and Ziolecka, A.,** A note on the protein content of the empty body of young Polish Black-and-White Lowland bulls, *Anim. Prod.,* 14, 119, 1972.
17. **Reid, J. T., Bensadoun, A., Bull, L. S., Burton, J. H., Gleeson, P. A., Han, I. K., Joo, Y. D., Johnson, D. E., McManus, W. R., Paladines, O. L., Stroud, J. W., Tyrrell, H. F., Van Niekerk, D. H., and Wellington, G. H.,** Some peculiarities in the body composition of animals, in *Body Composition of Animals and Man,* Publ. no. 1598, National Research Council, Washington, D.C., 1968, 19.
18. **Wilson, P. N.,** Growth analysis of the domestic fowl. 2. Effect of plane of nutrition on carcass composition, *J. Agric. Sci. Camb.,* 44, 67, 1954.
19. **McMeekan, C. P.,** Growth and development in the pig with special reference to carcass quality characters. I., *J. Agric. Sci. Camb.,* 30, 276, 1940.
20. **McMeekan, C. P.,** Growth and development in the pig with special reference to carcass quality characters. II. The influence of the plane of nutrition on growth and development, *J. Agric. Sci. Camb.,* 30, 387, 1940.
21. **McMeekan, C. P.,** Growth and development in the pig with special reference to carcass quality characters. III. Effect of the plane of nutrition on the form and the composition of the bacon pig, *J. Agric. Sci. Camb.,* 30, 511, 1940.
22. **Palsson, H. and Verges, J. B.,** Effects of plane of nutrition on growth and development of carcass quality in lambs. I. The effects of high and low planes of nutrition at different ages, *J. Agric. Sci. Camb.,* 42, 1, 1952.
23. **Wells, R. G.,** The relationship between dietary energy level, food consumption and growth in broiler chicks, *Br. Poult. Sci.,* 4, 161, 1963.
24. **Ryley, J. W., Moir, K. W., Pepper, P. M., and Burton, H. W.,** Effect of hexoestrol implantation and body size on the chemical composition and body components of chickens, *Br. Poult. Sci.,* 11, 83, 1970.
25. **Bixler, E. G., Combs, G. F., and Shaffner, C. S.,** Effect of protein level on carcass composition of turkeys, *Poult. Sci.,* 48, 261, 1969.
26. **Auckland, J. N. and Morriss, T. R.,** The effect of dietary nutrient concentration and calorie to protein ratio on growth and body composition of male and female turkey poults, *Br. Poult. Sci.,* 12, 305, 1971.
27. **Brody, S.,** *Bioenergetics and Growth,* Reinhold, New York, 1945.
28. **Godden, W.,** The relative efficiency of conversion of feeding stuffs by farm animals, *Agric. Prog.,* 23, 105, 1948.
29. **Leitch, I. and Godden, W.,** The efficiency of farm animals in the conversion of feeding stuffs to food for man, *Tech. Commun. Commonw. Bur. Anim. Nutr.,* No. 14, 1941.

30. **Lodge, G. A.,** Quantitative and qualitative control of proteins in meat animals, in *Proteins as Human Food,* Lawrie, R. A., Ed., Butterworths, London, 1970, 141.
31. **Holmes, W.,** Animals for food, *Proc. Nutr. Soc.,* 29, 237, 1970.
32. **Reid, J. T.,** The future role of ruminants in animal production, in *Physiology of Digestion and Metabolism in the Ruminant,* Phillipson, A. T., Ed., Oriel Press, Newcastle upon Tyne, 1970, 1.
33. **Kidwell, J. F. and McCormick, J. S.,** The influence of size and type on growth and development of cattle, *J. Anim. Sci.,* 15, 109, 1956.
34. **Wellington, G. H.,** Dairy beef, *J. Anim. Sci.,* 32, 424, 1971.
35. **Ziegler, J. H., Wilson, L. L., and Coble, D. S.,** Comparison of certain carcass traits of several breeds and crosses of cattle, *J. Anim. Sci.,* 32, 446, 1971.
36. **Callow, E. H.,** Comparative studies of meat. VII. A comparison between Hereford, Dairy Shorthorn and Friesian Steers on four levels of nutrition, *J. Agric. Sci. Camb.,* 56, 265, 1961.
37. **Branaman, G. A., Pearson, A. M., Magee, W. T., Griswald, R. M., and Brown, G. A.,** Comparison of the cutability and eatability of beef and dairy-type cattle, *J. Anim. Sci.,* 21, 321, 1962.
38. **Carroll, F. D., Clegg, M. T., and Kroger, D.,** Carcass characteristics of Holstein and Hereford steers, *J. Agric. Sci. Camb.,* 62, 1, 1964.
39. **Berg, R. T.,** Genetic and environmental influences on growth in beef cattle, in *Growth and Development of Mammals,* Lodge, G. A. and Lamming, G. E., Eds., Butterworths, London, 1968, 429.
40. **Mukhoty, H. and Berg, R. T.,** Influence of breed and sex on the allometric growth patterns of major bovine tissues, *Anim. Prod.,* 13, 219, 1971.
41. **Tulloh, N. M.,** Comparative breed studies of beef cattle. III. Carcass composition, *Aust. J. Agric. Res.,* 15, 333, 1964.
42. **Lawrie, R. A.,** Studies on the muscles of meat animals. I. Differences in composition of beef *longissimus dorsi* muscles determined by age and anatomical location, *J. Agric. Sci. Camb.,* 56, 249, 1961.
43. **Lawrie, R. A., Pomeroy, R. W., and Cuthbertson, A.,** Studies on the muscles of meat animals. III. Comparative composition of various muscles in pigs of three weight groups, *J. Agric. Sci. Camb.,* 60, 195, 1963.
44. **Butterfield, R. M.,** Relative growth of musculature of the ox, in *Carcass Composition and Appraisal of Meat Animals,* Tribe, D. E., Ed., C.S.I.R.O., Melbourne, 1963, Paper 7, 1.
45. **Butterfield, R. M.,** The effect of nutritional stress and recovery on the body composition of cattle, *Res. Vet. Sci.,* 7, 168, 1966.
46. **Butterfield, R. M. and Berg, R. T.,** A classification of bovine muscles based on their relative growth patterns, *Res. Vet. Sci.,* 7, 326, 1966.
47. **Butterfield, R. M. and Berg, R. T.,** Effect of nutrition on relative growth of muscles, *Proc. Aust. Soc. Anim. Prod.,* 6, 298, 1966.
48. **Butterfield, R. M. and Johnson, E. R.,** The effect of growth rate of muscle in cattle on conformation as influenced by muscle-weight distribution, in *Growth and Development of Mammals,* Lodge, G. A. and Lamming, G. E., Eds., Butterworths, London, 1968, 212.
49. **Rollins, W. C., Julian, L. M., and Carroll, F. D.,** A note on the body composition of a double-muscled female and a normal female from a linebred Aberdeen Angus herd, *Anim. Prod.,* 11, 111, 1969.
50. **Garrett, W. N.,** Energetic efficiency of beef and dairy steers, *J. Anim. Sci.,* 32, 451, 1971.
51. **Wiener, G.,** A comparison of the body size, fleece weight and maternal performance of five breeds of sheep kept in one environment, *Anim. Prod.,* 9, 177, 1967.
52. **Richmond, R. J. and Berg, R. T.,** Fat distribution in swine as influenced by liveweight, breed, sex and ration, *Can. J. Anim. Sci.,* 51, 523, 1971.
53. **Blendl, H. M.,** Results of full dissection in meat production testing of pigs, *Bayer. landwirt. Jahrb.,* 42, 941, 1965.
54. **Duckworth, J. E., Edge, T. M., Harrison, G., Olaniyan, O., Holmes, W., and Galazka, H.,** First report on trials with the Pietrain breed at Wye College, *Anim. Prod.,* 8, 356 (abst.), 1966.
55. **King, J. W. B.,** The interaction of genotype and environment in pig production, in *Pig Production,* Cole, D.J.A., Ed., Butterworths, London, 1972, 21.
56. **Kirsch, W., Fender, M., Rabold, K., Fewson, P., and Schoen, P.,** Comparative breeding, fattening and carcass trials with Improved Landrace, Pietrain and F1 crossbred pigs, *Zuchtungskunde,* 35, 254, 1963.
57. **McDougall, D. B. and Disney, J. G.,** Quality characteristics of pork with special reference to Pietrain, Pietrain x Landrace and Landrace pigs at different weights, *J. Food Technol.,* 2, 285, 1967.
58. **Turton, J. D.,** The effect of castration on meat production from cattle, sheep and pigs, in *Meat Production from Entire Male Animals,* Rhodes, D. N., Ed., Churchill, London, 1969, 1.
59. **Field, R. A.,** Effect of castration on meat quality and quantity, *J. Anim. Sci.,* 32, 849, 1971.
60. **Fredeen, H. T., Martin, A. H., and Weiss, G. M.,** Characteristics of youthful beef carcasses in relation to weight, age and sex. I. Organ weights, slaughter loss and cooler shrink in production of the dressed carcass, *Can. J. Anim. Sci.,* 51, 279, 1971.
61. **Fredeen, H. T., Martin, A. H., and Weiss, G. M.,** Characteristics of youthful beef carcass in relation to weight, age and sex. II. Carcass measurements and yield of retail product, *Can. J. Anim. Sci.,* 51, 291, 1971.

62. **Martin, A. H., Fredeen, H. T., and Weiss, G. M.,** Characteristics of youthful beef carcasses in relation to weight, age and sex. III. Meat quality attributes, *Can. J. Anim. Sci.*, 51, 305, 1971.
63. **Briedenstein, B. C., Briedenstein, B. B., Gray, W. J., Garrigan, D. S., and Norton, H. W.,** Comparison of carcass characteristics of steers and heifers, *J. Anim. Sci.*, 22, 1113 (abst.), 1963.
64. **Bradley, N. W., Cundiff, L. V., Kemp, J. D., and Greathouse, T. R.,** Effects of sex and sire on performance and carcass traits of Hereford and Hereford-Red Poll calves, *J. Anim. Sci.*, 25, 783, 1966.
65. **Wilson, L. L., Ziegler, J. H., Watkins, J. L., Thompson, C. E., and Purdy, H. R.,** Influence of sex and sire upon growth and carcass traits of beef cattle, *J. Anim. Sci.*, 28, 607, 1969.
66. **Prescott, J. H. D. and Lamming, G. E.,** The effects of castration on meat production in cattle, sheep and pigs, *J. Agric. Sci. Camb.*, 63, 341, 1964.
67. **Bailey, C. M., Probert, C. L., and Bohmann, V. R.,** Growth rate, feed utilization and body composition of young bulls and steers, *J. Anim. Sci.*, 52, 132, 1966.
68. **Berg, R. T.,** Genetic and environmental influences on growth in beef cattle, in *Growth and Development of Mammals,* Lodge, G. A. and Lamming, G. E., Eds., Butterworths, London, 1968, 429.
69. **Arthaud, V. H., Adams, C. H., Jacobs, D. R., and Koch, R. M.,** Comparison of carcass traits of bulls and steers, *J. Anim. Sci.*, 28, 742, 1969.
70. **Price, M. A.,** Infertile bulls versus steers. 3. Carcass characteristics, *J. Agric. Sci. Camb.*, 77, 317, 1971.
71. **Guilbert, H. R. and Gregory, P. W.,** Some features of growth and development of Hereford cattle, *J. Anim. Sci.*, 11, 3, 1952.
72. **Everitt, G. C. and Jury, K. E.,** Effects of sex and gonadectomy on the growth and development of Southdown x Romney cross lambs. Part I. Effects on live-weight growth and components of live-weight, *J. Agric. Sci. Camb.*, 66, 1, 1966.
73. **Everitt, G. C. and Jury, K. E.,** Effects of sex and gonadectomy on the growth and development of Southdown x Romney cross lambs. Part II. Effects on carcass grades, measurements and chemical composition, *J. Agric. Sci. Camb.*, 66, 15, 1966.
74. **Bradfield, P. G. E.,** Sex differences in the growth of sheep, in *Growth and Development of Mammals,* Lodge, G. A. and Lamming, G. E., Eds., Butterworths, London, 1968, 92.
75. **Bowland, J. P. and Berg, R. T.,** Influence of strain and sex on the relationship of protein to energy in the rations of growing and finishing bacon pigs, *Can. J. Anim. Sci.*, 39, 102, 1959.
76. **Charette, L. A.,** The effects of sex and age of male at castration on growth and carcass quality of Yorkshire swine, *Can. J. Anim. Sci.*, 41, 30, 1961.
77. **Buck, S. F., Harrington, G., and Johnson, R. F.,** The prediction of lean percentage of pigs of bacon weight from carcass measurements, *Anim. Prod.*, 4, 25, 1962.
78. **Blair, R. and English, P. R.,** Growth and carcass quality of uncastrated male pigs, *Anim. Prod.*, 5, 215 (abst.), 1963.
79. **Calder, A.,** Producing pork from boar pigs, *Rhodesian Agric. J.*, 60, 102, 1963.
80. **Lidvall, E. R., Burgess, C. R., Ramsey, C. B., and Cole, J. W.,** Performance and carcass characteristics of boars, barrows and gilts, *J. Anim. Sci.*, 23, 851 (abst.), 1964.
81. **Waldern, D. E.,** Influence of energy and protein level in rations for finishing market pigs on performance and carcass characteristics, *Can. J. Anim. Sci.*, 44, 168, 1964.
82. **Bell, J. M.,** Nutrient requirements for Canadian Yorkshire swine. V. A study on the lysine and protein requirements of finishing pigs weighing 100 to 200 lb, *Can. J. Anim. Sci.*, 45, 105, 1965.
83. **Hale, O. M., Johnson, J. C., and Warren, E. P.,** Influence of season, sex and dietary energy concentration on performance and carcass characteristics of swine, *J. Anim. Sci.*, 27, 1577, 1968.
84. **Young, L. G., Ashton, G. C., Forshaw, R. P., and Ingram, R. H.,** Relationship of dietary protein levels to performance and carcass merit of market swine, *Can. J. Anim. Sci.*, 48, 71, 1968.
85. **Teague, H. S., Plimpton, R. F., Cahill, V. R., Grifo, A. P., and Kunkle, L. E.,** Influence of diethylstilboestrol implantation on growth and carcass characteristics of boars, *J. Anim. Sci.*, 23, 332, 1964.
86. **Lodge, G. A. and Day, N.,** Sex effects on the performance of lightweight pork pigs, *Rep. Sch. Agric. Univ. Nottingham,* 1966-67, 62.
87. **Lodge, G. A., Hardy, B., and Lewis, D.,** Influence of energy and protein concentration in the diet on the performance of growing pigs. 4. Effects of sex on response to dietary protein level, *Anim. Prod.*, 14, 229, 1972.
88. **Blair, R., Dent, J. B., English, P. R., and Raeburn, J. R.,** Protein, lysine and feed intake effects on pig growth. 2. Effects on carcass composition and quality, *J. Agric. Sci. Camb.*, 73, 395, 1969.
89. **Patterson, R. L. S.,** Boar taint: its chemical nature and estimation, in *Meat Production from Entire Male Animals,* Rhodes, D. N., Ed., Churchill, London, 1969, 247.
90. **Elsley, F. W. H. and Livingstone, R. M.,** Effect of slaughter weight and feeding level on the incidence of boar taint, in *Meat Production from Entire Male Animals,* Rhodes, D. N., Ed., Churchill, London, 1969, 273.
91. National Research Council, Hormonal relationships and applications in the production of meats, milk and eggs, Natl. Res. Coun. Wash., Publ. no. 714, 1959.
92. **Preston, T. R., Greenhalgh, I., and McLeod, N. A.,** The effect of hexoestrol on growth, carcass quality, endocrines and reproductive organs of ram, wether and female lambs, *Anim. Prod.*, 2, 11, 1960.
93. **Aitken, J. N. and Crichton, J. A.,** The effect of hexoestrol implantation on growth and certain carcass characteristics of fattening steers, *Br. J. Nutr.*, 10, 220, 1956.

94. **Gee, I. and Preston, T. R.,** The effect of hexoestrol implantation on carcass composition and efficiency of feed utilization in fattening lambs, *Br. J. Nutr.*, 11, 329, 1957.
95. **Preston, T. R. and Gee, I.,** The influence of the route of administration on the effect of hexoestrol on fattening wether lambs, *Br. J. Nutr.*, 12, 158, 1958.
96. **Alder, F. E., Taylor, J. C., and Rudman, J. E.,** Hexoestrol implantation of steers fattened at pasture. II. Effects on empty weight, carcass weight and carcass quality, *Anim. Prod.*, 6, 57, 1964.
97. **Pomeroy, R. W.,** The effect of a sub-maintenance diet on the composition of the pig, *J. Agric. Sci. Camb.*, 31, 50, 1941.
98. **Wallace, L. R.,** The growth of lambs before and after birth in relation to the level of nutrition, *J. Agric. Sci. Camb.*, 38, 367, 1948.
99. **Wilson, P. N.,** The effect of nutrition on the growth and development of the East African dwarf goat, *J. Agric. Sci. Camb.*, 51, 4, 1958.
100. **Elsley, F. W. H., MacDonald, I., and Fowler, V. R.,** The effect of plane of nutrition on the carcasses of pigs and lambs when variations in fat content are excluded, *Anim. Prod.*, 6, 141, 1964.
101. **Fowler, V. R. and Livingstone, R. M.,** Modern concepts of growth in pigs, in *Pig Production,* Cole, D. J. A., Ed., Butterworths, London, 1972, 143.
102. **Hendrickson, R. L., Pope, L. A., and Hendrickson, R. F.,** Effect of rate of gain of fattening beef calves on carcass composition, *J. Anim. Sci.*, 24, 507, 1965.
103. **Butterfield, R. M., Johnson, E. R., and Pryor, W. J.,** A study of growth in calves. 1. Carcass tissues, *J. Agric. Sci. Camb.*, 76, 453, 1971.
104. **McNally, E. H.,** Calculation of the moisture and protein content of market chickens from the fat content, *Poult. Sci.*, 34, 152, 1955.
105. **Kondra, P. A., Richards, J. F., and Hodgson, G. C.,** The effect of sex, ration and strain on meat yield and its determination in chicken broilers, *Poult. Sci.*, 41, 922, 1962.
106. **Marion, J. E. and Woodroof, J. G.,** Composition and stability of broiler carcasses as affected by dietary protein and fat, *Poult. Sci.*, 45, 241, 1966.
107. **Tulloh, N. M.,** Comparative breed studies of beef cattle. 3. Carcass composition, *Aust. J. Agric. Res.*, 15, 333, 1964.
108. **Watson, D. M. S.,** Beef cattle in peace and war, *Emp. J. Exp. Agric.*, 11, 191, 1943.
109. **Callow, E. H.,** The food value of beef from steers and heifers, and its relation to dressing-out percentage, *J. Agric. Sci. Camb.*, 34, 177, 1944.
110. **Lohman, T. G.,** Biological variation in body composition, *J. Anim. Sci.*, 32, 647, 1971.
111. **Suess, G. G., Tyler, W. J., and Brungardt, V. H.,** Influence of weight and nutrition upon muscle growth and intramuscular fat deposition in Holstein steers, *J. Anim. Sci.*, 29, 410, 1969.
112. **Cooke, R., Lodge, G. A., and Lewis, D.,** Influence of energy and protein concentrations in the diet on the performance of growing pigs. 1. Response to protein intake on a high energy diet, *Anim. Prod.*, 14, 35, 1972.
113. **Lodge, G. A., Cundy, M. E., Cooke, R., and Lewis, D.,** Influence of energy and protein concentration in the diet on the performance of growing pigs. 2. Differing nutrient density at a constant energy:protein ratio, *Anim. Prod.*, 14, 47, 1972.
114. **Cooke, R., Lodge, G. A., and Lewis, D.,** Influence of energy and protein concentration in the diet on the performance of growing pigs. 3. Response to differences in levels of both energy and protein, *Anim. Prod.*, 14, 219, 1972.
115. **Lodge, G. A., Hardy, B., and Lewis, D.,** Influence of energy and protein concentration in the diet on the performance of growing pigs. 4. Effects of sex on response to dietary protein level, *Anim. Prod.*, 14, 229, 1972.
116. Anonymous, Nitrogen factors for pork, *Analyst* (London), 86, 557, 1961.
117. Anonymous, Nitrogen factors for beef, *Analyst* (London), 88, 422, 1963.
118. **Shrimpton, D. H.,** Eggs and poultry, in *Proteins as Human Food,* Lawrie, R. A., Ed., Butterworths, London, 1970, 225.
119. **Pudelkewicz, C., Gordon, H. W., and Kahlenburg, O. J.,** The effect of two different rations and two management practices on certain nutrients in poultry meat, *Poult. Sci.*, 42, 843, 1963.
120. **McReady, S. T. and Cunningham, F. E.,** Properties of salt-extractable proteins of broiler meat, *J. Sci. Food Agric.*, 22, 317, 1971.
121. **McReady, S. T. and Cunningham, F. E.,** Salt-soluble proteins of poultry meat. 1. Composition and emulsifying capacity, *Poult. Sci.*, 50, 243, 1971.
122. **Scott, M. L.,** Composition of turkey meat. 3. Essential amino acid composition, *J. Am. Diet. Assoc.*, 35, 247, 1959.
123. **Mountney, G. J.,** *Poultry Products Technology,* Avi Publishing Co., Westport, 1966, Chap. 4.
124. **Lawrie, R. A., Pomeroy, R. W., and Williams, D. R.,** Studies in the muscles of meat animals. IV. Comparative composition of muscles from 'doppelender' and normal sibling heifers, *J. Agric. Sci. Camb.*, 62, 89, 1964.
125. **Lawrie, R. A.,** Meat quality in the pig, in *Pig Production,* Cole, D. J. A., Ed., Butterworths, London, 1972, 163.
126. **Shorland, F. B., Czochanska, Z., Moy, M., Barton, R. A., and Rae, A. L.,** Influence of pasture species on the flavour, odour and keeping quality of lamb and mutton, *J. Sci. Food Agric.*, 21, 1, 1970.
127. **Park, R. J., Corbett, J. L., and Furnwal, F. P.,** Flavour differences in meat from lambs grazed on lucerne (Medicago Sativa) or phalaris (Phalaris tuberosa) pastures, *J. Agric. Sci. Camb.*, 78, 47, 1972.

128. **Rhodes, D. N.,** A comparison of the quality of meat from lambs reared intensively indoors and conventionally on grass, *J. Sci. Food Agric.,* 22, 667, 1971.
129. **Dawson, R. M. C. and Kemp, P.,** Biohydrogenation of dietary fats in ruminants, in *Physiology of Digestion and Metabolism in the Ruminant,* Phillipson, A. T., Ed., Oriel Press, Newcastle upon Tyne, 1970, 504.
130. **Hilditch, T. P. and Williams, P. N.,** *The Chemical Constitution of Natural Fats,* Chapman & Hall, London, 1964, Chap. 3.
131. **Kloze, A. A., Mecchi, E. P., Behman, G. A., Lineweaver, H., Kratzer, F. H., and Williams, D.,** Chemical characteristics of turkey carcass fat as a function of dietary fat, *Poult. Sci.,* 31, 354, 1952.
132. **Garton, G. A. and Duncan, W. R. H.,** Dietary fat and body fat: the composition of the back fats of pigs fed on a diet rich in cod-liver oil and lard, *Biochem. J.,* 57, 120, 1954.
133. **Machlin, L. J., Gordon, R. S., Marr, J., and Pope, C. W.,** Effect of dietary fat on the fatty acid composition of eggs and tissues of the hen, *Poult. Sci.,* 41, 1340, 1962.
134. **Marion, J. E. and Woodroof, J. G.,** The fatty acid composition of breast, thigh and skin tissues of chicken broilers as influenced by dietary fats, *Poult. Sci.,* 42, 1202, 1963.
135. **Isaacks, R. E., Davies, R. E., Ferguson, T. M., Reiser, R., and Couch, J. R.,** Studies on avian fat composition. 1. Effect of dietary fat on the fatty acids of the triglyceride and phospholipid fractions of the blood plasma and adipose tissue lipids of the laying hen, *Poult. Sci.,* 43, 105, 1964.
136. **Brooks, C. C.,** Fatty acid composition of pork lipids as affected by basal diet, fat source and fat level, *J. Anim. Sci.,* 33, 1224, 1971.
137. **Friend, D. W. and Cunningham, H. M.,** Growth, carcass, blood and fat studies with pigs fed once or five times daily, *J. Anim. Sci.,* 26, 316, 1967.
138. **Marchello, M. J., Fontenot, J. P., and Kelly, R. F.,** Effect of pre- and post-ruminal administration of corn oil on ovine fat, *J. Anim. Sci.,* 29, 874, 1969.
139. **Rumsey, T. S., Oltjen, R. R., Bovard, K. P., and Priode, B. M.,** Diet and breeding on fat composition of beef cattle, *J. Anim. Sci.,* 35, 196 (abstr.), 1972.
140. **Duncan, W. R. H., Ørskov, E. R., and Garton, G. A.,** Fatty acid composition of triglycerides of lambs fed on barley-based diets, *Proc. Nutr. Soc.,* 31, 19A, 1972.
141. **Garton, G. A., Hovell, F. D. DeB., and Duncan, W. R. H.,** Effect of dietary propionate on the fatty acid composition of lamb triglycerides, *Proc. Nutr. Soc.,* 31, 20A, 1972.
142. **Lough, A. K.,** Component fatty acids of plasma lipids of lambs with and without rumen ciliate protozoa, *Proc. Nutr. Soc.,* 27, 30A, 1968.
143. **Eadie, J. M. and Mann, S. O.,** Development of the rumen microbial population; high starch diets and instability, in *Physiology of Digestion and Metabolism in the Ruminant,* Oriel Press, Newcastle upon Tyne, 1970, 335.
144. **Leat, W. M. F. and Embleton, G. A.,** Adipose tissue fatty acids of young and mature Jersey cattle, *Proc. Nutr. Soc.,* 29, 48A, 1970.
145. **Link, B. A., Bray, R. W., Cassens, R. G., and Kauffman, R. G.,** Fatty acid composition of bovine subcutaneous adipose tissue lipids during growth, *J. Anim. Sci.,* 30, 722, 1970.
146. **Embleton, G. A. and Leat, W. M. F.,** Changes in the fatty acid composition of bovine adipose tissue associated with development, *Proc. Nutr. Soc.,* 31, 22A, 1972.
147. **Callow, E. H.,** Comparative studies on meat. Part VI. Factors affecting the iodine number of fat from the fatty and muscular tissue from lambs, *J. Agric. Sci. Camb.,* 51, 361, 1958.
148. **Tichenor, D. A., Kemp, J. D., Fox, J. D., Moody, W. G., and Deweese, W.,** Effect of slaughter weight and castration on ovine adipose fatty acids, *J. Anim. Sci.,* 31, 671, 1970.
149. **Crouse, J. D., Kemp, J. D., Fox, J. D., Ely, D. G., and Moody, W. G.,** Effect of castration, testosterone and slaughter weight on fatty acid content of ovine adipose tissue, *J. Anim. Sci.,* 34, 384, 1972.
150. **Terrell, R. N., Suess, G. G., and Bray, R. W.,** Influence of sex, liveweight and anatomical location on bovine lipids. 1. Fatty acid composition of subcutaneous and intermuscular fat depots, *J. Anim. Sci.,* 28, 449, 1969.
151. **Terrell, R. N., Suess, G. G., and Bray, R. W.,** Influence of sex, liveweight and anatomical location on bovine lipids. II. Lipid components and subjective scores of six muscles, *J. Anim. Sci.,* 28, 454, 1969.
152. **Link, B. A., Bray, R. W., Cassens, R. G., and Kauffman, R. G.,** Fatty acid composition of bovine skeletal muscle lipids during growth, *J. Anim. Sci.,* 30, 726, 1970.
153. **Terrell, R. N. and Bray, R. W.,** Influence of sex, liveweight and anatomical location on bovine lipids. III. Fatty acid composition of the neutral and phospholipid fractions from three muscles, *J. Anim. Sci.,* 29, 288, 1969.
154. **Duncan, W. R. H. and Garton, G. A.,** The fatty acid composition and intramolecular structure of triglycerides derived from different sites of the body in sheep, *J. Sci. Food Agric.,* 18, 99, 1967.
155. **Catchpole, C. and Lawrie, R. A.,** Influence of muscle location on fatty acid composition of total intramuscular lipids in the pig, *Anim. Prod.,* 14, 247, 1972.
156. **Mickleberry, W. C., Rogler, J. C., and Stadelman, W. J.,** The influence of dietary fat and environmental temperature upon chick growth and carcass composition, *Poult. Sci.,* 45, 313, 1966.
157. **Choo, S. H., Sell, J. L., and Kondra, P. A.,** The influence of dietary fat and strain of chicken on the fatty acid composition of egg yolk and body fat, *Poult. Sci.,* 46, 1245, 1967.

THE INCREASED AVAILABILITY OF NUTRIENTS FROM PLANT FOODSTUFFS THROUGH PROCESSING

M. L. Kakade
I. E. Liener

TABLE OF CONTENTS

Introduction 231
Physical Methods of Processing 232
Heat 232
Fractionation 232
Miscellaneous 234

Chemical Methods of Processing 235
Treatment with Water 235
Treatment with Acid and/or Alkali 235
Treatment with Organic Chemicals 236

Enzymatic Techniques 236
Fermentation 236
Proteolytic Enzymes 237
Carbohydrate-splitting Enzymes 237
Germination 237
Miscellaneous 238

Future Outlook 238

References 238

INTRODUCTION

For many people the very fact that a food item may have been processed before being offered for consumption carries with it the connotation that such a food has been "robbed" of nutrients. While it cannot be denied that processing may at times cause a destruction or elimination of essential nutrients, it is equally true that processing may enhance the nutritional quality of a foodstuff, for example, by destroying toxic constituents known to be present in many plant materials.[1] In fact, were it not for the simple expedient of cooking, it is doubtful whether the human species would have achieved the evolutionary superiority which it holds today. It was only after man had learned to use fire for cooking, about 40,000 years ago, that it became possible for him to take advantage of a greatly expanded food supply in the form of cooked vegetable foods. As pointed out by Leopold and Ardrey,[2] the rapid expansion of modern *Homo sapiens* coincided with the development of cooking which, by destroying the toxic substances of plants, brought a major evolutionary advantage to man. As the supply of animal protein fails to keep pace with the protein needs of an expanding world population, particularly in the lesser developed countries, man's continued survival may depend more than ever on an even greater use of plant foodstuffs as source of life-sustaining protein.

Although the application of heat is the most common form of processing to which most foods are subjected prior to consumption, it is by no means the only kind of treatment which a foodstuff may receive to improve its acceptability and nutritive properties. In addition to various forms of heat treatment, this chapter will show that such relatively simple techniques as fractionation on the basis of particle size, extraction with water or organic solvents, fermentation, etc. may also be effective means of increasing the availability of nutrients from plant proteins.

PHYSICAL METHODS

Heat

Osborne and Mendel[3] appear to be the first to report in 1917 that the nutritive value of a plant foodstuff, soybeans, was improved by heat treatment. They observed that rats fed raw soybeans as a source of protein did not grow nearly as well as those which were fed the cooked product. Innumerable reports have since appeared in the literature confirming and extending this observation to many other species of animals not only with soybeans but with many other legumes as well (see reviews by Liener[4,5]). In general, the degree of improvement effected by heat treatment is dependent on such variables as the temperature, duration of heat treatment, and moisture content. In the industrial processing of soybeans these conditions exert an effect which is reflected in the nutritive value of the final product. Various methods have been devised to provide a simple and rapid means of evaluating the efficacy of heat treatment with respect to the nutritional properties of soybeans. Perhaps the simplest and most commonly used technique is the one that measures the amount of protein which can be dispersed in water, the so-called "protein dispersibility index" or PDI. An inverse relationship is found between PDI and the nutritional value of commercial types of defatted soybean flours.[6] It is significant to note that rats fed commercially toasted samples of soybean flour obtained from various processors in the U.S. with PDI's ranging from 10 to 30 have consistently grown as well as those fed casein.[7] In general, the improvement in nutritive value effected by proper heat treatment of seed proteins is accompanied by an enhanced absorption of nitrogen and amino acids from the intestinal tract.[8,9]

An explanation for the beneficial effect of heat treatment on the nutritive value of most seed proteins has been the object of numerous studies; the literature dealing with this subject has been reviewed elsewhere.[1] Broadly speaking, it can be stated that the improvement in the nutritive value of many seed proteins effected by proper heat treatment is a consequence of the concomitant inactivation of specific heat-labile factors which are capable of eliciting untoward physiological responses in animals. For convenience these have been summarized in Table 1 along with information on their distribution in nature as well as their biological activities. In some cases (for example, the protease inhibitors and phytohemagglutinins of legumes, gossypol of cottonseed, goitrogens of rapeseed, cyanogens of cassava, etc.) these substances have been well characterized, but, in many other instances, their presence is recognized only by the deleterious effects that are produced in animals which have consumed foodstuffs containing them.

Preoccupation with attempts to correlate the beneficial effect of heat treatment with the destruction of these harmful substances has tended to obscure the favorable effect which heat might have on making the protein or carbohydrate more available independently of such factors. For example, it has been pointed out[11] that structural changes in the protein and possibly the carbohydrate constituents of foods induced by heat treatment may make them more susceptible to enzymatic attack. The enhanced vulnerability of denatured proteins to attack by proteolytic enzymes is well known to the enzymologist.

Fractionation

Mechanical separation on the basis of particle size to obtain high protein fractions from various seed proteins has been achieved by selectively grinding the meal followed by air classification or sifting.[12] In most cases, the final product also contains less fiber than the original material. Since fiber is known to interfere with protein utilization, such fractions should have improved nutritional characteristics. That this indeed is the case has been shown by a recent study[12] which demonstrated that the protein efficiency, N-retention, and protein digestibility of a wheat protein concentrate containing 3% fiber (prepared

TABLE 1

Antinutritional Factors Present in Plant Foodstuffs Which Are Destroyed or Eliminated by Processing[1,10]

Antinutritional factor	Common occurrence	Nutritional or biological effects
Protease inhibitors	Soybean, navy bean, lima bean, kidney bean, chick pea, cow pea, lentil, peanut, beet, potato, rice, wheat, corn	Decreased protein digestibility; pancreatic hypertrophy; increased requirement for S-amino acids
Hemagglutinins	Seeds belonging to *Leguminosae* (i.e., soybeans, kidney beans, navy beans, peanuts, etc.)	Interference with absorption of nutrients from intestines
Gossypol	Cottonseed	Increased requirement for protein and iron
Osteolathyrogens	*Lathyrus odoratus* (sweet peas)	Defect in collagen formation
Neurolathyrogens	*Lathyrus sativus* (chickling vetch), *Vicia sativa* (common vetch)	Neurotoxic effects
Cycasin	Cycads	Interference with synthesis of RNA
Goitrogens	Cabbage, turnip, rutabaga, mustard seed, rape seed, soybean	Interference with utilization of dietary iodine
Phytic acid	Seeds of mono- and dicotyledons (i.e., wheat, corn, rice, soybean, navy bean, peanut, etc.)	Interference with absorption of calcium, zinc, magnesium; increased requirement for vitamin D
Oxalic acid	Rhubarb, spinach, tea, cocoa	Increased requirement for calcium and vitamin D
Amylase inhibitor	Wheat, rye, barley, navy beans	Interference with digestion of carbohydrate
Ascorbic acid oxidase	Cabbage, cucumbers, pumpkin, lettuce, spinach, tomatoes, beets, potatoes, carrots, peaches	Destruction of vitamin C
Antivitamin D	Soybeans	Increased requirement for vitamin D
Antivitamin E	Kidney beans, alfalfa, peas	Increased requirement for vitamin E
Antipyridoxine	Linseed	Increased requirement for vitamin B_6

TABLE 1 (Continued)

Antinutritional factor	Common occurrence	Nutritional or biological effects
Antivitamin B_{12}	Soybeans	Increased requirement for vitamin B_{12}
Choline esterase inhibitor	Potatoes, broccoli, asparagus, eggplant, turnip, radish, celery, carrot, orange, apple	Interference with transmission of nerve impulse
Metal-binding constituents	Soybeans, sesame meal, peas	Increased requirement for zinc, manganese, copper, and iron
Lipoxidase	Soybeans	Increased requirement for vitamin A
Factors causing favism	*Vicia faba* (broad beans)	Hemolytic anemia
Oligosaccharides (raffinose, stachyose)	Most common legumes	Flatulence

by grinding and sifting shorts) were greater than those of the untreated shorts containing 10% fiber.

Woodham[13] has recently discussed the possibility of partitioning seed proteins into fractions which have superior nutritive quality because of their amino acid composition. For example, it has been demonstrated that particulate proteins of definite composition are isolable from peanut cotyledons by differential centrifugation[14] or by use of sucrose solutions of different strengths.[15] Other plants which are considered to be of inferior protein quality may in fact contain constituent proteins which are of excellent amino acid composition. For example, a glubulin fraction representing approximately one fifth of the total protein of barley – a cereal of poor overall amino acid composition – contains values for lysine, methionine, cystine, and threonine which are comparable to fresh meat protein.[13] Another example of the effectiveness of protein fractionation is the demonstration that the aleurone layer of the wheat kernel when combined with soybean flour has a biological value comparable to that of animal protein.[16]

Miscellaneous

There are numerous reports regarding the increased availability of nutrients as a result of processing techniques which cause a rupture of the plant cell walls and a dissolution of fibrous material. For example, Panalake and Murray[17] report that the quantity of crude carotene extractable from carrots was increased 70% by canning and 53% by cooking, presumably as a consequence of the increased accessibility of the carotene to the extracting solvent when the plant cells are ruptured. The availability of iron is also considerably increased by homogenizing plant foodstuffs in water by the "ultraturvax" process.[18] This effect may also be attributed to the comminution of the fibrous material of the plant since a similar effect was not observed in the case of dried skim milk. The improved growth response of chicks obtained with pelleted soybean diets has likewise been attributed to cellular disruption caused by the shearing force associated with pelleting.[19]

Particle size appears to play a role in the digestibility and absorption of fat. Mitchell et al.[20] have shown that fat is better digested by chicks as the particle size of roasted soybeans decreased. Stevens et al.[21] reported that rats grow better when fed a finely ground whole cereal meal than when the diet contained a coarser product. Ranhotra et al.[12] also point out that the growth of rats was greater on diets containing wheat shorts having a mesh size of 70 than a fraction which had a mesh size of 15, despite the fact that the fiber content was 10% in both cases. This indicates that the smaller size particles (70 mesh) are more efficiently utilized than particles of a larger size (15 mesh).

CHEMICAL METHODS OF PROCESSING

Water Treatment

Preliminary soaking of many plant materials prior to heat treatment, such as is employed in ordinary household cooking, is essential if optimum nutritive value is to be obtained. Examples of plant foodstuffs which require soaking before cooking are the various beans (kidney beans, lima beans, field beans), rapeseed, crambe seed, cycads, peas (especially those of the *Lathyrus* species), spinach, cabbage, and other leafy vegetables. In most cases, the soaking process serves simply to leach out water-soluble toxic substances, for example, the oxalic acid of rhubarb and spinach. Subsequent heat treatment may be necessary to reduce further any residual anti-nutritional factors such as the phytohemagglutinins of beans (*Phaseolus,* in particular).

An outstanding example involving soaking may be seen in the preparation of soybean milk which may be used as substitute for cow or human milk, particularly in the feeding of infants and children who are allergic to cow's milk or may be used where cow's milk is too expensive or unavailable. The traditional method for preparing soybean milk involves (1) soaking the beans overnight, (2) grinding to produce a slurry, (3) removal of the insoluble residue, and (4) boiling the extract for 20 to 30 min. Because of its low fiber content, the nutritional quality of soybean milk for infant feeding is quite comparable to that of cow's milk,[22,23] despite a deficiency of the sulfur amino acids revealed by rat growth studies.[24,25] This difference may be due to a less intense requirement for the sulfur amino acids by a growing child compared to the young rat, so that the low level of these amino acids in soybean milk may have little relevance to practical infant feeding.[26,27] The same consideration may apply equally as well to soybean meal or flour which has essentially the same amino acid composition as soybean milk.

It has been reported that the addition of water to animal diets exerted a significant improvement in the growth rate,[28-30] but the precise mechanism whereby this effect is produced remains to be elucidated.

One of the important considerations in the processing of rice is the retention of thiamine, particularly in those parts of the world where rice plays such a prominent role in the diet. The parboiling process (soaking and steaming) increases the thiamine content of rice, whereas steaming alone causes considerable destruction of this vitamin.[31]

Alkali and/or Acid Treatment

The isolation of proteins from protein-rich oil seeds has assumed considerable importance in recent years because of their potential for replacing proteins of animal origin which are apt to be in short supply in the not too distant future. The basic steps involved in the isolation process include solubilization of the crude protein by extraction with water or mild alkali, followed by precipitation of the protein at or near its isoelectric point, a step which requires the addition of acid to achieve a pH of 4 to 5. Such a preparation, containing about 90% protein, provides not only a rich source of protein but also has the nutritional advantage of being free of the carbohydrate fraction. The elimination of the insoluble fibrous carbohydrate fraction improves the overall digestibility as well as the utilization of the final product. The water-soluble fraction of carbohydrate, which is likewise absent from the soybean protein isolate, is known to contain the oligosaccharides, stachyose and raffinose, which have been implicated as causative factors of flatulence.[32] It is not surprising, therefore, that several investigators[33-35] have successfully used soybean protein isolates in the formulation of infant milk products. By replacing soybean flour with the protein isolate the disadvantages associated with the use of the former can be avoided; these include a disagreeable taste, the production of gas and colic, and frequent incidents of perianal dermititis.

Badenhop and Hackler[36] have reported that the presoaking of soybeans in 0.05 *N* NaOH produced a soybean milk product with a higher niacin content than is obtained by soaking the beans in water. Alkaline treatment apparently causes the release of niacin from a preexistent bound form of this vitamin. The flavor of the milk product was also improved as a result of this treatment. Presoaking of soybeans with 0.4 *M* sodium carbonate for 18 to 24 hr has been reported[37] to yield a milk product which had better flavor and body and a higher content of protein and fat than could be obtained by any other presoaking treatment including NaOH.

The importance of alkali treatment for enhancing the nutritive properties of corn is well recognized and has been generally attributed to an increased availability of niacin and certain essential amino acids.[28,38-41] Lime treatment also reduces the fiber content of corn and contributes significantly to the calcium intake of the population.[42]

An improvement in the nutritive value of fully toasted soy flour for calves and rats by pretreatment with alkali (pH 10.6 at 37° for 5 hr) or acid (pH 4 at 37° for 5 hr) has been reported by Colvin and Ramsey.[43] The authors suggest that these treatments somehow made certain nutrients more available from the soy flour. The experiments of Kakade et al.[44] point to the possible role of lecithin, which was present in the soy flour used in the study by Colvin and Ramsey, since this improvement was not observed by Kakade et al. with a non-lecithinated soy flour.

Delobez et al.[45] claim that the nutritive value of toasted soy flour is enhanced by pretreatment with alkali, an effect which they attribute to the destruction of a bound form of the trypsin inhibitor. Evidence for the existence of bound trypsin inhibitors in boiled soybeans has been recently reported by Wang et al.[46]

Treatment With Organic Chemicals

A variety of organic solvents, other than hexane which is most commonly used for the extraction of oil from soybeans, have been used for producing oilseed products having improved nutritional quality. For example, the gossypol of cottonseed meal can be reduced to very low levels by treatment with such solvents as aromatic and aliphatic amines, acetone, ethanol, and isopropanol or mixtures of solvents such as acetone-hexane-water.[47] Because of technical problems or economic considerations, however, their commercial application has met with little success. Recently a nonaqueous liquid classification process has been proposed for the removal of pigment glands which contain gossypol.[48] In this process defatted cottonseed flakes are ground in hexane to remove the pigment glands from the cellular tissue; the pigment glands are in turn separated from flour particles in a liquid centrifuge called a "liquid cyclone." The final product has been reported to contain 0.04% or less of free gossypol and less than 0.3% total gossypol.

Most of the plants belonging to the *Cruciferae* family contain goiterogenic substances (e.g., isothiocyanates, thiooxazolidones, etc.) which interfere with the metabolism of iodine.[49] It is obvious that the elimination or reduction of these goiterogenic substances greatly enhances the availability of dietary iodine. In addition to the application of heat and extraction with water, which are partially effective in reducing the goiterogenic content of most *Cruciferae*, extraction with cold acetone has also proved to be effective in removing these substances.[49]

Knowles et al.[50] found that by spraying fresh chopped alfalfa with an aqueous emulsion of the antioxidant, ethoxyquin (6-ethoxy-2,2,4-dimethyl-1,2-dihydroxyquinoline), the loss of carotenoids during subsequent dehydration and storage could be largely prevented.

PROCESSING INVOLVING ENZYMES

Fermentation

Although fermented bean products have been used for centuries in the Orient (e.g., tempeh, miso, and natto) and India (e.g., idli), until quite recently information concerning the nutritional properties of such foods has been quite scanty.

Tempeh is a soybean product popular in Indonesia which is prepared by soaking then boiling soybeans. The boiled beans are then fermented with the mold *Rhizopus* for about two days. Studies[51-56] have shown that as a result of this fermentation there was an increase in total soluble solids, vitamins, free fatty acids, soluble nitrogen, and free amino acids, whereas total nitrogen and total amino acids remained fairly constant. Experiments with rats, however, indicated that fermentation did not improve the growth-promoting property, protein efficiency ratio, nor digestibility of the soybean protein.[54,57] György,[58] however, did note considerable variation in the protein efficiency ratios of a number of tempeh preparations which had been processed under varying conditions; some of these did in fact have protein efficiency ratios which were higher than the unfermented control.

An increase in the levels of certain essential amino acids during fermentation has also been reported. For example, Sano[59] found an increase in several of the essential amino acid contents of natto, which is prepared by fermenting soybeans with *Bacillus subtilis*. Higher values for tryptophan and lysine have also been noted in natto by Standal.[60] Stillings and Hackler[55] also found a significantly higher level of tryptophan in tempeh which had been fermented for 24 hr. Radhakrishna Rao[61] likewise reported a 20% increase in methionine in idli which is prepared by fermenting a mixture of black gram (*Phaseolus mungo*) and rice. Studies by Wang et al.[62] on the protein quality of wheat and soybeans fermented with *Rhizopus oligosporus* indicate that the growth of rats fed the fermented wheat was significantly better than those fed the unfermented product. This improvement by fermentation was attributed to an increase in the availability of lysine as judged by in vitro digestibility studies. Their data also showed that, in addition to lysine, there is a general increase in the extent to which most of the other essential amino acids could be enzymatically released from the fermented wheat as compared to the control. No such improvement was observed in the case of soybeans, however.

The production of antibiotics by the mold *Rhizopus oligosporus* during the fermentation of Oriental soybean products has been reported by Wang et al.[63] The authors point out that antibiotics, in addition to minimizing infection, may exert growth-stimulating effects in animals, particularly if they are marginally deficient in one or more nutrients.[8,64,65]

Van Veen and Steinkraus[66] claim that the digestibility of soybean products for humans is greatly enhanced by fermentation. They also report an increase in certain of the vitamins as a result of fermentative action. Murata et al.[67] have also reported a two- to threefold increase in biotin and a four- to fivefold increase in total folate of tempeh during the 72-hr fermentation period. The increase in the latter nutrient was attributed to its release from a bound form. An increase in the availability of vitamin E in tempeh is believed to be due to the production of antioxidants during the fermentation process.[58,68] The increased availability of iron in bread[69] may also be a consequence of fermentation since it is known that yeast is capable of hydrolyzing phytic acid,[70] which would otherwise interfere with the availability of iron.

Proteolytic Enzymes

The "plastein" reaction (the reversal of enzymatic proteolysis) has been successfully used by a Japanese group[71-73] to effect an increase in the sulfur-containing amino acids of soybean protein. This provides a unique means for producing protein-like substances which have an amino acid composition resembling an ideal protein. The interested reader should consult the original references[71-73] for more detailed information on this novel method for enhancing the nutritive value of soybean protein.

The direct application of a proteolytic enzyme of microbial origin to heated soybeans causes an increase in nitrogen solubility as well as an enhanced susceptibility to peptic and tryptic digestion as measured in vitro.[74] This treatment also destroyed 33% of the lipoxygenase activity of the soybean.

Carbohydrate-splitting Enzymes

Many cellulases, generally of commercial origin, have been used to increase the nutritive value of plant foodstuffs for monogastric animals. By hydrolyzing indigestible cellulose and hemicellulose fractions of the plant cell wall, such enzymes would be expected to produce an increase in the available energy of plant materials. That this is indeed the case is illustrated by the recent studies of Saunders et al.[75] and Neudoerfer and Smith[76] which indicate that the availability of protein and sugar from wheat bran is considerably increased by treatment with cellulolytic enzymes following wet heating.

The oligosaccharides, stachyose and raffinose, of soy products have been implicated as factors responsible for the flatulence produced in many individuals who ingest beans.[32] Commercial preparations of α-galactosidase and invertase have been used to hydrolyze the oligosaccharides of soymilk,[77] but the effectiveness of such treatment in eliminating or reducing the flatulence problem remains to be determined.

Germination

Germination is known to result in an improvement in the nutritive value of various seed proteins such as the soybean,[78,79] black gram[80] (*Phaseolus mungo*), and chick pea[80] (*Cicer arietinum*). In general, there would appear to be little correlation between the effect of germination on the trypsin inhibitor content of seeds and their nutritive value; other factors affecting growth response are apparently involved. There is, however, a considerable increase in the level of certain amino acids (isoleucine, lysine, and valine) produced during the sprouting of soybeans.[60]

Miscellaneous

Many investigators have used enzyme preparations from various sources to improve the extractability of protein from plant materials.[81-83] Since these crude enzyme preparations are known to contain proteases as well as carbohydrases, plant foodstuffs so treated presumably owe their superior nutritional quality to increases in protein digestibility and available energy.

Rojas and Scott[84] were able to raise the level of metabolizable energy of cottonseed meal for chicks by treatment with a mold phytase preparation. This treatment also resulted in better utilization of phosphorus, zinc, and the proteins of cottonseed meal.

Since the starch component of various plant food materials is not well tolerated by many children, Buffa[85] has proposed that such foodstuffs should be pretreated with α-amylase to improve their digestibility and acceptability.

FUTURE OUTLOOK

To meet the protein needs of an ever-expanding world population, there is little doubt that much of this protein will have to come from plant sources. The most effective utilization of such protein will necessitate the employment of processing techniques which will optimize the quality as well as the yield of this protein. Because of their high protein content, the oil-bearing seeds and legumes will undoubtedly continue to be the focus of attention in this respect. We can look forward to major efforts on the part of the plant breeder to develop varieties with not only higher protein content but with protein of superior nutritional quality as well. At the same time ways and means of increasing the nutritive properties of the protein through improved methods of processing will no doubt receive more attention on the part of food technologists working in close cooperation with nutritionists. Conventional methods of processing involving heat treatment will probably be replaced to an ever-increasing extent by other forms of heat processing such as extrusion cooking,[86] microwave radiation,[87] and dielectric heating.[88] The fractionation of plant proteins by chemical or physical techniques in order to obtain protein-rich fractions having functional and nutritional properties comparable to meat protein has been realized in the case of soybeans[89] and remains to be explored with other plant proteins. Although fermentation has long been used in the Orient in the preparation of various plant foodstuffs for human comsumption, the full potential of this approach has yet to be realized in other parts of the world. What work has been done along these lines[90] has given promising indications that this age-old technique has much to offer in the future use of plant proteins.

REFERENCES

1. **Liener, I. E.,** *Toxic Constituents in Plant Foodstuffs,* Academic Press, New York, 1969.
2. **Leopold, A. C. and Ardrey, R.,** Toxic substances in plants and food habits of early man, *Science,* 176, 512, 1972.
3. **Osborne, T. B. and Mendel, L. B.,** The use of soybean as food, *J. Biol. Chem.,* 32, 369, 1917.
4. **Liener, I. E.,** Effect of heat on plant proteins, in *Processed Plant Protein Foodstuffs,* Altschul, A. M., Ed., Academic Press, New York, 1958, 79.
5. **Liener, I. E.,** Nutritional value of food protein products, in *Soybeans: Chemistry and Technology,* Smith, A. K. and Circle, S. J., Eds., Avi Publishing Co., Westport, Conn., 1972, 203.
6. **Horan, F. E.,** Defatted and full-fat soyflours by conventional processes, in *Soybean Protein Foods,* USDA/ARS Publication no. 71-35, 1967, 129.
7. **Kakade, M. L. and Thompson, R. T.,** unpublished observations, 1971.
8. **Kakade, M. L. and Evans, R. J.,** Growth inhibition of rats fed raw navy beans *(Phaseolus vulgaris), J. Nutr.,* 90, 191, 1966.
9. **de Muelenaere, H. J. H.,** Studies on the digestion of soybeans, *J. Nutr.,* 82, 197, 1964.
10. **Gontzea, I. and Sutzescu, P.,** *Natural Antinutritive Substances in Foodstuffs and Forages,* S. Karger, Basel, Switzerland, 1968.
11. **Grau, C. R. and Carroll, R. W.,** Evaluation of protein quality, in *Processed Plant Protein Foodstuffs,* Altschul, A. M., Ed., Academic Press, New York, 1958, 153.

12. **Ranhotra, G. S., Hepburn, F. N., and Bradley, W. B.,** Effect of fiber on availability of protein from wheat shorts, *Cereal Chem.,* 48, 9, 1970.
13. **Woodham, A. A.,** Oilseed protein: present and future, *World Rev. Nutr. Diet.,* 10, 44, 1969.
14. **Dieckert, J. W., Snowden, J. E., Moore, A. T., Heinzelman, D. C., and Altschul, A. M.,** Composition of some subcellular fractions from seeds of *Arachis hypogaea, J. Food Sci.,* 27, 321, 1962.
15. **Evans, W. J., Woodham, A. A., Carney, W. B., Dechary, J. M., and Altschul, A. M.,** Fractionation of particulate proteins of the peanut cotyledon, Proc. Seed Protein Conf., New Orleans, 1963, 218.
16. **Prier, R. F. and Derse, P. H.,** Nutritive value of a vegetable protein mixture, *J. Am. Diet. Assoc.,* 33, 1034, 1957.
17. **Panalake, T. and Murray, T. K.,** Effect of processing on content of carotene isomers in vegetables and peaches, *Can. Inst. Food Technol. J.,* 3, 145, 1970.
18. **Schlage, C. and Worstberg, B.,** Effect of hemogenization on the iron content of foods, *Z. Lebensm.-Unters. Forsch.,* 145, 97, 1971.
19. **Carew, L. B., Jr. and Nesheim, M. C.,** The effect of pelleting on the nutritional value of ground soybeans for the chick, *Poult. Sci.,* 41, 161, 1962.
20. **Mitchell, R. J., Waldrop, D. W., Hillard, C. M., and Hazen, K. R.,** Effects of pelleting and particle size on utilization of roasted soybeans by broilers, *Poult. Sci.,* 51, 506, 1972.
21. **Stevens, M. C., Sieburth, J. F., and McLaren, B.,** The effect of particle size on the nutritional characteristics of unrefined flour, *Food Res.,* 17, 74, 1952.
22. **Kay, J. L., Daeschmer, C. W., Jr., and Desmond, M. M.,** Evaluation of infants soybean and evaporated milk formulae from birth to 3 months, *Am. J. Dis. Child.,* 100, 264, 1960.
23. **Foman, J. J.,** Nitrogen balance studies with normal infants fed soybean protein, *Proc. Conf. Soybean Products for Protein in Human Foods,* U.S.D.A., Peoria, Ill., 1961, 175.
24. **Dutra de Olivira, J. E. and Scatena, L.,** Nutritional value of protein from a soybean milk powder, *J. Food Sci.,* 32, 592, 1967.
25. **Haskins, R. W. and Sarett, H. P.,** Method of comparing protein quality of soybean infant formulas in the rat, *J. Nutr.,* 91, 213, 1967.
26. **Block, R. J. and Mitchell, H. H.,** The correlation of the amino acid composition of proteins with their nutritive value, *Nutr. Abstr. Rev.,* 16, 249, 1946-1947.
27. **Block, R. J., Anderson, D. W., Howard, H. W., and Bauer, C. D.,** Effect of supplementing soybean proteins with lysine and other amino acids, *Am. J. Dis. Child.,* 92, 126, 1956.
28. **Lagune, J. and Carpenter, K. J.,** Raw versus processed corn in niacin deficient diets, *J. Nutr.,* 45, 21, 1951.
29. **Lepkovsky, S. and Furata, F.,** The effect of water treatment of feeds upon the nutritional value of feeds, *Poult. Sci.,* 39, 370, 1960.
30. **Keane, K. W., Smutke, C. J., Krieger, C. H., and Denton, A. E.,** The addition of water to purified diets and its effect upon growth and protein efficiency ratio in the rat, *J. Nutr.,* 77, 18, 1962.
31. **Subba Rao, P. V. and Bhattacharya, K. R.,** Effect of parboiling on thiamine content of rice, *J. Agric. Food Chem.,* 14, 479, 1966.
32. **Rackis, J. J., Sessa, D. J., Steggerda, F. R., Shimizu, T., Anderson, J., and Pearl, S. L.,** Soybean factors relating to gas production by intestinal bacteria, *J. Food Sci.,* 35, 634, 1970.
33. **Bates, R. D., Barrett, W. W., Anderson, D. W., Jr., and Saperstein, S.,** Milk and soy formulas, a comparative growth study, *Ann. Allergy,* 26, 577, 1968.
34. **Cowan, C. C., Jr., Brownlee, R. C., Jr., DeLoache, W. R., Jackson, H. P., and Mathews, J. P.,** A soy protein isolate formula in the management of allergy in infants and children, *South. Med. J.,* 61, 389, 1969.
35. **Wiseman, H. J.,** Comparison of two soy protein isolate infant formulas, *Ann. Allergy,* 29, 207, 1971.
36. **Badenhop, A. F. and Hackler, L. R.,** Effects of soaking soybeans in sodium hydroxide solution as pretreatment for soy milk production, *Cereal Sci. Today,* 15, 84, 1970.
37. **Khaleque, A., Bannatyne, W. R., and Wallace, G. M.,** Studies on the processing and properties of soy milk. I. Effect of processing conditions on the flavor and composition of soy milks, *J. Sci. Food Agric.,* 21, 579, 1970.
38. **Kodicek, E. R., Brande, S. K., Kon, S. K., and Mitchell, K. G.,** The effect of alkaline hydrolyses of maize on availability of its nicotinic acid to the pig, *Br. J. Nutr.,* 10, 51, 1956.
39. **Harper, A. E., Punekar, B. D., and Elvehjem, C. A.,** Effect of alkali treatment on the availability of niacin and amino acids on maize, *J: Nutr.,* 66, 163, 1958.
40. **Bressani, R. and Scrimshaw, N. S.,** Effect of lime treatment on *in vitro* availability of essential amino acids and solubility of protein fractions in corn, *J. Agric. Food Chem.,* 6, 774, 1958.
41. **Squibb, R. L., Braham, J. E., Arrogave, G., and Scrimshaw, N. S.,** Supplementation of low tryptophan-niacin deficient diets with beans and lime-treated corn in rats, *J. Nutr.,* 67, 351, 1959.
42. **Bressani, R., Paz y Paz, R., and Scrimshaw, N. S.,** Corn nutrient losses. Chemical changes in corn during preparation of tortillas, *J. Agric. Food Chem.,* 6, 770, 1958.
43. **Colvin, B. M. and Ramsey, A. A.,** Growth of young calves and rats fed soy flour treated with acid and alkali, *J. Dairy Sci.,* 52, 270, 1969.
44. **Kakade, M. L., Simons, N. R., and Liener, I. E.,** Nutritive value of acid treated soy flour – possible role of lecithin, *J. Dairy Sci.,* 54, 1705, 1971.

45. **Delobez, R. R., Duterte, R., and Rambaud, M.,** Determination of trypsin inhibitor of the soybean, *Rev. Fr. Corps Gras,* 18, 381, 1971.
46. **Wang, H. L., Vespa, J. B., and Hesseltine, C. W.,** Release of bound trypsin inhibitors in soybeans by *Rhizopus oligosporus, J. Nutr.,* 102, 1495, 1972.
47. **Berardi, L. C. and Goldblatt, L. A., Gossypol,** in *Toxic Constituents of Plant Foodstuffs,* Liener, I. E., Ed., Academic Press, New York, 1969, 212.
48. **Gastrock, E. A., D'Aquin, E. L., Eaves, P. H., and Cross, D. E.,** Edible flour from cottonseed by liquid classification using hexane, *Cereal Sci. Today,* 14, 8, 1969.
49. **Van Etten, C. H.,** Goitrogens, in *Toxic Constituents of Plant Foodstuffs,* Liener, I. E., Ed., Academic Press, New York, 1969, 103.
50. **Knowles, R. E., Livingston, A. L., Nelson, J. W., and Kohler, G. O.,** Stabilization of carotenoids by ethoxyquinon in harvested fresh alfalfa, *J. Agric. Food Chem.,* 16, 985, 1968.
51. **Steinkraus, K. H., Hwa, Y. B., Van Buren, J. P., Providenti, M. I., and Hand, D. B.,** Studies on tempeh – an Indonesian fermented soybean food, *Food Res.,* 25, 777, 1960.
52. **Wagenknecht, A. C., Mattick, L. R., Lewin, L. M., Hand, D. B., and Steinkraus, K. M.,** Changes in soybean lipids during tempeh fermentation, *J. Food Sci.,* 26, 373, 1961.
53. **Roelofson, P. A. and Talens, A.,** Changes in some B vitamins during molding of soybeans by *Rhizopus oryzae* in the production of tempeh kedelee, *J. Food Sci.,* 29, 224, 1964.
54. **Smith, A. K., Rackis, J. J., and Booth, A. N.,** Tempeh: nutritive value in relation to processing, *Cereal Chem.,* 44, 173, 1964.
55. **Stillings, B. R. and Hackler, L. R.,** Amino acid studies on the effect of fermentation time heat processing of tempeh, *J. Food Sci.,* 30, 1043, 1965.
56. **Murata, K. H., Ikehata, H., and Miyamoto, T.,** Studies on the nutritional value of tempeh, *J. Food Sci.,* 32, 580, 1967.
57. **Hackler, L. R., Steinkraus, K. H., Van Buren, J. P., and Hand, D. B.,** Studies on the utilization of tempeh protein by weanling rats, *J. Nutr.,* 82, 452, 1964.
58. **György, P.,** The nutritive value of tempeh, in *Meeting the Protein Needs of Infants and Children,* Natl. Acad. Sci., Natl. Res. Council Publ. 843, 1961, 281.
59. **Sano, T.,** Feeding studies with fermented soy products (natto and miso), in *Meeting the Protein Needs of Infants and Children,* Natl. Acad. Sci., Natl. Res. Council Publ. 843, 1961, 247.
60. **Standal, B. R.,** Amino acid studies in Oriental soybean foods, *J. Am. Diet. Assoc.,* 50, 397, 1967.
61. **Raddakrishna Rao, M. V.,** Some observations on fermented foods, in *Meeting the Protein Needs of Infants and Children,* Natl. Acad. Sci., Natl. Res. Council Publ. 843, 1961, 291.
62. **Wang, H. L., Ruttle, D. E., and Hesseltine, C. W.,** Protein quality of wheat and soybean after *Rhizopus oligosporus* fermentation, *J. Nutr.,* 96, 109, 1968.
63. **Wang, H. L., Ruttle, D. E., and Hesseltine, C. W.,** Antibacterial compound from a soybean product fermented by *Rhizopus oligosporus, Proc. Soc. Exp. Biol. Med.,* 131, 579, 1969.
64. **Kakade, M. L. and Evans, R. J.,** Effect of methionine, vitamin B_{12}, and antibiotic supplementation on protein nutritive value of navy beans, *Proc. Soc. Exp. Biol. Med.,* 115, 890, 1964.
65. **Kakade, M. L., Simons, N. R., and Liener, I. E.,** Nutritional effects induced in rats by feeding natural and synthetic trypsin inhibitors, *J. Nutr.,* 100, 1003, 1970.
66. **Van Veen, A. G. and Steinkraus, K. H.,** Nutritive value and wholesomeness of fermented products, *J. Agric. Food Chem.,* 18, 576, 1970.
67. **Murata, K., Miyamoto, T., Kokufu, E., and Snake, Y.,** Studies on the nutritional value of tempeh. III. Changes in biotin and folic acid during tempeh fermentation, *J. Vitaminol.,* 16, 281, 1970.
68. **György, P., Murata, K., and Ikehata, H.,** Antioxidants isolated from fermented soybeans (tempeh), *Nature,* 203, 870, 1964.
69. **Ranhotra, G. S., Hepburn, F. N., and Bradley, W. B.,** Availability of iron in enriched bread, *Cereal Chem.,* 48, 377, 1971.
70. **Leicher, J. and Joslyn, M.,** The state of iron in flour, dough, and bread, *Cereal Chem.,* 44, 346, 1967.
71. **Yamashita, M., Arai, S., Gonda, M., Kato, H., and Fujimaki, M.,** Enzymatic modification of proteins in foodstuffs. II. Nutritive properties of soy plastein and its bio-utility evaluation in rats, *Agric. Biol. Chem.,* 34, 1333, 1970.
72. **Yamashita, M., Arai, S., Matsuyama, J., Gonda, M., Kato, H., and Fujimaki, M.,** Enzymatic modification of proteins in foodstuffs. III. Phenomenal survey on α-chymotrypsin plastein synthesis from peptic hydrolyzate of soy protein, *Agric. Biol. Chem.,* 34, 1484, 1970.
73. **Yamashita, M., Arai, S., Tsai, S. J., and Fujimaki, M.,** Plastein reaction as a method for enhancing the sulfur-containing amino acid level of soybean protein, *J. Agric. Food Chem.,* 19, 1151, 1971.
74. **Arai, S., Noguchi, M., Yamashita, M., Kato, H., and Fujimaki, M.,** Applying proteolytic enzymes on soybeans. VII. Properties of soy protein treated with microbial acid protease (Molsin), *Agric. Biol. Chem.,* 34, 1338, 1970.
75. **Saunders, R. M., Connor, M. A., Edwards, R. H., and Kohler, G. O.,** Enzymatic processing of wheat bran: effects on nutrient availability, *Cereal Chem.,* 49, 436, 1972.

76. **Neudoerffer, T. S. and Smith, R. E.,** Enzymatic degradation of wheat bran to improve its nutritive value for monogastrics, *Can. J. Anim. Sci.,* 49, 205, 1969.
77. **Sugimoto, H. and Van Buren, J. P.,** Removal of oligosaccharides from soy milk by an enzyme from *Aspergillus saitoi, J. Food Sci.,* 35, 655, 1970.
78. **Everson, G., Steenbock, H., Cederquist, D. C., and Parsons, A. T.,** The effect of germination, the stage of maturity, and variety upon the nutritive value of soybean protein, *J. Nutr.,* 27, 225, 1944.
79. **Viswanatha, T. and De, S. S.,** Relative availability of cystine and methionine in the raw, germinated, and autoclaved soybeans and soybean milk, *Indian J. Physiol. Allied Sci.,* 5, 51, 1951.
80. **Chattapadhay, H. and Bannerjee, S.,** Effect of germination on biological value of proteins and trypsin inhibitor activity of common Indian pulses, *Indian J. Med. Res.,* 44, 185, 1953.
81. **Abdo, K. M. and King, K. W.,** Enzymatic modification of the extractability of protein from soybeans, *Glycin max, J. Agric. Food Chem.,* 15, 83, 1967.
82. **Chandrasekaran, A. and King, K. W.,** Enzymatic modification of the extractability of protein from coconuts *(Cocos mucifera), J. Agric. Food Chem.,* 15, 305, 1967.
83. **Sreekantriah, K. R., Ebine, A., Ohta, T., and Nakano, M.,** Enzymic processing of vegetable protein foods, *Food Technol.,* 23, 69, 1969.
84. **Rojas, S. W. and Scott, M. L.,** Factors affecting the nutritive value of cottonseed meal as a protein source in chick diets, *Poult. Sci.,* 48, 819, 1969.
85. **Buffa, A.,** Food technology and development. I. Processing low cost nutritious native foods for world's hungry children. Factors, formulas, processes, *Food Eng.,* 43, 79, 1971.
86. **Mustakas, G. C., Griffin, E. L., Jr., and Sohns, V. F.,** Full fat soybean flours by continuous extrusion cooking. World protein resources, *Am. Chem. Soc. Adv. Chem. Ser.,* 57, 101, 1966.
87. **Wang, R. W. and Alexander, J. C.,** The heating of soybean meals by microwave radiations, *Nutr. Rep. Int.,* 4, 387, 1971.
88. **Borchers, R., Manage, L. D., Nelson, S. D., and Stetson, L. E.,** Rapid improvement in nutritional quality of soybeans by dielectric heating, *J. Food Sci.,* 37, 333, 1972.
89. **Bressani, R., Viteré, F., Elias, L. G., De Zaghi, S., Alvarado, J., and Odell, A. D.,** Protein quality of a soybean protein textured food in experimental animals and children, *J. Nutr.,* 93, 349, 1967.
90. **Hesseltine, C. W. and Wang, H. L.,** Fermented soybean food products, in *Soybeans: Chemistry and Technology,* Smith, A. K. and Circle, S. J., Eds., Avi Publishing Co., Westport, Conn., 1972, 389.

FOOD FORTIFICATION

L. J. Teply

TABLE OF CONTENTS

Introduction . . . 243
Definition . . . 243
General Considerations . . . 243

Experience in Fortifying Foods with Various Nutrients . . . 244
General . . . 244
Vitamin A . . . 245
Vitamin D . . . 245
Thiamine, Riboflavin, and Niacin . . . 246
Vitamin C . . . 246
Iodine . . . 246
Iron . . . 246
Calcium . . . 247
Protein and Amino Acids . . . 247

Prospects for the Future . . . 247

References . . . 248

INTRODUCTION

Definition

For the purpose of this paper, the definition of "food fortification" is that adopted by the FAO/WHO Joint Expert Committee on Nutrition which met in Geneva in November, 1970.[1] It is the addition of specific nutrients to foods to maintain or improve dietary intakes of segments of a population or of a whole population. The nutrients may be added either as purified or synthetic materials or as concentrates from natural sources.

"Restoration" is the replacement of nutrients which have been lost in harvesting, storage, or processing of conventional foods. In the U.S. "enrichment" refers to the addition of nutrients in conformity to government standards for specific items. In both cases there is protection against nutritional imbalance. In the broader field of food fortification, regulation and control should protect against the addition of nutrients to too many vehicles or at unreasonably high levels.

General Considerations

It has been about a half century since goiter was shown to be preventable through addition of iodine compounds to salt, vitamin A concentrates were added to margarine to prevent severe vitamin A deficiency causing blindness, and vitamin D was added to milk to prevent rickets. Ever since those breakthroughs, with the identification of dietary deficiencies of additional vitamins and minerals and with newer knowledge of protein and amino acid nutrition, there has been an interest in many quarters in promotion of far more food fortification than is presently practiced. This paper will attempt to show that there is considerable scope for more food fortification, but that at the same time it is by no means a panacea.

Dozens of countries throughout the world have adopted policies for fortification of certain foods. Although there is general agreement that fortification is justified to combat specific deficiency diseases that are public health problems, there is a divergence of opinion when this is not the case. Some favor only restoration of nutrients lost in handling and processing of foods. On the other hand, for example, the Statements of General Policy in regard to Addition of Specific Nutrients to Foods of the Food and Nutrition Board, U.S. National Academy of Sciences, National Research Council and the Council of Foods and Nutrition, American Medical Association, jointly adopted first in 1953, and revised most recently in 1968,[2] endorse the principle of addition of specific nutrients to foods, provided that there is an advantage to a significant segment of the population, that appropriate food items are used as vehicles, and that the fortification does not interfere with the achievement of a diet good in other respects. The current statement also recommends continued efforts to develop new and improved formulated foods which may offer advantages in nutrition, acceptability, and economy.

There is general agreement that fortification should not be used to cover up poor practice in handling and processing of foods nor should it be used indiscriminately for promotion of certain foods.

The aforementioned FAO/WHO Joint Expert Committee on Nutrition,[1] a 1971 Technical Group Meeting of the Pan American Health Organization/Pan American Sanitary Bureau/ Regional Office of the World Health Organization,[3] and the Protein Advisory Group of the United Nations System[4] have considered the basic nutritional, technological, economic, and social factors that should be taken into account before deciding on a particular food fortification action; they are in agreement that the decision should be made on the basis of local circumstances and preferably within the context of a national food and nutrition policy, with alternative approaches being given appropriate consideration and priorities. In order to arrive at logical decisions, information must be obtained on the deficiency problems and responsiveness to added nutrients in target groups, the potential vehicles for the target groups, consumer acceptance, and costs of implementation, including costs of regulation and evaluation. It is generally true that fortification with most nutrients causes little or no change in the acceptability of the food. However, the overall costs may not be as low as is often assumed. In any case, there is some added cost and there may be reluctance on the part of consumers, governments, or commercial firms to bear this cost.

The newer nutritional knowledge of the 20th century with respect to vitamins, minerals, amino acids, proteins, and essential fatty acids enabled production in industrialized countries of nutritious (fortified) foods for infants without dependence on milk. This technology is now being applied as one means of meeting nutritional problems in the developing countries. Various supplementary foods, suitable for young children during the weaning period, have been produced and distributed through feeding programs and retail channels. These mixtures are usually based on cereal flours and are fortified with vitamins, minerals, protein concentrates, and sometimes with amino acids.[5]

EXPERIENCE IN FORTIFYING FOODS WITH VARIOUS NUTRIENTS

General

Historical information on food fortification is provided in many reviews.[1,3,6-9]

The fish liver oil concentrates used to fortify margarine with vitamin A eventually gave way to synthetic vitamin A when it could be produced at a competitive cost. Similarly, milk was first fortified with vitamin D by feeding materials containing vitamin D to cows or by irradiation of the milk. Eventually, purified vitamin D was added directly.

Shortly after the fortification of foods with vitamin A and D was established, fortification with the B vitamins thiamine, riboflavin, and niacin came to the fore. Again there were the following steps in the process: identification of the vitamin; establishment of requirement levels; accumulation of data on possible toxicity; development of appropriate technology, including assay methods for the control; and the synthetic production of the vitamin at reasonable cost. Somewhat similar steps took place in the case of iodine and iron.

An example of fortification with thiamine, riboflavin, and iron on a large scale is the addition of these nutrients to bakery-produced white bread and family white wheat flour which was introduced as a World War II order in the U.S. in 1941.[10] Similar "enrichment" of corn products followed.[11] During the same period the British Government investigated the possibilities of fortification. However, the main emphasis was placed on use of higher extraction flours. Eventually millers were allowed to choose their extraction rate but were required to fortify with thiamine, niacin, and iron to the level of 80% extraction flour. Bread and flour fortification are now permitted or required in many countries throughout the world.

With respect to amino acids, most of the basic steps were worked out at about the same time as for vitamins and minerals. However, the fortification of staple foods with amino acids has not developed as rapidly because the benefits are not as clear and the costs, so far, are relatively high.

Vitamin A

When margarine was substituted for butter in Denmark during World War I, some of the consumers developed "xerophthalmia" or "dry eye." In its more severe form blindness resulted. This could be attributed to deficiency of vitamin A; the desirability of fortifying margarine with vitamin A was obvious. This was first accomplished with fish liver oil concentrates but eventually synthetic vitamin A became available at a sufficiently low cost. Fortification of margarine with vitamin A is now standard practice in numerous countries.

The large-scale distribution of skim milk powder after World War II for supplementary feeding in developing countries that had vitamin A deficiency problems focused attention on the need to fortify the skim milk powder. UNICEF, with the cooperation of industry, supported work on the development of appropriate technology so that the product would be stable under the conditions of packaging and distribution.[12] The procedure of dry mixing stabilized "beadlets" into the powder was adopted. UNICEF made arrangements for initial production of the fortified powder going to countries with the most serious vitamin A problems and in the mid-1960's the U.S. adopted the policy of fortifying all skim milk powder provided for donation programs at a level of 5,000 I.U./100 g.

Other foods fortified with vitamin A include fluid milks, vegetable oils, and foods based on cereals.

A study in Jordan several years ago indicated that the best approach was fortification of flour. The technology was worked out but the program has not yet been implemented. Vitamin A is added to "modern bread" which has been promoted in India for several years.[13]

In Guatemala sugar has been selected as a vehicle for vitamin A.[14] Fortification of tea in India has been suggested.[15] This would offer advantages as far as reaching villages is concerned but more information is needed, for example, on the extent to which this would reach one of the main target groups – the younger children.

Vitamin D

Although it is difficult to separate the role of addition of vitamin D to milk from other factors such as use of vitamin D supplements or better pediatric care, pediatric authorities continue to be convinced that milk fortification is an important weapon in the control of rickets. Observations in a number of countries since vitamin D fortification of milk was instituted in the U.S. in the 1920's have indicated that, even though complete control has not been achieved, the prevalence of rickets declined markedly when the fortification was introduced and increases have been observed in periods of retrogression in the programs.

It had been known that high doses of vitamin D could produce toxicity but the practical problem in fortification programs emerged in the United Kingdom when increased incidence of hypercalcemia in infants was reported after the vitamin D content of the national dried milk was increased from 10 I.U./g to 18 I.U./g. Although the total number of cases was relatively small, in 1957 the Ministry of Health in the United Kingdom recommended that the levels of vitamin D in the national dried milk, in infant cereals, and in cod liver oil preparations be reduced. Canada allows addition of vitamin D only to milk and margarine. The Committee on Nutrition of the U.S. National Academy of Pediatrics has recommended a daily intake of 400 I.U. vitamin D and a limitation of foods fortified to milk and infant formulas.

In many developing countries, at least partly because infants are kept out of sunlight, rickets is a common disease.[16] Therefore, the skim milk powder in U.S. donation programs is fortified with 500 I.U. vitamin D/100 g.

Thiamine, Riboflavin, and Niacin

Certain diets may be particularly deficient in one B vitamin; for example, rice diets tend to be low in thiamine and maize diets in niacin. However, there is frequently a multiple deficiency and it is common practice to fortify with at least these three B vitamins.

The prevention of beriberi through rice fortification was shown in experiments in the Philippines in the 1940's. This was a culmination of a remarkable series of persevering efforts, particularly on the part of Dr. Robert R. Williams, starting with association of beriberi with deficiency of a dietary factor present in rice polishings to chemical synthesis of thiamine and development of satisfactory technology for fortification of rice. However, a national fortification program has not developed because of socioeconomic problems in implementation. Rice fortification programs have been implemented in Japan, Taiwan, and Korea. In some of the Asian countries fortification is difficult because of dispersal of milling among many small units. A project of Harvard University and the Government of Thailand, with support from AID, is testing the feasibility of fortification under these conditions.

Fortification of bread, white flour, and in particular, maize products was of particular interest in the U.S. because of the continued significant prevalence of pellagra, primarily due to niacin deficiency, in the southern part of the country. This disease was decreasing before the fortification programs were instituted so it is difficult to determine precisely what role the fortification played. However, it seems reasonable to assume that it made an appreciable contribution. Senti[18] has reviewed the impact of cereal grain product fortification on the nutrient content of the diet.

Pellagra and beriberi are still observed in some of the developing countries. These frank diseases are, of course, only the tip of the iceberg. Most of the developing world is covered with a blanket of dietary intakes of riboflavin that are lower than most nutrition authorities consider desirable. Biochemical tests and, in some cases, clinical signs substantiate this. Wherever these problems exist and it is feasible to fortify food items with these nutrients, this should be given serious consideration.

Vitamin C

Ascorbic acid is added to various products. It may be particularly useful when added to items, such as certain juices that have a relatively low content of vitamin C, which may replace good sources of vitamin C in the diet.

Iodine

The rich history of iodine and the prevention of goiter is summarized in a World Health Organization publication.[19] It seems that a relationship between iodine intake and goiter was suspected in the early 1800's; during the rest of that century several scientists suggested supplementation of diets with iodine for prevention of goiter. However, the first serious effort to establish iodization of salt occurred in the years following 1915 when Marine and Kimball demonstrated the effectiveness of this procedure in trials in Akron, Ohio. These investigators laid to rest many of the fears of "toxic effects" but some of these persist to this day. During the 1920's the use of iodized salt spread in European countries as well as in North America. Iodization has not been compulsory in the U.S. and over the years an increase in prevalence of goiter has been observed in certain areas where use of iodized salt declined for a time.

Lowenstein[20] summarized the progress in salt iodization in various parts of the world to 1965. Goiter continues to be a public health problem in many countries. In some areas the problem is of such severity that "cretinism" with impaired mental development is not uncommon. In some places where salt iodization is not feasible, periodic intramuscular injections of oil containing iodine are being tried, but this is a more expensive operation than salt fortification.

It has been found that iodate is more stable than iodide in the forms of salt and under the conditions of storage and handling of the salt in many of the developing countries. A convenient spray unit has been devised for adding iodate to crude forms of salt.[21] With assistance from UNICEF and the World Health Organization, this process has been introduced into Taiwan, India, Thailand, and Burma. Careful evaluations have shown a marked decline in prevalence of goiter where the iodated salt has been introduced.

Iron

Iron fortification programs have been operating in the U.S. and U.K. for prevention of iron deficiency anemia over many years. Only relatively recently have there been serious attempts to evaluate effectiveness. It appears that in at least some programs effect of iron added to bread and flour has been limited by the form of the iron added, the nature of the vehicle, and the composition of the rest of the diet. There have been proposals for raising the levels of the added iron. Although there does not seem to be a serious risk of toxic effects, a number of authorities have expressed a definite concern on this point. The Food and Nutrition Board of the U.S. National Academy of Sciences, National Research Council issued a Recommendation for Increased Iron Levels in the American Diet in November of 1969 and has continued to study the various aspects of iron fortification.[22] Goldsmith[23] has summarized some of the current developments on iron enrichment of bread and flour. In view of the prevalence of iron deficiency anemias throughout the world, the World Health Organization is continuing the study of various aspects of fortification of foods with iron as one approach to increasing dietary intakes.

Calcium

Calcium is added to various foods but information as to dietary needs and methodology for determining the nutritional status of individuals with respect to calcium is not sufficiently developed to allow definitive judgment as to the value of the fortification. It is quite possible that in certain areas with very low calcium intakes and where there is a high prevalence of osteoporosis, as in Japan and India, supplementation of the diet with an appropriate amount of calcium would have beneficial effects.

Protein and Amino Acids

Fortification of cereal-based foods with protein concentrates that improve nutritional quality and at the same time add some protein is a widely accepted procedure.[24] The proper balancing of amino acid content of foods and diets enables efficient use of protein which have an unsatisfactory nutritional value when used as the sole source of protein. In each situation a judgment must be made as to whether the diet that is being supplemented is deficient in protein, taking both quality and quantity into consideration, in relation to calories.[25] The alternative approach of adding limiting amino acids offers the potential advantage of minimal change in organoleptic properties; but there are other factors that must be considered. An international conference held at the Massachusetts Institute of Technology in 1969 considered possibilities for amino acid fortification.[26] The Protein Advisory Group of the United Nations System[5] also gave this subject serious attention. These considerations were summarized in a presentation to the Third Western Hemisphere Nutrition Congress in 1971.[27]

For amino acids it is more difficult to make a clear case for expected benefits to population groups than in the case of certain vitamins and minerals. Investigators in Japan have reported positive results from trials and some fortification with lysine is practiced in that country.[28] However, a school-feeding trial in Iran using a basic diet specifically designed to be low in lysine showed marginal results.[29] Harvard University, with support from AID, is conducting a large-scale field trial of fortification of wheat flour with lysine in Tunisia. It might be of interest to give more attention to the possibilities for fortification with other amino acids, such as methionine; this amino acid is already added to certain infant formulas based on soy.

Durrenmatt[30] has suggested that large-scale use of amino acids might reduce the cost markedly, as in the case of certain vitamins.

PROSPECTS FOR THE FUTURE

While food fortification is not a panacea, this should not detract attention from what appears to be vast possibilities for wider application of this approach. In many of the developing countries, besides protein-calorie malnutrition, various other deficiency diseases still exist as widespread public health problems. Tens of thousands of children go blind each year primarily from vitamin A deficiency. Iron deficiency anemias and anemias of pregnancy due to folate deficiency are common. Goiter is still unchecked in many areas. Along with other approaches, especially the promotion of production and consumption of conventional foods that provide adequate diets, food fortification can play a role in eliminating these deficiency diseases, even though some of the main target groups are sometimes difficult to reach through this approach, especially in the rural areas. It cannot be overemphasized that decision to invest resources in this approach should be made after considering alternatives and wherever feasible, it should be part of a national food and nutrition policy and development plan.

In most industrialized countries fortification of staple foods is fairly well established. For the future, formulated foods offer possibilities of providing convenient, acceptable, and nutritious foods at relatively moderate cost. Regulation and monitoring will be necessary to assure appropriate levels of various nutrients.[31]

It seems reasonable to expect that the science and technology of food formulation and fortification will gradually be applied in all countries of the world; hopefully this will promote a just distribution of the world's resources to provide a good diet for all.

REFERENCES

1. Joint FAO/WHO Expert Committee on Nutrition, Eighth Report, Food Fortification Protein-Calorie Malnutrition, World Health Organization Report Series No. 477, Geneva, 1971.
2. General Policies in regard to Improvement of Nutritive Quality of Foods, published jointly by the Council of Foods and Nutrition, American Medical Association, *J.A.M.A.*, 205(12), 868, 1968, and the U.S. Food and Nutrition Board, U.S. National Academy of Sciences, National Research Council, Washington, D.C., 1968.
3. Guidelines for Food Fortification in Latin America and the Caribbean, Report of a Technical Group Meeting, Pan American Health Organization, Pan American Sanitary Bureau, Regional Office of the World Health Organization, Washington, D.C., 1972.
4. Protein Advisory Group Statement No. 9, PAG Recommendation on Amino Acid Fortification of Foods, Protein Advisory Group, United Nations, New York, 1970.
5. **Orr, E.,** The Use of Protein-rich Foods for the Relief of Malnutrition in Developing Countries: An Analysis of Experience, Tropical Products Institute, London, 1972.
6. **Sebrell, W. H.,** The concept of fortification of foods with synthetic nutrients, in *Amino Acid Fortification of Protein Foods,* Part II, MIT Press, Cambridge, 1971, 63.
7. **Bauernfeind, J. C.,** Vitamin fortification and nutrified foods, in *Proceedings of Third International Congress of Food Science and Technology,* Institute of Food Technologists, Chicago, 1971, 217.
8. **Harris, R. S.,** Mineral fortification of foods and food products, in *Proceedings of Third International Congress of Food Science and Technology,* Institute of Food Technologists, Chicago, 1971, 200.
9. **Aylward, F. and Morton, I. D.,** Vitamin fortification of foods, in *Proceedings of Third International Congress of Food Science and Technology,* Institute of Food Technologists, Chicago, 1971, 192.
10. Enrichment of Flour and Bread. A History of the Movement, U.S. National Academy of Sciences National Research Council, Bulletin No. 110, Washington, D.C., November, 1944.
11. **Brooke, C. L.,** Enrichment and fortification of cereals and cereal products with vitamins and minerals, *Agric. Food Chem.,* 16(2), 163, 1968.
12. **Bauernfeind, J. C. and Allen L. E.,** Vitamin A and D enrichment of non-fat dry milk, *J. Dairy Sci.,* 46, 245, 1963.
13. **da Cunha, S.,** The modern bread story, in *Proceedings of the Third International Congress of Food Science and Technology,* Institute of Food Technologists, Chicago, 1971, 178.
14. **Arroyave, G.,** Distribution of vitamin A to population groups, in *Proceedings of the Western Hemisphere Nutrition Congress,* Futura Publishing Co., Mt. Kisco, N.Y., 1972, 68.
15. **Brooke, C. L. and Cort, W. M.,** Vitamin A fortification of tea, *Food Technol.,* 26, 6, 1972.
16. Joint FAO/WHO Expert Committee on Nutrition, Seventh Report, World Health Organization, Geneva, Technical Report Series, No. 377, 1967, 31.
17. Rice Enrichment in the Philippines, FAO Nutritional Studies No. 12, Rome, March, 1954.
18. **Senti, F. R.,** Impact of grain product fortification on the nutrient content of the U.S. diet, *Cereal Sci. Today,* 16, 92, 1971.
19. Endemic Goitre, World Health Organization, Monograph Series No. 44, Geneva, 1960.
20. **Lowenstein, F. W.,** Iodized salt in the prevention of endemic goitre: a world-wide survey of present programmes, *Am. J. Public Health,* 57, 1815, 1967.
21. **Hunnikin, C.,** The iodization of crude salt for the prophylaxis of goitre, *Food Technol.,* 18, 40, 1964.

22. Measures to Increase Iron in Foods and Diets, Proceedings of a workshop, Food and Nutrition Board, U.S. National Academy of Sciences, National Research Council, Washington, D.C., 1970.
23. **Goldsmith, G. A.,** Iron enrichment of bread and flour, *Am. J. Clin. Nutr.,* 26, 131, 1973.
24. **Milner, M., Ed.,** *Protein-enriched Cereals for World Needs,* American Association of Cereal Chemists, St. Paul, Minn., 1969.
25. The Protein Problem, Protein Advisory Group Statement No. 20, Protein Advisory Group, United Nations, New York, 1973.
26. **Scrimshaw, N. S. and Altschul, A. M., Eds.,** *Amino Acid Fortification of Protein Foods,* MIT Press, Cambridge, 1971.
27. **Teply, L. J.,** Amino acid fortification, in *Proceedings of the Third Western Hemisphere Nutrition Congress,* Futura Publishing Co., Mt. Kisco, N.Y., 1972, 37.
28. **Mitsuda, H.,** Approaches to amino acid and vitamin enrichment programmes in Japan, *Proceedings of the First Asian Congress of Nutrition,* Tulpule, P. G. and Rao, K. S. J., Eds., Nutrition Society of India, Hyderabad, 1972, 457.
29. **Hedayat, H., Shahbazi, H., Payan, R., and Donoso, J.,** Lysine field trial in Iran, *Progress in Human Nutrition,* Vol. 1, Margen, S., Ed., Avi Publishing Co., Westport, Conn., 1971, Chap. 4.
30. **Durrenmatt, K.,** in *Amino Acid Fortification of Foods,* Scrimshaw, N. S. and Altschul, A. M., Eds., MIT Press Cambridge, 1971, 528.
31. Report on an ad hoc meeting, Nutrition labeling, *Nut. Rev.,* 30, 247, 1972.

DEVELOPMENT OF NEW HIGHLY NUTRITIOUS FOOD PRODUCTS

R. Bressani
and
L. G. Elias

TABLE OF CONTENTS

Introduction 252

Available Sources 252
Vegetable Sources 253
Cereals 253
Legumes 253
Starchy Roots and Tubers 253
Nonconventional Foods 253
Oilseeds 253
Palm Kernel and Nuts 253
Leaf and Algae Protein 253
Yeast and Microbial Proteins 254
Nutrients 254
Amino Acids 254
Vitamins 254
Mineral Salts 254

Objectives of the Development of Highly Nutritious Foods 254

Applications 256
High Protein-containing Foods 256
Fortification 259
Synthetic Amino Acids 259
Protein Concentrates 259
Protein Concentrates Plus Amino Acids 260
Other Specific Nutrients (Vitamins and Minerals) 261
Other Important Aspects 261
Restoration 264
Enrichment 265
Replacement 267

Processing 267

Textured Vegetable Protein Foods 268

The Role of Genetics on the Development of Highly Nutritious Products 269

Significance and Role of Highly Nutritious Products 270

References 271

INTRODUCTION

Much interest has evolved on the subject of developing highly nutritious food products during the last decade, due to various reasons, among which the most important probably is the prevention of a nutrition crisis in developed and developing countries alike. It is well known that the nutrition problem is more acute in developing areas because of a constantly increasing population without parallel increases in food production. Furthermore, within the population of the developing countries, foods for the most vulnerable groups, such as weaning and pre-school children and pregnant women, require more attention, because such groups require foods with higher concentration of nutrients in the appropriate balance, for higher nutritional quality.

Among nutrients, one which has received particular attention is protein which, even if available in relatively large amounts, is not evenly distributed among the population within areas, with some getting foods of higher protein content than others.

Total protein is only part of the problem; more important is protein quality, that is, the concentration and balance of the essential amino acids in the protein. The usual protein foods which generally provide the needed protein quality in developed countries are milk, meat, and eggs. These foods are not easily obtained by the low socioeconomic groups in developing countries because of their low availability, high cost, and lack of appropriate transportation and storage facilities.

Although the quantity and quality of the nutrient, protein, have probably received more attention, nutritional and dietetic surveys have pointed out that other nutrients are also lacking in the diets of most people. These are vitamin A, riboflavin, and probably, iron. In particular cases, other nutrients can also be lacking, for example, niacin, vitamin D, calcium, iodine, ascorbic acid, and thiamine.

In view of the above, the development of highly nutritious foods can be a rather complex problem in which consideration must be given to the nutritional limitations of the food itself, as well as consideration of its role as a carrier of nutrients in relation to other foods consumed, the methods or ways in which it is prepared for consumption, nutrient requirements by specific population groups, stability of nutrients, economic and acceptability aspects, and many other points as well. The problem will not be solved by one group of scientists, but by all directly or indirectly concerned with foods, from the agronomist to the marketing specialist. However, a very important role is played by food scientists, technologists, and nutritionists, who are responsible for formulating such new or highly nutritious foods in terms of nutrient content, preservation during processing, and high standards of acceptability.

For efficient utilization of specific nutrients in a particular food, which is the principal aim of developing highly nutritious foods, consideration must be given to all nutrients which could be lacking in the food or diets. For example, little is accomplished by improving only protein quality if vitamins or minerals are also deficient. The present chapter summarizes some of the information available on the problem of the development of highly nutritious products, starting from the available nutrient sources, the objectives in developing highly nutritious foods, and the applications in terms of technologies at our disposal to provide mankind with highly nutritive and efficiently utilized food products.

AVAILABLE SOURCES

Animal and vegetable foods have been recognized through history to be the main sources of nutrients for mankind. However, as the world population increases, the supply of foods is becoming a crucial problem since food production has not increased in proportion to the growth of the population. The problem is even more serious in those areas of the world labeled underdeveloped, since in this case the challenge is not only to eliminate the shortage of foods, but also to improve their nutritional quality. In other words, this implies the utilization of the available resources with the highest degree of efficiency. On the other hand, it seems that among nutrients, the lack of protein ranks first, followed by calories, vitamins, and minerals. Unfortunately, meat, eggs, milk, and fish, considered to be the best natural sources of good quality protein, are either in short supply or expensive in the developing areas of the world. In general, vegetable sources such as cereals, legumes, oilseeds, and starchy roots constitute the main source of nutrients for those people. Such food commodities are considered to be of a relatively low nutritive value, as compared to the animal sources. However, the technology of this century has permitted the chemical and biological synthesis of many nutrients, such as amino acids and vitamins, that can be used to improve the nutritive value of many foods. From these introductory remarks, it can be concluded that the available food sources in this situation must be confined mainly to vegetable staple foods, to nonconventional sources, and to nutritional additives.

Vegetable Sources

Cereals

In general, this group of foods has low protein quantity and quality, lysine, tryptophan, and threonine being the most limiting amino acids. From the nutritional point of view, they must be regarded mainly as sources of calories, although this is not entirely true in practice due to their high intake which provides significant amounts of protein and of other nutrients.

Because they are bulky and low in protein, it is rather difficult to obtain an adequate protein intake with them.

Legumes

Leguminous seeds can be considered as natural supplements to cereals, since they contain adequate amounts of lysine;[2] they are generally deficient in the sulfur-containing amino acids,[3,4] which are in turn present in adequate levels in cereals. Another limitation is their low protein digestibility in many species and varieties[5,6] and the presence of adverse heat-labile physiological factors. However, these difficulties can be overcome by processing methods involving heat.[7] The antiphysiological factors can also be removed by protein extraction, giving products that can be useful in many preparations. Since legume foods have at least twice the protein content of cereals,[1] they can contribute significantly to the solution of the problem of protein quantity.

Starchy Roots and Tubers

As a source of nutrients, these groups of foods must be considered only as a source of calories; their protein content is very low,[8] although it must be recognized that potatoes, for example, have an attractive amino acid pattern.[9] Cassava roots have also been reported as a good source of calcium.[10]

Nonconventional Foods

Oilseeds

This group of resources can be considered as one of the best sources of both protein and calories. Their economic and nutritional properties constitute a valuable asset in the formulation of high nutritive foods.[1,11] The press cake left after oil extraction is a product with about five times more protein than the cereals and twice the amount present in the *Leguminosae* seed. The protein content can be further increased either by screening techniques, which separate the fiber,[12] or by precipitation of the protein after its extraction with adequate solvents.[13,14] In addition, they are relatively high sources of some essential amino acids, as for example, lysine and tryptophan in soybeans,[15-17] and methionine in both cottonseed,[11,18-21] and sesame protein.[16,22,23]

The presence of toxic factors in the oilseeds, such as gossypol in cottonseed[11] or trypsin inhibitors in soybeans,[24] can now be eliminated through appropriate processing techniques.[11,25] Soybeans can be considered as an exception in the group of oilseeds since they cannot be classified as a nonconventional food; their use as a natural source of nutrients in the Orient, mainly in the form of fermented foods,[26] is well known.

Palm Kernel and Nuts

This group must be regarded mainly as a source of calories or of essential fatty acids. Protein content can be increased either by oil extraction or by fiber removal. According to the particular product, it seems that lysine, methionine, and tryptophan are the most limiting amino acids.[27,28] More technological research and an increased availability must be attained in order to utilize them as a source of proteins.

Leaf and Algae Protein

The main drawback in the utilization of these materials as a source of protein has been from the economic and organoleptic points of view. The amino acid compositions indicate that the sulfur-containing amino acids are the most limiting in both cases.[29,30] In general, it can be said that they have a relatively good nutritive value, their low digestibility in some cases being their most important limitation.[31]

Yeast and Microbial Proteins

From the results of several studies,[1] it can be concluded that food yeasts (*Torulopsis utilis*) and brewers yeast should be good sources of proteins and vitamins of the B complex. Being rich sources of lysine with a protein content between 40 and 50% and also rich in vitamins, they are suitable materials to supplement many foods.[32,33] The main disadvantages of these products are a relatively high cost of production, the limited acceptability in human diets, and a high nucleic acid content.

The use of other microorganisms, mainly as a source of proteins and vitamins, should be encouraged. It is important to mention that some bacteria are able to synthetize vitamin B_{12}, which is not found in vegetable food sources.

Nutrients

Additional sources now available to improve the nutritive value of foods include some synthetic nutrients which can be used for the purpose of supplementation, enrichment, or fortification. They can be classified in three general groups; namely, amino acids, vitamins, and mineral salts.

Amino Acids

Among the amino acids, lysine and methionine are now available at a relatively low cost, permitting practical usage. Tryptophan and threonine, however, are not commercially available at a reasonable cost.

Vitamins

These important nutrients are now available commercially and are used in many instances to fortify different kinds of foods.

Mineral Salts

The most widely used mineral salts are iodine, iron, calcium, and phosphorus, in the form of their salts. These nutrients, together with the vitamins, play an important role in the efficient utilization of foods.

OBJECTIVES OF THE DEVELOPMENT OF HIGHLY NUTRITIOUS FOODS

The purpose of developing highly nutritious foods is probably different in technically advanced countries than in developing areas of the world. Since food is highly available and of greater variety in the developed countries, attention will be given here to foods already consumed in the latter areas which need nutritive quality improvement and to foods which are needed to supply the required nutrients for these populations because of the low availability and variety of the better quality foods of animal origin.

A highly nutritious food could be defined as one which is utilized by the animal organism with a minimum of waste, alone or with other foods, providing adequate amounts of the nutrients needed to meet the demands for the physiological functions of the organism. Therefore, the development of highly nutritious foods implies the improvement of the food not only in its protein component, but in the vitamin and mineral aspects of the food or diet as well. Of the three groups of nutrients, the protein component of the food probably represents the most difficult to correct when it is necessary to achieve high nutritious quality. This characteristic is best expressed as biological value, a figure which represents the amount of nitrogen absorbed which is retained by the organism to meet physiological demands.[34]

The biological value of the protein is determined by the essential amino acid content of the protein, which must be present in the correct balance[35] and in the appropriate proportions[35] for maximum and efficient utilization. These concepts have not been appreciated fully, and as a result, there is a great waste of nitrogen.

Improvement of the biological value of a protein must be carried out following the well-established concept of limiting amino acids. Consequently, the first limiting amino acid should be added in such concentration that the total amount of it in the food protein balances with that of the second limiting, as well as with other amino acids, according to the needs of the organism. This improvement can be brought about by different means; by adding protein, by adding the limiting amino acids, or by adding the correct mixture of the two.

As indicated above, the objective in developing high quality foods with respect to protein is to utilize protein efficiently, that is, with a minimum of waste. Even though higher intakes of protein may result in an appropriate intake of the essential amino acids, this is obtained at the expense of great waste, even if the organism is growing in apparently good nutrition (see Table 1). Results of

TABLE 1

Comparison Between the Protein Value and Amino Acid Intake of Opaque-2 and Normal Maize

	Opaque-2		Normal	
Maize intake to obtain nitrogen equilibrium, g/day	250*		547**	
Protein intake, g/day	27.9		43.8	
Biologic value of protein, %	82***		46.5**	
Protein retained, g	23		21	
Protein wasted	5		23	
Amino acid in protein retained	g/16 g N	% total EA int	g/16 g N	% total EA int
Isoleucine	1.01	8.63	2.00	10.53
Leucine	2.70	23.08	5.60	29.49
Lysine	1.34	11.45	1.25	6.58
Methionine	0.60	5.13	0.80	4.21
Cystine	0.55	4.70	0.56	2.95
Phenylalanine	1.33	11.37	1.96	10.32
Tyrosine	1.14	9.74	2.64	13.90
Threonine	1.10	9.40	1.72	9.06
Tryptophan	0.39	3.33	0.26	1.37
Valine	1.54	13.16	2.20	11.58
Total essential amino acids	11.70		18.99	

*(From Clark, H. E. et al., *Am. J. Clin. Nutr.*, 20, 825, 1967. With permission.)
**(From Kies, C. E. et al., *J. Nutr.*, 86, 350, 1965. With permission.)
***(From Young, V. R. et al., *J. Nutr.*, 101, 1479, 1971. With permission.)

Clark et al.[36] and Kies et al.[37] have shown that 250 g of Opaque-2 corn are sufficient for nitrogen equilibrium in adult humans, while 547 g of common corn are needed.

Assuming the same protein percentage in both foods, 27.9 g are ingested from Opaque-2 corn, while 43.8 g are ingested from common corn. Using a biological value of 82%[38] for Opaque-2 corn, about 23 g are retained of the 28 g protein ingested. This amount is similar to the amount of protein retained from common corn, around 21 g, with a biological value of 46.5%.[39] These figures indicate the great loss of nitrogen in common corn which is deficient in the essential amino acids, lysine and tryptophan,[39] and has a poor essential amino acid pattern. The loss of nitrogen from common maize amounts to 23 g, in contrast to 5 g lost from Opaque-2 maize. The respective essential amino acid intake is also shown in Table 1. These figures indicate that, with the exception of lysine and tryptophan, common corn provides greater intakes of other essential amino acids, which represent a load the body must eliminate contributing to the waste. These figures show that the amino acids absorbed are out of balance which further explains the poor biological value of common corn protein. The poor balance of essential amino acids is more obvious when amino acid intake is expressed as the percentage of the total essential amino acids ingested. This manner of expressing the values increases the deficiencies of lysine and tryptophan and magnifies the excesses of the other amino acids.

Protein quality is just one aspect of highly nutritious foods; other nutrients are also needed. This is emphasized by the results to be presented in proceeding sections (Table 8). They indicate that in order to obtain an improvement in protein quality through the addition of the two limiting amino acids of the maize-bean diet, vitamins and minerals are also required.[40]

APPLICATIONS

High Protein-containing Foods

High protein-containing foods were and are being developed throughout the world to meet the specific need for protein quality and quantity for population groups able to consume the usual high protein foods, such as milk, meat, and eggs. These high protein foods have been developed by combining, either from amino acid values or from the results of biological assays, various sources of proteins in such a way as to achieve higher concentration of protein as well as higher quality.[1,41-46]

In many cases, the ingredients used are exclusively of vegetable origin, and in others, variable amounts of animal protein sources, mainly milk powder or fish protein concentrate, have been included in the formulation. In such cases, the purpose has been to enhance protein quality as well as to indicate to the consumer that such foods contain animal food products, usually associated with good nutrition. The enhancement in protein quality can also be achieved by the addition of small amounts of synthetic amino acids.[35] The improvement in protein quality is necessary, particularly when the high protein food is made of vegetable protein sources which, as has already been indicated, have essential amino acid deficiencies even after various sources have been blended.

The high protein-containing foods with improved protein quality have been developed to be used as weaning foods or as protein supplements to low quantity and quality diets.[47,48] Although they provide good protein nutrition to people of all ages, they have been aimed at those population groups more susceptible to protein malnutrition; the weaning child, pre-school children, and pregnant and lactating mothers. The majority of these foods contain over 17% and up to 27.5% protein, with a protein efficiency ratio above 2.2. Many have been evaluated for their protein quality in biological assays with experimental animals and/or human subjects.[42,48,49] Some results, shown in Table 2, indicate that they are of a high protein quality in both species.

Table 3 summarizes some additional information on a few high protein foods. Observations of the ingredients show that most formulations are based on oilseed flours of a low fat content. These flours have been processed under well-controlled conditions to preserve the protein quality of the product. In some cases, the vegetable protein source utilized has been further processed to a higher concentration than the usual 50% commonly found in the oilseed flour. In some cases, flavoring agents have been added, while in others, they have been eliminated due to cost considerations, dietary habits, or preservation facilities. As previously indicated, some formulations contain small amounts of animal protein sources or essential amino acids. In most cases, the formulations have been supplemented with the vitamins

TABLE 2

Protein Quality of Some High Protein-containing Foods

Protein source	% casein* (rat)	Regression coefficient N absorbed to N retained** (children)
Whole egg	101	98
Whole milk	89	95
CSM	78	54
Superamine	93	67
TRL	83	76
IRL	85	76
Incaparina No. 9***	67	64
Incaparina No. 14	78	82
Incaparina No. 15	76	62

*Casein PER = 100
**Percentage of reference protein
***Without lysine
(From Viteri, F. E. and Bressani, R., *Bull. WHO,* in press. With permission.)

TABLE 3

Ingredient Composition of Some High Protein-containing Foods

High protein food	Incaparina No. 9	Incaparina No. 14	Incaparina No. 15	Soyacyt	Bal-Ahar Form A	Bal-Ahar Form E
Country	Guatemala and C.A.	Colombia	Colombia	Mexico	India	India
Soybean flour		X	X	X[1]		
Cottonseed flour	X		X			
Sunflower flour						
Peanut flour					X	X
Sesame flour						
Torula yeast	X					
Chickpea					X	
Lentil flour						
Skim milk				X		X
Fish Protein Concentrate						
Maize	X	X	X			
Wheat					X[2]	X[2]
Rice		X				
Teff						
Lysine	X					
Methionine						
Vitamins	X	X	X		X	X
Minerals	X	X	X	X	X	X
Flavoring agents				X		
Antioxidants						
Protein, %	25	25	25	21	24	21
PER	2.5	2.2	2.0	-	2.0	2.4
Main use	gruel	gruel	gruel	drink	gruel	gruel

High protein food	MPF Form A	Faffa SM 8 B	Pro Nutro	Superamine	Duryea	Leche Alim
Country	India	Ethiopia	S. Africa	Algeria	Colombia	Chile
Soybean flour			X		X	
Cottonseed flour						
Sunflower flour						X
Peanut flour	X	X				
Sesame flour						
Torula yeast						
Chickpea flour	X	X		X		
Lentil flour				X		
Skimmilk		X	X	X	X	X
Fish Protein Concentrate						X
Maize			X		X[5]	
Wheat			X[4]	X		X[6]
Rice						
Teff		X				
Lysine						
Methionine						
Vitamins	X			X	X	
Minerals	X			X	X	
Flavoring agents		X[3]		X		
Antioxidants						
Protein, %	42	13-14	22	21	28	27
PER	1.80	3.00	71*	2.40	2.40	-
Main use	protein supplement	-	cereal & soup mix	-	weaning food	drink

TABLE 3 (continued)

High protein food	CSM	VPM	Vitalia	Laubina 104	TRL	IRL
Country	world-wide	Middle East count.	Colombia	Lebanon		
Soybean flour	X	X	X		X	
Cottonseed flour						
Sunflower flour						
Peanut flour						
Sesame flour		X				
Torula yeast						
Chickpea flour		X		X	X	X
Lentil flour						X^9
Skimmilk	X			X	X	X
Fish Protein Concentrate						
Maize	X		X			
Wheat			X^8	X	X	X
Rice			X			
Teff						
Lysine						
Methionine						
Vitamins	X			X	X	X
Minerals	X			X	X	X
Flavoring agents				X		
Antioxidants						
Protein, %	19	37.8	17.8	16.8	21	18
PER	2.40	-	2.69	2.28	2.30	1.98
Main use	gruel	gruel	macaroni	weaning	weaning	weaning

X^1 = Full fat soybean flour
X^2 = Whole wheat flour
X^3 = Sugar and salt.
X^4 = Wheat germ
X^5 = Opaque-2 maize
X^6 = Toasted wheat flour
X^7 = Low fat soybean flour
X^8 = Wheat semolina
X^9 = Split pea flour
* = NPU (Net Protein Utilization)
/X/ = Either one

and minerals more deficient in the human dietary of the country or area where the food is being distributed and hopefully consumed. It should also be indicated that there are various formulations for the same product in many cases.

All these foods have many characteristics in common. They are of high nutritive value and were developed to meet specific nutrient needs and acceptability requirements since they resemble traditional accepted products with respect to taste, texture, and flavor. Furthermore, they are easy to handle and prepare for consumption and have a relatively long shelf life. At the beginning, in the formulation of high protein foods, the ingredients used in the formula were in a sense not well defined, even though the components met quality specifications.[47,50-52]

As research advanced, the ingredients utilized became more technologically sophisticated, permitting diversification of the form and uses of these high protein-containing foods. As animal proteins become less available and thus more expensive, in future years these high protein foods may be expected to take their place; this is already possible now, since plant protein is being processed into more acceptable forms than in previous years.

Fortification

In the last few years, attempts have been made to standardize the terminology used in the improvement of the nutritive value of foods. This has been a rather difficult task because of the interrelationship between the nutrients added and the food to be supplemented. Indeed, it is rather arbitrary to establish a definite boundary among the different approaches used to improve the nutritional quality of foods, as will be seen in the following discussion. However, efforts will be made, first, to define the scope covered by the different procedures and, second, to try to illustrate as much as possible, practical examples of each one of them.

Fortification will be defined here as the addition of specific nutrients in higher amounts than that found in natural foods. Fortification technology can be achieved by the addition of synthetic amino acids, protein concentrates, protein concentrates plus synthetic amino acids, and other specific nutrients (vitamins and minerals).

Synthetic Amino Acids

The production of some amino acids at a reasonable commercial cost has permitted their supplementary use to improve the protein quality of some important foods. Cereal protein, for example, can now be significantly improved by the addition of synthetic amino acids. Table 4 summarizes the results of several experiments carried out on the supplementation of lime-treated corn with its limiting amino acids.[53] Protein quality is more than doubled by the addition of lysine and tryptophan, thus changing a poorly utilized protein into a relatively high quality protein food. These results show the beneficial effect of the limiting amino acids, as well as the best ratio found for lysine and tryptophan as far as protein quality is concerned.

Similar improvement can be obtained with rice, wheat, oats, soybean, and other foods.[35]

Protein Concentrates

It is obvious that the addition of synthetic amino acids improves protein quality but does not change protein quantity. The second alternative, namely, the use of protein concentrates, has the advantage of not only supplying the deficient amino acids, but also of providing an increment in the total protein content. This is very important when the supplemented food is of a low protein concentration, as is the case of cereals. Table 5

TABLE 4

Supplementation of Lime-treated Corn with Amino Acids

Amino acids*	Average weight gain**	Protein efficiency ratio
Masa***	32	1.21
Masa + 0.31% lysine	41	1.51
Masa + 0.10% tryptophan	22	1.15
Masa + 0.31% lysine + 0.05% tryptophan	100	2.66
Masa + 0.31% lysine + 0.05% tryptophan + 0.20% threonine + 0.20% isoleucine + 0.15% methionine	112	2.69

*L-lysine HCl, DL-tryptophan, DL-methionine, DL-threonine, DL-isoleucine
**Average initial weight for all experiments: 48 to 52 g
***Masa dough prepared from lime-treated cooked corn
(From Bressani, R. et al., *Arch. Latinoamer. Nutr.*, 18, 126, 1968. With permission.)

TABLE 5

Optimum Levels of Protein Concentrates to Supplement Lime-treated Corn and Rice

	Corn		Rice	
Protein concentrate	Optimum level % in diet	Protein efficiency ratio	Optimum level % in diet	Protein efficiency ratio
–	–	1.00	–	1.73
Egg protein	3.0	2.24	–	–
Casein	4.0	2.21	6.0	3.22
Meat flour	4.0	2.34	–	–
Fish flour	2.5	2.44	6.0	2.70
Soya protein	5.0	2.30	–	–
Soya flour	8.0	2.25	8.0	2.88
Cottonseed flour	8.0	1.83	12.0	2.32
Torula yeast	2.5	1.97	8.0	3.29
Skim milk	–	–	12.0	3.16

(From Elías, L. G. et al., *Arch. Latinoamer. Nutr.*, 18, 35, 1968. With permission.)

shows an example of this fortification procedure, as applied to corn and rice proteins. The results show the optimum levels of each supplement necessary to obtain a maximum biological response when added to corn protein. It was found that the amounts of lysine and tryptophan in the supplements used correlated highly with the improvement in protein quality as measured by protein efficiency ratio (Figure 1).[32] Similar results are obtained with the supplementation of rice with protein concentrates.[54] In this case, a high correlation coefficient was obtained between PER (Protein Efficiency Ratio) and the amounts of lysine and threonine present in the supplements, since these two amino acids are the most limiting in rice protein. It should be noted that in some cases, the addition of protein supplements is used to provide the limiting amino acids plus additional protein, as in the case of cereal grains; in other cases, they are added only to provide the limiting amino acids, as for example, the addition of protein concentrates rich in lysine to cottonseed flour,[21] which is deficient in this amino acid and by-products from the wheat milling industry.[55]

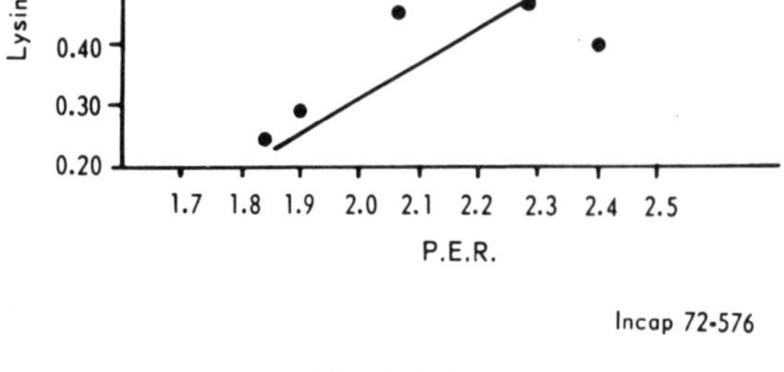

FIGURE 1.

Protein Concentrates Plus Amino Acids

Another procedure is the combination of the two alternatives previously mentioned, that is, the addition of a protein concentrate plus the complementary aggregate of the amino acid that the supplement does not provide in optimum amounts.

The results shown in Table 6 indicate that the addition of 0.1% lysine to corn supplemented with 8% soya flour increased utilizable protein as compared to the diet supplemented with amino acids or with 8% soya flour (Table 5). As a matter of fact, this additional improvement is a question of economy, since this increment could also be accomplished with a lower efficiency of utilization by raising the level of the protein concentrate used as the supplement.

TABLE 6

Effect of Various Supplements on the Nutritive Value of Corn[40]

Protein	Protein %	PER	Relative nutritive value** %	Utilizable protein %
Corn*	7.9	1.26	33.7	2.66
Corn* + 0.3% Lys + 0.1% Tryp	8.0	2.78	74.5	5.96
Corn* + Soya flour + 0.1% Lys	9.7	2.43	65.1	6.31
Casein	9.8	2.80	75.0	7.35

*Lime-treated corn
**Relative nutritive value to casein

Other Specific Nutrients (Vitamins and Minerals)

As has been mentioned elsewhere in this chapter, the lack of protein both in quality and in quantity is the most important problem in the developing areas of the world from the nutritional point of view. It must also be emphasized, however, that a well-balanced protein requires the presence of other micronutrients to perform its function with a higher efficiency of utilization. The need for these additional nutrients is not really appreciated in practice, in part, due to the obvious interrelationships among them or because the methodology used in protein evaluation must fulfill all those requirements to be valid. Since some of those other nutrients are also limiting in the daily diets of poor socioeconomic populations, it is important to take this aspect into consideration. This point is clearly shown in the results obtained by Bressani and Marenco[32] when supplementing tortilla flour with amino acids and vitamins. As illustrated in Table 7, the addition of the most limiting amino acids improved the quality of corn protein; however, a further significative increase was obtained when thiamin, riboflavin, and niacin were added to the amino acid-supplemented diet. Similar results were observed with vitamin A. As in the previous case, vitamin A has been reported as deficient in the diets of many parts of the world.

These concepts are even more important when the staple food is the one to be fortified, as for example, in the case of corn or rice which provides the main source of protein for large segments of populations. This aspect is illustrated in Table 8, which shows the effect of the individual addition of groups of nutrients on the quality of a corn-bean diet;[40] these two foodstuffs are the basic components of the daily diets of many low socioeconomic groups in Latin America.

From these data, it is clear that the addition of minerals as a group was the most important followed by the vitamins; of significance, however, was the fact that the addition of lysine and tryptophan in the absence of those nutrients showed no improvement as compared to the unfortified basal diet. Other important considerations are implicated in these results, as can be observed in Figure 2, which shows the weight gain of rats fed some of these diets for eight weeks; the tendency is that the differences in protein utilization become greater as the animals are kept under the same experimental conditions for a longer period of time. These results can be explained on the basis that, for its better utilization, a higher protein quality requires higher amounts of other nutrients which are normally limiting in these diets; these become even more limiting when the main protein deficiencies are corrected. Although these are experimental data obtained in well-controlled laboratory conditions, one is tempted to think that for people subsisting on poor protein quality diets, it is "fortunate," from the nutrition point of view, also to have inadequate amounts of other essential nutrients.

Other Important Aspects

If fortification technology is going to have an

TABLE 7

Effect of Adding Lysine, Tryptophan, and Vitamins on the Nutritive Value of Tortilla Flour*[32]

Nutrient added**, ***	Initial weight g	Weight gain g/28 days	Protein efficiency ratio
None	52	38	0.91
Riboflavin + Thiamine + Niacin	51	54	1.05
Lysine + Tryptophan	46	70	1.62
Lys + Try + B_1 + B_2 + Niacin	46	173	2.41
None	52	78****	
Lysine + Tryptophan	53	124****	
Vitamin A	53	80****	
Lysine + Tryptophan + Vitamin A	52	149****	

*Amount of tortilla flour: 90%
**Amount of riboflavin, thiamine and niacin added: 3 mg/100 g
***Amount of L-lysine HCl: 0.41%; DL-tryptophan: 0.10%.
****Weight gain in g/70 days

TABLE 8

Effect of the Individual Addition of Groups of Nutrients on the Quality of Corn-bean Diet*[40]

Treatment of corn-bean diet	Average food intake g/28 days	Average weight gain* g/28 days	PER
None	271 ± 8.8*****	26 ± 2.3*****	1.09 ± 0.07*****
+ Vitamins**	367 ± 18.7	49 ± 4.0	1.52 ± 0.06
+ Minerals***	388 ± 15.8	65 ± 4.3	1.91 ± 0.06
+ Lys + Try****	266 ± 14.4	26 ± 2.5	1.10 ± 0.08
+ Vit + Min	425 ± 10.5	70 ± 2.1	1.90 ± 0.04
+ Vit + Min + Lys + Try	484 ± 14.7	107 ± 4.9	2.55 ± 0.06

*72.4% corn + 8.10% bean
*Average initial weight: 44 g
**Recommended levels for lab rats: (B-complex and A, D, E, K)
***Recommended levels for lab rats
****0.25% L-lys Hcl and 0.025% DL-try
*****Standard error

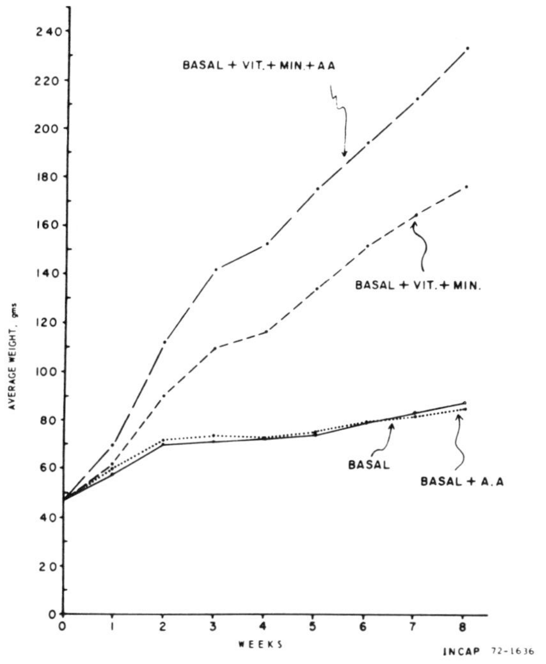

FIGURE 2. Effect of addition of lysine and Tryptophan to a corn-bean diet in the presence and absence of vitamins and minerals.

impact in providing nutritious foods, the following additional points must be taken into consideration.

The criteria in selecting the nutrients to be added, as well as their level, must be related not only to the food itself, but also to its contribution to the whole diet usually consumed. The results in Table 9 illustrate this point; the daily diets of a large group of people in Latin American countries are based on corn and beans which are of low protein content and quality due to the fact that they contain higher amounts of corn as compared to beans. If fortification is applied to bean protein by the addition of methionine, no improvement in the nutritional quality is observed. However, the use of a high protein bean with a higher lysine and tryptophan content almost doubles the protein utilization of the basal diet, since these two amino acids are the most limiting in this diet.

The nutrient(s) added should not change the physical and organoleptic properties of the supplemented food. The yellow color of cottonseed flour or the particular taste of *torula* yeast has probably been the disadvantage of the use of those protein concentrates as supplements. On the other hand, soybean flour has been successfully accepted by its favorable characteristics. For example, tortilla

TABLE 9

Effect of Fortified Beans on the Performance of Rats and Quality of Corn-bean Diets

Dietary treatment	Average weight gain, g/28 days	PER
72.4% maize + 8.1% beans	69	2.11
72.4% maize + 8.1% beans + 0.30% L-Lys HCl + 0.10% DL-Try	103	2.64
72.4% maize + 8.1 % beans + 0.30% DL-Met	66	1.93
72.4% maize + 8.1% beans + 0.30% L-Lys HCl + 0.10% DL-Try + 0.30% DL-Met	108	2.69
	Average weight gain, g/28 days	Utilizable protein %
87% Maize + 13% Beans (23% Prot)	48	4.54
87% Maize + 13% Beans (35% Prot)	72	5.87

flour does not change its common color by the addition of soybean flour, wheatshorts, or glandless cottonseed flour; however, the addition of edible cottonseed flour from common cottonseed gives a light-yellow color to the supplemented tortilla. Other acceptability trials must also be carried out to meet the requirements set by the consumers.

The added nutrient(s) must be stable to the normal processing conditions used in the preparation of the food to be supplemented. In general, foodstuffs are submitted to heat treatment before they are consumed to improve their texture, palatability, and sometimes, digestibility. Furthermore, it is important to carry out stability studies to assure that the added nutrients are not destroyed or inactivated during processing and storage.

Large-scale processing techniques for the preparation of the supplemented food are also of the utmost importance because in the developing countries foods are generally homemade, constituting a problem for the successful application of fortification technology. Adequate methods for the addition of the nutrients to the food at an industrial level must be studied. Since in these areas of the world food industries are generally located in urban centers, it is also important to recommend adequate methods of transportation to the rural areas, where undernutrition is more prevalent. Industrial processing also insures a more homogeneous product available all the time and in different convenient food forms. Although there are many problems to be solved on the implementation of the fortification technology, it represents a valuable way to improve the shortage of nutritious foods in the world.

Restoration

Restoration can be defined as the addition of a nutrient to a particular food to restore its original chemical composition. In a broader sense, restoration can also mean the total or partial replacement of a processed food by another food. In both cases, the purpose is to recover and/or improve the nutritive value or the physical and organoleptic properties altered during processing. Sometimes restoration technology aims at economic aspect, as for example, the replacement of wheat flour by a flour prepared from cassava or sweet potatoes without paying attention to the nutritive value of the product. However, in this section, emphasis will be placed only on the nutritive aspects of restoration; examples of this technology can be found in the literature. Tortillas, a staple foodstuff in some Latin American countries, can be improved by using this technique. In this case, part of the tortilla flour was replaced by wheat shorts, a by-product of the wheat milling industry. The amount replaced ranged from 0 to 30% and the results obtained are shown in Table 10. In this case, the significant improvement obtained in the nutritive value of tortilla is due to the amounts of lysine and tryptophan present in the wheat shorts, as well to an increment in protein content of the mixture.[23] Organoleptic tests were carried out in the tortillas made from this mixture; the results indicated that the appearance and texture were

TABLE 10

Effect of Replacing Lime-treated Corn Flour by Various Levels of Wheat Short on Nutritive Value

Amount of lime-treated corn-flour, %	Amount of wheat short flour, %	Protein in diet, %	Average weight gain, g	PER	Relative Nut. value to casein %	Utilizable protein, %
70	–	7.0	18	1.07	29.7	2.08
70	10	9.0	36	1.42	39.4	3.55
70	20	11.0	72	1.88	52.2	5.74
60	30	12.0	93	2.06	57.2	6.86
90	–	9.0	31	1.10	30.5	2.74
Casein	–	10.0	120	2.70	–	–

Average initial weight: 47g
Biological value of casein: 75%

(From Bressani, R., *Proceedings Western Hemisphere Nutrition Congress III*, 1972, 374. With permission.)

not affected by such a replacement, although a characteristic flavor of bread was detected. Consumer preference tests, however, were positive for the supplemented tortilla.

Similar reports have been made by Ranhotra[56] using a wheat protein concentrate (WPC) to partially replace wheat flour for the preparation of bread. This author studied the nutritive value as well as the rheological and baking characteristics of the different mixtures of wheat flour and WPC. He found that the improvements obtained in the protein quality and quantity were directly proportional to the levels of WPC added. He explained these results on the basis of the lysine content of the WPC. As far as baking characteristics were concerned, he found that the loaf volume was most affected by the addition of this supplement.

Encouraging improvement has also been obtained with this product in the preparation of chapatties,[57] a type of bread consumed in India and with other wheat-based foods.[58] Breads made with cassava flour and peanut or soybean flour have a higher nutritive value compared to those made with wheat flour only, as has been reported by Kim and De Ruiter.[59] Cassava flour has also been used to replace wheat flour in the preparation of some breads;[60] to improve the protein quantity and quality of this mixture, 6% of soybean flour is added. In these last two examples, the economic aspect is also favored, since cassava flour is less expensive and more available than wheat flour.

This approach can also be used to extend the availability of some higher nutritious foods; for example, Dutra de Oliveira and Da Silva[61] have suggested the partial replacement of common maize by Opaque-2 maize to improve the protein quality of the former.

Enrichment

Enrichment technology is concerned with the addition of nutrient(s) to a specific food to utilize it as a carrier for this nutrient(s). In general, the nutrient(s) added is not a component normally expected in the food and as a consequence, its supplementary value is improved; however, in some cases, the nutritive value of the particular food is enhanced. As the definition implies, the enrichment procedure must be employed only under well-controlled conditions to avoid undesirable effects; this means that both the vehicle and nutrients added should be well characterized in terms of the quality and quantity they will provide to the diet of the population group for which they are intended. Perhaps the most important consideration in relation to this procedure is the selection of the appropriate vehicle for the nutrient(s), that is, their suitability to fulfill the nutritional function in terms of stability, processing conditions, and consumption, both in frequency and amount, and in relation to the flavor and appearance of the product.

Obviously, in the case of the nutrient added, minimum levels of tolerance must be determined, as well as its interrelationship with the other nutrients present in the diets, this last requirement perhaps being the most difficult to foresee in practice.

Due to the relatively complicated mechanism, examples of enrichment technology as related to protein nutrition are scarce, as compared to restoration and fortification technology. The use of cassava flour as a carrier for the amino acid methionine has been proposed by Dutra de Oliveira and Menezes Salata for the northern and northeastern parts of Brazil.[62] In that country, cassava flour is eaten with common beans (*Phaseolus vulgaris*); the nutritive value of this mixture is of low protein quality because common beans, although relatively high in protein content, are limiting in methionine.[1]

Table 11 shows the results of the experiment carried out by these authors to illustrate this point. As expected, in all three combinations used, the addition of methionine to the cassava flour improved the nutritive value of the diets; the difference in weight gain observed among the combinations is due to the higher amounts of protein provided by common beans.

Although these results are clear and the principle is sound, other questions should be answered before it can be useful in practice. For example, it is essential to know the amount of beans usually consumed in the diet, as well as if other foods are also consumed with cassava flour. These are important points in relation to the level of methionine that should be added and the degree of improvement expected.

Table 12 shows the results obtained when the ratio of cassava to beans in the diet is higher[63] than that used in the experiment of Dutra de Oliveira and Menezes Salata.[62] As can be seen, the supplementary effect of methionine is ob-

TABLE 11

Protein Quality of Manioc Flour with and without Methionine Addition Mixed with Various Levels of Beans*

Dietary treatment	Protein, % in diet	Average weight gain, g	PER
65% manioc flour + 35% bean flour	8.04	7.7	0.78
65% manioc flour + 0.6% methionine + 35% bean flour	8.85	68.2	2.70
55% manioc flour + 45% bean flour	9.97	14.2	0.96
55% manioc flour + 0.6% methionine + 45% bean flour	10.09	66.8	2.68
45% manioc flour + 55% bean flour	12.17	31.7	1.28
45% manioc flour + 0.6% methionine + 55% bean flour	12.23	71.0	2.27

(From Dutra de Oliveira, J. E. and Menezes Salata, E.B.Z., *Nutr. Pre. Int.*, 3, 291, 1971. With permission.)

TABLE 12

Effect of Adding Methionine on the Nutritive Value of Various Cassava-beans[63] Mixtures

Dietary treatment	% Protein in diet	Weight changes g/28 days	PER	Cassava/bean ratio
Cassava (100)	1.9	–16.0	–	–
Cassava (87) bean (13)	4.3	–10.0	–	6.7
Cassava (87) bean (13) + methionine*	4.1	–7.0	–	6.7
Cassava (74) bean (26)	6.4	–6.4	–	2.8
Cassava (74) bean (26) + methionine*	6.7	+29.0	1.78	2.8
Cassava (61) bean (39)	8.8	+11.0	0.66	1.56
Cassava (61) bean (39) + methionine*	9.0	+67.0	2.42	1.56

*Figures in parenthesis refer to amounts, in grams, in the diets
**Amount added: 0.03 g of DL-Methionine per gram of bean protein

served only when the ratio of cassava to beans is similar to that reported in their study.[62]

Other examples of enrichment technology include the addition of vitamins and minerals, as for instance, the addition of vitamin D in milk to fight rickets in infants, the use of salt as carrier of iodine or iron to help in the prevention of goiter or anemia, and the addition of vitamin A in margarine and in sugar.[64]

Although these last examples are not directly related to protein nutrition, they are contributing to making a variety of foods convenient sources of essential nutrient, thus solving many nutritional deficiencies.

The addition of nutrients to foods that are not natural sources for such nutrients is a matter which has different implications for populations with a relatively high state of nutrition, such as those in developed countries in contrast to populations in developing countries. In these, there are groups of people consuming diets that are nutritionally as good as those consumed in developed countries, as well as the majority of people who consume diets of poor nutritive quality, deficient in more than one nutrient.

In such a common situation, consideration must be given to various factors. If the diet is deficient in three or four nutrients, enrichment with only one may cause greater undesirable effects than those occurring without it. This is even more meaningful if the nutrient added is related to one present in the diet. On the other hand, if the nutrient added is related metabolically to one not added at the same time or absent in the diet, the effect from it can be less than expected or none at all. The level of the nutrient to be added is also significant. If it is high, it may cause problems for those already ingesting adequate amounts of it.

The choice of the carrier is also of importance in the case of enrichment programs for developing countries. In the opinion of the authors, it is not advisable to choose a universal carrier, such as salt or sugar, because it is consumed by the entire population of such a country. Such approaches have been proposed for vitamin A in sugar[64] and iron in salt.[65] The case of vitamin A in sugar probably better illustrates the implications of such an approach. While sugar is consumed by all groups of people, in developing countries sugar consumption follows a gradient based on dietary habits, economic status, and diversity of foods reaching the dining room table. Therefore, those people with nutrient deficiencies may not ingest enough of the nutrient because they consume less of the carrier. Those without nutrient deficiencies will ingest more of the nutrient because they consume more of the carrier from various sources, including vitamin pills.

It would appear that for developing countries, enrichment should be done on a carrier which provides other nutrients as well and is consumed with a greater frequency by the population which is deficient in the nutrient in question. Although this approach has its limitations, it has more advantages and is less risky for the overall population.

Replacement

From time to time during the last few years, it has been indicated that world milk supplies are constantly decreasing with little hope of equaling the amounts of 10 years ago. Vegetable protein sources have become very useful in increasing the availability of dried milk supplies, particularly if the vegetable protein isolate has the functional properties and physical and organoleptic characteristics required to extend milk supplies.

Over the last few years, a product known as toned milk became popular in India.[66] This product contained 50% reconstituted skim milk powder and 50% fresh whole milk standardized to 3% fat. The milk powder was imported, making it relatively expensive and possibly incapable of continuously producing the tone milk. A substitute was developed containing 50% animal milk and 50% vegetable milk, prepared from peanut protein isolate and dextro maltose. Similar types of preparations have been described by Bressani;[45] however, the vegetable product used consisted of very fine cottonseed or soybean flour and carbohydrate sources. These products have a high protein quality, but lack the physical characteristics of toned milk, as indicated above. Similar products containing 25% milk powder and peanut and cereal flours supplemented with methionine have also been described.[67] These, however, could be reconstituted as fluid milk and had a protein efficiency ratio of 2.70.

The same approach for other food preparations has also been reported. For example, skim milk added to soybean milk has been made into cheese by lactic fermentation, yielding a product with a good flavor and with a possible high protein quality, depending on the amount of skim milk used.[68,69]

Along the same lines, a soy cheese whey protein preparation has been described. The mixture used consisted of three parts of soy protein to one part whey protein. The product was obtained by heating at 98°C at a pH of 4.7, was used with corn grits, giving a food product with a protein quality superior to that of soy protein-corn or casein-corn mixtures.[70]

PROCESSING

Oil-containing seeds have been extremely useful in the preparation of a variety of highly nutritious foods, the most common of which is the oil-free flour, as has already been mentioned. They have also served as raw materials for the preparation of protein isolates; however, special processing techniques have made it possible to produce high protein foods from the native kernel. For example, Lawhon, Cater, and Mattil[71,72] have described a process for the preparation of a high-protein nut-like food from glandless cottonseed kernels. The food product known as Tamunuts could be produced by oven roasting, toast-steam, pressure steaming-oven roast, or deep-fat frying. Protein content of cottonseed kernels produced by any technique varied from 33 to 37% with at least 79 to 94% of it in insoluble form. Oil content varied from 38 to 43%. The authors indicated that consumer response to the food items from Tamunuts was highly favorable in acceptance tests. By applying high pressures at various temperatures, times, and moisture levels, Pominski, Pearce, and Spadaro[73] prepared partially defatted peanuts. High protein full-fat products have been produced from soybeans by extrusion cooking.[74] Flours of high protein quality, flavor, and good stability were prepared by dehulling and preheating the extracted soybean meats to inactivate lipoxidase, premixing with water to add moisture, extruding, cooling, drying, and grinding. The product contained about 41% protein with 22.5% fat and its protein efficiency ratio was 1.98, adjusted to a 2.5 value for casein.

Soybean milk has been prepared for a long time in the Orient by soaking beans in water for several hours, followed by grinding with water, filtration, and cooking. Although this process method is relatively simple, soymilks obtained from such a process usually have a bland or undesirable aroma.

Wilkens, Mattick, and Hand[75] and Hand et al.[76] described a process using a high temperature, rapid hydration grinding process that gave a nearly bland soymilk. The process consists of grinding unsoaked, dehulled soybeans with water at temperatures between 80 and 100°C and maintaining the temperature for 10 min to completely inactivate the lipoxidase enzyme system, the primary factor in off-flavor production.

Fermentation has been very useful in preparing better quality foods in the Orient with the soybean, alone or in mixtures with rice and other foods.[1]

TEXTURED VEGETABLE PROTEIN FOODS

The high cost of meat, resulting mainly from the relatively low efficiency with which the animal is able to transform vegetable protein into muscle, has been one of the factors which stimulated the development of what is known today as "textured vegetable protein foods."[77,78] These foods had their origin from the advances made in protein isolation techniques together with synthetic fiber technology, which permitted the development of protein food with the physical, organoleptic, and nutritional characteristics associated with meat. The textured vegetable protein foods are made from oilseed or cereal products, and processed in the form of fibers, cubes, chunks, chips, or granules. The isolated protein converted into filaments provides textured products which are blended with fat, flavor, coloring stabilizers, and supplemental nutrients. All of these components are then bound together with a heat-coagulable protein.

These foods can also be made by thermoplastic extrusion, in which a mixture of soybean flour, flavoring and coloring components, and water is subjected to heat and pressure for specific periods of time. After cooking, the mass is extruded into atmospheric pressure which causes expansion. By the use of the appropriate size and shape of dyes, different forms can be made.

Since they are man-made, these textured foods may be converted into highly nutritious foods. In most cases, the protein base has been derived from soybean, which is low in sulfur-containing amino acids, but the addition of other components can overcome such a deficiency. For example, egg albumin is the most widely used binding agent and it is one of the highest quality proteins. The nutritive value of this textured food can be high and some results are shown in Table 13. In this case, the textured food was a simulated ground beef.[79] The performance of the animal species used to evaluate its protein quality is quite good, comparable to natural beef or casein. Likewise, the results in children show it to be a food of a relatively high protein value.

As indicated above, the nutritive value can be improved even further if there is any need to do so. These foods offer great stability, uniformity, organoleptic variety, nutritional control, and, eventually, economy.

TABLE 13

Protein Quality of Soybean Textured Food in Rats, Dogs, and Children

Protein food	Protein quality in rats		
	Protein in diet, %	Average weight gain, g	PER
Soybean protein textured food	11.6	125	2.69
Casein	11.7	116	2.66
Dehydrated beef	12.2	123	2.66

	Nitrogen balance in dogs Nitrogen					
	Intake	Fecal	Urine	Absorbed	Retained	Retention % intake
	mg/kg/day					
Soybean textured food	261	55	138	206	68	26.0
Dehydrated beef	292	69	149	223	74	25.3

	Nitrogen balance in children Nitrogen					
	Intake	Fecal	Urine	Absorbed	Retained	Retention % intake
	mg/kg/day					
Soybean textured food	312	46	183	266	82	26.6
Milk	342	52	210	290	80	23.4

(From Bressani, R., *J. Nutr.*, 92, 357, 1967. With permission.)

THE ROLE OF GENETICS ON THE DEVELOPMENT OF HIGHLY NUTRITIOUS PRODUCTS

For some time, food chemists and some plant breeders have known that protein concentration and even amino acid content, as well as other nutrients in cereals, legumes, and other products of vegetable origin, vary widely, depending on genetic and environmental factors. This variation was, however, not fully appreciated until 1964, when Mertz, Bates, and Nelson[80] reported that a strain of maize homozygous for the recessive mutant gene, Opaque-2, had a significantly higher lysine and tryptophan content than normal maize. This research has produced a major breakthrough in plant genetics and it constitutes what could be a very formidable approach to the development of highly nutritious food products, particularly in those more often consumed by the great majority of the world population, that is, cereal grains and legume foods. This approach to better nutritive food products could be named *genetic fortification.*

In the particular case of maize indicated above, the Opaque-2 gene caused an increase in the essential amino acids, lysine and tryptophan, by reducing the concentration of alcohol soluble proteins in maize and increasing the concentration of the sodium hydroxide protein fraction, richer in the two amino acids. Although little appreciated, the Opaque-2 gene also caused a reduction in the amino acid leucine which, being in high concentration in normal maize protein, may contribute to the low protein quality of normal maize and could also be related to the development of pellagra, or niacin deficiency.[81,82] In terms of nutritional value, Opaque-2 maize has a biological value in human adults and children of 92 and 72%, respectively, as compared to egg protein with a value of 96% for adults, and milk with 80% for children.[38,83] The role of genetics in developing better nutritive quality foods has also been demonstrated with other food crops or sources of protein.

Through genetic manipulation, it was possible to develop cottonseed varieties free of the pigment gossypol in 1953. These varieties were called glandless to indicate that they did not contain the glands which hold the gossypol pigments. It has been known for some time that gossypol is a toxic substance for monogastric animals[84] and the presence of this substance in cottonseed has limited its use in nutrition. Furthermore, upon processing to remove the oil from the seed, gossypol pigments are responsible to a large degree in the characteristic color of cottonseed flour. Upon processing, glandless cottonseed yields a flour as light in color as soybean flour. The nutritive value of the protein from glandless cottonseed is superior to that from common cottonseed. Similar results are also being reported for other protein sources. For example, some varieties of rapeseed low in erucic acid as well as a variety of the same seed low in glucosinolate have been found. Genetic improvement is not limited to protein quality or freedom from toxic substances. Research has also indicated that through genetic selection, the quality of vegetable oils can be changed to contain desired concentrations of oleic and linoleic acids in safflower, soybean, and other oils from oil-containing seeds.[85,86] Vitamin content can also be modified by genetic means.

SIGNIFICANCE AND ROLE OF HIGHLY NUTRITIOUS PRODUCTS

The idea of upgrading the nutritional quality of the foods consumed by man is really not one developed within the last 15 or 20 years, but one which evolved since early in this century. The need for such upgrading was really not world-wide, but rather for specific population groups who suffered from vitamin deficiency caused by consumption of foods that processing had degraded from the nutritional point of view, although upgraded in terms of acceptability. The addition of the nutrients eliminated during processing improved their nutritional quality and eliminated the deficiencies found in the human population consuming them.[87]

Upgrading the nutritional quality of foods today and in future years is more pressing because of factors already discussed and well accepted; the objective is to achieve the highest utilization efficiency of the food consumed. This concept of efficiency of utilization is not well understood or applied, but it may be as important to the world as increasing food production.

One of the aspects in agricultural research which receives particular attention is that of increasing yield of a food crop per unit area, rather than increasing yield by expanding the total area of cultivation. In this way, production is more efficient in terms of utilizing to the maximum possible the nutrients from the soil, the available water, and carbon dioxide and the solar energy. Similarly, in animal production, the objective is to produce a maximum of a product with the minimum feed at the lowest cost, emphasizing again the efficiency of production. Human populations are of course not plants or animals and their nutrition is really not for the same purpose; however, because of increasing populations, dietary habits, food availability and, possibly, other factors, it is becoming increasingly necessary for foods to be utilized with the greatest efficiency. This increased efficiency of nutrient utilization is the significance of improving the quality of food supplies and of developing highly nutritious foods.

Increased food production has taken place in the world in previous years by improved varieties and hybrids, control of soil fertility and of insects, and by various other agronomic developments. The more recent of the impacts of agricultural research is the *green revolution,* which was achieved by the use of improved varieties responding to the application of fertilizers and water. The emphasis has been on the cereal grains; it is hoped that soon the same result will be accomplished also with legume foods. The consumption of both cereal and legume grains has probably kept many populations in a certain degree of nutritional health, providing them protein diets of higher quality than those from cereals alone. But increased production of legume grains will provide even better protein nutrition when consumed with cereal grains. This may be also considered as the development of highly nutritious foods.

The new technology can be of significant help to the expanded production derived from the *green revolution*. This will increase as greater numbers of people move from rural to urban areas, depending more and more upon processed foods. Through the *green revolution* it is possible to produce greater amounts of foods, and it will be possible to develop better nutritive quality foods through food technology. Examples of this have already been given in previous sections. From the standpoint of protein nutrition, animal products are and have been the main source of protein for developed populations, and even for primitive civilization when population and economic pressures were not as great as they are today and will be in future years. The role, therefore, of the highly nutritious foods, whether from the efforts of agronomy or from food technology, would be to replace the animal food products that are inefficiently produced in most cases, particularly if they are produced from foods which may be or are also consumed by humans.

REFERENCES

1. **Bressani, R. and Elías, L. G.,** Processed vegetable protein mixtures for human consumption in developing countries, *Adv. Food Res.,* 16, 1, 1968.
2. **Bressani, R. and Elías, L. G.,** Legume foods, in *New Protein Foods,* Vol. I, Altschul, A. M., Ed., Academic Press, to be published.
3. **Bressani, R., Elías, L. G., and Navarrete, D. A.,** Nutritive value of Central American beans. IV. The essential amino acid content of samples of black beans, red beans, rice beans and cowpeas of Guatemala, *J. Food Sci.,* 26, 525, 1961.
4. **Elías, L. G., Colindres, R., and Bressani, R.,** The nutritive value of eight varieties of cowpeas *(Vigna sinensis), J. Food Sci.,* 29, 118, 1964.
5. **Patwardhan, U. N.,** Pulses and beans in human nutrition, *Am. J. Clin. Nutr.,* 11, 12, 1962.
6. **Jaffé, W. G.,** Protein digestibility and trypsin inhibitors activity of legume seeds, *Proc. Soc. Exp. Biol. Med.,* 75, 219, 1950.
7. **Bressani, R., Elías, L. G., and Valiente, A. T.,** Effect of cooking and of amino acid supplementation on the nutritive value of black beans *(Phaseolus vulgaris, L), Br. J. Nutr.,* 17, 69, 1963.
8. **Munsell, H. E., Louis, O., Williams, L., Quild, P., Troescher, B., Nightingale, G., and Harris, R. S.,** Composition of food plants of Central America. I. Honduras, *Food Res.,* 14, 144, 1949.
9. **Mc Coy, O. M.,** The nutritive value of potatoes, in *Potato Processing,* Talburt, W. F. and Smith, O., Eds., The Avi Publishing Co., New York, 1959, 187.
10. **Jaraj, A. P., Joseph, K., Rao, M. N., Bhagavan, R. K., Swaminathan, M., and Subrahmanyan, U.,** Effect of varying levels of protein and calcium in the diet on the structure and composition of liver rats. 1. The effect of supplementation of diets based on rice and rice-tapioca with calcium on the growth and structure and composition of liver of albino rats, *Ann. Biochem. Exp. Med.,* 20, 341, 1960.
11. **Bressani, R., Elías, L. G., and Braham, J. E.,** Cottonseed protein in human foods, in *World Protein Resources.* A symposium sponsored by the Division of Agricultural and Food Chemistry at the 150th Meeting of the American Chemical Society, Atlantic City, N. J., Sept. 13-15, 1965, Altschul, A. M., Symposium Chairman, American Chemical Society, Washington, D. C., 1966, 75 (Advances in Chemistry Series 57).
12. **Bressani, R., Jarquín, R., and Elías, L. G.,** Cottonseed flour. Free and total gossypol, epsilon amino lysine, and biological evaluation of cottonseed meals and flours in Central America, *J. Agric. Food Chem.,* 12, 278, 1964.
13. **Anson, M. L.,** Potential uses of isolated oilseed protein in foodstuffs, in *Processed Plant Protein Foodstuffs,* Altschul, A. M., Ed., Academic Press, New York, 1958, 277.
14. **Anson, M. L.,** Oilseed proteins in foods, *Arch. Biochem. Biophys.,* Supp. 1, 68, 1962.
15. **Flodin, N. W.,** Amino acids and proteins. Their place in human nutrition problems, *J. Agric. Food Chem.,* 1, 222, 1953.
16. **Almquist, H. J. and Grau, C. R.,** Mutual supplementary effect of the proteins of soybean and sesame meals, *Poult. Sci.,* 23, 341, 1944.
17. **Waddel, J.,** Supplementation of plant proteins with amino acids, in *Processed Plant Protein Foodstuffs,* Altschul, A. M., Ed., Academic Press, New York, 1958, 307.
18. **Allison, J. B., Wannemacker, R. W., Jr., and Mc Coy, J. R.,** The determination of the nutritive value of cottonseed flour, in *Proceedings of a Conference on Cottonseed Protein for Animal and Man, New Orleans, 1960,* U.S.D.A., New Orleans, April 1962, 1. (USDA, ARS 72-24).
19. **Elías, L. G., Sánchez, S., and Bressani, R.,** Estudio comparativo de diferentes métodos para evaluación del valor proteínico de harinas de semilla de algodón, *Arch. Latinoamer. Nutr.,* 19, 279, 1969.

20. **Braham, J. E., Elías, L. G., and Bressani, R.,** Factors affecting the nutritional quality of cottonseed meals, *J. Food Sci.,* 30, 531, 1965.
21. **Elías, L. G. and Bressani, R.,** Amino acid and protein supplementation of defatted cottonseed flour, *Arch. Latinoamer. Nutr.,* 21, 149, 1971.
22. **Krishnamorthy, K., Tasker, P. K., Ramakrishnan, T. N., Rajagopalan, R., and Swaminathan, M.,** Studies on the nutritive value of sesame seeds. I. The amino acids composition of the proteins and the chemical composition of sesame seeds and meal, *Ann. Biochem. Exp. Med.,* 20, 73, 1960.
23. **Elías, L. G.,** Utilización de sub-productos ricos en proteínas, in *Recursos Proteínicos en América Latina,* Béhar, M. and Bressani, R., Eds., Memorias de una Conferencia de nivel latinoamericano celebrada en el Instituto de Nutrición de Centro América y Panamá (INCAP), ciudad de Guatemala, del 24 al 27 de febrero de 1970. Talleres Gráficos del INCAP, Guatemala, C. A., 1971, 396.
24. **Liener, I. E.,** Effect of heat on plant proteins, in *Processed Plant Protein Foodstuffs,* Altschul, A. M., Ed., Academic Press, New York, 1958, 79.
25. **Bressani, R. and Elías, L. G.,** Cambios en la composición química y en el valor nutritivo de la proteína de la harina de semilla de algodón durante su elaboración, *Arch. Latinoamer. Nutr.,* 18, 319, 1968.
26. **Sakurei, Y. and Nakano, M.,** Production of high protein food from fermented soybean products, in Progress in Meeting Protein Needs of Infants and Pre-school Children, Proc. Internat. Conf., NRC Pub. 843, Washington, D.C., 1960, 251.
27. **Elías, L. G. and Bressani, R.,** The nutritive value of the Brazil nut oil, *J. Oil Chem. Soc.,* 38, 450, 1961.
28. **Squibb, R. L., Aguirre, A., and Bressani, R.,** African and Mbocayá palm meals as substitutes for sesame oil meal in baby chick rations, *Turrialba,* 8, 24, 1958.
29. **Duckworth, J. and Woodman, A. A.,** Leaf protein concentrates. I. Effect of source of raw material and method of drying on protein value for chicks and rats, *J. Sci. Food Agric.,* 12, 5, 1961.
30. **Cooke, B. B., Law, E. W., and Bailey, B. M.,** The protein quality of waste-grown green algae. I. Analysis of protein in mixtures of algae non-fat powdered milk and cereals, *J. Nutr.,* 81, 23, 1963.
31. **Waterlow, J. E.,** The absorption and retention of nitrogen from leaf protein by infants recovering from protein malnutrition, *Br. J. Nutr.,* 16, 531, 1962.
32. **Bressani, R. and Marenco, E.,** The enrichment of lime-treated corn with proteins, lysine and tryptophan, and vitamins, *J. Agric. Food Chem.,* 11, 517, 1963.
33. **Elías, L. G. and Bressani, R.,** Valor nutritivo de la proteína de la levadura torula y como complemento de concentrados proteínicos, *Arch. Latinoamer. Nutr.,* 20, 135, 1970.
34. **Allison, J. B.,** Biological evaluation of proteins, *Physiol. Rev.,* 35, 664, 1955.
35. **Bressani, R., Elías, L. G., and Gómez Brenes, R. A.,** Improvement of protein quality by amino acid and protein supplementation, in *International Encyclopaedia of Food and Nutrition,* Bigwood, E. J., Ed., Vol. 11, Pergamon Press, Oxford, 1972, 475.
36. **Clark, H. E., Allen, P. E., Meyers, S. M., Tuckett, S. N., and Yamamura, Y.,** Nitrogen balances of adults consuming Opaque-2 maize protein, *Am. J. Clin. Nutr.,* 20, 825, 1967.
37. **Kies, C., Williams, E., and Fox, H. M.,** Determination of first limiting nitrogenous factor in corn protein for nitrogen retention in human adults, *J. Nutr.,* 86, 350, 1965.
38. **Young, V. R., Ozalp, I., Cholakos, B. V., and Scrimshaw, N. S.,** Protein value of colombian Opaque-2 corn for young adult men, *J. Nutr.,* 101, 1475, 1971.
39. **Bressani, R.,** The importance of corn for human nutrition in Latin America and other countries, in Proceedings of the Conference on Nutritional Improvement of Corn, Institute of Nutrition of Central America and Panama (INCAP), Guatemala, 1972.
40. **Elías, L. G. and Bressani, R.,** Nutritional value of the protein of tortilla flour and its improvement by fortification in Central America, in Proceedings of the Conference on Nutritional Improvement of Corn, Institute of Nutrition of Central America and Panama, (INCAP), Guatemala, 1972.
41. **Matoth, Y., Elian, E., and Gruenberg, E.,** Evaluation of a protein-rich mixture based on vegetable foods of middle eastern countries, *Am. J. Clin. Nutr.,* 21, 226, 1968.
42. **Bressani, R.,** Formulation and testing of weaning and supplementary foods containing oilseed proteins, in *Protein-Enriched Cereal Foods for World Needs,* Milner, M., Ed., Am. Assoc. Cereal Chemists, St. Paul, Minn., 1969, 49.
43. **Parpia, H. A. B.,** Protein foods of India based on cereals, legumes and oilseed meals, in *Protein-Enriched Cereal Foods for World Needs,* Milner, M., Ed., Am. Assoc. Cereal Chemists, St. Paul, Minn., 1969, 129.
44. **Senti, F. R.,** Formulated cereal foods in the U.S. Food for peace program, in *Protein-Enriched Cereal Foods for World Needs,* Milner, M., Ed., Am. Assoc. Cereal Chemists, St. Paul, Minn., 1969, 246.
45. **Bressani, R.,** Application of food science and technology to the exploitation of new protein sources, in *Proceedings Western Hemisphere Nutrition Congress III,* August 30-September 2, 1971, Miami Beach, Fla., Futura Publishing Co., Mount Kisko, N.Y., 1971, 368.
46. **Elder, A. and Weisber, S. M.,** High nutrition - low cost foods; their impact in developing countries, in Proceedings of the III International Congress of Food Science and Technology, SOS/70, Washington, D.C., 1970.

47. FAO/WHO/UNICEF Protein Advisory Group, *PAG Guideline on Mixtures for Use on Weaning Foods*, Protein Advisory Group of the United Nations System, United Nations, New York, 1971 (PAG Guideline No. 8).
48. FAO/WHO/UNICEF Protein Advisory Group, *Human Testing of Supplementary Food Mixtures*, FAO/WHO/UNICEF Protein Advisory Group, United Nations, New York, 1970 (PAG Guideline No. 7).
49. **Viteri, F. E. and Bressani, R.**, The human testing of new sources of protein with emphasis on protein quality, *Bull. WHO*, in press.
50. FAO/WHO/UNICEF Protein Advisory Group, *Edible Heat Processed Soy Grits and Flour*, FAO/WHO/UNICEF Protein Advisory Group, United Nations, New York, 1969 (PAG Guideline No. 5).
51. FAO/WHO/UNICEF Protein Advisory Group, *Preparation of Edible Cottonseed Protein Concentrate*, FAO/WHO/UNICEF Protein Advisory Group, United Nations, New York, 1970 (PAG Guideline No. 4).
52. FAO/WHO/UNICEF Protein Advisory Group, *Preparing Food Quality Groundnut Flour*, FAO/WHO/UNICEF Protein Advisory Group, United Nations, New York, 1970 (PAG Guideline No. 2).
53. **Bressani, R., Elías, L. G., and Braham, J. E.**, Suplementación, con aminoácidos, del maíz y de la tortilla, *Arch. Latinoamer. Nutr.*, 18, 123, 1968.
54. **Elías, L. G., Jarquín, R., Bressani, R., and Albertazzi, C.**, Suplementación del arroz con concentrados proteicos, *Arch. Latinoamer. Nutr.*, 18, 27, 1968.
55. **Elías, L. G. and Bressani, R.**, Valor proteínico de los subproductos de la industria del trigo. II. Complementación y suplementación del granillo de trigo con concentrados proteínicos, *Arch. Latinoamer. Nutr.*, to be published.
56. **Ranhotra, G. S.**, Supplemental effect of wheat-protein-concentrate upon the protein quality of white wheat flour, in *Proceedings Western Hemisphere Nutrition Congress III*, August 30-September 2, 1971, Miami Beach, Fla., Futura Publishing Co., Mount Kisko, N.Y., 1971, 378.
57. **Hedges, N. J. and Tinklin, G. L.**, Chapatti quality as affected by wheat protein concentrate, *Cereal Sci. Today*, 14, 344, 1969.
58. **Tosello, A.**, Considerações nutricionais na formulação de farinhas de trigo com outras farinhas, in *Recursos Proteínicos en América Latina*, Béhar, M. and Bressani, R., Eds., Memorias de una Conferencia de nivel latinoamericano celebrada en el Instituto de Nutrición de Centro América y Panamá (INCAP), ciudad de Guatemala, del 24 al 27 de febrero de 1970. Talleres Gráficos del INCAP, Guatemala, C.A., 1971, 388.
59. **Kim, J. C. and De Ruiter, D.**, Bread from non-wheat flour, *Food Technol.*, 22, 867, 1968.
60. **Bacigalupo, A.**, Protein-rich cereal foods in Peru, in *Protein-Enriched Cereal Foods for World Needs*, Milner, M., Ed., Am. Assoc. Cereal Chemists, St. Paul, Minn., 1968.
61. **Dutra de Oliveira, J. E. and Da Silva, L. P.**, Valor nutritivo de milho Opaco-2 e de mixturas do milho hibrido e Opaco-2 producidos no Brasil. Resumen de temas libres presentados en la I Reunión Científica de la Sociedad Latino Americana de Nutrición, Caracas, Venezuela, 1968.
62. **Dutra de Oliveira, J. E. and Menezes Salata, E. B. Z.**, Methionine fortified manioc flour to combat protein malnutrition, *Nutr. Rep. Int.*, 3, 291, 1971.
63. **Elías, L. G. and Bressani, R.**, unpublished data.
64. **Arroyave, G.**, Distribution of vitamin A to population groups, in *Proceedings Western Hemisphere Nutrition Congress III*, August 30-September 2, 1971, Miami Beach, Fla., Futura Publishing Co., Mount Kisko, N.Y., 1971, 68.
65. **Levison, F. J. and Berg, A. D.**, With a grain of fortified salt, *Food Technol.*, 23, 1174, 1969.
66. **Parpia, H. A. B.**, Food technology problems in India and other developing countries, *Food Technol.*, 22, 62, 1968.
67. **Chandrasekhara, M. R., Shurpalekar, S. R., Rao, B. H. S., Kurien, S., and Shurpalekar, K. S.**, Development of infant foods based on soybean, *J. Food Sci. Technol.*, 3, 94, 1966.
68. **Hang, Y. D. and Jackson, H.**, Preparation of soybean cheese using lactic starter organisms. I. General characteristics of the finished cheese, *Food Technol.*, 21, 1033, 1967.
69. **Hang, Y. D. and Jackson, J.**, Preparation of soybean cheese using lactic starter organisms. II. Effect of addition of rennet extract and skimmilk, *Food Technol.*, 21, 1035, 1967.
70. **Loewnstein, M. and Paulraj, V. K.**, Preparation and growth producing evaluation of a concentrated coprecipitate of soy-cheese whey protein, *Food Prod. Dev.*, 5, 56, 1972.
71. **Lawhon, J. T., Cater, C. M., and Mattil, K. F.**, Preparation of a high-protein low-cost nut-like food product from glandless cottonseed kernels, *Food Technol.*, 24, 701, 1970.
72. **Lawhon, J. T., Cater, C. M., and Mattil, K. F.**, Influence of the deep-fat frying medium on the acceptability and stability of glandless cottonseed kernels for use as a high-protein, low-cost edible nut, *Food Technol.*, 24, 817, 1970.
73. **Pominski, J., Pearce, H. M., Jr., and Spadaro, J. J.**, Partially defatted peanuts – factors affecting oil removal during pressing, *Food Technol.*, 24, 716, 1970.
74. **Mustakas, G., Albrecht, W. J., Book Walter, G. N., McGhee, J. E., Kwolek, W. F., and Griffin, E. L., Jr.**, Extruder-processing to improve nutritional quality flavor and keeping quality of full fat soyflour, *Food Technol.*, 24, 1290, 1970.
75. **Hand, D. B., Steinkraus, K. H., Van Bureau, J. P., Hackler, L. R., Rawis, I., and Pallesen, H. R.**, Pilot plant studies on soy milk, *Food Technol.*, 18, 139, 1964.

76. **Wilkens, W. F., Mattick, L. R., and Hand, D. B.,** Effect of processing method on oxidation off-flavors of soybean milk, *Food Technol.,* 21, 1630, 1967.
77. **Thulin, W. W. and Kuramoto, S.,** Bontrae – a new meat-like ingredient for convenience foods, *Food Technol.,* 21, 168, 1967.
78. **Johnson, D. W.,** Oilseed proteins. Properties and applications, *Food Prod. Dev.,* 3, 78, 1970.
79. **Bressani, R., Viteri, F. E., Elías, L. G., Zaghi, S. de, Alvarado, J., and Odel, A. D.,** Protein quality of a soybean protein textured food in experimental animals and children, *J. Nutr.,* 93, 349, 1967.
80. **Mertz, E. T., Bates, L. S., and Nelson, E. R.,** Mutant gene that changes protein composition and increases lysine content of maize endosperm, *Science,* 145, 279, 1964.
81. **Kies, C. and Fox, H. M.,** Interrelationships of leucine with lysine, tryptophan, and niacin as they influence protein value of cereal grains for humans, *Cereal Chem.,* 49, 223, 1972.
82. **Bressani, R., Elías, L. G., and Gómez Brenes, R. A.,** Protein quality of Opaque-2 corn evaluation in rats, *J. Nutr.,* 97, 173, 1969.
83. **Bressani, R., Alvarado, J., and Viteri, F. E.,** Evaluación en niños de la calidad de la proteína del maíz Opaco-2, *Arch. Latinoamer. Nutr.,* 19, 129, 1969.
84. **Miravalle, R. J.,** The plant geneticists' contribution toward changing the lipid and amino acid composition of cottonseed, *J. Am. Oil Chem. Soc.,* 49, 15, 1972.
85. **Knowless, P. F.,** The plant geneticists' contribution toward changing lipid and amino acid composition of safflower, *J. Am. Oil Chem. Soc.,* 49, 27, 1972.
86. **Howell, R. W., Brim, C. A., and Rinne, R. W.,** The plant geneticists' contribution toward changing lipid and amino acid composition of soybeans, *J. Am. Oil Chem. Soc.,* 49, 30, 1972.
87. **Sebrell, W. H.,** Enrichment: good gift of yesterday, *Cereal Sci. Today,* 11, 228, 1966.

NEED FOR FOOD AND NUTRITION POLICIES

M. Ganzin, J. Périssé and P. François

TABLE OF CONTENTS

Introduction 275

Present Trends in Food Consumption in the 1970's 276

Food and Nutrition Policy 277
Definition 277
Methodological Aspects 277
Data Requirements 278
Food Balance Sheets 278
Food Consumption and Household Budget Surveys 278
Models 278
Integration of Food and Nutrition Policies in Agricultural Planning 280

Components of a Food and Nutrition Policy 281
Analysis of the Situation by Socioeconomic Groups 281
Analysis of the Situation by Products 282

Implementation of Food and Nutrition Policies 283
Educational Measures 283
Economic and Administrative Measures 284
Technological Measures 285
Legislative Measures 285

Conclusions 285

References 286

INTRODUCTION

In a statement to the press on the world food situation on February 3, 1973, the Director-General of FAO, Mr. A. H. Boerma, described the unusually bad harvests in the previous two years which were mainly due to droughts. He announced that these bad harvests resulted in massive purchases of grains by a few highly populated countries which in turn depleted international wheat stocks and led to a tremendous increase in world wheat prices amounting to some 80%. He entreated before concluding his statement, "In the name of reason can this world of the 1970's with all its scientific prowess and its slowly growing sense of common purpose, go on enduring a situation in which the chances of enough decent food for millions of human beings may simply depend on the whims of one year's weather? Is this a tolerable human condition? Emphatically not." He went on to propose two ways of tackling the problem: first, "to give much more serious and concentrated attention to the longer-term problem of food production in the developing countries" and second, that "we have reached the point where there must be some sort of reserves of food stocks to meet emergencies."[1]

At a first glance both proposals may not appear to be in the sphere of the nutritionist. Yet the experience gained during the past 25 years makes it universally accepted that quantitative or qualitative nutritional deficiencies are primarily the result of poverty and of the social constraints which poverty imposes, such as ignorance and poor health. In fact, it was poverty that prevented many countries from making the same unprecedented purchases of grain which were made by the few, for "a great number of poor countries far less able to afford to import food, have also been seriously affected,"[1] and this was aggravated by the rise of prices. This is why reserve food stocks are necessary not only for emergency relief but also to maintain the prices at a level accessible to the poor.

The longer-term problem of food production in the developing world is of great concern since "the main increase in agricultural production was in the developed market economies of the western world — an increase of some six per cent — while in the developing countries taken together the increase was only between one and two per cent."[2] This is a depressingly small increase, well below the previous year's figure of 3% for the developing countries. It is well below their rise in population of about 2.5% a year, thus evoking the specter of possible famine in parts of the developing world.

The problem is, therefore, complex: food production inadequate to face the demographic expansion; poverty which both impairs production and does not allow for imports; hard climatic conditions which enhance the previous factors; high rate of demographic expansion which aggravates the deficiencies and increases the demand; urgent need for social investments which competes with economic and agricultural investments, etc. Generally speaking, there is the lack of a planning system which can take all these factors into consideration. Governments and politicians are primarily concerned with the energy (calories) problem which is the most sensitive because lack of food could lead to famine, and an excessive increase in the prices of the staple crops might overthrow a government. Meanwhile, qualitative deficiencies that generate malnutrition are scientific questions which bother governments only when they become public health problems with political implications. Under these conditions food supply problems, as well as malnutrition problems, are usually tackled emotionally rather than scientifically, i.e., at policy level.

The planner is working with Food Balance Sheets and Gross National Products figures which hide poverty because they do not show the variations in consumption levels with populations where poverty is a key factor; the nutritionist, using vital or medical statistics, tries to convince the first of the value of a satisfactory diet in the economic development process, but not always with reliable convincing facts or data.

For instance, the protein gap has been unduly emphasized. There is mainly an economic gap and because of the uneven distribution of income there is also an excess demand at national and/or international levels for certain products (meat, for instance) in relation to the supply which has increased the food injustice. And, there is no substitute for the elimination of poverty.

Up to the present time, the planner on the one hand and the nutritionist on the other have each proposed his own solution without or with very little integration between the two because their concepts, language, objectives, and approaches are different. The studies made during the preparation of the Indicative World Plan (IWP) were the first attempt to find a definition or a methodology for the formulation of food and nutrition policies at a national level; they have led to a set of techniques that we propose to call "nutrimetrics." It is, in a sense, equivalent in the field of food planning to "econometrics" in economic development.

The purpose of this chapter is to explain briefly the present trends in food consumption as related to agriculture and food production and to describe the main elements of a food and nutrition policy and the requirements for its formulation and implementation on a national scale to improve the food and nutrition situation for a given population.

PRESENT TRENDS IN FOOD CONSUMPTION IN THE 1970's

Over the past decade world agriculture has kept pace with population growth but has been unable to outstrip it. A slight improvement has taken place in the average per caput consumption in the developing countries, for example, in Asia and the Far East, especially regarding calories and vegetable protein. Animal protein consumption, however, has remained stationary in most developing countries while it has risen rapidly in the developed countries. In nutritional terms, the previous differences in consumption levels between these two groups of countries have become slightly more pronounced in the case of protein and fats, and have slightly decreased for calories because developed countries are approaching a saturation point. In 1972, however, for the reason explained before, the rate of demographic expansion has been superior to the annual food production increase.

In developing countries the output of animal products has only just kept level with the increase of population. As the per caput consumption of animal proteins remained virtually unchanged during the decade, even though household income in some regions rose, it must be assumed that the increase in potential demand for meat, eggs, fish, and milk products did not materialize and that adjustment by price occurred.* The production constraints for products of animal origin identified during the IWP study, therefore, appear to be borne out. In other regions such as Africa, the increase in per caput income was too small to stimulate demand beyond the rate of population increase.

It is likely that in most developing countries higher prices have led to increased disparities in food consumption between socioeconomic groups to the detriment of the poorer classes, just as disparities between rich and poor countries have increased. In eight years the rich countries have succeeded in raising their per caput animal protein intake by the same amount as is now available to the poor countries.

This is a problem which calls for urgent measures, and action has already been taken to counteract the trend of increasing disparities. Some developing countries have undertaken agrarian reforms, while other have instituted rationing of food distribution so as to effect a fairer sharing of the means of food production or of their slender food resources. However, most governments appear to have been unable to produce a marked drop in income inequalities, to ward off agricultural disasters, or to bring about a rapid settlement of conflicts that cause famines. There is, therefore, reason to think that the percentage of people suffering from undernourishment and malnutrition has not decreased significantly. Furthermore, as world population grew by 680 million during the decade, and the average dietary level remained virtually unchanged, the number of these people is possibly higher in absolute terms than it was and nutritional problems may be even more acute than when the decade opened.

FOOD AND NUTRITION POLICY

Definition

A food and nutrition policy can be defined as being a complex of educational, economic, technical, and legislative measures designed to reconcile, at a level judged feasible by the planner, projected food demand, forecasted food supply, and nutritional requirements. These measures are not only of economic but also of social impact. They are directed at palliating distortions detrimental to the public interest between what the consumer desires, what he can obtain, and what he needs physiologically. This is an interdisciplinary exercise in which the politician has the last word on the choice of priorities.

Methodological Aspects

In view of current trends in population and technology that oblige countries to face rapid changes and the complex interrelationships between economic growth and social objectives, common sense measures or the advice of a single expert is no longer sufficient. It has been a mistake to view food policy as a simple list of measures to be taken. The real problem is to bring about the technical conditions and level of information which will allow the formulation of various alternatives, to furnish a knowledge of the implications of the various choices proposed, to integrate them in national development plans, and to assist in their implementation following a well-defined strategy.

If, for example, the legislator decides by decree, on the advice of food technologists, to introduce 10% of a local cereal into imported wheat flour

*A significant part of the increase in per caput income at the national level is the result of a rapid transfer of population from the low-income rural sector to an urban sector of relatively high income. However, the increase in consumption of animal proteins accompanying this transfer is markedly less than the increase in income.

during bread-making, the repercussions will be many and various. By this means, a pattern of consumption is enforced on the consumers which does not reflect their current food preferences. The forecasts of wheat demand must, therefore, be revised downward, while the demand for local cereal will increase above the earlier expected rate. In the economic field the effect will be a drop in imports and a transfer of money resources to the rural world. From the viewpoint of agricultural policy and supply analysis, a spur to production and marketing is created which will speed up the transition to a market economy. This means that one must estimate the employment effects, the agricultural inputs, and the marketing and storage facilities needed to meet this new demand for local cereal. As far as nutrition is concerned, this measure will only affect consumers who, according to the survey, are in a market economy for bread products. If this market is large and allows vulnerable groups to be reached, supplementary legislation may provide for the enrichment of these products by appropriate nutrients.

Data Requirements

Food Balance Sheets

The information available for food planning is generally very limited. Food balance sheets showing uses for human consumption are prepared from production/utilization accounts for agricultural products. Essentially these accounts put statistics on production and foreign trade into a consistent framework. In such a process the final utilization corresponding to food is obtained only as a balance since direct data on consumption are generally not available. However, an overall feasibility study of the results in nutritional terms usually avoids excessive errors which would be made. Although the statistical data available are often poor and insufficient, the consistent framework is satisfactory and even essential to the planner. The food balance sheets make it possible to compare overall consumption with levels of food production and processing, thus giving an overall picture on a product-by-product basis that constitutes a fundamental element in the analysis of the food situation and allows the construction of supply/demand models. In the future, by applying adequate investigation techniques, one may hope to produce a marked improvement in the quality and variety of data, so that each element in the balance sheets will come sufficiently close to reality to be a guide for action at the overall national level.

Food Consumption and Household Budget Surveys

However, even assuming such a future improvement in the content of the balance sheets, an overall analysis framework that identifies only an average national diet is not a sufficiently refined tool for formulating specific action programs and making choices. To keep only to consumption, variations in income and welfare levels between socioeconomic groups or disparities in the quality of the environment exert such an influence that the present food situation must be known in distribution terms if specific actions are to be planned for the future. Increased efforts have, therefore, to be made to measure food inequalities within a population group and define the factors responsible (ecology, rural/urban, family size, income level, etc.). The promotion of integrated food consumption and household budget surveys that are directed toward these two objectives, and assistance to countries in this respect must be greatly intensified. Such surveys furnish the elements for an analysis of the basic situation in various sectors (demography and employment, structure of the food budget, levels of income, food consumption, nutrition, and education). Suitable processing of the information thus obtained will then furnish the planner with the elements he needs (projections of population, household income, food demand, and nutritional requirements). (See Table 1.)

Models

On the basis of these data, econometric and nutrimetric models can be developed which will not only identify with sufficient accuracy the population groups subject to food stress but also plan possible future improvements and their cost according to various assumptions regarding development and redistribution of income. Obviously, this level of analysis would consider not only quantitative but also fundamental qualitative factors such as food choices and preferences by households, so as to enable the formulation of more functional action programs.

In short, the planner must possess a coherent frame at national level and comprehensive data from household surveys. Jointly they form a basis for policies to reduce gaps and inequalities

TABLE 1

Basic Information to be Derived from a Food Consumption and Household Budget Survey

Demography and employment	Food consumption	Income and expenditures
Pyramid of age Size of family Composition of family Height and weight per person Educational level Migrations Occupation, employment Birth rate, fertility rate Mortality rate	Quantity per family, per caput: Weight Calories, nutrients Monetary value Distribution and frequency Origin of products: Subsistence Barter, purchase Gifts Domestic preparation: Processing Refuse, waste Behavioral pattern: Menu, weaning Preferences, taboos	Expenditure for food and nonfood items: By family By product In quantity In value Agricultural in- and outputs Sources of income: Monetary Nonmonetary Frequency distribution of income

Variables Used for Stratification and Correlation of Data

Geographical area, ecological zone, season
Rural/urban, level of income, access to markets
Profession, ethnic group, educational level, size of household

Elements {
For analysis of food situations
For food and agricultural planning
For food and nutrition policies

Population	Agricultural and food production	Food economy	Nutrition	Home economics
Identification of vulnerable groups Demographic projections	Production/utilization accounts Food balance sheets Supply projections and agricultural inputs Policy on food industry Agricultural calendar	Cost of living index Market study Demand projection Redistribution of income Price policy Policy on trade and employment	Consumption requirement analysis Food disparities Food additive control and legislation Policy on trade and employment Consumer protection	Family budgets Housing, kitchen Food processing Ability to change Nutrition education

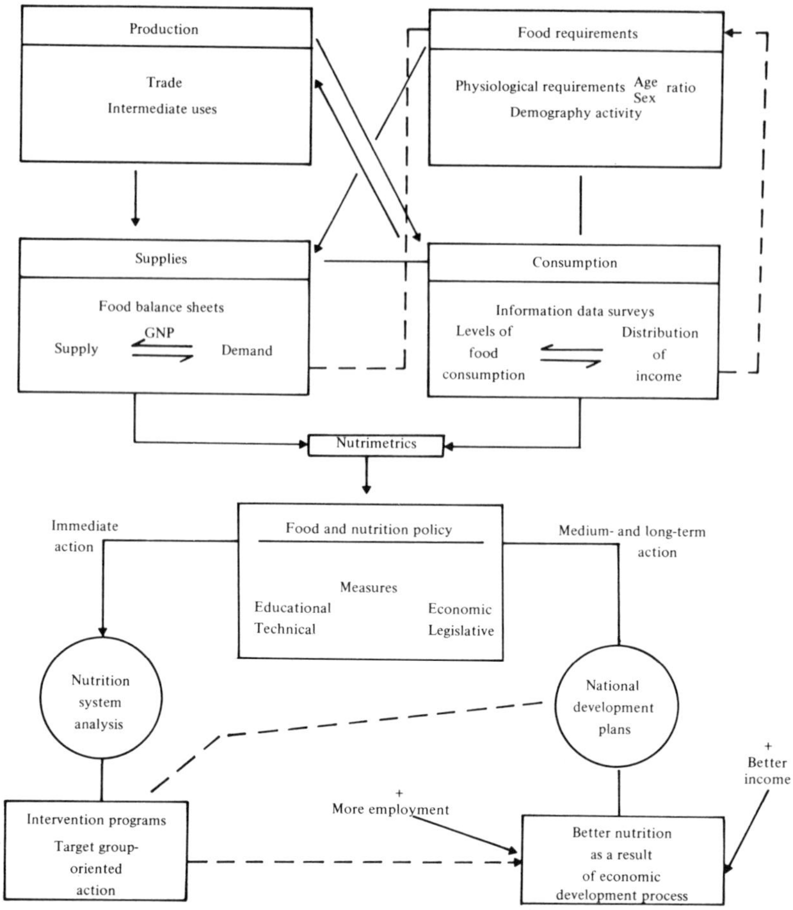

FIGURE 1

identified during the process of economic growth and for specific programs aimed, according to priority, at groups at risk (see Figure 1).

Integration of Food and Nutrition Policies in Agricultural Planning

The nutritionist has the means to estimate physiological requirements for calories and nutrients, but for the supply of these nutrients there is an almost infinite number of food combinations. The approach consisting in building up standard diets is highly satisfactory from the point of view of physiology, but it ignores economic constraints and gives only subjective consideration to consumer attitudes. The econometrics of demand endeavor to quantify changes in behavior by introducing income as an explanatory variable.*

The nutritionist wants to know whether the laissez-faire policy implicit in the demand model is capable of eventually improving the nutritional situation. It is obvious that the increase of supplies and the diversification of the diet achieved due to the economic expansion of the developed countries have, in general, made it possible in the nutrition field to solve most problems of underfeeding and malnutrition.**

Changes imposed on production in developed

*Income is only one of the explanatory variables of behavior changes; its value lies in the fact that it is measurable, but it is only the resultant, for consumption, of a number of economic and sociocultural factors which, being closely interwoven, cannot be separately isolated and quantified at the moment.

**It may be objected that such diets, judging by the frequency of obesity, diabetes, and cardiovascular ailments, do not represent a nutritional optimum.

countries by the evolution of consumption have not been rapid because they took place against the background of a small population increase, thus allowing a smooth adjustment between demand and supply. During this decade, problems in the developing countries will be of quite a different dimension and will require recourse to planning aimed at eventually producing a given economic situation by a compromise between what is possible and what is desirable. The concern for consistency implies the simultaneous estimate of objectives, resources, and instruments. Hence the necessity to perform an overall analysis, of which the demand model is one of the indicators.

This overall analysis stage is only the first in an agricultural and food planning study. Measures to be taken in regard to agricultural and food policies cannot be truly formulated until production and market specialists know the level of supply for each product. It will then be possible to judge, in economic and nutritional terms, the impact of possible constraints on the average diet. After that, products that have a favorable or unfavorable effect on diet balance can be identified and the emphases that appear desirable can be formulated in qualitative terms. By a process of reiteration, alternative and adjustment by-products can be proposed which will be designed to meet either economic considerations (concerning employment, trade, etc.) or social considerations (improved satisfaction of this or that nutritional requirement). The purpose of the measures to be taken will be, depending on the case, to create consumption or production incentives or to introduce constraints into consumer or producer behavior so as to adjust the supply or demand for each product in the desired direction.

COMPONENTS OF A FOOD AND NUTRITION POLICY

Any culture constitutes an integrated whole with its own logic. It is certainly by a process of gradual substitution, which allows time for adaptation, that the sociocultural balance is maintained. But the countries are today beset with abrupt and spectacular upheavals: Better health and sanitation upset the primeval equilibrium between man and his land; schooling and urbanization superimpose new cultural patterns; and the profit motive is emerging as a rival to the traditional concept of mere self-sufficiency. In this context of disrupted equilibria, difficulties in various socioeconomic groups and problems in food commodities arise, clamoring for the attention of public authorities.

Analysis of the Situation by Socioeconomic Groups

Experience shows that in weakly monetarized countries the traditional rural environment is still dependent on subsistence production for most of its food. In fact, higher income affects nutrition only if accompanied by changes in the economic and social scene (marketing, dietary habits, etc.). The phenomenon of accelerated urbanization, aided by influx from the countryside, leads to disorderly urban growth and to the creation of shantytowns. The lengthening of the distance between residence and place of work is leading to the breakdown of the consumer group at the same time as underemployment and unemployment lead to an increasing dependence on the breadwinners in the family. Urban consumers have access to a more diversified diet than is available in the countryside, but often obsolete and inefficient marketing and distribution systems tend to keep prices high when goods are sold in the small quantities that the poor consumers can typically afford at any given time. This practice penalizes the low-income groups so that the nutritional status of the urban poor is at least as low as that of the least well-off of their rural counterparts. In fact, a renewal of malnutrition is observed in the towns. However, the mingling of people, the multiplication of intercultural contacts, and the preponderant role acquired by cash income tend to give rise to a distinctive and dynamic urban culture and a dietary pattern which the majority generally finds attractive and adopts.

Between rural people living in a pure subsistence economy and newly urbanized people suddenly plunged into a market economy lies the immense majority of the rural world which is gradually acquiring a growing cash income. The regulatory effect that family financial resources may have on the diet is largely offset by the seasonal nature of money income. When such income occurs at times of food difficulty the consumer is obliged to use his cash supplies to purchase staple foods. As soon as this seasonal demand appears, prices rise steeply because of the inadequacy of trade channels and storage facilities. When income coincides with the period of food plenty the consumer starts spending money on prestige items which will meet his social obligations and buys the most necessary agricultural inputs (tools, etc.) as well as consumer goods which will show his social success. This competition between consumer goods and food products leads the family into dietary improvisations that are bound to upset the precarious balance of traditional diets.

Access to a market economy is, therefore, not in itself the answer to all nutritional problems, being rather a precondition for any food policy than a solution as such. The analysis of economic development in relation to food consumption shows that the transition to a money economy ultimately accentuates dietary inequalities during the first development phases. To counteract this trend would require means to harmonize the distribution of resources and income, town and country planning to avoid the creation of large urban complexes around a rural vacuum, and even the pursuit of a land-use planning policy. Such harmonious development, in which mankind would not be sacrificed, is still a utopian dream in view of the variety of sociocultural situations and the diversity of interests involved in building an industrial society, but laissez faire in this field is proving to be only a makeshift solution.

Analysis of the Situation by Products

Analysis of the situation on a product-by-product basis shows that compared with export crops, the development of domestic staple foods has received relatively little attention from governments. In 1965 these products supplied 60% of the calories and proteins in the diet for the developing countries as a whole and represent in value, at the farm-gate price, 62% of food supplies of vegetable origin.

Efforts have been made from the production stage to storage on the farm, but the most important step has been the introduction of high-yielding varieties. For the moment, these varieties are benefiting the rural inhabitants in a significant way only in a limited number of countries such as Mexico, Pakistan, India, the Philippines, Arab Republic of Egypt, and Turkey. Even in these countries they tend to favor farmers living in fertile agricultural areas who are in a position to adapt themselves technically and to buy the inputs (fertilizers, pesticides) required by these new cultural techniques. For cultivators of marginal land, the race with these privileged farmers runs the risk of being lost before it starts. Their economic and dietary situation is liable to get worse owing to the foreseeable drop in cereal prices. There is, therefore, a danger that the flow of less skilled laborers to the city will accelerate.

Rice and wheat eating countries have processing industries. In countries consuming millet, sorghum, maize, or roots and tubers, and pulses, industries to process these products are at best at the experimental pilot project stage. The processing operations involved, namely, sorting, grinding, winnowing, peeling, fermentation, drying, preservation and packing, etc., are simply added to the farming activities of rural families or are carried out by local craftsmen using primitive methods. For the housewife, in particular, this involves physically strenuous and unrewarding tasks as well as losses of time which could be better employed attending to the family and looking after the children. These activities are seldom measured in terms of value added and their economic value is underestimated in national accounts.

Animal products play an essential part from the point of view of quality of the diet. In the developing countries they supply only 9% of calories and 20% of proteins but in value they account for 34% of food supplies. Owing to their inherently high unit price, which enables them to bear the cost of transport, and the lack of mixed farming, they are the subject of active marketing. These prestige products are marketed by highly organized and often oligopolistic channels. For this reason the intake of products of animal origin is closely connected with cash income per caput.

The total protein intake is the reflection of two phenomena: one relating to vegetable proteins and more closely linked to ecology and the other relating to animal proteins and associated with the income of households and their effective demand. This means that even in cities the poor reach the protein level imposed on them by their ecological environment, while the rich attain the protein level permitted them by their income.

The constraints on production of animal products that have become evident over the past decade and can be predicted in the medium term will bring about a price increase to the disadvantage of the less affluent groups. To palliate these inequalities, it would be necessary for supplies of pulses and oilseeds to meet at least the demand objectives, i.e., to grow faster than supplies of cereals. This is very difficult because extension programs of cereals urgently needed to face the population increase risk altering crop rotations at the expense of these products. If these objectives cannot be achieved, the poor classes will be hard put to improve the protein quality of their diets, and constraints on oilcake production will slow down animal protein production programs short of the demand perspectives.

In view of the priority to be given to satisfying calorie requirements and the need to supply the vulnerable groups with a protein diet of high biological quality, these three food groups (cereals, animal products, pulses) are of priority interest both for agricultural development planning and for food policy formulation.

Analysis of the distribution curves of consumption and requirements shows that average per caput supplies equal to the average requirement do not mean a satisfactory consumption level for everyone. If the task of substantially improving consumption levels is left to economic expansion, the time needed, on the assumption of continuous population growth, will be such that it will be impossible to contain extremely serious social movements.

IMPLEMENTATION OF FOOD AND NUTRITION POLICIES

In accordance with the definition of the policy given in the section, "Food and Nutrition Policy," the measures to be taken can be classified into educational, economic, technological, and legislative. The description that follows is only illustrative and sketchy and not intended to be exhaustive. The purpose of the paper is a first attempt to explain the approach to policy formulation and to show the level of information and the methodological frame needed to obtain coherent discussions and coordinated action. Adequacy and value of the measures vary from country to country, according to the resources that can be mobilized. They depend also on the ability to identify the explanatory variables of food inequalities and on the relative weight given by the government to economic vs. social development.

Educational Measures

Among groups living in a subsistence economy there is little stimulus to change, and economic measures can be of only limited effect. The application of educational measures that will lead to better use of potential resources appears to be the best solution. The agronomist and the agricultural extension staff must learn about human nutritional requirements and how these can be met from foods that can be produced locally to advise farmers on what to grow for home consumption; provision should also be made for educational programs in nutrition and home economics aimed at mothers, through agricultural extension, community development, and other services. The teaching of nutrition should also be introduced into the school curriculum. Likewise a series of practical actions, such as the development of school and home gardens or the production of poultry, fish, and small animals, can be envisaged.

Examples of educational programs that have been effective in modifying dietary practices with a resultant improvement in the pattern of food consumption are found in the Philippines, Korea, Lesotho, Swaziland, Colombia, St. Lucia, Paraguay, and Bolivia. In both Lesotho and Swaziland, for instance, the taboo on feeding eggs to children has been practically overcome, while one project in Bolivia provides an interesting illustration of the outreach into the community of a school-centered nutrition education and school garden program. Simple drying techniques were taught in schools to preserve surplus vegetables from the school gardens. These techniques were adopted by housewives in the community with the result that vegetables became available throughout the year, instead of for a very limited season.

For newly urbanized populations, efforts should be made to reconstitute a community which on the whole is fairly close to that found in the countryside, using the techniques available through the social sciences, followed up by a home economics program with a strong nutrition education bias. Endeavors should also be made to integrate into city life people living on its margin by making them receptive to the practices of the population already assimilated.

The use of effective methods of communication is essential to the success of nutrition education programs. The use of modern audio-visual aids, e.g., radio, television, and other mass media at the community level, seems promising and might be decisive in bringing about desirable dietary changes.

To provide the necessary infrastructure for nutrition education there must be an adequate reservoir of trained personnel at various levels and within the various services. Agronomists, economists, and statisticians concerned with planning must have a good background in nutrition; nutrition advice is needed in agricultural planning to test in terms of calories and nutrients the consistency of the demand supply models, to help, in an interdisciplinary approach, formulate policies and implement programs. A major effort is needed at the community level since women take an active part in the management of home resources and in food preparation and utilization. One of the issues to be solved is how to provide improved education in nutrition for women, more especially during the transition from a subsistence economy to a money economy, so that this hitherto unused potential – as food producers, consumers, home managers, and "producers of producers" – is fully exploited. How best can this be done through a massive program of assistance to nutrition education?

Economic and Administrative Measures

A number of economic and administrative measures can be envisaged as a part of a food and nutrition policy. The aim is to promote, by affecting either the supply or demand, the consumption patterns and levels in the desired direction. For these measures to be effective, it must be possible to identify the consumer groups capable of obtaining access to this market and the producers who can satisfy it. Where this has not been done the response has exceeded expectations and serious surpluses or deficits have occurred.

A particular problem arises from the apparent conflict between, on the one hand, policies providing producers with sufficient incentives to increase the production of the desired foodstuffs and, on the other hand, the necessity to keep the price to consumers sufficiently low to make possible increased consumption, and to keep the general level of prices from rising too rapidly.

There are various ways of overcoming this. They include price stabilization measures at the producer level, so as to ensure that consumer prices remain reasonable at preharvest periods or in years of low harvests, or when, in the case of exporting countries, world market prices are high or domestic supplies limited. Buffer stock operations and control over imports and exports are used frequently. In other cases it has been found necessary to subsidize consumer prices, either for all quantities of specified products sold (especially in urban markets) or for specific quantities (e.g., Sri Lanka rice rations) or consumer groups (e.g., civil servants and other fixed income groups, or indigent families). A variant form of food subsidy is the "fair price shops" operating in several Indian states, or the use of other authorized outlets to sell specified food at controlled prices (e.g., the "carros tienda" of Colombia). In many countries, institutional feeding schemes (schools, hospitals, factory canteens, and other institutions) are being supplemented with food provided by WFP, Food for Peace, and other programs.

For potential demand to materialize, it is important to create adequate channels of distribution. Thus, a concerted program of intensifying trade between ecologically different areas may be very effective despite the barriers due to ethnic habits and cultural regionalisms. The surpluses that may be produced in small scattered areas may not be large enough to justify setting up modern marketing facilities that will be economically profitable in a short time. It should be the function of marketing boards to support these facilities in the early phase and to help mitigate the seasonal fluctuations of prices for staple foods in the preharvest period.

It will not be enough to tackle problems from the producing areas to the wholesale markets. It will be necessary to work out a rational marketing network stretching from the central markets to the peripheral areas where the poorest groups live. Likewise, rationalization of the retail market (from supermarket to street stall) and large-scale feeding facilities will be equally necessary (canteens, community restaurants) and decisive in altering the consumer's attitude in the direction of a better diet.

In addition, food aid used in institutional feeding schemes is a means of developing infrastructure projects involving human investment. It also mitigates the paradoxical problems of food superabundance and food want existing side by side. It promotes paths of economic and social development particularly beneficial to vulnerable population groups through feeding projects, leading to an improvement in the quality of the labor force and expansion of employment opportunities. Food aid is acceptable where, by reason of its scope, it does not restrict production incentives. It plays a decisive part in natural disaster and in cases of crop failure provided relief is rapidly mobilized.

Can a suitable strategy be evolved to optimize returns from investment on government-sponsored nutrition feeding programs with reference to the most vulnerable classes and areas?

Technological Measures

Transfers of technology resulting from genetic researches and applied to production will have more impact among the weakly monetarized rural classes from the nutritional viewpoint than the improvements that can be expected from increased per caput income. For the farmer the best incentive is high yields. This criterion is much closer to the peasant's reach than one based on nutritional quality. Selection must, therefore, extend to other cereals (maize, sorghum, millet) to obtain varieties which are even more productive, especially in the marginal areas. However, the criteria for selection of varieties must also take account of nutritional value following the line of research adopted for maize of the "opaque 2" type, and must be accompanied by acceptability tests. For roots and tubers likewise, productivity must take account of the starch and protein content. For pulses, the highest nutritional gains that can be expected will be derived much more from selecting varieties having a high protein digestibility than from seeking high-protein varieties.

Between production and consumption there is considerable room on the market for local foods and drinks which take account of cultural patterns but on which technology would confer the prestige and ease of use they lack. This requires an advanced level of technology, investment in research, and extensive specialization. Such food industries, by turning regional produce to account, would benefit from a strongly expanding urban market. They would generate employment and partly block the flight to the large cities. Protein-rich formulated foods for vulnerable groups are part of this activity and from the social viewpoint are of a priority nature for the prevention of malnutrition.

Legislative Measures

Faced with the growing pollution of the environment and its effects on the food chain, governments must realize the value of food control to protect the consumer and develop trade. The adoption of new technical solutions must be accompanied by the framing of suitable legislation. It should cover the adoption of standards for food products and additives in conformity with those established by the FAO/WHO Codex Alimentarius Commission and rules concerning marketing (weights and measures, labeling regulations, etc.). Where industrially processed food products enter a market economy and become commonly used, one may consider supplementation programs and take legislative steps to produce an enriched diet.

CONCLUSIONS

There have been and there will always be in the world food and nutrition problems: undernutrition, overnutrition, and malnutrition. Yet, we still do not seem to know who is primarily responsible for properly feeding a given population: the politician, the economist, or the producer? Or is the responsibility with the food industries, market, and trade? Or do we believe that it is the sole responsibility of the consumer living within his social, economic, or ecological constraints? The fact is that a food policy is no more than an element in the overall economic and social policy; an important element that brings together all parameters, which were dealt with separately in the past and which could be a means for correctly assigning the responsibilities for feeding a nation properly.

The formulation of a food and nutrition policy integrated in national development plans aims at securing an adequate diet to each consumer in the near future, irrespective of his income level. From national food and nutrition policies, we should be able to draw up international policies aiming at the reduction of injustices between nations. At the same time it will be essential to identify specific nutrition problems and the best alternatives for solving them. In the past, nutrition problems have been tackled by means of nutrition activities. By using a more systematic approach (nutrition systems analysis), we should now be able to propose the best objective alternative for solving a well-defined problem on a cost/benefit or a cost/efficiency basis. This is of paramount importance because it gives the nutritionist not only his right place in the identification of the problem and in proposing the solutions, but it also gives the right person, whoever he is, the responsibility of solving it. For instance, employment policy, fiscal and legislative measures, or some agricultural programs might better solve a nutrition problem which nutrition programs would never have solved, but only temporarily alleviated.

In other words, as is everything that affects man, the food problem is complex. It is only by means of national consumption and household budget surveys that one could come to grips with the problem, to identify the various causal variables of food inequalities, and the human groups affected by them. To assess the value and effectiveness of a food and nutrition policy measure, the resulting effects must be quantifiable at the planning level in a consistent framework of production and utilization accounts in costs, quantities, and values. If the impact of such a measure is found to be negligible according to economic or social criteria, it can be rejected knowingly and other alternatives can be proposed. There may be many solutions, but they must be coherent and actions must be coordinated.

Governments that intend to include food and nutrition policies in their development plans need to have a planning body with sufficient authority to identify the measures, to coordinate the activities of the many different ministries involved, and possibly to propose readjustments during the development plan, if it is not possible to formulate their food and nutrition policies when elaborating a new development plan.

REFERENCES

1. **Boerma, A. H.,** Statement to the press on the world food situation, FAO Director-General's Bulletin, 73/4, Rome, 1973.
2. **Boerma, A. H.,** The world food situation and its implications, Address to the Washington Institute of Foreign Affairs, October 1972.

ABBREVIATIONS AND SYMBOLS

AA	Amino acid(s)
AID	Agency for International Development (US)
ATPase	Adenosine triphosphatase
a_w	Water activity
BHA	Butylated hydroxyanisole
BHT	Butylated hydroxytoluene
BMR	Basal metabolic rate
C	Centigrade
CA	Central America
CAB	Commonwealth Agricultural Bureaux
cal	Calorie
CIMMYT	Centro Internacional de Mejoramiento del Maiz y Trigo (International Maize and Wheat Improvement Center)
cm	Centimeter
CSIRO	Commonwealth Scientific and Industrial Research Organisation
CSM	Corn-soy milk
2,4-D	2,4-Dichlorophenoxyacetic acid
DBC	Dye-binding capacity
DDT	Dichlorodiphenyltrichloroethane
EA	Essential amino acid(s)
EBW	Ingesta-free, wool-free body weight
EEC	European Economic Community
E_h	Oxidation-reduction potential
ERS	Economic Research Service (USDA)
F	Fahrenheit
FAO	Food and Agriculture Organization (UN)
ft	Foot (or feet)
g	Gram
GE	Gross energy
GNP	Gross National Product
ha	Hectare
HMSO	His (or Her) Majesty's Stationary Office
hr	Hour
ICNND	Interdepartmental Committee on Nutrition for National Defense (US)
INCAP	Institute de Nutrición de Centro América y Panama
INEAC	Institut National pour l'Étude Agronomique du Congo
IU	International Unit
IWP	Indicative World Plan
JAMA	Journal of the American Medical Association
kcal	Kilocalorie
kg	Kilogram
km	Kilometer
LAI	Leaf area index
lb	Pound
m	Meter
ME	Metabolizable energy
mg	Milligram
min	Minute
ml	Milliliter
mm	Millimeter
ND_pCal	Net dietary protein calories
NPN	Nonprotein nitrogen
NPR	Net protein retention
NPU	Net protein utilization
OECD	Organization for Economic Cooperation and Development
O-R	Oxidation-reduction
PAG	Protein Advisory Group (UN)
PCM	Protein-calorie malnutrition
PDI	Protein dispersibility index
PER	Protein efficiency ratio
pH	Hydrogen-ion concentration
ppm	Parts per million
RH	Relative humidity
RNA	Ribonucleic acid
UK	United Kingdom
UN	United Nations
UNCTAD	U.N. Conference on Trade and Development
UNICEF	U.N. International Children's Emergency Fund
U.S.	United States
USAID	U.S. Agency for International Development
USDA	U.S. Department of Agriculture
U.S.S.R.	Union of Soviet Socialist Republics
WFP	World Food Program
WHO	World Health Organization (UN)
WPC	Wheat protein concentrate

TABLES AND FIGURES

Tables

Mortality due to Nutritional Deficiency (as an Underlying Cause) in Children under Five Years of Age . 3
Pattern of Nutritional Deficiency in Mortality of Infants under One Year of Age 4
Pattern of Nutritional Deficiency in Mortality of Children 1–4 Years of Age 5
Range of % Prevalence of PCM in Community Surveys (1963–1972) 6
Range and Median of % Prevalence of PCM in Community Surveys (Selected Surveys with More than 1,000 Children Examined) 6
Regional Differences in the Pattern of PCM (Hospital Cases) 8
% Prevalence of Kwashiorkor and Nutritional Marasmus in Young Children: Community Surveys . . . 9
Different Levels of Cereal Consumption per Capita in Countries in Different Regions of the World . . 17
Different Levels of Starchy Food Consumption per Capita in Countries in Different Regions of the World 21
Different Levels of Pulses, Vegetables, and Fruit Consumption per Capita in Countries in Different Regions of the World 23
Different Levels of Meat, Egg, and Fish Consumption per Capita in Countries in Different Regions of the World 27
Different Levels of Milk and Cheese Consumption per Capita in Countries in Different Regions of the World 29
Different Levels of Fat, Sugar, and Beverage Consumption per Capita in Countries in Different Regions of the World 31
Major Components of World Food Production, 1969 35
World Area and Production of Major Crops and Groups of Crops, 1948–52 and 1966–70 36
Summary of Major Food Crops by Region and Area, 1948–52 and 1966–70 38–39
Summary of Major Food Crops by Region – Production, 1948–52 and 1966–70 40–41
Major Uses of Land by World Regions 43
Arable Land and Population by World Regions as of 1970 43
Estimated Potentially Arable Land in the World 46
Total Population and Expectation of Life 57
Crude Birth Rates, Crude Death Rates, and Gross Reproduction Rate 58–59
Estimated Population of Selected Countries 60
Age Distribution Population Size: Annual Growth Rate of Age Groups: Percentage Distribution of Age Groups 61
Urban and Rural Population: Number and Rate of Growth 1960–2000 62–63
Calorie Requirements of Men Aged 20–29, Central Africa 66
Children's Calorie Requirements per Day 66
Calorie and Reference Protein Requirements per Day 68–69
Calorie and Reference Protein Standards 70
Average Calorie Intake, Total Protein and Animal Protein Intake – Asia, Africa, Latin America . .71–72
Farm Value Income Elasticities of Total Food as Computed from FAO Projections 73
Value and Quantity Income Elasticities in Venezuela, India, and the Philippines, for Selected Commodities, Compared with FAO 74
Estimated Fertilizer Rates and Yield Responses for Corn for Two Selected Agricultural Subregions in the U.S. 98
U.S. Average Yields of Selected Crops for the Years Indicated (1930, 1960, 1970) 104
Yield Increase Compared to Farmed Area Increase between 1950 and 1970 in Percentage 111
Yields in 100 kg/ha and Yield Increases of Food Crops between 1950 and 1970 by Region 112
Yields in 100 kg/ha and Yield Increases by Country 117
Mean Monthly Global Solar Radiation in cal cm^{-2} day^{-1} 120

Potential Yields in Tons and Calories of Grains, Roots, or Tubers per ha per Year 121
Realized Record Yields in Tons/ha 122
Targets for Yield Increases in Percentage per Year between 1962 and 1985 124
The Mean Productivity of Farm Livestock in Different Regions of the World Expressed in Terms of the Daily Production of Protein per Person in the Population 128
The Farm Animal Population of the World 129
Crude Productivity of Cattle and Buffalo by World Regions 130
Crude Productivity of Pigs by World Regions 130
The Productivity of Beef Cattle in South Africa Showing Superiority of a New Breed Including Indigenous and Exotic Blood 142
Production of Meat and Milk per Head of Cattle Population in Major Regions 1966/67, in Kilograms per Head per Year 151
Approximate Freezing Point of Selected Foods 178
Optimal Storage Temperatures and Relative Humidities of Commodities Susceptible to Cold Injury when Improperly Stored 183
Sources of Carbon for Human Food 194
World Production of Seeds Yielding a Protein-rich Residue 196
The Three Products Made by Fractionating a Fresh Leafy Crop 198
Chemical Composition of the Pig at Successive Stages of Prenatal Life 216
Chemical Composition of the Pig at Successive Stages of Postnatal Life 217
Range in Body Composition of Cattle, Sheep, and Pigs 218
Overall Efficiencies of Protein Production from Meat-Producing Species 219
Breed Differences in Body Composition of Sheep at Successful Slaughter Weights 220
Sex Effects on Chemical Composition of Carcass Weight Changes in Lambs 221
Relative Effects of Age and Weight on Body Composition of Sheep 223
Composition of the Middle Section of Pigs Slaughtered at 59 kg/Liveweight Following Different Energy and Protein Intakes 224
Antinutritional Factors Present in Plant Foodstuffs which are Destroyed or Eliminated by Processing . . . . 233 – 234
Comparison between the Protein Value and Amino Acid Intake of Opaque-2 and Normal Maize . . . 255
Protein Quality of Some High Protein-containing Foods 256
Ingredient Composition of Some High Protein-containing Foods . . . . 257 – 258
Supplementation of Lime-treated Corn with Amino Acids 259
Optimum Levels of Protein Concentrates to Supplement Lime-treated Corn and Rice 260
Effect of Various Supplements on the Nutritive Value of Corn 261
Effect of Adding Lysine, Tryptophan, and Vitamins on the Nutritive Value of Tortilla Flour 262
Effect of the Individual Addition of Groups of Nutrients on the Quality of Corn-bean Diet 262
Effect of Fortified Beans on the Performance of Rats and Quality of Corn-bean Diets 263
Effect of Replacing Lime-treated Corn Flour by Various Levels of Wheat Short on Nutritive Value . . 264
Protein Quality of Manioc Flour with and without Methionine Addition Mixed with Various Levels of Beans 266
Effect of Adding Methionine on the Nutritive Value of Various Cassava-bean Mixtures 266
Protein Quality of Soybean Textured Food in Rats, Dogs, and Children 269
Basic Information to be Derived from a Food Consumption and Household Budget Survey 279

Figures

A Small-scale Soil Map of the World Based on the Soil Classification Current in the U.S. from about 1950 to 1965 82
Soils of the World. Distribution of Orders and Suborders. A Small-scale Soil Map of the World Based on the Current System of Soil Taxonomy in the U.S. 83
Cutting a Tree in the Tropical Rain Forest at Ground Level 86

"Stinger" on Blade Splits Large Tree in Tropical Forest 86
Piling Brush and Logs after Cutting Trees in Tropical Rain Forest 87
In Kerala State, India, a Man Rests while Cutting the Doughy Laterite into Potential Bricks 88
A Typical Acid Sulfate Clayey Soil with Rushes in the Delta of the Mekong River not far from Saigon . 89
Graph Showing Potassium Accumulation in Corn for the Whole Plant and Plant Parts 94
The Influence of Soil pH on the Relative Availability of Certain Nutrients 96
Economic Benefits from Three Combinations of Improved Management Practices Used to Achieve Increased Corn Production in Kenya 104
Ranges of Potential Rice Yields for a Modern Nonlodging Variety with a Constant Growth Cycle at Different Latitudes and in Different Seasons 121
Calculated and Obtained Wheat Yields in the Netherlands since 1965 122
World Distribution of Foot-and-Mouth Disease Classified according to Type of Virus 134
Amounts of Calories, Total Protein, and Animal Protein in National Food Supplies of 90 Countries . 148
Amounts of Total Protein and Proportions of Animal and Plant Protein in Food Supplies of 90 Countries 149
Amounts of Animal Protein in Food Supplies of 90 Countries 149
Amounts of Milk, Meat, Eggs, and Fish in the Food Supplies of 90 Countries 150
Chart Showing the Relationship between Levels of Income and Supplies of Animal Protein per Person in 30 Countries 154
Devastating Effect of Lethal Yellowing Disease on Tall Coconut Palms in Jamaica 168
A Swarm of Desert Locust Invading an Airport in Somalia 170
A Solid Carpet of Locust Feeding on Grasses during an Invasion in Morocco 170
Outbreak and Invasion Areas of the African Migratory Locust 171
Distribution of the Desert Locust and Spread of its Invasion Area 172
Trend in Herbicide Use in Rice Growing in Japan 173
Yearly Reduction in Man's Working Hours in Rice Fields Resulting from Mechanization and Herbicide Use 173
Average Rice Production in Japan and Major Causes of Yield Reduction over a 40-Year Period . . . 173
Average Crop Losses Caused by Pests and Diseases in Rice over the Period 1949-1965 174
Temperature Relations for Growth and Survival of Microorganisms 180
pH Values of Foods 181
Comparison of Water Activity Values for Various Meats with those Limiting the Germination of Growth of Microorganisms 182
E_h Conditions for an Aerobe and an Anaerobe 185
Effect of Initial Bacterial Populations on Storage Life of Sliced and Ground Beef 186
Relationship between PER and Lysine 260
Effect of Addition of Lysine and Tryptophan to a Corn-bean Diet in the Presence and Absence of Vitamins and Minerals 263

AUTHOR INDEX

Numbers in parentheses indicate reference numbers.

A

Abbott, G. W., 54 (2, 3)
Abdel Hak, T., 176 (26)
Abdo, K. M., 241 (81)
Adams, J. R., 97, 107(7)
Aguirre, A., 272 (28)
Aitken, J. N., 228 (93)
Alberda, Th., 124 (12)
Albertazzi, C., 273 (54)
Albrecht, W. J., 273 (74)
Alder, F. E., 229 (96)
Aldrich, S. A., 107 (10)
Aldrich, S. R., 107 (1, 2)
Alexander, G. I., 146 (15)
Alexander, J. C., 241 (87)
Alexander, L. T., 89 (7)
Allaway, W. H., 211, 213 (24)
Allen, L. E., 248 (12)
Allen, P. E., 272 (36)
Allison, J. B., 271 (18), 272 (34)
Almquist, H. J., 271 (16)
Altschul, A. M., 239 (14, 15), 249 (26)
Alvarado, J., 241 (89), 274 (79, 83)
Anderson, B. M., 214 (40)
Anderson, D. W., 239 (27)
Anderson, D. W., Jr., 239 (33)
Anderson, J. R., 54 (6), 239 (32)
Anson, M. L., 271 (13, 14)
Antonovics, J., 214 (67)
Arai, S., 240 (71, 72, 73, 74)
Ardrey, R., 231, 238 (2)
Arriaga, E. E., 12 (6)
Arrogave, G., 239 (41)
Arroyave, G., 248 (14), 273 (64)
Arthaud, V. H., 228 (69)
Ascoli, W., 12 (8)
Ashbel, O. D., 124 (3, 4)
Ashcroft, M. T., 65, 76 (11)
Ashton, G. C., 228 (84)
Auckland, J. N., 226 (26)
Austin, A., 214 (64)
Aykroyo, W. R., 1, 11, 12 (1), 124 (5)
Aylward, F., 248 (9)
Ayres, J. C., 188 (7)

B

Bacigalupo, A., 273 (60)
Badenhop, A. F., 235, 239 (36)
Bailey, B. M., 272 (30)
Bailey, C. M., 228 (67)
Baker, D. E., 206, 213 (26, 27, 28, 29)
Banerjea, 76 (18)
Bannatyne, W. R., 239 (37)
Bannerjee, S., 241 (80)
Barber, W. D., 211, 214 (68)
Barghoorn, E. S., 176 (1)
Barley, K. P., 213 (25)
Barrett, W. W., 239 (33)
Barton, R. A., 226 (11), 229 (126)
Basu, D., 72, 77 (40)
Bates, L. S., 274 (80)
Bates, R. D., 239 (33), 269
Bauer, C. D., 239 (27)
Bauernfeind, J. C., 248 (7, 12)
Beeson, K. C., 208, 214 (41, 45)
Beevers, L., 214 (70)
Behman, G. A., 230 (131)
Bell, J. M., 228 (82)
Bengoa, J. M., 2, 7, 12 (5, 7, 13, 14) 13 (38, 56)
Bennett, M. K., 65, 76 (9)
Bennett, O. L., 213 (19)
Bensadoun, A., 226 (17)
Berardi, L. C., 240 (47)
Berg, A. D., 273 (65)
Berg, R. T., 219, 227 (39, 40, 46, 47, 52), 228 (68, 75)
Bhagavan, R. K., 217 (10)
Bhattacharya, K. R., 239 (31)
Bigelow, W. D., 188 (8)
Biskas, A. K., 77 (52)
Bixler, E. G., 226 (25)
Black, C. A., 107 (3)
Black, C. C., 124 (6)
Black, J. N., 213 (36)
Blair, R., 221, 228 (78, 88)
Blaxter, K. L., 146 (3), 226 (8)
Blendl, H. M., 227 (53)
Block, R. J., 239 (26, 27)
Boerma, A. H., 275, 286 (1, 2)
Bohmann, V. R., 228 (67)
Bonner, J., 124 (7)
Book Walter, G. N., 273 (74)
Booth, A. N., 240 (54)
Borchers, R., 241 (88)
Borrie, W. D., 60, 76 (3)
Bose, D. W., 77 (52)
Bould, C., 204, 213 (10)
Bourgeois-Pichat, J., 76 (4)
Bovard, K. P., 230 (139)
Bowland, J. P., 228 (75)
Bradfield, P. G. E., 228 (74)
Bradley, N. W., 228 (64)
Bradley, W. B., 239 (12), 240 (69)
Bradshaw, A. D., 214 (67)
Braham, J. E., 239 (41), 271 (11), 272 (20), 273 (53)
Branaman, G. A., 227 (37)
Brande, S. K., 239 (38)
Bray, R. W., 230 (145, 150, 151, 152, 153)
Bressani, R., 239 (40, 42), 241 (89), 256, 259, 261, 264, 269, 271 (1, 2, 3, 7, 11, 12, 19), 272 (20, 21, 25, 27, 28, 32, 33, 35, 39, 40, 42, 45), 273 (49, 53, 54, 55, 63), 274 (79, 82)
Briedenstein, B. B., 228 (63)
Briedenstein, B. C., 228 (63)

Briggs, M. H., 146 (14)
Brim, C. A., 274 (86)
Brock, 11
Brody, S., 226 (27)
Brooke, C. L., 248 (11, 15)
Brooks, C. C., 226 (5), 230 (136)
Brougham, R. W., 124 (8)
Brouwer, R., 124 (1)
Brown, G. A., 227 (37)
Brown, L. R., 162 (14)
Brown, L. W., 153
Brown, R. G., 2, 12 (9)
Brown, R. H., 124 (6)
Brownlee, R. D., Jr., 239 (34)
Brungardt, V. H., 226 (15), 229 (111)
Buck, S. F., 228 (77)
Buddenhagen, I. W., 176 (22)
Buffa, A., 238, 241 (85)
Bull, L. S., 226 (17)
Bull, T. A., 124 (9)
Bunting, A. H., 146 (22)
Buol, S. W., 107 (4)
Burgess, A. P., 12 (26, 27)
Burgess, C. R., 228 (80)
Burgess, H. J. L., 12 (21, 22, 23, 26, 27, 28)
Burkholder, P. R., 211, 214 (66)
Burton, G. W., 214 (60)
Burton, H. W., 226 (24)
Burton, J. H., 226 (17)
Butterfield, R. M., 219, 226 (12), 227 (44, 45, 46, 47, 48), 229 (103)

C

Cady, J. G., 89 (7)
Cahill, V. R., 228 (85)
Calder, A., 228 (79)
Callow, E. H., 227 (36), 229 (109), 230 (147)
Calloway, D. H., 67, 77 (33)
Cannon, H. L., 214 (40)
Carew, L. B., 239 (19)
Carlton, B. C., 188 (3)
Carney, W. B., 239 (15)
Carpenter, F. M., 176 (2)
Carpenter, K. J., 210, 214 (51), 239 (28)
Carroll, F. D., 227 (38, 49)
Carroll, R. W., 238 (11)
Carter, W., 176 (9)
Cassens, R. G., 230 (145, 152)
Catchpole, C., 230 (155)
Cater, C. M., 268, 273 (71, 72)
Cathcart, P. H., 188 (8)
Cederquist, D. C., 241 (78)
Chalmers, A. W., 146 (7)
Chandler, R. F., Jr., 107 (5), 125 (10)
Chandrasekaran, A., 241 (82)
Chandrasekhara, M. R., 273 (67)
Charette, L. A., 228 (76)
Chattapadhay, H., 241 (80)
Chen, T. M., 124 (6)
Chiang, H. C., 176 (17)
Chiarappa, L., 176 (16, 17, 27)
Cholakos, B. V., 272 (38)
Choo, S. H., 230 (157)
Clark, C. G., 66, 67, 70, 72, 76 (15), 77 (25, 27, 29, 41, 50, 51), 146 (2)
Clark, H. E., 255, 272 (36)
Clausen, H., 216, 226 (13)
Clegg, M. T., 227 (38)
Clements, H. F., 205, 213 (11)
Coble, D. S., 227 (35)
Cole, J. W., 228 (80)
Cole-King, S. M., 12 (21)
Colindres, R., 271 (4)
Collander, R., 213 (37)
Colvin, B. M., 236, 239 (43)
Combs, G. F., 226 (25)
Connor, M. A., 240 (75)
Cook, R., 12 (29)
Cooke, B. B., 272 (30)
Cooke, G. W., 107 (6), 125 (11)
Cooke, R., 229 (112, 113, 114)
Corbett, J. L., 229 (127)
Corry Mann, H. C., 202 (4)
Cort, W. M., 248 (15)
Couch, J. R., 230 (135)
Cowan, C. C., Jr., 239 (34)
Crane, H. L., 213 (8)
Cravioto, J., 12 (15)
Crichton, J. A., 228 (93)
Cross, D. E., 240 (48)
Crouse, J. D., 230 (149)
Croy, L. I., 213 (17)
Cullumbine, 65
Cundiff, L. V., 228 (64)
Cundy, M. E., 229 (113)
Cunningham, F. E., 229 (120, 121)
Cunningham, H. M., 230 (137)
Cuthbertson, A., 227 (43)
Czochanska, Z., 229 (126)

D

da Cunha, S., 248 (13)
Daeschmer, C. W., Jr., 239 (22)
D'Aquin, E. L., 240 (48)
Darby, W. J., 13 (53)
Da Silva, L. P., 265, 273 (61)
Davies, R. E., 230 (135)
Davis, K., 12 (6)
Dawson, R. M. C., 230 (129)
Day, N., 221, 228 (86)
De, S. S., 241 (79)
Dechary, J. M., 239 (15)
DeLoache, W. R., 239 (34)
Delobez, R. R., 236, 240 (45)
de Muelenaere, H. J. H., 238 (9)
Dent, J. B., 228 (88)
Denton, A. E., 239 (30)
Derse, P H., 239 (16)
De Rulter, D., 265, 273 (59)
Desmond, M. M., 239 (22)

deVos, N. M., 125 (31)
de Vries, C. A., 125 (32)
Deweese, W., 230 (148)
DeWit, C. T., 124 (1), 125 (36, 37, 38)
Dexter, S. T., 213 (21)
De Zaghi, S., 241 (89)
Dhar, R. D., 214 (65)
Dieckert, J. W., 239 (14)
Dimbleby, G. W., 146 (12)
Disney, J. G., 227 (57)
Donoso, J., 249 (29)
Doron, E., 124 (4)
Driessen, F., 12 (22)
Duckham, A. N., 146 (4)
Duckworth, J. E., 272 (29), 227 (54)
Dudley, J. W., 213 (7, 16)
Duffield, R. D., 213 (17)
Duncan, W. G., 213 (20)
Duncan, W. R. H., 230 (132, 140, 141, 154)
Dunn, K. M., 214 (50)
Durrenmatt, K., 247, 249 (29)
Duterte, R., 240 (45)
Dutra de Oliveira, J. E., 239 (24), 265, 266, 273 (61, 62)
Dykstra, W. A., 188 (6)

E

Eadie, J. M., 230 (143)
Eastin, J. D., 213 (12)
Eaves, P. H., 240 (48)
Ebine, A., 241 (83)
Edge, T. M., 227 (54)
Edwards, R. H., 240 (75)
Eilrich, G. L., 209, 214 (55)
El Baradi, T. A., 124
Elder, A., 272 (46)
Elian, E., 272 (41)
Elías, L. G., 241 (89), 260, 271 (1, 2, 3, 4, 7, 11, 12, 19), 272 (20, 21, 23, 25, 27, 33, 35, 40), 273 (53, 55, 63), 274 (79)
Elsley, F. W. H., 222, 226 (4), 228 (90), 229 (100)
Elvehjem, C. A., 239 (39)
Ely, R. E., 214 (50)
Embleton, G. A., 230 (144, 146)
English, P. R., 228 (78, 88)
Enrüdi, G., 125 (25)
Epstein, E., 213 (14)
Escapini, H., 13 (44)
Evans, D. E., 13 (58)
Evans, R. J., 238 (8), 240 (64)
Evans, W. J., 239 (15)
Everitt, G. C., 221, 228 (72, 73)
Everson, G., 241 (78)
Eviatar, A., 124 (4)

F

Fender, M., 227 (56)
Ferguson, T. M., 230 (135)
Ferguson, T. U., 125 (13)
Ferguson, W., 146 (21)
Ferwerda, J., 125 (32)
Fewson, P., 227 (56)
Field, R. A., 220, 227 (59)
Flach, M., 125 (32)
Flodin, N. W., 271 (15)
Foman, J. J., 239 (23)
Fontenot, J. P., 226 (5), 230 (138)
Forshaw, R. P., 228 (84)
Fowler, V. R., 222, 226 (2), 229 (100, 101)
Fox, H. M., 65, 66, 69, 70, 76 (19), 272 (37), 274 (81)
Fox, J. D., 230 (148, 149)
Fredeen, H. T., 227 (60, 61), 228 (62)
Frenk, S., 12 (15)
Friend, D. W., 230 (137)
Fujimaki, M., 240 (71, 72, 73, 74)
Fukunaga, K., 176 (30)
Furata, F., 239 (29)
Furnwal, F. P., 229 (127)

G

Gaastra, P., 125 (14)
Galazka, H., 227 (54)
Galvan, Ramos, R., 11, 12 (5), 13 (57)
Ganor, E., 124 (4)
Garret, W. N., 227 (50)
Garrigan, D. S., 228 (63)
Garton, G. A., 230 (132, 140, 141, 154)
Gastrock, E. A., 240 (48)
Gee, I., 229 (94, 95)
Geertz, C., 77 (46)
Gelland, M., 146 (11)
Giesberger, G., 124
Gilbert, J. H., 204, 213 (5)
Gleeson, P. A., 226 (17)
Godden, W., 226 (28, 29)
Goldblatt, L. A., 240 (47)
Goldin, E., 125 (15)
Goldsmith, G. A., 247, 249 (23)
Gómez Brenes, R. A., 272 (35), 274 (82)
Gomez, F., 5, 12 (15)
Gonda, M., 240 (71, 72)
Gontzea, I., 238 (10)
Goodall, D. W., 213 (1)
Gopalan, C., 10, 13 (35), 67, 70, 77 (28)
Gordon, H. W., 229 (119)
Gordon, J. E., 2, 12 (8), 13 (51)
Gordon, R. S., 230 (133)
Gorsline, G. W., 213 (27, 28, 29)
Gossypol, 240 (47)
Graham, P. P., 226 (5)
Grau, C. R., 238 (11), 271 (16)
Gray, W. J., 228 (63)
Greathouse, T. R., 228 (64)
Greenhalgh, I., 228 (92)
Gregory, F. G., 213 (1)
Gregory, P. W., 228 (71)
Griffin, E. L., Jr., 241 (86), 273 (74)
Grifo, A. P., 228 (85)
Griswald, R. M., 227 (37)
Groves, T. D. D., 226 (6)

Grube, W. E., 213 (29)
Gruenberg, E., 272 (41)
Guilbert, H. R., 228 (71)
György, P., 236, 240 (58, 68)

H

Hackler, L. R., 235, 237, 239 (36), 240 (55, 57), 273 (75)
Hafez, E. S. E., 146 (10)
Hafiz, A., 176 (23, 26)
Hageman, R. H., 209, 213 (7, 16), 214 (55, 70)
Haines, R. B., 188 (4, 5)
Hale, O. M., 228 (83)
Hall, A. D., 204, 213 (3)
Hammond, J., 216, 222, 226 (1)
Han, I. K., 226 (17)
Hand, D. B., 240 (51, 52, 57), 268, 273 (75), 274 (76)
Hang, Y. D., 273 (68, 69)
Hansen, J. D. L., 13 (58)
Hansen, N. W., 188 (9)
Hardenburg, R. E., 183, 188 (1)
Hardy, B., 228 (87), 229 (115)
Harper, A. E., 239 (39)
Harrington, G., 228 (77)
Harris, P. L., 214 (47)
Harris, R. S., 214 (48), 248 (8), 271 (8)
Harrison, G., 227 (54)
Har-Tzook, A., 125 (15)
Haskell, P. T., 176 (28)
Haskins, R. W., 239 (25)
Haswell, M., 66, 72, 76 (15), 77 (25, 41), 146 (2)
Hatch, M. D., 125 (16)
Haynes, P. H., 125 (13)
Hazen, K. R., 239 (20)
Hedayat, H., 249 (29)
Hedges, N. J., 237 (57)
Hegsted, D. M., 67, 69, 70, 77 (26)
Heinzelman, D. C., 239 (14)
Henderlong, P. R., 213 (19)
Hendrickson, R. L., 229 (102)
Henry, J., 89 (6)
Hepburn, F. N., 239 (12), 240 (69)
Hesseltine, C. W., 240 (46, 62, 63), 241 (90)
Hewitt, L. F., 188 (11)
Hilditch, T. P., 225, 230
Hillard, C. M., 239 (20)
Hishikura, H., 173, 174, 176 (5)
Hodgson, G. C., 229 (105)
Hodgson, J. F., 213 (23)
Hohler, G. O., 214 (61)
Hole, F. D., 107 (4)
Hollingsworth, D., 214 (49)
Holmes, W., 227 (31, 54)
Hopkins, H. T., 214 (47)
Horan, F. E., 238 (6)
Hori, M., 173, 174, 176 (29)
Hornicke, H., 226 (14)
Houston, D. F., 214 (61)
Hovell, F. D., DeB, 230 (141)
Howard, H. W., 239 (27)
Howard, L. O., 176 (14)
Howell, R. W., 274 (86)
Hsu, T. Y., 153, 162 (10)
Hunnikin, C., 248 (21)
Hunt, P., 176 (20)
Hurd, E. A., 176 (32)
Huskell, 170
Hutcheson, J. K., 13 (42)
Hutcheson, R. H., 13 (42)
Hwa, Y. B., 240 (51)

I

Ibach, D. B., 97, 107 (7)
Idso, S. B., 125 (17)
Ignatieff, V., 89 (4)
Ikehata, H., 240 (56, 68)
Indian, 65
Ingram, R. H., 228 (84)
Isaacks, R. E., 230 (135)

J

Jackson, H. P., 239 (34), 273 (68)
Jackson, J., 273 (69)
Jacobs, D. R., 228 (69)
Jaffé, W. G., 271 (6)
Jakobsen, S. T., 205, 213 (13)
Jaraj, A. P., 271 (10)
Jarquín, R., 271 (12), 273 (54)
Jarrell, A., 213 (26)
Jelliffe, D. B., 7, 12 (7, 16, 31)
Johnson, D. E., 226 (17)
Johnson, D. W., 274 (78)
Johnson, E. R., 226 (12), 227 (48), 229 (103)
Johnson, J. A., 214 (59)
Johnson, J. C., 228 (83)
Johnson, R. F., 228 (77)
Johnson, R. G., 152, 162 (9)
Johnson, T. O., 65, 76 (13)
Johnson, V. A., 214 (53, 54, 57)
Jones, G. T., 65, 72, 73, 77 (22, 40)
Joo, Y. D., 226 (17)
Joseph, K., 271 (10)
Joshi, N. R., 152, 153, 162 (7, 8)
Joslyn, M., 240 (70)
Julian, L. M., 227 (49)
Jurion, F., 89 (6)
Jury, K. E., 221, 228 (72, 73)

K

Kahlenburg, O. J., 229 (119)
Kakade, M. L., 236, 238 (7, 8), 239 (44), 240 (64, 65)
Kaldy, M. S., 208, 214 (44)
Kato, H., 240 (71, 72, 74)
Kauffman, R. G., 230 (145, 152)
Kaul, A. K., 214 (64, 65)
Kawano, K., 125 (29)
Kay, J. L., 239 (22)

Keane, K. W., 239 (30)
Keet, M. P., 13 (58)
Kellogg, C. E., 89 (1, 2)
Kelly, F. C., 10, 13 (45)
Kelly, R. F., 230 (138)
Kemp, J. D., 228 (64), 230 (148, 149)
Kemp, P., 230 (129)
Kennedy, J. F., 189
Khaleque, A., 239 (37)
Khan, A. A., 125 (39)
Khan, M. N. A., 214 (59)
Kidwell, J. F., 227 (33)
Kies, C. E., 255, 272 (37), 274 (81)
Kim, J. C., 265, 273 (59)
King, J. W. B., 227 (55)
King, K. W., 241 (81, 82)
Kirsch, W., 227 (56)
Kirton, A. H., 226 (11)
Kloze, A. A., 230 (131)
Knowles, R. E., 236, 240 (50)
Knowless, P. F., 274 (85)
Koch, R. M., 228 (69)
Kodicek, E. R., 239 (38)
Kohler, G. O., 240 (50, 75)
Kokufu, E., 240 (67)
Kon, S. K., 239 (38)
Kondra, P. A., 229 (105), 230 (157)
Kramer, S. N., 176 (3)
Kratzer, F. H., 230 (131)
Krieger, C. H., 239 (30)
Krishnaji, N., 77 (48)
Krishnamorthy, K., 272 (22)
Kroger, D., 227 (38)
Kunkle, L. E., 228 (85)
Kuramoto, S., 274 (77)
Kurien, S., 273 (67)
Kwolek, W. F., 273 (74)
Kyle, R., 156, 162 (19)

L

Lagune, J., 239 (28)
Lambert, R. J., 213 (7)
Lamming, G. E., 228 (66)
Latham, M. C., 12 (17)
Law, E. W., 272 (30)
Lawhon, J. T., 268, 273 (71, 72)
Lawrie, R. A., 227 (42, 42), 229 (124, 125), 230 (155)
Leat, W. M. F., 230 (144, 146)
LeGros Clark, F., 202 (1)
Lehmann, C., 65, 76 (17)
Lehmann, G., 33 (6)
Leicher, J., 240 (70)
Leitch, I., 226 (29)
Leng, E. R., 107 (1), 213 (16)
Leopold, A. C., 231, 238 (2)
Lepkovsky, S., 239 (29)
Levison, F. J., 273 (65)
Lewin, L. M., 240 (52)
Lewis, D., 228 (87), 229 (112, 113, 114, 115)
Lidvall, E. R., 228 (80)
Liener, I. E., 214 (58), 232, 238 (1, 4, 5), 239 (44), 240 (65), 272 (24)
Lineweaver, H., 230 (131)
Ling, J., 76 (11)
Link, B. A., 230 (145, 152)
Linlithgow, Lord, 153
Livingston, A. L., 240 (50)
Livingstone, R. M., 228 (90), 229 (101)
Lodge, G. A., 221, 227 (30), 228 (86, 87), 229 (112, 113, 114, 115)
Loewnstein, M., 273 (70)
Lohman, T. G., 223, 229 (110)
Loomis, R. S., 125 (19)
Lough, A. K., 230 (142)
Louis, O., 271 (8)
Lovell, H. G., 76 (11)
Lowenstein, F. W., 246, 248 (20)
Lutz, J. M., 183, 188 (1)

M

MacArthur, M., 65, 77 (20)
MacDonald, I., 229 (100)
McDougall, D. B., 227 (57)
Machlin, L. J., 230 (133)
Mack, R., 146 (8)
Macy, P. F., 204, 213 (4)
Magee, W. T., 227 (37)
Mahadevana, P., 146 (18)
Maletnlema, T. N., 12 (26, 27)
Manage, L. D., 241 (88)
Mangelsdorf, P. C., 208, 214 (42)
Mann, S. O., 230 (143)
Maramorosch, K., 176 (20)
Marchello, M. J., 230 (138)
Marenco, E., 261, 272 (32)
Marion, J. E., 229 (106), 230 (134)
Mariscal, C., 13 (57)
Marr, J., 230 (133)
Marshall, L. E., 213 (26)
Martin, A. H., 227 (60, 61), 228 (62)
Martin, P. E., 214 (49)
Martin, W. P., 107 (10)
Martineaud, M. L. L., 12 (20, 25)
Masefield, G. B., 146 (4)
Mathews, J. P., 239 (34)
Mathias, E. L., 213 (19)
Matoth, Y., 272 (41)
Matrone, G., 214 (46)
Matsuyama, J., 240 (72)
Mattern, P. J., 214 (54, 57)
Mattick, L. R., 240 (52)
Mattick, L. R., 268, 274 (76)
Mattil, K. F., 268, 273 (71, 72)
Maynard, L. A., 207, 209, 213 (33, 34)
McCormick, J. S., 227 (33)
McCoy, J. R., 271 (18)
McCoy, O. M., 271 (9)
McCracken, R. J., 107 (4)
McFie, J., 65, 76 (10)
McGhee, J. E., 273 (74)

McKeown, T., 2, 12 (9, 10)
McLaren, B., 239 (21)
McLaren, D. S., 12 (18), 13 (44), 67, 77 (32)
McLaughlin, E. A., 152, 153, 162 (8)
McLeod, N. A., 228 (92)
McManus, W. R., 226 (17)
McMeekan, C. P., 222, 226 (19, 20, 21)
McNally, E. H., 229 (104)
McReady, S. T., 229 (120, 121)
McVeigh, I., 211, 214 (66)
Mecchi, E. P., 230 (131)
Mendel, L. B., 232, 238 (3)
Menezes Salata, E. B. Z., 265, 266, 273 (62)
Meridith, H. V., 65, 76 (12)
Mertz, E. T., 269, 274 (80)
Mertz, W., 213 (38)
Mevers, S. M., 272 (36)
Miall, W. E., 76 (11)
Michael, G., 214 (63)
Mickleberry, W. C., 230 (156)
Miller, D. S., 67, 77 (31)
Milner, M., 249 (24)
Miravalle, R. J., 274 (84)
Mitchell, H. H., 239 (26)
Mitchell, K. G., 239 (38)
Mitchell, R. J., 234, 239 (20)
Mitchell, R. L., 107 (8)
Mitsuda, H., 249 (28)
Miyamoto, T., 240 (56, 67)
Moir, K. W., 226 (24)
Monteith, J. G., 125 (21)
Moodie, A. D., 11, 13 (58)
Moody, W. G., 230 (148, 149)
Moore, A. T., 239 (14)
Morriss, T. R., 226 (26)
Morton, I. D., 248 (9)
Morwood, R. B., 176 (18)
Mountney, G. J., 229 (123)
Moy, M., 229 (126)
Moyer, R. T., 152, 162 (9)
Mukhoty, H., 219, 227 (40)
Munger, H. M., 125 (33), 213 (15)
Munoz, A., 13 (52)
Munsell, H. E., 271 (8)
Murata, K. H., 237, 240 (56, 67, 68)
Murray, T. K., 234, 239 (17)
Mustakas, G. C., 241 (86), 273 (74)
Myers, A. T., 213 (8)
Myrdal, G., 77 (46)

N

Naik, M. S., 214 (64)
Nakano, M., 241 (83), 272 (26)
Navarrete, D. A., 271 (3)
Nelson, E. R., 274 (80)
Nelson, J. W., 240 (50)
Nelson, L. B., 213 (32)
Nelson, O. E., 214 (56)
Nelson, S. D., 241 (88), 269
Nesheim, M. C., 239 (19)
Neudoerfer, T. S., 237, 241 (76)
Nightingale, G., 271 (8)
Nikiforoff, C. C., 207, 213 (30)
Noda, T., 73, 77 (42, 45)
Noguchi, M., 240 (74)
Norton, H. W., 228 (63)

O

Ocfemia, G. O., 176 (19)
Odell, A. D., 241 (89), 274 (79)
Ohta, T., 241 (83)
Olaniyan, O., 227 (54)
Oltjen, R. R., 230 (139)
Oomen, H. A. P. C., 13 (44)
Orlob, G. B., 176 (6)
Orr, E., 248 (5)
Orr, L. E., 189
Ørskov, E. R., 230 (140)
Ortiz, P. B., 13 (57)
Orvedal, A. C., 89 (2)
Osborne, B. T., 232, 238 (3)
Osinska, Z., 226 (16)
Osmond, C. B., 125 (16)
Ozalp, I., 272 (38)
Ozbun, J. L., 213 (15)

P

Padwick, G. W., 176 (13)
Page, H. J., 89 (4)
Paladines, O. L., 226 (17)
Palleson, H. R., 273 (75)
Palsson, H., 226 (2, 22)
Panalake, T., 234, 239 (17)
Papp, C. S. E., 214 (40)
Paris, Q., 73, 77 (44, 45)
Park, R. J., 229 (127)
Parker, F. W., 213 (32)
Parpia, H. A. B., 272 (43), 273 (66)
Parsons, A. T., 241 (78)
Patterson, R. L. S., 228 (89)
Patwardban, V. N., 10, 13 (53), 271 (5)
Paulraj, V. K., 273 (70)
Pawley, W. H., 107 (9)
Payan, R., 249 (29)
Payne, P. R., 67, 77 (31)
Paz y Paz, R., 239 (42)
Pearce, H. M., Jr., 268, 273 (73)
Pearl, S. L., 239 (32)
Pearson, A. M., 227 (37)
Pellet, P. L., 67, 77 (32)
Pepper, P. M., 226 (24)
Perez, C., 12 (7)
Perpillou, A. V., 146 (5)
Peterson, C. E., 188 (3)
Peterson, H. B., 107 (16)
Phillips, P. G., 65, 66, 76 (14)
Phillips, R. W., 152, 153, 161, 162 (4, 5, 6, 7, 8, 9, 10, 23)
Pierre, W. H., 107 (10)

Pinto, F. F., 176 (32)
Pirie, N. W., 202 (1, 7, 8)
Plavšić-Banjac, B., 176 (20)
Plimpton, R. F., 228 (85)
Plouidy, G., 11
Poehlman, J. M., 107 (11)
Pomeroy, R. W., 227 (43), 229 (97, 124)
Pominski, J., 268, 273 (73)
Pope, C. W., 230 (133)
Porritt, S. W., 188 (2)
Porter, J. R., 188 (11)
Poulsen, K. K., 176 (25)
Prescott, J. H. D., 228 (66)
Preston, T. R., 228 (92), 229 (94, 95)
Pretorius, P. J., 10, 13 (54)
Price, M. A., 228 (70)
Prier, R. F., 239 (16)
Priode, B. M., 230 (139)
Probert, C. L., 228 (67)
Providenti, M. I., 240 (51)
Pryor, W. J., 229 (103)
Pudelkewicz, C., 229 (119)
Punekar, B. D., 239 (39)
Purdy, H. R., 228 (65)

Q

Quild, P., 271 (8)
Quisenberry, K. S., 107 (12)

R

Rabold, K., 227 (56)
Rachie, K. O., 214 (60)
Rackis, J. J., 239 (32), 240 (54)
Raddakrishna Rao, M. V., 240 (61)
Rae, A. L., 229 (126)
Raeburn, J. R., 228 (88)
Ragland, J. L., 213 (29)
Rajagopalan, R., 272 (22)
Ramakrishnan, T. N., 272 (22)
Rambaud, M., 240 (45)
Ramsey, A. A., 236, 239 (43)
Ramsey, C. B., 228 (80)
Ranhotra, G. S., 239 (12), 240 (69), 265, 273 (56)
Rao, B. H. S., 273 (67)
Rao, M. N., 271 (10)
Rao, N. P., 13 (36)
Rao, R., 237
Rawis, I., 273 (75)
Read, W. W. C., 12 (18)
Rechcigl, M., 212
Record, R. G., 2, 12 (10)
Reed, A. D., 176 (12)
Reid, J. T., 217, 219, 222, 223, 226 (17), 227 (32)
Reiser, R., 230 (135)
Rendel, J. M., 146 (20)
Reynolds, H. T., 176 (31)
Rhodes, D. N., 230 (128)
Richards, J. F., 229 (105)
Richmond, R. J., 227 (52)
Riemann, H., 188 (9)
Rijtema, P. E., 125 (25)
Rinne, R. W., 274 (86)
Robinson, R. A., 176 (33)
Roelofson, P. A., 240 (53)
Rogler, J. C., 230 (156)
Rojas, S. W., 238, 241 (84)
Rollins, W. C., 227 (49)
Rollinson, D. H. L., 146 (19)
Rostron, H., 125 (26)
Roth, H. H., 162 (18)
Rudman, J. E., 229 (96)
Rudolph, L., 77 (47)
Rudolph, S., 77 (47)
Rumsey, T. S., 230 (139)
Russell, E. W., 107 (13)
Rutishauser, I. H. E., 12 (30)
Ruttle, D. E., 240 (62, 63)
Ryley, J. W., 226 (24)

S

Sakurei, Y., 272 (26)
Salmon-Legagneur, E., 226 (7)
Salunkhe, D. K., 214 (71)
Sanchez, C. R. S., 214 (59)
Sánchez, S., 271 (19)
Sano, T., 237, 240 (59)
Saperstein, S., 239 (33)
Sarett, H. P., 239 (25)
Saunders, R. M., 237, 240 (75)
Scatena, L., 239 (24)
Schaefer, A. E., 202 (2)
Schertz, L. P., 153, 162 (15)
Schlage, C., 239 (18)
Schlehuber, A. M., 204, 213 (6)
Schmidt, J. W., 214 (53, 54, 57)
Schoen, P., 227 (56)
Schultze, L., 176 (7)
Scott, G. R., 146 (7)
Scott, M. L., 229 (122), 238, 241 (84)
Scott, W. J., 188 (10)
Scrimshaw, N. S., 70, 77 (34), 239 (40, 41, 42), 249 (26), 272 (38)
Sebrell, W. H., 248 (6), 274 (87)
Seiler-Kelbitsch, H., 214 (63)
Sell, J. L., 230 (157)
Senti, F. R., 248 (18), 272 (44)
Seoane, N., 12 (17)
Sessa, D. J., 239 (32)
Shaffner, C. S., 226 (25)
Shahbazi, H., 249 (29)
Shear, C. B., 213 (8)
Sherwood, F. W., 214 (46)
Shimizu, T., 239 (32)
Shorland, F. B., 229 (126)
Shrimpton, D. H., 229 (118)
Shurpalekar, K. S., 273 (67)
Shurpalekar, S. R., 273 (67)
Sibma, L., 125 (27)

Sieburth, J. F., 239 (21)
Simons, N. R., 239 (44), 240 (65)
Singh, B., 212, 214 (71)
Singh, D., 13 (36)
Slatyer, R. O., 125 (16)
Smart, W. W. G., Jr., 214 (46)
Smith, A. K., 237, 240 (54)
Smith, C. B., 213 (29)
Smith, E. L., 213 (17)
Smith, F. H., 214 (46)
Smith, R. E., 241 (76)
Smith, R. F., 176 (17, 24, 31)
Smutke, C. J., 239 (30)
Snake, Y., 240 (67)
Snedden, W. W., 10, 13 (45)
Snowden, J. E., 239 (14)
Sohns, V. F., 241 (86)
Spadaro, J. J., 268, 273 (73)
Specht, A. W., 204, 213 (9)
Spector, H., 67, 77 (33)
Sprague, G. F., 107 (14, 15)
Squibb, R. L., 239 (41), 272 (28)
Sreekantriah, K. R., 241 (83)
Srikantia, S. G., 10, 13 (51)
Standal, B. R., 237, 240 (60)
Starr Chester, K., 176 (8)
Steenbjerg, F., 205, 213 (13)
Steenbock, H., 241 (78)
Steggerda, F. R., 239 (32)
Steinkraus, K. H., 237, 240 (51, 57, 66), 273 (75)
Steinkraus, K. M., 240 (52)
Stetson, L. E., 241 (88)
Stevens, M. C., 239 (21)
Stevens, R. D., 77 (39)
Stevenson, E. H., 214 (47)
Stewart, D. M., 176 (26)
Stillings, B. R., 237, 240 (55)
Stout, G. L., 176 (11)
Stroud, J. W., 226 (17)
Subba Rao, P. V., 239 (31)
Subrahmanyan, U., 271 (10)
Suess, G. G., 223, 229 (111), 230 (150, 151)
Sugimoto, H., 241 (77)
Sukhatme, P. V., 67, 70, 77 (24, 30)
Sundrum, R. M., 76 (6)
Sutzescu, P., 238 (10)
Swaminathan, M. C., 13 (36), 210, 214 (52, 64, 65), 271 (10), 272 (22)

T

Talens, A., 240 (53)
Tanaka, A., 125 (29, 30)
Tasker, P. K., 272 (22)
Taylor, J. C., 229 (96)
Teague, H. S., 228 (85)
Tegeler, H. H., 54 (4)
Temple, R. S., 246 (17)
Teply, L. J., 249 (27)
Terrell, R. N., 230 (150, 151, 153)
Thai, 65
Theophrastus, 176 (4)
Thijsse, Ir., J. P., 124
Thomas, H. R., 226 (5)
Thomas, W. I., 211, 213 (26, 29), 214 (68)
Thompson, C. E., 228 (65)
Thompson, R. T., 238 (7)
Thorne, D. W., 107 (16)
Thulin, W. W., 274 (77)
Tichenor, D. A., 230 (148)
Tinklin, G. L., 273 (57)
Tolbert, N. E., 188 (3)
Tomes, M. L., 214 (62)
Tosello, A., 273 (58)
Toutain, G., 176 (21)
Troescher, B., 271 (8)
Trowell, H. C., 65, 76 (16)
Tsai, S. J., 240 (73)
Tucker, B. B., 204, 213 (6)
Tuckett, S. N., 272 (36)
Tulloh, N. M., 219, 222, 223, 227 (41), 229 (107)
Turner, R. G., 214 (67)
Turton, J. D., 220, 227 (58)
Tyler, S. A., 176 (1)
Tyler, W. J., 226 (15), 229 (111)
Tyrrell, H. F., 226 (17)

U

Ucko, P. J., 146 (12)
Underwood, E. J., 146 (6)
Usher, D., 77 (45)

V

Valiente, A. T., 271 (7)
Vallega, J., 176 (27)
Van, Veen, A. G., 240 (66)
Van Buren, J. P., 240 (51, 57), 241 (77), 273 (75)
van der Zijl, C. E., 125 (41)
vanDobben, W. H., 124 (1), 125 (12)
Van Etten, C. H., 240 (49)
vanIttersum, A., 125 (18)
Van Niekerk, D. H., 226 (17)
Veen, V., 237
Verges, J. B., 226 (22)
Verhaar, G., 124
Vespa, J. B., 240 (46)
Viets, F. G., Jr., 213 (22)
Viniegra, A., 13 (57)
Vipperman, P. E., 226 (5)
Viswanatha, T., 241 (79)
Viteré, F., 241 (89)
Viteri, F. E., 256, 273 (49), 274 (79, 83)
Von Losecke, H., 214 (48)

W

Waddel, J., 271 (17)
Wagenknecht, A. C., 240 (52)

Waldern, D. E., 228 (81)
Waldman, R. C., 226 (15)
Waldrop, D. W., 239 (20)
Wallace, A. T., 214 (60)
Wallace, D. H., 125 (33), 205, 211, 213 (5)
Wallace, G. M., 239 (37)
Wallace, L. R., 222, 226 (10), 229 (98)
Wang, H. L., 236, 237, 240 (46, 62, 63), 241 (90)
Wang, R. W., 241 (87)
Wannemacker, R. W., Jr., 271 (18)
Ward, G. M., 214 (50)
Warner, R. L., 204, 213 (7)
Warren, E. P., 228 (83)
Wassink, E. C., 125 (34)
Waterlow, J. C., 12 (19)
Waterlow, J. E., 272 (31)
Watkins, J. L., 228 (65)
Watson, D. J., 125 (35)
Watson, D. M. S., 229 (108)
Weaver, E., 214 (50)
Weisber, S. M., 272 (46)
Weiss, G. M., 227 (60, 61), 228 (62)
Weldon, V., 214 (46)
Wellington, G. H., 226 (17), 227 (34)
Wells, R. G., 226 (23)
Wheeler, E., 12 (23)
Whitehead, R. G., 12 (30)
Wiener, G., 227 (51)
Wilkens, W. F., 268, 274 (76)
Williams, D. R., 225, 229 (124), 230 (131)
Williams, E., 272 (37)
Williams, L., 271 (8)
Williams, P. N., 230 (130)
Williams, R. R., 246
Williams, W. A., 125 (19)
Wilson, J., 13 (43)
Wilson, L. L., 227 (35), 228 (65)
Wilson, P. N., 218, 222, 226 (18), 229 (99)
Wise, G. H., 214 (46)
Wiseman, H. J., 239 (35)
Wit, F., 124 (1)
Wittmann, W., 13 (58)
Wood, A. J., 226 (6)
Woodham, A. A., 234, 239 (13, 15)
Woodman, A. A., 272 (29)
Woodroof, J. G., 229 (106), 230 (134)
Worstberg, B., 239 (18)
Wu, M. T., 214 (71)
Wyon, J. B., 12 (8)

Y

Yamamura, Y., 272 (36)
Yamashita, M., 240 (71, 72, 73, 74)
Young, L. G., 228 (84)
Young, V. R., 255, 272 (38)

Z

Zaghi, S. de, 274 (79)
Zaman, M. B., 125 (39)
Zelitch, I., 125 (40)
Ziegler, J. H., 227 (35), 228 (65)
Ziolecka, A., 226 (16)

SUBJECT INDEX

A

Achatina, as a source of human food, 197
Achromobacter, 182
effect of temperature on, 179
Acid treatment, increase in nutritive value of plant foods by, 235–236
Adipose tissue of livestock
effect of diet on, 225
fatty composition of, 225
Administrative measures for implementation of food and nutrition policy, 284–285
Aerobic bacteria, 184
Afghanistan
animal protein in food supplies of, 149
calories
total protein and animal protein in food supplies of, 148
total protein and animal protein intake in, 71
crop yields in, 116–117
milk, meat, eggs, and fish in food supplies of, 150
total protein and proportions of animal and plant protein in food supplies of, 149
Africa
arable land and population of, 43
birth rate, death rate, and reproduction rate in, 58
bovine pleuropneumonia in, control of, 138
calorie and reference protein requirements in, 68–69
calorie requirements of children in, 66
calorie, total protein, and animal protein intake in, 71
cereal consumption in, 17
crop yield increase compared to farm area increase in 1950 and 1970, 111
crop yields and crop yield increases in 1950 and 1970,
crop yields in 1950 and 1970, 112
114–115
farm animal population in, 129
food consumption trends in, 277
food taboos in, 16
iron deficiency anemia in, 8
kwashiorkor and marasimus in, 9
land in, major uses of, 43
livestock diseases in, 134
livestock losses due to rabies in, 134
losses caused to agriculture by locust, 170–171
malnutrition in,
prevalence of, 6
population and expectation of life for 1960 and 2000, 57
potential for increases in animal production in, 160–161
potentially arable land in, 44
production of major food crops in, 39, 41
productivity of cattle and buffalo in, 130
productivity of farm livestock in, 128
productivity of pigs in, 130
reason for low animal production in, 151
rinderpest in,
control of, 137
epidemic of, 134
solar radiation in, 120
Southeast, maize consumption in, 19
starchy food consumption in, 21
targets for crop yield increases between 1962 and 1985 in, 124
tsetse fly, effect of on cattle production in, 156
tsetse fly, eradication effect of on animal production in, 134
trypanosomiasis in, 138
urban and rural population of, 62
wildlife as a source food in, 156
African Migratory Locust, 170
outbreak and invasion areas of, 171
African swine fever, 134
Africander cattle
cross with Hereford stock, 142
Age, effect on body composition of various breeds of sheep, 220
Agricultural development, conditions necessary for, 52–53
Agricultural extension, role of in implementation of food and nutrition policies, 283
Agricultural planning, integration of food and nutrition policies in, 280–281
Agricultural policies, and livestock production, 144–145
Agricultural production
development of new land for, 52
value of, 42
Agricultural systems, 45–52, 80
collective, 51
commercial, 48–49
Agricultural wastes, solid, use of in feeding, 197
Agriculture
animal, in different regions of the world, 151
as contrasted to farming, 80
commercial and surplus food production, 48
economic incentives in, 54
effect of industrial revolution on, 80
four major systems and subtypes of, 46–47
history of, 80
in U.S., reason for changes in, 51
intensive, sedentary, and food production, 48
nature of, 79–80
primitive, sedentary, and food production, 47
relation to other sectors, 54
subsistence and food production, 47–48
systems of, *see* Agricultural systems
technological innovations in, 53
use of land resources for, 42
Agropyron sp., 211
Agrostis sp., 211
Agrostis stolonifera, 211
Agrostis tenuis, 211
AID, 212
fortification studies supported by, 246
lysine fortification studies supported by, 247
Air velocity, effect on animal production, 135
Albania
animal protein in food supplies of, 149

calories, total protein, and animal protein in food supplies of, 148
crop yields in, 114, 115
milk, meat, eggs, and fish in food supplies of, 150
total protein and proportions of animal and plant protein in food supplies of, 149
Alcaligenes, effect of temperature on, 179
Alcohol, as antimicrobial agent in beverages, 186
Alcoholism, as causative factor in pellagra, 10
Alfalfa, antivitamin E in, 233
Algae, green, *see* Green algae
Algae protein, use in formulation of new nutritious food products, 253
Algeria
animal protein in food supplies, 149
bayoud disease of date palm in, 168
calorie and protein intake in, 71
calories, total protein, and animal protein in food supplies of, 148
crop yields in, 114–115
milk, meat, eggs, and fish in food supplies of, 150
total protein and proportions of animal and plant protein in food supplies of, 149
Alkali disease of livestock, 133
Alkali treatment
destruction of trypsin inhibitor in soy flour by, 236
increase in nutritive value of plant foods by, 235–236
increased availability of niacin and essential amino acids in corn by, 236
increased availability of niacin in soybean milk by, 235–236
Aluminum, in grasses, breeding against toxic levels, 211
Aluminum uptake, by plants, effect of lime on, 211
Amaranthus, as source of food protein, 193
American Medical Association, 190
Amino acid, concept of limiting, 254, 259, 260
Amino acid fortification, 247, 259, 260
MIT conference on, 247
reasons for slow development of, 245
Amino acid imbalance, pellagra from, 10
Amino acids
content of, effect on biological value of protein, 254
essential content of beans, effect of fermentation on, 236–237
in corn, increased availability by alkali treatment, 236
in meat, content of, 224
in plant sources, deficiency of, 200–201
requirements by man, 200
sulfur-containing, in soybean protein, enhancement by "plastein" reaction, 237
synthesis of, 200
Ammonia, utilization by plants, 93
L-Amylase, improvement of starch digestibility in plant foodstuffs by, 238
Amylase inhibitor, in plant foodstuffs, 233
Anemia
iron deficiency, 247
megaloblastic, 8
nutritional, 7–8
public health significance of, 8
of pregnancy, 247
prevention of, with iron enriched salt, 266
Angola
calorie and protein intake in, 71
crop yields in, 114–115
Angoumois grainmoth, food deterioration due to, 187
Animal breeding, 141–143
effect on animal production, 152–153
control of
enzootic diseases, 137–138
local disease and parasitism, 138–139
effect on animal production, 133–135
Animal diseases
control of
enzootic, 133
epizootic, 133
Animal foods
inhibitory substances in, 186–187
susceptibility to rancidity, 179
Animal industry, emergence of, for food production, 131
Animal population, farm, in various regions of world, 129
Animal production
advances in, 136
agricultural policies relating to, 144–145
areas that can be devoted to increased output of, 161
difficulties hindering progress in expansion of, 144
factors limiting increases in, 147
in developing countries, reason for low levels of, 152
intensification of, 161–162
key programs for increasing, 137
methods of augmenting, 136–144
most productive regions for, 132
numbers vs. productivity, 152
potentials for increases in difference regions, 157–161
Africa, 160–161
Europe, 157–158
Far East, 159
Latin America, 158–159
Near East, 160
North America, 158
Oceania, 158
potentials for increasing, 154–162
farm animals, 154–155
fisheries, 156–157
wildlife, 155–156
relative potential of specific meat-producing animals, 147–162
restraints on, 132–136
animal disease, 133–135
climate, 135
land and water resources, 132–133
social, religious, and cultural factors, 135–136
technical measures for increasing, 127–146
variations in different countries, 148
Animal production systems, complexity of, 136
Animal products
as source of protein, 109
effect of taboos on consumption of, 135
role of, in developing countries, 282
supply of
reasons for variations in, 151–154
general, 151–152
genetic levels of productivity, 152–153
numbers vs. productivity, 152
relation of economic levels to demands for animal

products, 153–154
Animal protein
amounts in national food supplies of 90 countries, 148, 149
and income levels in 30 countries, 154
and plant protein in food supplies of 90 countries, 149
consumption of, developing countries vs. developed countries, 277
four major sources of, 150
intake of
in China, India, Indonesia, and Nigeria as compared to that in U.S., 109
in developing regions of the world, 71–72
production of
estimation of, 128
in various regions of the world
from cattle and buffalo, 130
from pig, 130
supplies of,
in 90 countries, 150
in relation to annual income, 153
Animal reproduction, role in augmenting animal production, 141–143
Animal trypanosomiasis, effect on animal production, 133
Animal Virus Research Institute (UK), 137
Animals
and plants, as food sources for man, 130–132
body composition of
breed differences, 218–220
nutritional influences on, 221–224
sex differences, 220–221
species differences, 217–218
contribution to man's food supply and nutritional quality of diet, 147
conversion of vegetable protein to animal protein by, 196–198
improving nutrient composition of, 215–230
nutritional influences on body composition of, 221–224
nutritive value of carcass, 224–225
patterns of normal growth of, 216–217
Annual crops, major limitation to high yields of, 119
Antarctic krill, as source of human food, 197
Antelope, as source of food, 156
Antibiotics, produced by fermentation, growth-stimulating effects of, 237
Antienzymes, in foods, 187
Antimicrobial agents, in foods, 186–187
Antinutritional factors, in plant foodstuffs, 233–234
Antioxidants
production of, in fermentation, 237
use of
in formulation of nutritious food products, 257–258
prevention of rancidity by, 184
Antipyridoxine, in plant foodstuffs, 233
Antivitamin B_{12}, in plant foods, 234
Antivitamin D, in plant foodstuffs, 233
Antivitamin E, in plant foodstuffs, 233
Antivitamins
in foods, 187
in plant foodstuffs, 233–234
Aphids
development of resistance in alfalfa to, 103
food deterioration due to, 187
Apple, metal-binding constituents in, 234
Arable land, *see* Land, arable
Arachis, as source of protein, 193
Arachnids, food deterioration due to, 187
Arboviruses, livestock diseases caused by, 134
Area, world, planted to cereals, root crops, pulses, oilseeds, and vegetables, 109
Argentina
animal protein in food supplies of, 149
calorie and protein intake in, 72
calories, total protein, and animal protein in food supplies of, 148
cattle production in, 159
crop yields in, 116–117
milk, meat, eggs, and fish in food supplies of, 150
total protein and proportions of animal and plant protein in food supplies of, 149
Arid areas
management of, for cattle and sheep grazing, 140
restraints on animal production in, 132
Arsenicals, use against Colorado beetle, 164
Artificial insemination, in developing countries, 142
Artocarpus communis L., 166
Ascrobic acid, *see also* Vitamin C
low intake in developing countries, 252
prevention of browning by, 186
prevention of rancidity by, 184
Ascorbic acid oxidase, in plant foodstuffs, 233
Ash content, of pig during prenatal and postnatal stages of life, 216, 217
Asia
calorie and reference protein requirements in, 68–69
calorie, total protein, and animal protein intake in, 71
crop yields and crop yield increases in 1950 and 1970 in, 116–117
food consumption, trends in, 277
iron deficiency anemia in, 8
kwashiorkor and marasmus in, 9
livestock losses due to rabies in, 134
malnutrition in, prevalence of, 6
number of farm animals vs. animal productivity, 152
reason for low animal production in, 151
targets for crop yield increases between 1962 and 1985, 124
Aspergillus glaucus, 182
Aspergillus niger, 182
Australia
animal protein in food supplies of, 149
calories, total protein, and animal protein in food supplies, 148
cobalt and copper deficiency diseases in cattle in, 133
crop yields in, 116–117
livestock deficiency diseases in, on mineral deficient soils, 133
meat production in, 158
milk, meat, eggs, and fish in food supplies of, 150
pastoral farming in, 140
selenium poisoning of livestock in, 133
total protein and proportions of animal and plant

protein in food supplies of, 149
Australia and New Zealand
crude birth rates, death rates, and gross reproduction rates in, 59
total population and expectation of life in, 57
urban and rural population in, 63
Austria
animal protein in food supplies of, 149
calories, total protein, and animal protein in food supplies of, 148
crop yields in, 114, 115
milk, meat, eggs, and fish in food supplies of, 150
total protein and proportions of animal and plant protein in food supplies of, 149
Auxins, effect on protein synthesis of plants, 212
Avidin, in raw egg white, 187
Azores, crop yields in, 114–115

B

Bacillus, 180
Bacillus cereus, 182
Bacillus mycoides, 182
Bacillus stearothermophilus, 179, 180
effect of temperature on, 179
Bacillus subtilis, use in food fermentation, 237
Bacillus thermoacidurans, effect of temperature on, 179
Bacteria
growth of
effect of pH on, 179
effect of temperature on, 179
effect of water activity on, 183, 184
size of population, effect on storage life of beef, 185, 186
symbiotic, nitrogen fixation by, 93
Bacterial wilt of bananas, *see* Moko disease
Bal-Ahar, ingredient composition of, 257
Bananas, diseases of, 168–169
Barbados
crop yield in, 116–117
prevalence of kwashiorkor and marasmus in children in, 9
Barley
area and production by region, 38–41
consumption in different regions of the world, 17, 19
high nitrogen varieties, 193
threshold optimum nitrogen level in, 204
world area and production of, 36
yields and yield increases by region, 112
Barley protein, nutritionally superior fraction, 234
Barley-rich diet, effect on adipose tissue composition of lambs, 225
Barrier vaccination, against foot-and-mouth disease, 137
Basal metabolism, 70
Basella, as source of food protein, 193
Bayoud disease, of date palm, 167–168
Beans
nutritive value of
effect of fortification on, 263
effect on fortification with lysine and tryptophan on, 263
Beef
consumption of, 27, 28
effect of religious beliefs on, 151
demands for, in developed countries vs. those in developing countries, 155
effect of taboos on consumption of, in Hindus, 135
production and consumption
in Africa, 160
in Europe, 157
in Far East, 159
in Latin America, 159
in North America, 158
in Oceania, 158
production of, in major regions, 151
storage life of, effect of population size of bacteria on, 185, 186
Beef cattle, productivity of, in South Africa, 142
Beer
as source of vitamins, 191
consumption of, 32
Beetles, food deterioration due to, 187
Belgium
animal protein in food supplies of, 149
calories, total protein, and animal protein in food supplies of, 148
crop yields in, 114, 115
milk, meat, eggs, and fish in food supplies of, 150
total protein and proportions of animal and plant protein in food supplies of, 149
Benzoic acid, as yeast inhibitor, 186
Beriberi, 11
in developing countries, 246
prevention of, 246
Bermuda, crop yields in, 116–117
Berseem, use of, in Egypt, 139
Berundi
calorie and protein intake in, 72
crop yields in, 114–115
Beverages
alcoholic, inhibitory substances in, 186
consumption in different regions of world, 31, 32
Biological value
of corn protein, 255
of protein, definition of, 254
Biomass, 199
Biotin, destruction by avidin, 187
Birds, food deterioration due to, 188
Birth rates, crude, in major regions of world for 1965 to 2000, 58–59
Biuret, as source of nonprotein nitrogen, its use in pastoral farming, 140
Black beans, hemagglutinin in, 187
Black gram
nutritive value of, effect of germination on, 237
preparation of idli from, 237
Blight, damage caused by, history of, 163
Blind staggers, 133
Blindness, due to vitamin A deficiency, 245, 247
Blue grass, yield of, effect of slope orientation on, 206
Blue-green algae, as source of human food, 198
Blue tongue, of cattle, 134

Body composition
close relationship to body weight, 222
of different species of animals, range in, 218
of lamb, sex differences in, 221
of livestock
breed differences in, 218–220
nutritional influences on, 221–224
relationship between growth rate and, 223
set differences in, 220–221
species differences in, 217–218
of pig
at birth, 216
during postnatal growth, 216, 217
during prenatal life, 216
effect of energy and protein intake on, 224
of sheep, breed differences in, 200
Body fat composition, of ruminants vs. nonruminants, 224–225
Body tissues
of pig, differences between breeds, 220
relative proportions in various species, 218
Body weight
close relationship of body composition to, 222
effect on calorie requirements, 64
Body weight data, for various regions, 65
Bolivia
animal protein in food supplies of, 149
calorie and protein intake in, 71
calories, total protein, and animal protein in food supplies of, 148
cretinism in, 10
crop yields in, 116–117
milk, eggs, and fish in food supplies of, 150
total protein and proportions of animal and plant protein in food supplies of, 149
Boll weevil, losses caused by, effect on farmer, 166
Boophilus sp., 142
Boran cattle, 142
Boron
application of, to soil, 211
in soil, effect of pH on availability of, 96
requirement by plants, 93
Bos indicus, 141, 142
different types of, 142
prevalence of, 141
Bos taurus, 141, 142
prevalence of, 141
Botswana
calorie and protein intake in, 71
crop yields in, 114–115
Bovine pleuropneumonia, control of, 138
Brazil
animal protein in food supplies of, 149
calorie and protein intake in, 71
calories, total protein, and animal protein in food supplies of, 148
cattle production in, 159
crop yields in, 116–117
livestock losses due to infectious and parasitic diseases in, 135
milk, meat, eggs, and fish in food supplies of, 150
total protein and proportions of animal and plant protein in food supplies of, 149
Bread
iron in, increased availability by fermentation, 237
use of protein concentrates in preparation of, 265
Bread fortification
with B vitamins, 246
with iron, 247
with vitamin A, 245
Breadfruit
consumption in Jamaica, 22
Pingalap disease of, 166–167
Breed differences
in body composition
of animals, 218–219
of pigs, 220
of sheep, 220
British Honduras, crop yields in, 116–117
British Solomon, crop yields in, 116–117
Broad beans, consumption of, 23
Brown Swiss cattle, 142
cross with Red Sindhi cattle, 142
Brunei, crop yields in, 116–117
Buckwheat, as source of food protein, 195
Buffalo, African, as source of food, 156
Buffalo meat, consumption of, 28
Bulgaria
animal protein in food supplies of, 149
calories, total protein, and animal protein in food supplies of, 150
total protein and proportions of animal and plant protein in food supplies of, 149
Burma
calorie and protein intake in, 71
crop yields in, 116–117
salt iodination in, 246
Bush sickness, of livestock, 133
Butter fat, consumption of, 30
Butylated hydroxyanisole, prevention of rancidity by, 184
Butylated hydroxytoluene, prevention of rancidity by, 184
By-products
of crop production, use in livestock feeding, 131
of fishing industry, use in livestock feeding, 131
of industrial processing, use in livestock feeding, 131
surplus of, use of in livestock industry, 140

C

Cacao, consumption of, 23
Cadang-cadang, effect on coconut palm production, 167
Cadelle, food deterioration due to, 187
Cajanus, 195
Cajanus cajan, improvement of, 211
Calcium
absorption of, interference of phytic acid with, 233
in corn, content of, effect of lime on, 236
in lespedeza hay, content of, effect of lime on, 208
in soils,
content of, 94
effect of pH on availability of, 96

intake in developing countries, 252
requirement by plants, 93, 94
supplementation, 191
Calcium fortification, 247
Calf, body composition of, 216
Calorie, and reference protein requirements, in developing regions of world, 68–69
Calorie intake
effect on nitrogen balance, 67
in developing regions of world, 71–72
Calorie-protein interaction, 67–70
Calorie requirements, 67–67
effect of body weight on, 64–67
effect of work on, 65
estimated by FAO, 64
functional, 64
of children, 66
of man, daily, 109
of men aged 20 to 29 in Central Africa, 66
Calorie standards, at a given age, 70
Calories
in national food supplies of 90 countries, 148
produced by various crops, 121, 122
supplies of, in relation to annual income, 153
Cambodia, calorie and protein intake in, 71
Camel meat, consumption of, 28
Cameroon
animal protein in food supplies of, 149
calorie and protein intake in, 71
calories, total protein, and animal protein in food supplies of, 148
crop yields in, 114–115
milk, meat, eggs, and fish in food supplies of, 150
total protein and proportions of animal and plant protein in food supplies of, 149
Canada
animal protein in food supplies of, 149
arable land and population of, 43
calories, total protein, and animal protein in food supplies of, 148
crop yields in, 116–117
major uses of land in, 43
milk, meat, eggs, and fish in food supplies of, 150
production of major food crops in, 38, 40
total protein and proportions of animal and plant protein in food supplies of, 149
Canning, increased extractability of carotene by, 234
Cape St. Paul Wilt, 167
Cape Verde, crop yields in, 114–115
Capital, effect on agricultural development, 52–53
effect on crop yields, 119
Carbohydrates
as source of energy, 109
as substrates for microbial growth, 199
availability of, increase by heat treatment, 232
digestion of, interference of amylase inhibitor with, 233
from plants, 191
in foods, 185–186
Carbon dioxide concentration, effect on crop yields, 118
Carbon sources, for human food, 193, 194
Carcass, *see* Body composition
Carcass components, of livestock, nutritive value of, 224–225
Carcass composition, factors affecting, 217
Caribbean
calorie and reference protein requirements in, 68, 69
calorie, total protein, and animal protein intake in, 72
crude birth rates, crude death rates, and gross reproduction rates in, 59
lethan yellowing disease of coconut in, 167
total population and expectation of life, 57
urban and rural population in, 63
Carotene
destruction by lipoxidase, 187
in alfalfa, prevention of its loss by ethoxyguin, 236
in carrots, increased extractability by canning, 234
in tomatoes, content of, effect of breeding on, 210
leaves as source of, 193
Cash inputs, for seed, fertilizer, and pesticides, dependence of agricultural productivity on, 106
Casein, optimum level to supplement lime-treated corn and rice, 260
Cassava
see also Root crops
area and production by region, 38–41
consumption in different regions of world, 20–22
reason for small yields of, 122
world area and production of, 36
yield increase compared to farmed area increase by region, 111
yields
and yield increases by country, 114, 116
and yield increases by region, 112
potential, 121
realized record of, 122
Cassava-bean mixture, nutritive value of, effect of methionine on, 266
Cassava flour
as carrier for methionine, 265
bread made from, 265
Castor, world production of, 196
Castration, effects of, on growth and carcass characteristics, 220
Cat clays, 88
Cattle
adipose tissue in, effect of diet on, 225
and buffalo
crude productivity of, by world regions, 130
population of, in major regions of world, 129
world productivity of, in terms of daily production of protein per person, 128
body composition of, 217, 218
differences between species, 219
effect of sex differences on, 219
breed replacement, problems in, 142
breeds immune to trypanosomes, 138
death of, due to rabies, 133
European, 141
compared to other types, 142
heat tolerance of, 142
introduction into developing countries, 141
feed lot fattening, in developed countries, 139
muscle, distribution of, in various breeds, 219
production

effect of tsetse fly on, 160
in Africa, 160
factors limiting, 155
resistant to ticks, 142
Cattle productivity, variations in, in different regions, 152
Cellulases, increase of nutritive value of plant foodstuffs by, 237
Cellulose, hydrolysis by cellulases, 237
Central Africa, calorie requirements of men aged 20 to 29 in, 66
Central African Republic
calorie and protein intake in, 71
crop yields in, 114–115
Central America
calorie, total protein, and animal protein intake in, 72
crop yields and crop yield increases in 1950 and 1970 in, 116–117
death in cattle caused by rabies, 133
maize consumption in, 19
plantain consumption in, 22
use of Incaparina in, 201
Cephalopod, as source of human food, 197
Cereal-based foods, fortification of, with protein concentrates, 247
Cereal crops
antinutritional factors in, 233–234
arable land used for production of, 27
development of new varieties of, 270
inverse relation between grain yield and grain protein in, 209
yields and yield increases by country in 1950 and 1970, 114, 116
Cereal flour, fortification of, 244
Cereal grain, nonessential amino acids in, 210
Cereal products, preparation of textured vegetable protein foods from, 268
Cereal protein
amino acid imbalance in, 210
fortification with amino acids, 259
Cereal seeds, as source of protein, 193
Cereals
as source of calories, 109
as source of protein, searching for new varieties, 193
consumption of, 16–20
maize, 19
other grain, 19–20
rice, 18
wheat, 18–19
edible dry matter produced by, 119
fortification of
with protein concentrates, 259
with vitamin D, 245
new varieties, effect on livestock farming, 139
potential and target yields of, in temperate regions and tropics, 121
potential of, 120
production by region, 38–41
rachitogenic properties of, 187
surpluses of, in developing countries, development of intensive livestock industries from, 139
total area planted to, 110
use of, in formulation of new nutritious food products, 253
world area and production of, 36
yield increase compared to farmed area increase in 1950 and 1970, 111
yield increases by regions in 1950 and 1970, 112
Ceylon
animal protein in food supplies of, 149
calorie intake, total protein, and animal protein intake in, 71
calories, total protein, and animal protein in food supplies of, 148
crop yields in, 116–117
milk, meat, eggs, and fish in food supplies of, 150
total protein and proportions of animal and plant protein in food supplies of, 149
Chapatties, use of wheat protein concentrate in preparation of, 265
Cheese, consumption of, 29–30
Cheese skipper, food deterioration due to, 187
Chemical reactions, food deterioration due to, 177
Chemopharyngodon, 198
Chenopodium seeds, as staple in Europe, 195
Chick peas, *see also* Legume crops
consumption of, 23, 24
farmed area increase of region, 111
in formulation of nutritious food products, 257–258
nutritive value, effect of germination on, 237
yield increase compared to farmed area increase by region, 111
yields and yield increases by region, 112
Chickens, protein content of, 218
Children
death of, due to malnutrition, 2–3
FAO scale of calorie requirements for, 65
mortality of
decline in, 2
in Latin America, 3–5
rickets and osteomalacia in, 10
xerophthalmia in, 9
Chile
animal protein in food supplies of, 149
calorie and protein intake in, 72
calories, total protein, and animal protein in food supplies of, 148
crop yields in, 116–117
milk, meat, eggs, and fish in food supplies of, 150
protein-calorie malnutrition in, 8
total protein and proportions of animal and plant protein in food supplies, 149
China
arable land and population of, 43
calorie, total protein, and animal protein intake in, 71
crop yields in, 116–117
crude productivity of cattle and buffalo in, 130
crude productivity of pigs, 130
farm animal population in, 129
major uses of land in, 43
mean productivity of farm livestock in, 128
production of major food crops in, 39, 41
Chinese grass carp, as source of human food, 198
Chlorella, 198
as source of human food, 198
Chlorine, requirement by plants, 93

2-Chloro-4,6,bis (ethylamino)-S-triazine, *see* Simazine
Chlorosis in plants
nitrogen deficiency due to, 93, 97
sulfur and iron deficiency due to, 97
Choline esterase, inhibition by solanine, 187
Choline esterase inhibitor, in plant foodstuffs, 234
Cicer, 195
Cicer arietinum, 237
improvement of, 211
Citric acid, in foods, 186
Citrus fruits, consumption of, 26
Citrus pulp, use in livestock industry, 140
Climate
as constraint on food production, 275–276
as restraint on animal production, 133
cold, environmental control in livestock production in, 143
effect on livestock production, 135
effect on soil, 92
temperate, dry matter production of crops at, 121
Clostridium botulinum, 179, 180, 182, 184
growth of
effect of moisture on, 184
effect of pH on, 179
Clostridium nigrificans, 180
Clostridium perfringens, 179, 180
growth of, effect of pH on, 179
Clostridium thermosaccharolyticum, 180
Cloudiness, effect on radiation in different parts of the world, 120
Coast disease, of livestock, 133
Cobalt deficiency diseases, of livestock, 133
Cobalt, soil deficiency of, as restraint on animal production, 133
Cobalt uptake, by plants, effect of irrigation on, 212
Cockroaches, food deterioration due to, 187
Coconut
consumption of, 24
unknown diseases of, 167
world production of, 196
Coconut palm, uses of, 167
Coconut protein concentrate, preparation of, 195–196
Coconut water, use of, in food fermentation, 199
Cocos nucifera L., 167
Coliforms, 179
Collagen formation, defect in, due to osteolathyrogens, 233
Colombia
animal protein in food supplies, 149
calorie and protein intake in, 71
calories, total protein, and animal protein in food supplies of, 148
crop yields in, 116–117
goiter in, 10
milk, meat, eggs, and fish in food supplies of, 150
total protein and proportions of animal and plant protein in food supplies of, 149
Colorado beetle, control of, 164
Commitee on Nutrition of the National Academy of Pediatrics (U.S.), 245
Commodities, selected, income elasticities in Venezuela, India, and Philippines for, 74
Communication, methods of, in nutrition education, 283
Comore Island, crop yields in, 114–115
Confused flour beetle, food deterioration due to, 187
Congo
calorie and protein intake in, 71
crop yields in, 114–115
Conventional foods, 191
Cooking, effect on nutritional value of foods, 231
Copper
application of, to soil, 211
in soil
deficiency of, effect on animal production, 133
effect of pH on availability of, 96
Copper deficiency disease, in cattle, 133
Copper requirement
by plants, 95
effect of metal-binding constituents on, 234
Corn, *see also* Cereals
average yield in U.S., 104
comparison between protein value and amino acid intake of, 255
estimated fertilizer rates and yield responses in two agricultural subregions in U.S., 98
fortification of, with protein concentrates plus amino acids, 261
high-yielding varieties of, in Kenya, 161
in Kenya, factorial trials with, 103–104
lime-treated
effect of amino acid supplementation of protein quality, 259
fortification of
with lysine and tryptophan, 259
with protein concentrates, 260
nitrogen, genetic control of, 211
nutritive value of, increase by alkali treatment, 236
phosphate content, genetic control of, 211
yields
realized record of, 122
relation of nitrate reductase activity to, 204
targets for increase in, 124
yields and yield increase by country in 1950 and 1970, 114
zinc deficiency in, 211
Corn-bean diet
effect of lysine and tryptophan in presence or absence of vitamins and minerals, 263
nutrition value of
effect of fortification on, 263
effect of fortification with lysine, tryptophan, minerals, and vitamins on, 262
Corn flour, lime-treated, nutritive value of, effect of replacement with wheat shorts on, 264
Corn production
in Kenya, economic benefits from combinations of improved management practices used to increase, 104
U.S. soil management practices in, 92
Corn protein
biological value of, 255
quality of
effect of vitamins and minerals on, 255, 263
relation to lysine content, 260
Corn-soy-milk mixture, 190

Costa Rica
animal protein in food supplies of, 149
calorie and protein intake in, 71
calories, total protein, and animal protein in food supplies of, 148
crop yields in, 116–117
milk, meat, eggs, and fish in food supplies of, 150
total protein and proportions of animal and plant protein in food supplies of, 149
Cottonseed
gossypol-free, development of genetic variety of, 270
gossypol in, 233
use of in preparation of Ineaparina, 201
world production of, 196
Cottonseed flour
fortification of, with lysine-rich protein concentrates, 260
milk products substitutes made from, 267
optimum level to supplement lime-treated corn and rice, 260
use as protein concentrate, 263
use of, in formulation of nutritious food products formulation, 257–258
Cottonseed meal
increased availability of nutrients by phytase treatment, 238
metabolizable energy of, increase by phytase, 238
reduction of gossypol in, 236
Cottonseed oil, consumption of, 31
Cottonseed protein concentrate, preparation of, 195
Council of Foods and Nutrition (AMA), policy on food fortification by, 244
Cowpeas, *see also* Legume crops
consumption of, 24
yield increase compared to farmed area increase by region, 111
yields and yield increases by region, 112
Cresylic compounds, in foods, 186
Cretinism, 10
due to iodine deficiency, 246
Crop breeding programs, establishment of, developments necessary for, 103
Crop improvement, 103–106
objective of, 103
use of
cross-pollinating species, 104–105
in increasing crop yields, 103–106
population improvement, 105–106
self-pollinating species, 103–104
Crop "logging," 205, 212
Crop losses
development of methods for assessment of, 166
effect on consumer, 166
effect on farmer, 166
effect on state finances, 166
examples of
Bayoud disease of date palm, 167–168
Moko disease of bananas, 168–169
new wheats and old pathogens, 169
Pingalap disease of breadfruit, 166–169
unknown disease of coconut, 166–167
history of, 163–165
identification and qualification of, 165–166
information on their magnitude, 166
in Japan, caused by pests and disease in rice, 174
reduction of 163–176
promises of future, 174–175
selected examples of actual and potential, 166–169
strategies for effective control, 169–174
types of, 165
Crop pests
and diseases, control of, reasons for slow progress in, 164–165
control of, in Japan, 172–174
great flexibility of, 165
lack of appreciation of amount of losses caused by, 165
Crop preharvest losses, *see* Crop losses
Crop production
by-products of, use in livestock feeding, 131
disease control in, 102–103
evolution in, 110
for livestock production, 42
increase in, effect of using improved varieties and management practices on, 103–104
limiting constraints in, 92
technical measures to increase, 91–107
Crop production practices, 99–103
Crop productivity, as incentive for farmer, 285
Crop protection, in soil management, 84
Crop residues
handling of, role in control of plant diseases, 102
soil organic matter from, 95, 96
utilization of, in tillage operation, 99–100
Crop rotation
as plant disease control measure, 102
role of, 92
Crop yield
effect of photosynthetic efficiency on, 118
factors determining, 113, 118–119, 123
genetic component of, 205
physiological components of, 205
role in food production, 110
Crop yields
and yield increases by country, 114–117
differences in, between various countries, 114–117, 119
expected increases in, 123–124
increases of the past, 110–113
compared to farmed area increase in 1950–1970, 111
targets for various crops, 124
targets set by Indicative World Plan for, 123–124
potential, 113–123
and target of various crops, in temperate regions and in tropics, 121
in future, 123
methods for calculation of, 120
realized record for various crops, 122
technical measures for increasing
crop improvement, 103–106
infrastructure, 106–107
production practices, 99–103
soil management, 92–99
up to 19th century, 110
Cropland, *see also* Land, arable
potential, and soil quality, 47
Crops

choice of, in soil management, 84
contribution to world food production, 35
development of
new varieties, resistant to pathogens, 102
resistance to insects in, 102–103
efficient
food crops belonging among, 118
photosynthetic efficiency of, 120
estimated fertilizer rates and yield responses of, 97, 98
fertilization of, and water availability, 101
genetic potential of, fertility and management, 103
growth and yield of
factors determining, 203
use of tissue analysis in defining optimal conditions for, 205
inorganic elements in, genetic control of, 211
new varieties, effect on increased food production, 53
nonefficient, photosynthetic efficiency of, 120
nutritional value of, effect of fertilizers on, 209
pests and diseases of, history of, 163–165
principal varieties grown for food, 36
processing industries for, developing countries, 282
protein quality of, genetic upgrading of, use of screening techniques for, 211
relative potential of specific, 109–124
crop yield increases in past, 110–113
crops in man's food supply, 109–110
expected yield increases, 123–124
potential yields, 113–123
sources of
development of nutritious food products from
cereals, 253
legumes, 253
starchy roots and tubers, 253
temperature requirement of, variation and specificity in, 100
world area and production of, 36
Crossbreeding, of cattle, 141
Cross-pollinating species, improvement of, plant breeding practices in, 104–105
Cruciferae, goitrogenic substances in, 236
Crucifers, 193
CSM, ingredient composition of, 258
Cuba
calorie and protein intake in, 72
crop yields in, 116–117
use of molasses and urea in livestock feeding in, 140
Culicoides, blue tongue transmission by, 135
Cultivation, as weed control method, 100
Customs, effect on animal production, 151
Cyanogens, of cassava, 232
Cycads, antinutritional factor in, 233
Cycasin, in plant foodstuffs, 233
Cyprus, crop yields in, 116–117
Cystine, sulfur supplied by, 95
Czechoslovakia, 148, 149, 150
crop yields in, 114, 115
food supplies of
animal protein in, 148
calories, total protein, and animal proteins in, 148
milk, meat, eggs, and fish in, 150
total protein and proportion of animal and plant protein in, 149

D

Dahomey
calorie and protein intake in, 71
crop yields in, 114–115
Dairy cattle production
environmental control in, 143
in Africa, 160
Dairying
commercial, 50
major areas of, 50
Dairying industries, in developed countries, 139
Date palm, Bayoud disease of, 167–168
DDT, control of tsetse fly by, 138
Death rates
due to malnutrition, 2–3
in major regions of world for 1965 to 2000, 58–59
trends in, age-specific, 2
Deficiency disease, world, historical review of, 1
Demography and employment, information on, derived from household budget surveys, 279
Denmark
animal protein in food supplies of, 149
calories, total protein, and animal protein in food supplies of, 148
crop yields in, 114, 115
development of xorophthalmia from margarine, 245
milk, meat, eggs, and fish in food supplies of, 150
total protein and proportions of animal and plant protein in food supplies of, 149
Desalinization, of sea water, 47, 87
Desert locust, 170
distribution of and spread of its invasion area, 172
Desert plants, as source of human food, 199
Developed countries
agricultural productivity of, effect of infrastructure on, 106
animal protein consumption in, 277
birth date, death rate, and reproduction rate in, 57–58
nutrition problems in, 280
population and life expectancy in, 57
population in, age structure of, 60, 61
Developing countries
agricultural productivity of, effect of infrastructure on, 106
animal production in, causes of low levels of, 152
animal protein consumption in, 277
beriberi in, 246
calorie and reference protein requirements per day in, 68–69
calorie, total protein, and animal protein intake in, 71–72
crops in
expected demand for, 123
importance of population improvement, 106
decline in mortality among children, 2
factors limiting cattle production in, 155
farm value income elasticities of total food in, 73
fertilizer trials to evaluate plant nutrient needs and responses in, 97
food consumption trends in, 276–277
food enrichment programs in, 267
food production vs. population growth in, 276
livestock production, reasons for differences between developed countries and, 144

need for development of highly nutritious foods in, 254
pellagra in, 246
political, institutional, social, and economic restraints on animal production in, 144–145
population
age structure of, 60, 61
aggregate rate of growth in, 64
birth rate, death rate, and reproduction rate in, 57–58
population and life expectancy in, 57
prospects for food fortification in, 247–248
rickets in, 245
value and quality income elasticities for selected commodities in, 74
vitamin A deficiency in, 245
vulnerable groups in, requirement of food by, 252
2,4-Dichlorophenoxyacetic acid, effect on protein synthesis of plants, 212
Dieldrin, control of tsetse fly by, 138
Diet, ideal, 67
Dietary effects, on body fat composition of ruminants, 225
Digestibility, of soybean products, enhancement by fermentation, 237
Diptera, effect of temperature on hatching of eggs of, 135
Disease control
effect on crop yields, 118
in crop production, 102–103
Diseases
communicable, death of livestock due to, 133
food-borne, pests transmitting, 187
of crops, damage caused by, history of, 163–165
Distribution of food, its relation to hunger and future food policy, 76
Dogs, rabies transmitted by, 134
Dominican Republic
animal protein in food supplies of, 149
calorie and protein intake in, 72
calories, total protein, and animal protein in food supplies of, 148
crop yields in, 116–117
milk, meat, eggs, and fish in food supplies, 150
total protein and proportions of animal and plant protein in food supplies of, 149
Double cropping, 44
Drought
effect on plant appearance, 97
effect on wheat prices, 275
effect on world food supply, 275
Drought injury, in plants due to nitrogen deficiency, 93
Drugs, against trypanosomasis, 138
Dry beans, *see also* Legume crops
consumption of, 23, 24
yield increase, compared to farmed area increase by region, 111
yields
and yield increases by country in 1950 and 1970, 115, 117
and yield increases by region, 112
potential, 121
Dry farming, 42
Dry matter
differences between crop varieties, 119
distribution of, in different crop varieties, 119
edible, relative amounts produced by different types of crops, 119
production of, in crops in temperate climates, 121
Dry peas, *see also* Legume crops
consumption of, 23
yield increase, compared to farmed area increase by region, 111
yields
and yield increase by country, 115, 117
and yield increase by region, 112
potential, 121
Duryea, ingredient composition of, 257
Dye-binding capacity, 211

E

East Africa, animal production in, improvements of, 161
East Asia
crude birth rate, crude death rate, and gross reproduction rate for 1960 and 2000, 58
population and expectation of life for 1960 and 2000, 57
urban and rural population of, 62
East Europe, *see also* Europe
cereal consumption in, 18
collective agriculture in, 51
Econometric models, use of in formulation of food and nutrition policy, 278
Econometrics of demand, 280
Economic factors, effect on livestock production, 141, 144
Economic gap, effect on nutritional status, 276
Economic measures, for implementation of food and nutrition policies, 284–285
Economics, effect on malnutrition, 190
Ecuador
animal protein in food supplies of, 149
calorie and protein intake in, 71
calories, total protein, and animal protein in food supplies of, 148
crop yields in, 116–117
milk, meat, eggs, and fish in food supplies of, 150
total protein and proportions of animal and plant protein in food supplies of, 149
Edible plants, *see* Plants, edible
Educational measures, for implementation of food and nutrition policies, 283–284
Educational programs, effective, in modifying dietary practices, 283
Egg protein, optimum level to supplement lime-treated corn, 260
Egg white, raw, avidin in, 187
Eggs
amounts in food supplies of 90 countries, 150
as source of protein, 127
consumption in different regions of world, 25, 30
effect of taboos on consumption of, in Mashona tribe, 136
production of
effect of temperature on, 135
in Africa, 161
in developing countries vs. U.S.,153
in Europe, 157
in Latin America, 159

Egypt
calorie and protein intake in, 71
crop yield in, 114–115
pellagra in, 10
El bayoud, *see* Bayoud disease
Eland, as source of human food, 156
Elements
content of in plants, mechanism controlling, 204
major and minor, required by plants, 93
Eleucine coracana, 118
Eleucine sp., 210
Elephant, as source of food, 156
El Salvador
animal protein in food supplies of, 149
calorie and protein intake in, 71
calories, total protein, and animal protein in food supplies of, 148
crop yields in, 116–117
milk, meat, eggs, and fish in food supplies of, 150
total protein and proportions of animal and plant protein in food supplies of, 149
Employment, and demography, information on, derived from household budget surveys, 279
Employment, relation to hunger and future food policy, 76
Endemic goiter, 10
Energy requirement, *see* Calorie requirement
Energy value
of diet
effect on fat content of pig, 223
effect on muscle growth of pig, 224
England, foot-and-mouth disease in livestock in, 134
English sparrow, food deterioration due to, 188
Enteric disease, effect on animal production, 133
Enteric pathogens, 179
Environment, safeguard of, concern over, 174
Environmental control, in livestock industry, 143–144
Enzootic diseases, 133
control of, 137–138
Enzyme activity
factors affecting, 179
increased availability of nutrients from plant foodstuffs by, 236–238
of food, food deterioration due to, 177
use in food to improve digestibility, 199
Epizootic diseases, 133
effect on animal production in Africa, 151
Equatorial Guinea, crop yields in, 114–115
Erucic acid, rapeseed variety low in, 270
Escherichia coli, 180
growth of, effect of moisture on, 184
Eskimos, effect of food taboos on consumption of caribou by, 136
Estrogen, effect of growth rate and carcass characteristics of livestock, 221
Ethiopia
animal protein in food supplies of, 149
calorie and protein intake in, 72
calories, total protein, and animal protein in food supplies of, 148
crop yields in, 114–115
milk, meat, eggs, and fish in food supplies of, 150
total protein and preparations of animal and plant protein in food supplies of, 149
Ethoxyquin, prevention of carotene loss from alfalfa by, 236
Ethylene
adverse effects of, 179
production during ripening of fruits, 179
Europe
agriculture in, reliance on manure, 49
animal production in, 151
potential for increases, 157–158
cattle and buffalo in, productivity of, 130
cereal consumption in, 17
consumption of pulses, nuts, and seeds in, 23
crop yields and crop yield increases in 1950 and 1970, 114–115
farm livestock in
population of, 129
productivity of, 128
food crop production in, 38, 40
goiter in, 10
iron deficiency anemia in, 8
land, arable, and population of, 43
land, major uses of, 43
pigs in, productivity of, 130
population
and expectation of life for 1960 and 2000, 57
birth rate, death rate, and reproduction rate of, 58
growth in, 110
urban and rural, 62
solar radiation in, 120
starchy food consumption in, 21
European Economic Community, 53
Expenditures and income, information on, derived from household budget surveys, 279
Extension service, dependence of agricultural productivity on, 107
Extrusion cooking, 268

F

Facultative organisms, 184
Faffa, ingredient composition of, 257
Fagopyrum, 195
Fair price shops, 284
Falling disease, of livestock, 133
Famine
crop pests as factor in bringing about, 166
in Ireland, due to potato blight epidemic, 164
of Bengal, crop losses as factor in, 166
FAO, 33, 42, 74, 81, 128, 129, 130, 137, 153, 161, 162, 166, 176, 189, 286
Agricultural Commodities Projection by, 73
estimates of calorie requirement by, 64
fertilizer trials in developing countries sponsored by, 97
Food Balance Sheets, 16, 70, 72, 276, 278
Indicative World Plan of, 123, 154, 159, 160, 162, 193, 197, 202
Production Yearbooks, 35, 36, 41, 43, 54, 111, 112, 116,
scale of calorie requirement for children by, 65
State of Food and Agriculture, 35, 146, 148, 155, 156, 162

statement on world food situation by, 275
strategy on locust control, 172
symposium on crop losses, 166
FAO/WHO
Codex Alimentarius Commission, 285
Joint Expert Committee on Nutrition, 2, 4, 7, 8, 70, 243, 244
Far East
animal production in, potential for increases, 159
cattle and buffalo in, productivity of, 130
cereal consumption in, 17
crop yield increase compared to farmed area increase in 1950 and 1970, 111
crop yields in 1950 and 1970, 112
farm animal population in, 129
farm livestock in, mean productivity of, 128
fowl consumption trends in, 277
land, arable, and population of, 43
land in, arable, 44–45
land in, major uses of, 43
pigs in, productivity of, 130
solar radiation in, 120
starchy food consumption in, 21
xerophthalmia in, 8
Farm animals, potentials of, for increasing animal production, 154–155
Farm production practices, use of, in increasing crop yields, 99–103
Farm value elasticities, FAO estimates of, 73
Farmed area increase, compared to crop yield increase in 1950–1970, 111
Farmer
effect of crop losses on, 166
incentives for, 285
Farming
as occupation, 190
development of new lands for, 79–89
grain, 49
intensive, effect of, on pest control, 165
mixed crop and livestock, 49
Fat
as source of energy, 109
content of carcass
in ruminants vs. nonruminants, 224–225
interrelationship between body water and, 217
of Holstein steer, 217
content of livestock, effect of nutrition on, 223
content of pigs, during prenatal and postnatal stages of life, 216, 217
content of poultry, 218
content of sheep, breed differences in, 220
in plants, synthesis of, 191
production of, emphasis of early livestock breeders on, 215
Fat-bone ratio, in livestock, effect of nutrition on, 222
Fat-muscle ratio, in livestock, effect of nutrition on, 222
Fats and oils, consumption in different regions of world, 30–31
Fatty acid composition, of adipose tissue, in ruminants vs. nonruminants, 224–225
Favism causing factors, in plant foodstuffs, 234
Feed lot fattening of cattle, 139
Fermentation
antibiotic production by, 237
enhancement of digestibility of soybean products by, 237
increased availability of nutrients from plant foodstuffs by, 236–237
nature of, 200
use in food production, 199
use in preparation of highly nutritious foods, 268
Fermented bean products, 236
Fertility
of livestock, effect on animal production, 152
of soils, *see* Soils, fertility of
Fertilization of crops, and water availability, 101
Fertilizer requirements and response, 97–98
assessment of economic value, 97
ways of estimating, 97
Fertilizers
chemical, use of, in U.S. in corn production, 92
crop yield increase by use of, 113, 118
effect on nutritional value of crops, 209
reliance of agriculture on, in U.S., 49
use of, in soil management, 85
Fiber, interference with protein utilization by, 232
Field crop engineering, 205
Fiji, crop yields in, 116–117
Filth, in food, pests transmitting, 187
Finland
animal protein in food supplies of, 149
calories, total protein, and animal protein in food supplies of, 148
crop yields in, 114, 115
milk, meat, eggs, and fish in food supplies of, 150
total protein and proportions of animal and plant protein in food supplies of, 149
Fish
as source of human food, 197–198
by-products of, use in livestock feeding, 131
consumption in different regions of world, 25, 30
contribution to world food production, 35
herbivorous, as source of human food, 198
in food supplies of 90 countries, 150
inhibitory substances in, 186–187
potential for increasing animal production, 156
production of, factors limiting, 156–157
raw, thiaminase in, 187
Fish farming, fresh water, 198
Fish flour, optimum level to supplement lime-treated corn and rice, 260
Fish liver oil concentrate, fortification of margarine with, 244
Fish protein concentrate, use of, in formulation of nutritious food products, 257–258
Fish sausage, 201
Fisheries
amount of catch
in Africa, 161
in Europe, 158
in Far East, 159
in Latin America, 159
in Near East, 160
in Oceania, 158
in U.S., 158
world, output of, 156

Flatulence
causative factors of, 235
due to oligosaccharides, 234
Flavobacterium, 179
Flavor, of meat, effect on acceptability, 224
Flavoring agents, use of, in formulation of nutritious food products, 257–258
Flies, food deterioration due to, 187
Flour
fortification of
with iron, 247
with vitamin A, 245
with vitamin B complex, 245
wheat, fortification with lysine, 247
Floury-2 corn, 209
Fluorine poisoning, of livestock, 133
Fluorine, supplementation, 191
Folic acid deficiency
anemias of pregnancy due to, 247
megaloblastic anemia due to, 8
Food
distribution of, its relation to hunger and future food policy, 76
principal sources of, 35–37
sources of carbon for, 194
synthetic, 200
Food aid, importance of, 284
Food and Nutrition Board
of National Academy of Sciences (U.S.), 247
(NAS), policy on food fortification, 244
Food and nutrition policy, 275–286
components of, 281–283
definition of, 276, 277
formulation of
data requirements for, 278–280
definition and methodology by Indicative World Plan, 276
use of models in, 278
implementation of, 283–285
integration of, in agricultural planning, 280–281
methodological aspects of, 277–278
Food Balance Sheets (FAO)
see also FAO, *Food Balance Sheets*
preparation of, 278
Food commodities situation, analysis of, as component of food and nutrition policy, 282–283
Food consumption
and household budget surveys, 278
basic information derived from, 279
determining factors of, 64
effect of income on, 70
inequalities within a population group, factors responsible for, 278
information on, derived from food consumption surveys, 279
of animal products, effect of taboos on, 135
patterns
improvement of, by educational programs, 283
world, 15–33
relationship between income and, 72
trends in, at present, in relation to agriculture and food production, 276
trends in the 1970's, 276–277
world
beverages, 32
cereals, 16–20
eggs and fish, 30
fats and oils, 30–31
fruits, 26–27
meat, 27–28
milk and milk products, 28–30
pulses, nuts, and seeds, 22–24
starchy foods, 20–22
sugar, 31–32
vegetables, 24–26
Food crops, arable land used for production of, 37
Food decomposition, signs of, 177
Food distribution, 284
Food enrichment, 265–267
definition of, 243, 265
Food enrichment programs
choice of carrier in, 267
in developed vs. developing countries, 267
Food for Peace Program, 284
Food fortification, 243–249, 259–264
definition of, 243, 259
experience with various nutrients, 244–247
general background on, 243–247
historical reviews on, 244
policies on, 244
prospects for the future, 247–248
with amino acids, 247, 259,
with calcium, 247
with iodine, 246
with iron, 246–247
with minerals, 246–247, 261
with protein concentrates, 247, 259–260
with protein concentrates plus amino acids, 260–261
with vitamin A, 245
with vitamin B complex, 246
with vitamin C, 246
with vitamin D, 245
with vitamins, 244–246, 261
Food habits
difficulty in changing, 201
Western type, societies aspiring to, 132
Food intake, of major part of world population, 113
Food losses, postharvest, due to pests, 187–188
Food needs
future estimate of, 72
world
and future population growth, 55–77
in year 2000, 55
Food poisoning organisms, effect of pH on, 179
Food processing
increased availability of nutrients from plants through, 231–241
chemical methods, 235–236
enzymatic techniques, 236–238
future outlook, 238
physical methods, 232–235
Food production
breakthroughs in, 52

development of new land for, 52
effect of new technology of, 53
effect on food supply, 16
from animals, present situation, 128–130
from soils, ways to increase, 79–89
in developed vs. developing countries, 276
increase in, by enlarging cultivated area, 110
increase in, realization through yield increases, 110, 113
influence of agricultural system on, 45
need for long-term policy on, 275
of crops, technical measures to increase, 91–107
policy on, 75–76
relative potential of meat-producing animals in increasing, 147–162
state of world
agricultural systems, 45–52
increasing world food population, 52–54
principal sources of food, 35–37
trends and patterns in food production, 37–42
use of land resources, 42–45
surplus, areas of, 48
trends and patterns in, 37–38
under commercial system of agriculture, 48
under intensive sedentary subsistence system of agriculture, 48
use of unconventional sources for, 189–202
world
barriers to changing status of, 54
main components of, 35
prospects for increasing, 52
state of, 35–54
Food products
new highly nutritious, formulation of, 251–274
standards for, as established by FAO/WHO, 285
Food replacement, 267
Food restoration, 265–266
definition of, 243, 264
Food spoilage
and deterioration, 177–188
factors involved in, 177–188
inhibitory substances, 187–188
nutrients, 186–187
oxygen tension, 184–185
pests, 185–186
pH, 179–181
temperature, 178–179
time, 177–178
water activity, 181–184
due to microorganisms, 177
factors affecting, 177
Food supply
available sources of, 252–
effect on food consumption, 16
of 90 countries
animal protein in, 149
calories, total protein, and animal protein in, 148
milk, meat, eggs, and fish in, 150
total protein and proportions of animal and plant protein in, 149
role of crops in, 109–110
Food taboos, effect on food consumption, 16
Foods
high acid, 179
high protein, natural, 256
highly nutritious, use of processing in preparation 267–268
high-protein containing
development of, 256–259
quality of, 256
ingredient composition of, 257–258
high-protein quality, lack in developing countries of, 252
low acid, 179
nutritional quality of, upgrading of, 270
perishable, 177
plant, improving nutritional quality of, 203–214
priority in, by developing countries, 283
stable, 177
storage life of, 178
unconventional, *see also* Unconventional foods
unconventional, 189–202
conventionalizing of, 201
for whom should they be made, 190–191
need for, 191–192
nutritional value of, 200–201
possible sources of, 192–200
sources of
for nutritious food products, 253–254
leaf and algae protein, 253
oilseed, 253
palm kernel and nuts, 253
yeast and microbial protein, 254
Foot-and-mouth disease, 133, 151
control of, 137
responsible for, 137
vaccination against, 137
world distribution of, 134
Forest areas, in Near East, 160
Formaldehyde, in foods, 186
Formulation, of highly nutritious food products, 251–274
Fractionation, of plants, 195
France
crop yields in, 114, 115
food supplies of
animal protein in, 149
calories, total protein, and animal protein in, 148
milk, meat, eggs, and fish in, 150
total protein and proportions of animal and plant protein in, 149
Freezer burn, in frozen foods, 178
Freezing, effect on food deterioration, 178
Freezing point, of selected foods, 178
French Guiana, crop yields in, 116–117
French Polynesia, crop yields in, 116–117
Frozen foods, deterioration of, 178
Fruit farming, commercial, 50
Fruit flies, food deterioration due to, 187
Fruits
arable land used for production of, 37
as source of vitamins, 109
consumption in different regions of world, 23, 26–27
inhibitory substances in, 186–187
Fungal spoilage, food losses due to, 141

Fungi
as source of human food, 199
history of, on earth, 163
responsible for potato blight, 164
Fungicides, use of, in control of plant diseases, 102
Fusarium oxysporum f.s. albedinis, 168

G

Gabon
calorie and protein intake in, 71
crop yields in, 114–115
food supplies of
animal protein in, 149
calories, total protein, and animal protein in, 148
milk, meat, eggs, and fish in, 150
total protein and proportions of animal and plant protein in, 149
L-Galactosidase, use in hydrolysis of oligosaccharides of soy milk, to reduce flatulence, 237
Gambia
food supplies of
animal protein in, 149
calories, total protein, and animal protein in, 148
milk, meat, eggs, and fish in, 150
total protein and proportions of animal and plant protein in, 149
Game management, for meat production, 155
Game ranching, 156
Genetic control, of crop yield, 205
Genetic improvement, of livestock, in temperate countries, 142
Genetic potential, of crops, and fertility and management, 103
Genetics
effect on animal productivity, 152–153
effect on egg production, 153
effect on milk production, 153
Genetics, role of, in development of highly nutritious foods, 269–270
Genotypes, within animal species, differences between, 218

Germany
crop yields in, 114–115
food supplies of
animal protein in, 149
calories, total protein, and animal protein, 148
milk, meat, eggs, and fish in, 150
total protein and proportions of animal and plant protein in, 149
Germination
improvement in nutritive value of seed proteins by, 237
of crops, variation of temperature requirement for, 100
Ghana,
calorie and protein intake in, 71
crop yields in, 114–115
food supplies of
animal protein in, 149
calories, total protein, and animal protein in, 148
milk, meat, eggs, and fish in, 150
total protein and proportions of animal and plant protein in, 149
poultry industry in, 139
Giant snail, as source of human food, 197
Giraffe, as source of food, 156
Glossina, see also Tsetse fly, *Glossina* sp.
Glossina sp., 138
Glucosinolate, rapeseed variety low in, 270
Gnats, food deterioration due to, 187
Goat meat, consumption of, 27, 28
Goiter
endemic, 10
in U.S., 246
prevalence of, 247
prevention of, 243
with iodine, 246
with iodine-enriched salt, 266
Goitrogens
in plant foodstuffs, 233
in rapeseed, 232
interference of, with metabolism of iodine, 236
Gossypol
development of genetic variety of cottonseed free of, 270
in cottonseed, 232
removal of, 195
in cottonseed meal, reduction by chemical treatment, 236
in plant foodstuffs, 233
Grain farming, mid-latitude, 49
Grain, inverse relation between yield and protein content of, 204
Grass tetany, in cattle, 95
Grazing, control of, 140
Great Britain, *see also* United Kingdom
leaf protein production in, 196
malnutrition in, 190
Greece
crop yields in, 114–115
food supplies of
animal protein in, 149
calories, total protein, and animal protein in, 148
milk, meat, eggs, and fish in, 150
total protein and proportions of animal and plant protein in, 149
Green algae, as source of human food, 198
Green revolution
crop vulnerability due to, 169, 175
future of, 174
risks of, 169
role in food production, 270–271
Groundnut oil, consumption of, 31
Groundnuts, *see also* Legume crops
as source of protein, 193
consumption of, 24
world production of, 196
yield increase compared to, farmed area increase by region, 111
yields
and yield increase by country in 1950 and 1970, 115, 117
and yield increases by region, 112
potential, 121
realized record in, 122
targets for increase in, 124

Growth, animal, patterns of normal, 216–217
Growth rate
as criterion of protein quality, 208
of livestock, relationship between body composition and, 223
Guadeloupe, crop yields in, 116–117
Guam, Pingalap disease of breadfruit in, 166–167
Guatemala, 10
calorie and protein intake in, 71
crop yields in, 116–117
food supplies of
animal protein in, 149
calories, total protein, and animal protein in, 148
milk, meat, eggs, and fish in, 150
total protein and proportions of animal and plant protein in, 149
vitamin A fortification in, 245
Guinea
calorie and protein intake in, 71
crop yields in, 114–115
Guyana
calorie and protein intake in, 71
crop yields in, 116–117
prevalence of kwashiorkor and marasmus in children in, 9

H

Haiti
calorie and protein intake in, 72
crop yields in, 116–117
Hard-pan, formation of, in soils, 99
Health, poor, nutritional deficiencies due to, 276
Heat treatment
destruction of plant inhibitors by, 232
effect on nutritive value of plant foodstuffs, 232
increased availability of plant protein and carbohydrate by, 232
Helicopter, use of, for controlling rice pests and diseases in Japan, 173
Helminthosporium maydis, as cause of epidemic of Southern Corn Leaf Blight, 165
Hemagglutinnis
in plant foodstuffs, 233
in raw legumes, 187
Hemoglobin concentration, as criterion of iron deficiency anemia, 7
Hemolytic anemia, in favism, 234
Hemorrhagic septicemia, in livestock, 138
Herbage, improvement of, by application of nonprotein nitrogen, 140–141
Herbicide, effect of, in improving protein content of plants, 212
Herbicides
specificity of, 100
use of
for controlling rice pests and diseases in Japan, 173
in weed control, 100
Hereford cattle
development of Bonsmara breed from, 142
introduction to North and South America, 141
Hessian fly, crop resistance to, 103
High acid foods, 179
High protein containing feeds, *see* Foods, high protein containing
High protein foods, natural, 256
High-yielding varieties, impact of, in developing countries, 282
Hindus, taboos of, effect on consumption of beef, 135
Hippopotamus, as source of food, 156
Hoggett ill thrift, 133
Homestead Act, 53
Honduras
calorie and protein intake in, 71
crop yields in, 116–117
food supplies of
animal protein in, 149
calories, total protein, and animal protein in, 148
milk, meat, eggs, and fish in, 150
total protein and proportions of animal and plant protein in, 149
prevalence of kwashiorkor and marasmus in children, 9
Honey, spoilage of, by yeasts, 184
Hong Kong, crop yields in, 116–117
Horizontal resistance
as approach to control plant disease through breeding, 175
nature of, 175
Horse meat, consumption of, by Kazak of Turkestan, 136
Household budget surveys
and food consumption, 278
basic information derived from, 279
Household refuse, in livestock feeding, 131
Housing, in livestock production, 143
Humid tropics, restraints on animal production in, 132–133
Humidity
effect on animal production, 135
relative, effect on microbial growth, 183
Hungary
crop yields in, 114–115
food supplies of
animal protein in, 149
calories, total protein, and animal protein in, 148
milk, meat, eggs, and fish in, 150
total protein and proportions of animal and plant protein in, 149
Hunger, income as causative factor in, 75
Hybrid maize, development in U.S., 105
Hybridization, use of, in improvement of cross-pollinating species, 105
Hybrids, of self-pollinating crops, development of, 105
Hydrogen ion concentration, as factor in food spoilage, 179–181
Hypercalcemia, in infants, 245

I

Idli, 236
methionine content of, increase by fermentation, 237
Ignorance
effect on food consumption, 16

nutritional deficiencies due to, 276
Immunity, in cattle, to trypanosomes, 138
Inbreeding, of cross-pollinating species, function of, 105
INCAP, development of cottonseed as human food by, 195
Incaparina, 201
ingredient composition of, 257
Income
as explanatory variable of behavior change, 280
calorie level and animal protein supplies in national food supplies in relation to, 153
distribution of, effect on food consumption, 70
effect on demand for animal products and fodder crops, 123
inequalities of, in developing countries, undernutrition and malnutrition due to, 277
relation to hunger and future food policy, 75
relationship between food consumption and, 72
uneven distribution of, in relation to food supply, 276
Income and expenditures, information on, derived from household budget surveys, 279
Income and supplies of animal protein in 30 countries, 154
Income elasticity
farm value of total food, 73
major source of data, 73
types of, 70
urban vs. rural, 73–74
value and quantity, in Venezuela, India, and Philippines, 74
India
calorie, total protein, and animal protein, intake in, 71
crop yields in, 116–117
fluorine poisoning of cattle in, 133
food supplies of
animal protein in, 149
calories, total protein, and animal protein in, 148
milk, meat, eggs, and fish in, 150
total protein and proportions of animal and plant protein in, 149
leaf protein production in, 196
osteoporosis in, 247
pellagra in, 10
prevalence of kwashiorkor and marasmus in children in, 9
salt iodization in, 246
use of by-products in livestock industry, 140
Indian Agricultural Research Institute, 195, 210
Indian meal-moth, food deterioration due to, 187
Indicative World Plan (FAO), 123, 276
Indonesia
Indonesia
calorie and protein intake in, 71
crop yields in, 116–117
food supplies of
animal protein in, 149
calories, total protein, and animal protein in, 148
milk, meat, eggs, and fish in, 150
total protein and proportions of animal and plant protein in, 149
use of fermented soy and groundnut as human food in, 199
Industrial processing, by-products, use in livestock feeding, 131
Industrial revolution, effect on agriculture, 80
Industrialization, in developing countries, 145
Infant formulas, fortification of, with vitamin D, 245
Infant milk products, formulation of, use of soybean protein isolate in, 235
Infant mortality in Latin America, pattern of nutritional deficiency in, 4
Infantile beriberi, 11
Infection, effect on animal production,133
Infectious diseases, malnutrition associated with, 11
Infrastructure
as limiting factor in developing potentially arable soils, 88
precision of, for nutrition education, 284
role of, in increasing crop production, 106–107
Inhibitory substances, in foods, effect on food spoilage, 186–187
Inorganic elements
content of crops, genetic control of, 211
in leaves, relation to crop performance, 204
Insect eggs, as source of human food, 197
Insect pests, control of, 102–103
Insects
dissemination of bacterial wilt disease of bananas by, 169
grain infestation by, food losses due to, 141
history of, on earth, 163
wastage of food due to, 177
Institutional factors, as restraint on livestock production, 144–145
Integrated control, in controlling insects, 175
Inter-American Investigation of Mortality in Childhood, 2, 3, 4, 5
Interdepartmental Committee on Nutrition for National Defense, 10
Intermediate technology, 191
International Biological Program, 196
International Rice Research Institute, 212
International Vegetable Research Institute, 193
Invertase, use in hydrolysis of oligosaccharides of soy milk, to reduce flatulence, 237
Invertebrates, as source of human food, 197
Iodate, its use in salt fortification, 246
Iodine
enrichment of salt with, 266
fortification of salt with, prevention of goiter by, 243
low intake of, in developing countries, 252
metabolism of, interference of goitrogenic substances with, 236
prevention of goiter by, 246
supplementation of foods with, 191
utilization of, interference of goitrogens with, 233
Iodized oil, use in goiter control, 10
Iodized salt, use in goiter control, 10, 246
Iran
calorie, total protein, and animal protein intake in, 71
crop yields in, 116–117

food supplies of
animal protein in, 149
calories, total protein, and animal protein in, 148
milk, meat, eggs, and fish in, 150
total protein and proportions of animal and plant protein in, 149
lysine fortification study in, 247
PCM in, 8
selenium poisoning of cattle in, 133
Iraq
calorie and protein intake in, 71
crop yields in, 116–117
food supplies of
animal protein in, 149
calories, total protein, and animal protein in, 148
milk, meat, eggs, and fish in, 150
total protein and proportions of animal and plant protein in, 149
Ireland
crop yields in, 114–115
food supplies of
animal protein in, 149
calories, total protein, and animal protein in, 148
milk, meat, eggs, and fish in, 150
total protein and proportions of animal and plant protein in, 149
potato blight epidemic in, 164
selenium poisoning of cattle in, 133
IRL, ingredient composition of, 258
Iron
application of, to soil, 211
in bread, increased availability by fermentation, 237
in plants, increased availability by homogenization, 237
in soil, effect of pH on availability of, 96
low intake in developing countries, 252
Iron deficiency anemia, 7
prevalence of, 247
prevention of, 247
Iron deficiency, of plants, symptoms of, 97
Iron enrichment, of salt, 266, 267
Iron fortification
of bread, 244
of bread and flour, 247
of foods, 246–247
of white flour, 245
Iron requirement
of man
effect of gossypol on, 233
effect of metal binding constituents on, 234
of plants, 93
Irradiation, of milk, 244
Irrigation
arable land under, 42
as source of water in crop production, 118
effect on uptake by plants of cobalt and molybdenum, 211–212
importance of land-water-drainage scheme in, 98
Israel
calorie and protein intake in, 71
crop yields in, 116–117
food supplies of
animal protein in, 149
calories, total protein, and animal protein in, 148
milk, meat, eggs, and fish in, 150
total protein and proportions of animal and plant protein in, 149
selenium poisoning of cattle in, 133
Italy
crop yields in, 114–115
food supplies of
animal protein in, 149
calories, total protein, and animal protein in, 148
milk, meat, eggs, and fish in, 150
total protein and proportions of animal and plant protein in, 149
Ivory Coast
crop yields in, 114–115
food supplies of
animal protein in, 149
calories, total protein, and animal protein in, 148
milk, meat, eggs, and fish in, 150
total protein and proportions of animal and plant protein in, 149

J

Jamaica
calorie and protein intake in, 72
crop yields in, 116–117
devastating effect on lethal yellowing disease on tall coconut palms in, 168
food supplies of
animal protein in, 149
calories, total protein, and animal protein in, 148
milk, meat, eggs, and fish in, 150
total protein and proportions of animal and plant protein in, 149
PCM in, 8
prevalence of kwashiorkor and marasmus in children in, 9
Jams and jellies, spoilage of, by mold, 184
Japan
animal production in, 159
birth rates, death rates, and reproduction rates in, 58
crop yields in, 116–117
food supplies of
animal protein in, 149
calories, total protein, and animal protein in, 148
milk, meat, eggs and fish in, 150
total protein and proportions of animal and plant protein in, 149
increase in rice production in, 118
lysine fortification study in, 247
osteoporosis in, 247
population
total, and expectation of life, 57
urban and rural, 62
rice fortification programs in, 246
strategy on intensive use of plant protection measures in, 172–174
Jersey cattle
cross with Red Sindhi cattle, 142
in Ghana, 143

Jews, taboos of, effect on consumption of pork, 135
Joint FAO/WHO Expert Committee on Nutrition, 2, 4, 7
Jordan
calorie and protein intake in, 71
crop yields in, 116–117
food supplies of
animal protein in, 149
calories, total protein, and animal protein in, 148
milk, meat, eggs, and fish in, 150
total protein and proportions of animal and plant protein in, 149
PCM in, 8
vitamin A fortification in, 245
Juices
fortified with vitamin C, 246
plant, inhibitory substances in, 186

K

Kaincopé, effect on coconut production, 167
Kazak of Turkestan, effect of taboos on consumption of meat in, 136
Kenke, 19
Kenya
artificial insemination of cattle in, 142
calorie and protein intake in, 72
crop yields in, 114–115
effect of high-yielding varieties of corn on animal production in, 161
factorial trials with maize in, 103–104
food supplies of
animal protein in, 149
calories, total protein, and animal protein in, 148
milk, meat, eggs, and fish in, 150
total protein and proportions of animal and plant protein in, 149
losses due to insect damage of maize in, 141
starvation caused by rinderpest epidemic in, 134
surpluses of maize in, development of beef production system from, 139
Keratomalacia, 8
Khiner Republic, crop yields in, 116–117
Kidney beans
consumption of, 23
hemagglutinins in, 187
Korea
calorie, total protein, and animal protein intake in, 71
crop yields in, 116–117
food supplies of
animal protein in, 149
calories, total protein, and animal protein in, 148
milk, meat, eggs, and fish in, 150
total protein and proportions of animal and plant protein in, 149
Kwashiorkor, 2, 7
in community surveys, prevalence of, 9
infant mortality due to, 3
in Latin America, 4, 5
symptoms of, 4

L

Lactic acid, in food, 186
Lactic acid bacteria, wine deterioration due to, 186
Lactobacilli, 179
Lactobacillus thermophilus, effect of temperature on, 179
Lamb
body composition of, 216
sex differences in, 221
carcass composition of, chemical effect of sex differences on, 221
production and consumption
in Europe, 157
in Latin America, 159
in North America, 158
in Oceania, 158
Land
agricultural, effect of transportation system on development of, 52
and water resources, effect on animal production, 132–133
arable
and population by world regions, 43
changes in area of, 44
distribution of, 42
estimated potential in world, 46
expansion of, 44
extending the area of, to expand farm production, 79–89
potential for further expansion of, 45
quality of, 42
use for producing animal fodder, 197
uses of, 37
uses of, by world regions, 43
Land clearing
methods of, 85
need for, in development of potentially arable soils, 85
Land reform, 52
Land resources, use of, 42–45
in livestock production, 42
Land tenure system, effect on livestock production, 145
Land utilization, for wildlife production, 155
Laos
calorie and protein intake in, 71
crop yields in, 116–117
Laterite
as hazard in tropical soils, 88
use of, 88
Lathyrus odoratus, 233
Lathyrus sativus, 233, 235
improvement of, 211
Latin America
animal production in, 151
arable land and population of, 43
arable land in, 45
birth rate, death rate, and reproduction rate in, 59
calorie and reference protein requirements, 68–69
calorie, total protein, and animal protein intake in, 72
cereal consumption in, 17
corn-bean diet in, 262–263

crop yield increase compared to farmed area increase in 1950 and 1970, 111
crop yields in 1950 and 1970, 112
food restoration in, 264
investigation of mortality in childhood in, 2, 3
kwashiorkor and marasmus in, 9
major uses of land in, 43
malnutrition in, prevalence of, 6
population and expectation of life for 1960 and 2000, 57
potential for increases of animal production in, 158–159 158–159
production of major food crops in, 38, 40
protein from plant sources in, 154
solar radiation in, 120
starchy food consumption in, 21
tortillas in, 264
urban and rural population of, 62–63
Latitude, calculation of potential yield of crops for different, 120
Laubina, ingredient composition of, 258
Leaf area index, 119
Leaf protein, use in formulation of new nutritious food products, 253
Leaf protein concentrate, 201
preparation of, 196
Leafy crop, fractionation of, 198
Leafy vegetables, as source of problem, 193
Leaves
as source of proteins, 193
chemical analysis of, use in monitoring the nutritional status of plants, 205
inorganic elements in, relation to crop performance, 204
Lebanon
calorie and protein intake in, 71
crop yields in, 116–117
food supplies of
animal protein in, 149
calories, total protein, and animal protein in, 148
milk, meat, eggs, and fish in, 150
total protein and proportions of animal and plant protein in, 149
Leche Alim, ingredient composition of, 257
Lecithin, effect on nutritive value of soy flour, 236
Legislative measures, for implementation of food and nutrition policies, 285
Legislator, role of, in formulation in food and nutrition policy, 277–278
Legume crops
as protein source, 109
potential and target yields of temperate regions and in tropics, 121
yield increase compared to farmed area increase in 1950 and 1970, 111
yield increases by region in 1950 and 1970, 112
yields and yield increases by country in 1950 and 1970, 115, 117
Legume seeds, 201
as source of protein, potential production, 195
Legumes
antinutritional factors in, 233–234
as source of food protein, 193
consumption of, 22–24
deep-rooted, effect on hard-pan, 99
hemagglutinin in, 187
inhibitory substances in, 187
making use of atmospheric nitrogen by, 93
nutritional improvement of, by genetic means, 210
nutritive value of, effect of heat on, 232
use of, in formulation of new nutritious food products, 253
Leguminosae, 233, 253
Lentil flour, use of, in nutritious food products, 257–258
Lentils
consumption of, 23
yields and yield increases by region, 112
Lesotho
calorie and protein intake in, 71
crop yields in, 114–115
Lethal yellowing disease of coconut, damage caused by, 167
Lethal yellowing, effect on coconut production, 167
Leuconostoc, 179
Liberia
calorie and protein intake in, 71
crop yields in, 114–115
Libya
calorie and protein intake in, 71
crop yields in, 114–115
food supplies of
animal protein in, 149
calories, total protein, and animal protein in, 148
milk, meat, eggs, and fish in, 150
total protein and proportions of animal and plant protein in, 149
Life expectancy, in major regions of world in 1960 and 2000, 57
Light, effect in crop production, 99
Light intensity, effect on crop yields, 118
Lime
effect on calcium content of corn, 236
effect on soil pH and crop production in area of highly leached lateritic soils, 97
effect on soil pH and crop production in temperate regions, 96
increased uptake by plants of trace elements due to, 211
Lime fertilizer, effect on calcium and phosphorus content of lespedeza hay, 208
Linoleic acid, in oil seeds, effect of genetics on, 270
Linseed
antipyridoxine in, 233
world production of, 196
Lipids
autoxidation of, rancidity of fats due to, 184
in foods, 185–186
Lipoxidase, in raw soybeans, 187
Lipoxygenase activity, of soybean, destruction by proteolytic enzymes, 237
Liver, rachitogenic property of, 187
Livestock and crops, as human food, their supplementary value, 131
Livestock
body composition of
effect of sex differences on, 220–221
nutritional influences on, 221–224
carcass components of, nutritive value of, 224–225

chemical composition of, differences in species, 218
contribution to world food production, 35
different types of, as result of natural and artificial selection of, 141
domesticated
as source of human food, 127
uses of, 127
efficiency of protein production in, 219
improving nutrient composition of, 215–230
productivity of, 128
estimation of, 128
measured in terms of daily production of protein per person, 128
Livestock breeders, early, emphasis on fat production by, 215
Livestock farming
effect of new varieties of cereals on, 139
mixed crop and, 49
Livestock feed
need for, in developing countries, 154–155
technical measures for increasing,
nonpastoral livestock, 139–140
pastoral farming, 140–141
Livestock industry
intensive
based on cereals, 139
in developing countries, 139
of developed countries, intensification of, 139
Livestock production
agricultural policies and, 144–145
reasons for differences between developed vs. developing countries, 144
role in agricultural sector
in Africa, 160–161
in Far East, 159
in Near East, 160
in Oceania, 158
separation of primary production from secondary production, 131
use of crops for, 42
world, value of, 42
Livestock productivity, potential, estimation of, 129
Livestock ranching, 50–51
major regions of, 51
Locust
as source of human food, 197
control of, overall strategy developed by FAO, 172
damage caused by, history of, 163
losses caused to agriculture by, 170–171
Locusta migratoria migratoroides, 170
Lolium sp., 211
Low acid foods, 179
Lupines, consumption of, 23
Luxembourg
crop yields in, 114–115
food supplies of
animal protein in, 149
calories, total protein, and animal protein in, 148
milk, meat, eggs, and fish in, 150
total protein and proportions of animal and plant protein in, 149
Lysine
as first limiting amino acid in cereals, 210
effect on nutritive value of corn-bran diet in presence and absence of vitamins and minerals, 263
fortification, of cottonseed flour with protein concentrates rich in, 260
improvement of quality of cereal protein by, 259
in wheat, increased availability by germination, 237
in wheat protein concentrate, effect on nutritive value of wheat flour, 265
maize varieties containing high levels of, 193
use of, in nutritious food products, 257–258
Lysine content
effect on protein quality of corn and rice, 260
of cereals, 209
of opaque and floury-2 corn, 209
of pearl millet, effect of nitrogen fertilizer on, 211
of wheat, effect of fertilizer on, 210
Lysine deficiency, of corn, 255
Lysine fortification
of corn, 259
of corn-bean diets, 262, 263
of tortilla flour, 262
studies on, 247

M

Madagascar
calorie and protein intake in, 72
crop yields in, 114–115
food supplies of
animal protein in, 149
calories, total protein, and animal protein in, 148
milk, meat, eggs, and fish in, 150
total protein and proportions of animal and plant protein in, 149
Madeira, crop yields in, 114–115
Magnesium
content of clover, effect of magnesium on, 204
content of rose clover, relation between yield and, 204
deficiency in animal symptoms of, 95
in soil, availability of, effect of pH on, 96
interaction with potassium, importance in plant and animal nutrition, 94
requirement by plants of, 93, 94
Magnetism, absorption of, interference of phytic acid with, 233
Maize, *see also* Corn
area and productivity by region, 38–41
as causative factor in pellagra, 10
consumption in different regions of world, 17, 19
high lysine varieties of, 193
use of, in formulation of nutritious food products, 257–258
world area and production of, 36
yield increase compared to farmed area increase by country, 111
yields
and yield increases by country, 114, 116
and yield increases by region, 112
potential, 121
Maize diets, low niacin content of, 246
Malabsorption, folate deficiency precipitated by, 8
Malawi

calorie and protein intake in, 72
crop yields in, 114–115
development of intensive cattle industry in, 139
prevalence of kwashiorkor and marasmus in children, 9
Malaysia
calorie and protein intake in, 71
crop yields in, 116–117
food supplies of
animal protein in, 145
calories, total protein, and animal protein in, 148
milk, meat, eggs, and fish in, 150
total protein and proportions of animal and plant protein in, 149
Mali
food supplies of
animal protein in, 149
calories, total protein and animal protein in, 148
milk, meat, eggs, and fish in, 150
total protein and proportions of animal and plant protein in, 149
Malic acid, in foods, 186
Malnutrition
as associated cause of death in children in Latin America, 2–3
as underlying cause of death in children in Latin America, 2–3
degree of, 5
difficulties and limitations encountered in identification of, 1
in affluent countries, 190
intermediate form of, infant mortality due to, 3
lack of concern by governments for, 276
livestock losses due to, 135
moderate forms of, 2
nutritional structure of diet in, 67
severe form of, 2
Malta, crop yields in, 114–115
Manatee, as source of human food, 198
Manganese
application of, to soil, 211
in grasses, breeding against toxic levels, 211
in soil, availability of, effect of pH on, 96
requirement by plants, 93
requirement, effect of metal-binding constituents on, 234
Manganese uptake, by plants, effect of lime on, 211
Manioc flour, protein quality of, with and without methionine addition mixed with beans, 266
Manure
reliance of agriculture on, in Europe, 49
use of, in corn production, 92
Manure crops, green, use of, in crop production, 92
Marasmus, 2, 7
in community surveys, prevalence of, 9
in Latin America, 4, 5
infant mortality due to, 3
symptoms of, 4
Margarine
consumption of, 30
development of xerophthalmia from, 245
enrichment of, with vitamin A, 266
fortification of
with vitamin A, 243, 244, 245
with vitamin D, 245
Marine animals, as source of human food, 197–198
Market economy, access to, as precondition for food and nutrition policy, 282
Market opportunities, as factor in livestock production, 145
Market system, provision for, and agricultural productivity, 106
Marketing, 284
Martinique, crop yields in, 116–117
Masai, supplementation of, with amino acids, 259
of Kenya
customs of, 151
effect of social structure on animal production in, 136
starvation of, by rinderpest epidemic, 134
Mashona tribe
effect of social structure on animal production in, 136
effect of taboos on consumption of eggs in, 136
Mass selection, use of, in improvement of cross-pollinating species, 105
Mauritania
calorie and protein intake in, 71
crop yields in, 114–115
Mauritius
calorie and protein intake in, 72
crop yields in, 114–115
food supplies of
animal protein in, 149
calories, total protein, and animal protein in, 148
milk, meat, eggs and fish in, 150
total protein and proportions of animal and plant protein in, 149
Meat
acceptability of, factors determining, 224
amounts in food supplies of 90 countries, 150
as source of protein, 127
consumption in different regions of world, 25, 27–28
inhibitory substances in, 186
production of, estimated needs for, by year 2000, 132
Meat flour, optimum level to supplement lime-treated corn, 260
Meat-producing animals
see also Animals, meat-producing
relative potential of, 147–162
Meats, water activity values of, 181, 182
Mediterranean countries, wheat consumption in, 18
Mediterranean flour-moth, food deterioration due to, 187
Melanesia
crude birth rates, crude death rates and gross reproduction rate in, 59
total population and expectation of life in, 57
urban and rural population in, 63
Melanesian people, effect of taboos on consumption of pork in, 135–136
Melon seeds, consumption of, 24
Mesophilic bacteria, temperature relations for growth and survival of, 180
Mesophilic organisms, 179
Metabolizable energy, of cottonseed meal, increase by phatase, 238
Metal-binding constituents, in plant foodstuffs, 234
Methionine
as first limiting amino acid to man, 210

content of beans, 265
content of idli, increase by fermentation, 237
content of soybean, protein heterogeneity of different fractions in, 210
effect on nutritive value of cassava-beans mixture, 266
plant sources of, 201
sulfur supplied by, 95
use of, in formulation of nutritious food products, 257–258
Methionine fortification, 247
of corn-bean diet, 263
Metmyoglobin, formation from myoglobin, 184
Mexico
calorie and protein intake in, 71
crop yields in, 116–117
food supplies of
animal protein in, 149
calories, total protein, and animal protein in, 148
milk, meat, eggs, and fish in, 150
total protein and proportions of animal and plant protein in, 149
Mice
food deterioration due to, 188
in U.S., 188
Microbes, as factor in food spoilage, 177
Microbial protein, use in formulation of new nutritious food products, 254
Micrococous roseus, 182
Micronesia, *see* Polynesia and Micronesia
Micronutrients, requirements by plants, 93, 95
Microorganisms
oxidation-reduction potential favorable for aerobic and anaerobic, 185
role in food production of, 199
temperature relationship for growth and survival of, 180
Microrelief, 206
Midge larvae, as source of human food, 197
Migration
effect on usage of arable soil, 87
from rural to urban areas, 60
Mildew, damage caused by, history of, 163
Milk
amounts in food supplies of 90 countries, 150
as source of protein, 127
consumption in different regions of world, 28–30
enrichment of, with vitamin D, 266
fortification of, with vitamin D, 243, 244, 245
Milk production
estimated need for, by year 2000, 132
impact of commercial dairying on, 50
in developing countries vs. U.S., 153
in major regions, 151
in various regions of world, 130
Milk products
inhibitory substances in, 186
substitute of, use of vegetable protein sources in preparation of, 267
Milk yield, effect of temperature on, 135
Millet, *see also* Cereals
area and production by region, 38–41
consumption in Africa, 19
consumption in different regions of world, 17, 19
targets for yield increases in, 124
world area and production of, 36
yield increase compared to farmed area increase by region, 111
yields
and yield increases by region, 112
potential, 121
"Milpa" system of primitive agriculture, 92
Mineral deficiency, of soil, as restraint in animal production, 133
Mineral fortification
of corn-bean diet, 262
of food, 261
of tortilla flour, 262
Minerals
effect on protein quality of corn, 255, 263
in foods, 185–186
sources of, 191
use of, in formulation of nutritious food products, 257–258
Miso, 236
Mites
food deterioration due to, 187
wastage of food due to, 177
Mixed crop and livestock farming, 49
Moisture, as factor in food spoilage, 185
Moko disease, of bananas, 168–169
Molasses, use in livestock industry, 140
Molds
as source of vitamin B_{12}, 191
growth of
effect of pH on, 179
effect of temperature on, 179
effect of water activity on, 183, 184
temperature relations for growth and survival of, 180
Molybdenum
application of, to soil, 211
in soil, availability of, effect of pH on, 96
requirement by plants, 93
uptake by plants, effect of irrigation on, 212
Mongolia, crop yields in, 116–117
Monocultures, 118
Morocco
crop yields in, 114–115
damage caused by bayoud disease of date palm in, 168
food supplies of
animal protein in, 149
calories, total protein, and animal protein in, 148
milk, meat, eggs, and fish in, 150
total protein and proportions of animal and plant protein in, 149
locust feeding on grasses during invasion in, 170
Mortality
due to anemia, 8
of children in Latin America, due to nutritional deficiency, 3
Mortality rates, of children, as indicator of nutritional state, 2
Mozambique
calorie and protein intake in, 72
crop yields in, 114–115
food supplies of
animal protein in, 149
calories, total protein, and animal protein in, 148

milk, meat, eggs, and fish in, 150
total protein and proportions of animal and plant protein in, 149
MPF, ingredient composition of, 257
Mulch, use of crop residues in, 99
Musa, disease of, 168–169
Muscle
distribution of
in various breeds of cattle, 219
in various breeds of sheep, 219
skeletal, constancy of, 222
weight, in various breeds of animals, in relation to other tissues, 219
Muscle-bone ratio, in livestock, constancy of, 222
Muslims, taboos of, effect on consumption of pork, 135
Mussels, as source of human food, 197
Mutation breeding, of cereals, 211
Mutton
and lamb, consumption of, 27, 28
production and consumption
in Europe, 157
in Far East, 159
in Latin America, 159
in North America, 158
in Oceania, 158
Mycoplasma, as factor in coconut disease, 167
Myoglobin
formation of metmyoglobin from, 184
reaction with nitric oxide, 184

N

Nagana, effect on animal production, 134
Nairobi sheep disease, 134
Namibia
calorie and protein intake in, 71
crop yields in, 114–115
National development plans, integration of food and nutrition policy with, 285
Natto, 236
essential amino acids in increase by fermentation, 237
Natural selection, of cattle, 141
Near East
arable land and population of, 43
cereal consumption in, 17
crop yield increase compared to farmed area increase in 1950 and 1970, 111
crop yields in 1950 and 1970, 112
crude productivity of cattle and buffalo in, 130
crude productivity of pigs in, 130
farm animal population in, 129
land in, major uses of, 43
losses caused in agriculture by locust, 170–171
mean productivity of farm livestock in, 128
potential for increases in animal production in, 160
production of major food crops in, 39, 41
solar radiation in, 120
starchy food consumption in, 21
targets for crop yield increases between 1962 and 1985, 124
Nepal
calorie, total protein, and animal protein intake in, 71
cretinism in, 10
crop yields in, 116–117
Nerve impulse, transmission of, interference of choline esterase inhibitor with, 234
Net protein retention, 208
Net protein utilization, 208
Netherlands
crop yields in, 114–115
food supplies of
animal production in, 149
calories, total protein, and animal protein in, 148
milk, meat, eggs, and fish in, 150
total protein and proportions of animal and plant protein in, 149
Netherlands Antilles, crop yields in, 116–117
Neurolathyrogens, in plant foodstuffs, 233
Neurotoxic effects, of neurolathyrogens, 233
New Caledon, crop yields in, 116–117
Newcastle disease, 133
New Guinea, crop yields in, 116–117
New Zealand, *see also* Australia and New Zealand
cobalt and selenium deficiency disease in cattle in, 133
crop yields in, 116–117
food supplies in
animal protein in, 149
calorie, total protein, and animal protein in, 148
milk, meat, eggs, and fish in, 150
total protein and proportions of animal and plant protein in, 148
livestock deficiency diseases in, on mineral deficient soils, 133
meat production in, 158
Niacin
availability in corn, increase by alkali treatment, 236
content of soybean milk increase by alkaline treatment, 235
low intake in developing countries, 252
Niacin deficiency, 246
Niacin fortification, 244, 245
in U.S., 246
of food, 261
of tortilla flour, 262
of white flour, 245
Nicaragua
calorie and protein intake in, 71
crop yields in, 116–117
food supplies of
animal protein in, 149
calories, total protein, and animal protein in, 148
milk, meat, eggs, and fish in, 150
total protein and proportions of animal and plant protein in, 149
Niger
calorie and protein intake in, 71
crop yields in, 114–115
Nigeria
calorie and protein intake in, 71
crop yields in, 114–115
food supplies of
animal protein in, 149
calories, total protein, and animal protein in, 148
milk, meat, eggs, and fish in, 150
total protein and proportions of animal and plant

protein in, 149
kwashiorkor and marasmus in children in, prevalence of, 9
Nitrate reductase activity
effect of 2,4-dichlorophenoxyacetic acid on, 212
effect of Simazine on, 212
in bluegrass, 206
in corn, relation to corn yields, 204
Nitrate, utilization by plants, 93
Nitric oxide, in foods, 184
Nitrite burn, 184
Nitrogen
atmospheric, use of, by legumes, 93
content of barley, effect of nitrogen on, 204
content of soil organic matter, 95
effect on nitrogen composition of barley, 204
food, sources of, 193
in soils
availability of, effect of pH on, 96
content and availability of, 93
use of, by plants, 93
inorganic, conversion by microorganisms to protein, 199
losses of, under "Milpa" system of primitive agriculture, 92
nonprotein, use in pastoral farming, 140
organic, mineralization of, 93
requirement by plants, 93
threshold optimum level of, existence in grain, 204
Nitrogen balance, effect of calorie intake on, 67
Nitrogen balance index, 208
Nitrogen deficiency
of plants, 93
of plants, symptoms of, 97
Nitrogen fertilizer, effect on protein content of wheat, 209
Nitrogen fixation, 206
Nitrosohemochromogen, 184
Nitrosomyoglobin, 184
Nomadism, 140
Nonruminants, wastes and by-products for feeding, 197
North Africa
fluorine poisoning of cattle in, 133
rickets in, 10
North America
animal production in, 151
area sown with wheat and corn, 110
birth rate, death rate, and reproduction rate for 1965 and 2000, 59
cereal consumption in, 17
consumption of pulses, nuts, and seeds, 23
crop yield increase, compared to farmed area increase in 1950 and 1970, 111
crop yields, and crop yield increases in 1950 and 1970, 116–117
crop yields in 1950 and 1970, 112
crude productivity of cattle and buffalo in, 130
crude productivity of pigs in, 130
farm animal population, 129
mean productivity of farm livestock in, 128
population and expectation of life for 1960 and 2000, 57
population growth in, 110
population of, urban and rural, 62
potential for increases of animal production in, 158
selenium poisoning of livestock in, 133
solar radiation in, 120
starchy food consumption in, 21
Norway
crop yields in, 114–115
food supplies of
animal protein in, 149
calories, total protein, and animal protein in, 148
milk, meat, eggs, and fish in, 150
total protein and proportions of animal and plant protein in, 149
Nutrients
absorption of, interference of hemagglutinins with, 233
availability of, effect on crop products, 113, 118
in soil, availability of, effect of pH on, 96
fortification of foods with
calcium, 247
experience in, 244–247
general, 244
iodine, 246
iron, 246
protein and amino acid, 247
thiamine, riboflavin, and niacin, 246
vitamin C, 246
vitamin D, 244–245
from plant foodstuffs, increased availability through processing, 231–241
in foods, 185–186
in soil, availability of
effect of organic matter on, 95
effect of pH on, 96
main sources of, 252
Nutrimetric model
scheme of, 280
use of, in formulation of food and nutrition policy, 278
Nutrimetrics, 276
Nutrition, and food policy, *see* Food and nutrition policy
Nutrition
effect on body composition of livestock, 221–224
in developed countries, problems of, 280
knowledge of, dependence of food and nutrition policy on, 284
world
state of, 1–13
beriberi, 11
death rates due to malnutrition, 2–3
endemic goiter and cretinism, 10
nutritional anemias, 7–8
pellagra, 10
protein-calorie malnutrition, 3–7
rickets and osteomalacia, 10–11
scurvy, 10
trends in age-specific death rates, 2
xerophthalmia, 8–9
Nutrition systems analysis, 285
Nutritional anemias, *see* Anemias, nutritional
Nutritional deficiency
in children in Latin America, pattern of, 3–5
poverty as primary cause of, 276
Nutritional marasmus, *see* Marasmus
Nutritional quality, of foods and feeds of plant origin, 207–209

Nutritional requirements
analysis of, based on food consumption surveys, 279
of farm livestock, research in developed countries on, 139
Nutritional status, of plants, role of field experiments to evaluate, 97
Nutritious food, definition of, 254
Nutritious foods
formulation of
available source for, 252–254
factors affecting, 252
objectives of, 254–256
role in, 269–270
Nutritious food products
applications, 256–267
available sources of, 252–254
formulation of, 251–274
objectives of development of, 254–255
processing, 267–268
role of genetics on development of, 269–270
significance and role of, 270–271
textured vegetable protein foods, 268–269
Nutritious fortified foods, development of, 244
Nuts
consumption of, 22
use in formulation of new nutritious food products, 253

O

Oats
area and production by region, 38–41
consumption in different regions of world, 17, 19
high nitrogen varieties, 193
world area and production of, 36
yields and yield increases by region, 112
Oceania
arable land and population of, 43
cereal consumption in, 17
crop yield increase, compared to farmed area increase in 1950 and 1970, 111
crop yields in 1950 and 1970, 112
crude birth rate, crude death rate, and gross reproduction rate for 1965 and 2000, 59
crude productivity of cattle and buffalo, 130
crude productivity of pigs, 130
farm animal population in, 129
land in, major uses of, 43
population and expectation of life for 1960 and 2000
potential for increases of animal production in, 158
in, 57
production of major food crops in, 39, 41
productivity of farm livestock in, 128
solar radiation in, 120
starchy food consumption in, 21
urban and rural population of, 63
Odor, absorption by foods during storage, 179
OECD, 16, 24, 25
Oil crops
arable land used for production of, 37
production by region, 38–41
world area and production of, 36
Oil seeds
antinutritional factors in, 233–234
formulation of high-protein food products based on, 253, 256
genetic improvement of, 270
oleic acid content of, effect of genetics on, 270
preparation of highly nutritious foods from, 267
preparation of protein isolates from, 268
preparation of textured vegetable protein foods from, 268
residues of, use in livestock industry, 140
yielding a protein residue, world production of, 196
Oils, consumption of, 30–31
Oleic acid, content in oil seeds, effect of genetics on, 270
Oligosaccharides
as causative factors of flatulence, 235
in plant foodstuffs, 234
in soy products, as causative factors of flatulence, 237
Olive oil, consumption of, 31
Opaque-2 corn, 209
comparison between protein value and amino acid intake of, 255
nutritive value of, 269–270
replacement of corn with, 265
Orange, metal-binding constituents in, 234
Organic chemicals, increase availability of nutrients in plant foodstuffs by treatment with, 236
Organic matter, soil
definition of, 95
effect in soil tilth, 95–96
influence on availability of micronutrients, 95
Organic solvents, increased availability of nutrients from plant foodstuffs by use of, 236
Ornithosis, transmitted by birds, 188
Oryza sativa, 211
Osteolathyrogens, in plant foodstuff, 233
Osteomalacia, 10–11
Osteoporosis, prevention of, 247
Overnutrition, 11, 16
Oxalic acid
in foods, 186
in plant foodstuffs, 233
in rhubarb and spinach, leaching out of, 235
Oxidation-reduction potential
condition for aerobic and anaerobic organisms, 184–185
definition of, 184
of various foods, 184–185
Oxidation-reduction reactions, 184
Oxidative deterioration, in frozen foods, 178
Oxygen tension, as factor in food spoilage, 184–185

P

Pacific Islands
crop yields in, 116–117
Pingalap disease of breadfruit in, 166–167
Pakistan
calorie, total protein, and animal protein intake in, 71
crop yields in, 116–117
food supplies of

animal protein in, 149
calories, total protein, and animal protein in, 148
milk, meat, eggs, and fish in, 150
total protein and proportions of animal and plant protein in, 149
kwashiorkor and marasmus in children in, prevalence of, 9
wheat consumption in, 19
Palm kernel, use in formulation of new nutritious food products, 253
Palm oil, consumption of, 31
Panama
calorie and protein intake in, 71
crop yields in, 116–117
food supplies of
animal protein in, 149
calories, total protein, and animal protein, 148
milk, meat, eggs, and fish in, 150
total protein and proportions of animal and plant protein in, 149
kwashiorkor and marasmus in children in, prevalence of, 9
Pan-American Foot and Mouth Disease Commission (FAO), 137
Pan American Health Organization, 2, 3, 4, 5
policy on food fortification by, 244
Panicum miliaceum, 118, 210
Papua, crop yields in, 116–117
Paraguay
calorie and protein intake in, 72
crop yields in, 116–117
food supplies of
animal protein in, 149
calories, total protein, and animal protein in, 148
milk, meat, eggs, and fish in, 150
total protein and proportions of animal and plant protein in, 149
Parasitic diseases
as restraint on animal production, 135
control of, 138–139
Parasitic nematodes, effect of temperature on, 135
Particle size, of food, effect on digestibility, 234
Paspalum sp., 210
Pasteurellosis, in livestock, 138
Pastoral farming, 131, 140–141
Pastoral life, in Old World vs. New World, 135
Pastoral people, effect of social structure on animal production in, 136
Pasture improvement, 140
Peaches, ascorbic acid oxidase in, 233
Peanut flour, in nutritious food products, 257–258
Peanut protein isolate, milk products substitutes made from, 267
Pear decline disease, losses caused by, 165
Pearl millet
lysine content of, 210
nutritive value of, 210
prolamine content of, effect of nitrogen fertilizer on, 211
Pellagra
due to niacin deficiency, 246
in developing countries, 246
prevalence of, 10
Pennisetum typhoides, 210, 211
Peroxidase, darkening of fruits due to, 184
Peru
calorie and protein intake in, 71
crop yields in, 116–117
food supplies of
animal protein in, 149
calories, total protein, and animal protein in, 148
milk, meat, eggs, and fish in, 150
total protein and proportions of animal and plant protein in, 149
Pest control
alternative approaches to, 174
effect on crop yields, 118
horizontal resistance, 175
integrated approach to, 175
strategies for effective, 169–174
Pesticides
availability of, and crop production, 106
undesirable effects of, 175
Pests
damage caused to crops by, 163
food deterioration due to, 187–188
post-harvest food losses due to, 187–188
pH, of soil
importance of, 96
influence on availability to plants of micronutrients, 95, 96
pH value of foods, 181
Phaseolus, 195
as source of food protein, 195
Phaseolus aureus, 211
Phaseolus mungo, 237
Phaseolus vulgaris, 265
Phenanthridinium compounds, as prophylactics against trypanosomiasis, 138
Phenolic compounds, in foods, 186
Philippines
beriberi in, 11
cadang-cadang disease of coconut in, 167
calorie and protein intake in, 71
coconut diseases losses in, 167
crop yields in, 116–117
food supplies of
animal protein in, 149
calories, total protein, and animal protein in, 148
milk, meat, eggs, and fish in, 150
total protein and proportions of animal and plant protein in, 149
Phoenix dactylifera L., 167
Phosphate fertilizer, effect on uptake by plants of trace elements, 211
effect on yield of soybean forage and phosphate concentration in forage, 208
Phosphorous, in soils
availability of, 94
effect of pH on, 96
content and availability of, 93
Phosphorus content
of corn, genetic control, 211
of lespedeza hay, effect of lime on, 208
of plants, relation to available supply of phosphorus and crop yield, 93

of soil organic matter, 95
of soybean forage, effect of phosphate fertilizer on, 208
Phosphorus deficiency
of plants, symptoms of, 94
of soil
as restraint on animal production, 133
improvement of pastoral farming by correcting, 140
Phosphorus requirement, by plants, 93
Photosynthetic efficiency
effect on crop yields, 118
maximum gross, 120
maximum net, 120
of plants, two categories of, 118
Photosynthetic efficient crops, 118, 122
Physical factors, food deterioration due to, 177
Physiological components, of crop yield, 205
Phytase, mold, increase in metabolizable energy of cottonseed meal by, 238
Phytic acid
in bread, hydrolysis by yeast, 237
in plant foodstuffs, 233
Phytohemagglutinins, of legumes, 232
Pig
adipose tissue in, effect of diet on, 225
as efficient food converter, 154
body composition of, 217, 218
effect of energy and protein intake on, 224
effect of sex differences on, 221
breeds, with ability to convert carbohydrate into fat, 215
chemical composition of
at successive stages during postnatal life, 217
during prenatal life, 216
effect of disease on production of, 133–135
effect of energy value of diet on muscle growth, 224
industry, intensive, in developed countries, 139
population, in major regions of world, 129
productivity of
by world regions, 130
in Far East, 129
in terms of daily production of protein per person, 128
proportion of body tissues in, breed differences, 220
Pigeon, food deterioration due to, 188
Pigeon peas
consumption of, 24
yields and yield increases by region, 112
Pingalap disease, of breadfruit, 166–167
Pisum, 195
Planning, in food and nutrition, lack of, 276
Plant breeding, 103–106
effect on crop yields, 119
for horizontal resistance to control plant diseases, 175
in control of plant diseases, 102
in cross-pollinating species, 104–105
in self-pollinating species, 103–104
of tomatoes, increase in carotene content by, 210
of wheat, increase in protein content by, 209
Plant cytokinins, regulation of size of barley grain by, 210
Plant density, optimum, variables involved in, 101
Plant diseases
control of, 102–103
progress in therapy of, 102
Plant foods and feeds, nutritional quality of, 207–209
Plant foodstuffs
antinutritional factors in, 233–234
increased availability of nutrients through processing from, 231–241
Plant germ plasm, sources of, useful for human food, 208
Plant lice, food deterioration due to, 187
Plant nutrients
classification of, 93
lack of, low yields due to, 113
supply of, in soil management, 84
Plant nutrition, 203–214
Plant parasitic nematodes, yearly losses caused by, 165
Plant pathogens, adaptation to local environment and increased infectivity of, 102
Plant pathogens, control of, 102
Plant pathogens, eradication of, 102
Plant pathology, 102–103
Plant production *see* Crop production
Plant production, future of, 174–175
Plant protection, programs in Japan, factors responsible for success of, 174
Plant protection, strategy developed in Japan, 172–174
Plant protein
and animal protein in food supplies of 90 countries, 149
digestibility of, enhancement by enzyme treatment, 238
extractability of, enhancement by enzymes, 238
production in Latin America, 154
Plantain, 168
consumption in different regions of world, 21, 22
Plantation agriculture, in U.S., transformation of, 49
Plantation crops, 49
Plantations, role in food production, 48–49
Planting, time of, effect on crop yield, 100
Plants
and animals, as food sources for man, 130–132
chemical analyses of, estimation of fertilizer requirements and response by, 97
deficiency in minerals, as restraint on animal production, 133
edible
as source of protein, 193–195
seeds, 193–195
underground parts, 195
vegetables, 193
element composition of, 203–205
element composition of, as indicator of element availability to plant roots, 204
inhibitory substances in, 186–187
nutrient composition of, improving, 203–214
nutrient deficiencies of, characteristic symptoms of, 97
nutrients in
increased availability through processing, 231–232
chemical methods, 235–236
enzymatic methods, 236–238
future outlook, 238
physical methods, 232–235
Plants, nutritional quality of, improving, 203–214
Plants, nutritional status of, 203–205
indicators of, 97
Plants, nutritive composition of
element composition and, 203–205

improving of, 209–212
nutritional quality of plants, 207–209
soil and other site factors in relation to, 205–207
protein content of, effect of herbicides on, 212
nutritive requirement of, 92
species used in feeding people, 208
tissue analysis of, as criterion in defining mineral needs and soil management practice required for growth and yield of specific crops, 205
unconventional photosynthesis, as source of human food, 198–199
Plastein reaction, 237
Plinthite, 88
Poa pratensis L., 206
Poland
crop yields in, 114–115
food supplies of
animal protein in, 149
calories, total protein, and animal protein in, 148
milk, meat, eggs, and fish in, 150
total protein and proportions of animal and plant protein in, 149
Policies
agricultural, affecting progress in animal production, 144–145
food and nutrition, *see also* Food and nutrition policy
food and nutrition, 76–77
need for, 275–286
Political factors, effect on livestock production, 144
Politician, role of, in formulation of food and nutrition policy, 277
Pollution, effect on food chain, need for legislative measures on, 285
Polynesia and Micronesia
crude birth rates, death rates, and gross reproduction rates in, 59
total population and expectation of life in, 57
urban and rural population in, 63
Population
age structure of, in less developed vs. more developed regions, 60, 61
and arable land by world regions, 43
farm animal vs. human in various regions of world, 129
growth
aggregate rate of, in developing countries, 64
in developing countries, compared to food production, 276
in the 1960's in relation to world agriculture, 276
world, and future food trends, 55–77
growth rate
during 19th century, 56
in future, 56
in various regions, 56
since 1950, 56
humans vs. farm animal population in various regions of world, 129
in India, Indonesia, Pakistan, and China from 1965 to 1985, 60
in major regions of world for 1960 to 2000, 57
projections of, based on household budget surveys, 279
rural, number and rate of growth for 1960 to 2000, 62–63
rural tropics, poor nutritional status of, 191
steady-state, definition of, 60
urban, number and rate of growth for 1960 to 2000, 62–63
vulnerable groups, 252
world, 109
in 1970 and 2000, 55
rate of growth in 19th century, 110
rate of growth up to 19th century, 110
Population density, of plants, effect on crop yield, 101–102
Population improvement, in crops, 105–106
Pork
consumption of, 27, 28
effect of taboos on consumption of
in Melanesia, 136
on Muslims and Jews, 135
production and consumption
in Africa, 160
in Europe, 157
in Far East, 159
in Latin America, 159
in North America, 158
in Oceania, 158
Port Guinea, crop yields in, 114–115
Port Timor, crop yields in, 116–117
Portugal
crop yields in, 114–115
food supplies of
animal protein in, 149
calories, total protein, and animal protein in, 148
milk, meat, eggs, and fish in, 150
total protein and proportions of animal and plant protein in, 149
Potassium
accumulation in corn, 94
deficiency in plants, 94
in soil
availability of, effect of pH on, 96
content and availability of, 94
interaction of magnesium with, importance in plants and animal nutrition, 94
requirement by plants, 94
uptake by plants, effect of lime on, 211
Potato blight, epidemic of 1845–46, 164
Potato mosaic virus, economic losses caused by, 165
Potato production, effect of potato latent mosaic virus on, 165
Potato protein, biological value of, 208
Potatoes
see also Root crops
area and production by region, 38–41
as causative factor in scurvy, 10
as source of food protein, 195
average yield in U.S., 104
consumption in different regions of world, 20–22
inhibitors in "green," 187
world area and production of, 36
yield increase compared to farmed area increase by region, 111
yields
and yield increases by country, 114, 116
and yield increases by region, 112
potential, 121

realized record of, 122
Poultry
adipose tissue in, effect of diet on, 225
as efficient converters of cereals to human food, 139
as efficient food converters, 154
body composition of, 218
constancy of muscle-bone ratio in, 222
consumption of, 27, 28
effect of disease on production of, 133–135
genetically superior breeds, distribution of, 143
inhibitory substances in, 186
population of, in major regions of world, 129
Poultry industry
in developed countries, 139
in developing countries, 139
Poultry production
and consumption
in Africa, 160–161
in Far East, 159
in Latin America, 159
in Near East, 160
effect of temperature on, 135
environmental control in, 143
Poverty
as cause of malnutrition, 190
as cause of nutritional deficiencies, 276
Precipitation, lack of, and low yields, 42
Pregnancy
anemias of, due to folate deficiency, 247
folate deficiency during, 8
Price
of food, increased disparities in food consumption between socioeconomic groups due to higher, 277
of food, relation to hunger and future food policy, 75–76
Price ratios, input-output, effect on crop yields, 119
Price stabilization, as factor in implementation of food and nutrition policies, 284
Processed vegetables, consumption of, 25
Processing, plants requiring, 195
Processing industries, in developing countries, 282
Prolamine
content of
cereal grains, reduction of, 210
pearl millet, effect of nitrogen fertilizer on, 211
Pro Nutro, ingredient composition of, 257
Protease inhibitors, 232
in plant foodstuffs, 233
Protein
availability of, increase by heat treatment, 232
daily requirement of, 109
food, plants and animals as source of, 130–131
from unconventional sources of food, 192
gap of, emphasis on, 276
high quality, livestock as source of, 215
indigestible, in plants, 195
Protein, intake
effect on energy production, 70
effect on nitrogen balance at different level of calorie intake, 67–70
in developing regions of world, 71–72
plant
concentration of, 195
conversion to animal protein by animals, 196–198
situation, analysis of, and food and nutrition policy, 282–283
sources of food, in developed vs. developing countries, 271
total amounts and proportions of animal and plant protein in food supplies of 90 countries, 149
total amounts in national food supplies of 90 countries, 148
Protein Advisory Group (UN), 192
policy on food fortification by, 244
statement on amino acid fortification by, 247
Protein-calorie malnutrition
associated with xerophthalmia, 9
definition of, 3–4
five forms of, 4
in community surveys, pattern of, 7
moderate, prevalence of, 6
prevalence of, 4–7
in 3 continents, 6
severe, prevalence of, 6
Protein concentrates, 195
fortification of cereal-based foods with, 247
fortification of cereals with, 259
fortification of corn with, plus amino acids, 260, 261
fortification of food with, 259–260
plus amino acids, 260
fortification of lime-treated corn and rice with, 260
content
of carcass, of Holstein steers, 217
of cereal crops, inverse relation between grain yield and, 209
of cereals, increase by fortification with protein concentrate, 259
of grain, inverse relation between yield and, 204
of livestock
effect of nutrition on, 223
species differences in, 217
of pig during prenatal and postnatal stages of life, 216, 217
of plants, effect of herbicides on, 212
of poultry, 218
of rice varieties, effect of environmental factors on, 210
of sheep, breed differences in, 220
of wheat, effect of fertilizers on, 209
of wheat cultivars, effect of environmental vs. genetic factors on, 210
Protein deficiency, role of calorie deficiency in, 70
Protein digestibility, interference of protease inhibitors with, 233
Protein dispersibility index, 232
Protein efficiency ratio, 208
of cassava bean mixture supplemented with methionine, 266
of corn and rice supplemented with protein concentrates, 260
of fortified beans and of corn-bean diets, 263
of fortified corn-bean diet, 262
of fortified tortilla flour, 262
of lime-treated corn flour replaced with wheat short, 264

of lime-treated corn supplemented with amino acids, 259
of manioc flour with and without methionine addition mixed with beans, 266
of selected high protein-containing foods, 257–258
Protein fortification, 247
Protein malnutrition, population groups susceptible to, 256
Protein needs of people, contribution of farm livestock to, 130
Protein production
daily, from farm livestock, 128
efficiency of, from various meat-producing animals, 219
Protein quality
of carcass, livestock, 224
of corn, effect of vitamins and minerals on, 255, 263
of foods, as problem in developing countries, 252
of foods, evaluation of, 208
of some high protein-containing foods, 256
of soybean textured food, 269
Protein requirements, 67, 192
effect of gossypol on, 233
reference, in developing regions of world, 68–69
Protein-rich foods
animal products as source of, 127
use of, for relief of malnutrition, 244
Protein utilization, interference of fiber with, 232
Proteins
from plants, 191
in foods, 185–186
possible sources of, 192–201
unconventional, sources of, 192–200
edible plants, 193–195
microbial conversions, 199–200
plant products requiring processing, 195–198
synthesis, 200
unconventional photosynthetic plants, 198–199
Proteolysis, enzymatic, 237
Proteolytic enzymes
destruction of lipoxygenase in soybeans by, 237
increased availability of amino acids from plant foodstuffs by, 237
Pseudomonas, 182
effect of temperature on, 179
Pseudomonas solanacearum, Moko disease of bananas, caused by, 169
Psychroduric bacteria, temperature relations for growth and survival of, 180
Psychrophilic organisms, 179
Public health measures, decline in mortality of children due to, 2
Public health significance, of nutritional anemia, 8
Puccinia graminis f. sp. *tritici,* 169
Puerto Rico
calorie and protein intake in, 72
crop yields in, 116–117
Pulses
antinutritional factors in, 233–234
arable land used for production of, 37
consumption in different regions of world, 22–24
production by regions, 38–41
production of edible dry matter by, 119
targets for yield increases in, 124
world area and production of, 36

Q

Quantity income elasticity
computation of, 72
for selected commodities, 74
Quarantine measures, to control plant diseases, 102
Queensland, pastoral cattle farming in, 140, 141
Quinapyramine salts, as prophylactic against trypanosomiasis, 138
Quinoa, use as human food, 195

R

Rabies, paralytic, in cattle, 133
Rachitogenic foods, 187
Radiation, available for photosynthesis, 120
Raffinose
as causative factor of flatulence, 235, 237
in plant foodstuffs, 234
Rainfall
areas of limited, water management practices in, 98
effect on crop yields, 118
seasonal, as restraint on animal production, 133
Ranching, 156
Rancidity, susceptibility of fat-containing animal products to, 179
Range land, in Near East, 160
Rapeseed
varieties low in erucic acid and glucosinolate, 270
world production of, 196
Rats, food deterioration due to, 188
Red Sindhi cattle, 142
cross with European breeds, 142
Reference man, 64, 65
Reference protein, 67
and calorie requirements, in developing regions of world, 68–69
Reference protein standards, at given age, 70
Refuse, town, use of, in food fermentation, 199
Relative humidities, and storage temperatures of commodities susceptible to cold injury when improperly stored, 183
Religious beliefs
effect on animal production, 136
effect on food consumption, 151
Religious customs, effect on food consumption, 16
Reproduction rate, gross, in major regions of world for 1965 to 2000, 58–59
Research information, and agricultural productivity, 107
Respiration, magnitude of, 120
Restoration, of nutrients in foods, 264
Reunion, crop yields in, 114–115
Rhizopus oligosporus, use in food fermentation, 237
Rhizopus, use in fermentation of beans, 236
Rhodesia
calorie and protein intake in, 72
crop yields in, 114
Riboflavin, low intake in developing countries, 252

Riboflavin deficiency, in developing countries, 246
Riboflavin fortification, 245
of bread, 244
of food, 261
of tortilla flour, 262
Rice
see also Cereals
area and production by region, 38–41
as causative factor in beriberi, 11
average yield in U.S., 104
calculation of potential yield of, 120
consumption in different regions of world, 17, 18
diets, low thiamine content of, 246
fortification of
with protein concentrates, 260
with thiamine, 246
genetic improvement of, 210
maximum photosynthetic efficiency of, 120
parboiling of, effect on thiamin retention, 235
use of herbicides and helicopters in Japan for controlling pests and diseases affecting, 173
varieties, protein content of, effect of environmental factors on, 210
world area and production, 36
yields
and yield increases by country in 1950 and 1970, 114, 116
and yield increases by region, 112
increase in
compared to farmed area increase by region, 111
by use of fertilizer, 118
potential, at different latitudes and different seasons, 121
realized record of, 122
targets for increases in, 124
Rice production
in Japan
and major causes of yield reduction over 40-year period, 173
effect of plant protection measures on, 173–174
Rice protein concentrate, preparation of, 195
Rickets, 10–11
in developing countries, 245
prevalence of, 10
prevention of, 243
with vitamin D enriched milk, 266
Rift Valley fever, 134
Rinderpest, 151
control of, 137–138
epidemic in Africa, 134
vaccination against, 137
Ring vaccination, against foot-and-mouth disease, 137
RNA synthesis, interference by casein with, 233
Robigalia, 164
Rodent damage, food losses due to, 141
Rodents, food deterioration due to, 188
Romania
crop yields in, 114–115
food supplies of
animal protein in, 149
calories, total protein, and animal protein in, 148
milk, meat, eggs, and fish in, 150
total protein and proportions of animal and plant protein in, 149
Root crops
antinutritional factors in, 233–234
as source of calories, 109
edible dry matter produced by, 119
use in formulation of new nutritious food products, 253
yield increases by region in 1950 and 1970, 112
yields
and yield increases, by country in 1950 and 1970, 114–117
increase in, compared to farmed area increase in 1950 and 1970, 111
potential and target, in temperate regions and in tropics, 121
Root growth, effect of hard-pan on, 99
Rose clover, relation between yield and magnesium concentration, 204
Rothamsted, leaf protein production at, 196
Ruminant production, factors limiting, 155
Ruminants
effect of disease on production of, 133–135
fatty acid composition of, 225
use of wastes and by-products for feeding, 197
Rural population, *see* Population, rural
Rust, history of, 163–164
Rwanda
calorie and protein intake in, 72
consumption of plantains and bananas in, 22
crop yields in, 114–115
food supplies of
animal protein in, 149
calories, total protein, and animal protein in, 148
milk, meat, eggs, and fish in, 150
total protein and proportions of animal and plant protein in, 149
kwashiorkor and marasmus in, prevalence of, 9
Rye
area and production by region, 38–41
consumption in different regions of world, 17, 19
world area and production of, 36
yield and yield increases by region, 112
Ryukyu Islands, crop yields in, 116–117

S

Sabah
calorie and protein intake in, 71
crop yields in, 116–117
Saccharum officinarum L., 205
Safflower, genetic improvement of, 270
Sahara, Bayoud disease of date palm in, 167–168
Sahiwal cattle, 142
Salicylic acid, in foods, 186
Salmonella, 180
growth of, effect of pH on, 179
Salmonellosis, transmitted by birds, 188
Salt
enrichment with iodine, 266
enrichment with iron, 266, 267

fortification of, with iodine, 243
iodization of, first efforts, 246
Saudi Arabia
calorie and protein intake in, 71
crop yields in, 116–117
food supplies of
animal protein in, 149
calories, total protein, and animal protein in, 148
milk, meat, eggs, and fish in, 150
total protein and proportions of animal and plant protein in, 149
Santa Gertrudis, breed of cattle, 141
São Tomé and Principe, crop yields in, 114–115
Sarawak,
calorie and protein intake in, 71
crop yields in, 116–117
Saw-toothed grain beetle, food deterioration due to, 187
Schistocerca gregaria, 170
Scurvy, occurrence of, 10
Sea water, desalinization of, 47, 87
Season, effect on nitrogen composition of plants, 204
Seasonal labor, availability of, and crop production, 106–107
Seed production and distribution, adequacy of, and crop production, 106
Seed proteins
fractionation of, into fractions of superior nutritive value, 234
nutritive value of, beneficial effect of heat treatment on, 232
Seeds
as source of food protein, 193
consumption of, 22–24
Selenium
effect on selenium content of plants, 211
soil deficiency of, as restraint on animal production, 33
uptake by plants, effect of sulfate on, 212
Selenium deficiency
in cattle, 133
of soils, 211
Selenium poisoning, in livestock, 133
Self-pollinating species, improvement of, plant breeding practices in, 103–104
Senegal
calorie and protein intake in, 71
crop yields in, 114–115
PCM in, 8
Sesame, world production of, 196
Sesame meal, metal binding constituents in, 234
Sesame seeds, consumption of, 24
Setaria italica, 118
Setaria sp., 210
Sex differences, effect on body composition of livestock, 220–221
Sex hormones, effect on growth and carcass characteristics of livestock, 221
Seychelles, crop yields in, 114–115
Sheep
body composition of, 217–218
breed differences in, 220
constancy of, 222
effect of sex differences on, 220–221
relative effects of age and weight on, 223
fat tailed, prevalence of, 141
haired, prevalence of, 141
muscle distribution in, in various breeds, 219
Sheep and goats
population of, in major regions of world, 129
world productivity of, in terms of daily production of protein per person, 128
Shelter, importance of, for livestock production in severe climates, 143
Shigellae, 180
Sierra Leone
calorie and protein intake in, 71
crop yields in, 114–115
Simazine
effect on enzyme activities of bean leaves, 212
effect on protein content of pea seeds, 212
Singapore,
calorie and protein intake in, 71
crop yields in, 116–117
Skim milk
use of
in nutritious food products, 257–258
optimum level to supplement lime-treated corn and rice, 260
Skim milk powder, 190
fortification of, with vitamin A, 245
Slash and burn system, of primitive agriculture, 92
Social constraints, effect on food production, 276
Social factors
as restraint on livestock production, 144–145
effect on livestock production, 144
Social, religious, and cultural restraints, on livestock production, 135–136
Social structure, effect on animal production, 136
Socioeconomic analysis, as component of a food and nutrition policy, 281–282
Soil
acidity of, effect of calcium, on, 94
addition of trace elements to, 211
arable, effect of migration on usage of, 87
buffering capacity of, effect of organic matter on, 95
effect of climatic factors on, 92
effect on nutrient composition of plants, 205–207
mineral deficiencies of
as restraint on animal production, 133
as restraint on pastoral farming, 140
nature of, effect on crop yields, 113
potentially arable
in various parts of world, 85–86
reason for little use of, 85
water and nutrients supplied by, 92
water holding capacity of, 98
Soil aeration, effect on crop yield, 101
Soil blowing, control of, 85
Soil erosion, control of, 85
Soil inventories, nature of, 206
Soil management, 47
four aspects of, 84
objectives of, 92
use of
in increasing crop yields, 92–99

in fertilizer requirements, 97–98
in organic matter, 95–96
in pH, 96–97
in plant nutrients, 93–95
in water management, 98–99
Soil management practices, in tropical areas, 206
Soil management systems, 206
Soil map
of world, 81–83
uses of, 81–84
Soil quality, and potential cropland, 47
Soil surveys, 81
Soil survey maps, use of, 206
Soil taxonomy, new system of, 81
Soil tilth
effect of organic matter on, 95
effect of tillage on, 99
Soils
acid-sulfate, hazard of, 88
calcium content of, 94
chemical analysis of, estimation of fertilizer requirements and response by, 97
extending area of, to expand farm production, 79–89
fertility of, differences in, 93
lateritic, effect of lime on, 97
organic matter in, 95–96
phosphorous content of, 94
potassium content of, and availability in, 94
selenium deficiency of, 211
structure of, loss due to cultivation, 99
study of, history, 81
world, distribution of orders and principal suborders, 83
Solanine, as cholinesterase inhibitor, 187
Solar radiation, by region, 120
Somalia
calorie and protein intake in, 71
crop yields in, 114–115
food supplies of
animal protein in, 149
calories, total protein, and animal protein in, 148
milk, meat, eggs, and fish in, 150
total protein and proportions of animal and plant protein in, 149
Sorghum, *see also* Cereals
area and production by region, 38–41
as causative factor in pellagra, 10
consumption in Africa, 19
consumption in different regions of world, 17, 19
high nitrogen varieties of, 193
low water requirement of, 113
world area and production of, 36
yield increase compared to farmed area increase, by region, 111
yields
and yield increases by country, 114, 116
and yield increases by region, 112
potential, 121
realized record of, 122
targets for increases, 124
Sorghum shoot fly, crop resistance to, 103
Sorghum vulgare, 211
South Africa
calorie and protein intake in, 71
crop yields in, 114–115
development of Bonsmara breed from indigenous Africander and imported Hereford breeds, 141–142
food supplies of
animal protein in, 149
calories, total protein, and animal protein in, 148
milk, meat, eggs, and fish in, 150
total protein and proportions of animal and plant protein in, 149
PCM in, 8
pellagra in, 10
productivity of beef cattle in, 142
South America
crop yields and crop yield increases in 1950 and 1970 in, 116–117
crude productivity of cattle and buffalo in, 130
crude productivity of pigs, 130
death in cattle caused by rabies, 133
farm animal population in, 129
foot-and-mouth disease in, 134
iron deficiency anemia in, 7
mean productivity of farm livestock in, 128
targets for crop yield increases between 1962 and 1985, 124
wheat consumption in, 19
South Asia
anticipated increase in population, 56
crude birth rates, crude death rates, and gross reproduction rate for 1960 and 2000, 58
population and expectation of life for 1960 and 2000, 57
urban and rural population of, 62
Southeast Asia
eradication of rinderpest in, 137
pasteurellosis of livestock in, 138
Southern Corn Leaf Blight, epidemic of, 165
Soviet Union, *see* U.S.S.R.
Soyacyt, ingredient composition of, 257
Soybean flour
milk products substitutes made from, 267
use of
as protein concentrate, 263
as protein supplement of lime-treated corn and rice, 260
in bread making, 265
in development of high protein foods, 257–258
in nutritious food products, 257–258
Soybean milk, 267
deficiency of sulfur amino acids in, 235
preparation of, 235
improvement in, 268
Soybean products, digestibility of, enhancement by fermentation, 237
Soybean protein
biological value of, 208
sulfur amino acids in, enhancement by "plastein" reaction, 237
Soybean protein isolate
absence of oligosaccharides in, 235

use of, in formulation of infant milk products, 235
Soybean textured food, protein quality of, 269
Soybeans, *see also* Legume crops
Soybeans, 201
antinutritional factors in, 233–234
average yield in U.S., 104
consumption of, 24
fermented, use of, in Far East, 199
genetic improvement of, 270
increase in nutritive value by alkali treatment, 235
lipoxygenase activity of, destruction by proteolytic enzymes, 237
nutritive value of
effect of germination on, 237
effect of heat on, 232
preparation of fermentation products from, 236
raw, lipoxidase in, 187
sprouting of, increase in amino acids due to, 238
world production of, 196
yield increase compared to farmed area increase by region, 111
yields
and yield increases by country, 115, 117
and yield increases by region, 112
potential, 121
realized record, 122
Soy cheese whey protein mixture, 267
Soy flour
consumption of, 23
destruction of trypsin inhibitor by alkali in, 236
nutritive value of, improvement by alkali treatment, 236
Soymilk, oligosaccharides in, hydrolysis by enzymes to reduce flatulence, 237
Spain
crop yields in, 114–115
food supplies of
animal protein in, 149
calories, total protein, and animal protein in, 148
milk, meat, eggs, and fish in, 150
total protein and proportions of animal and plant protein in, 149
Species, animal, differences in body composition of, 217–218
Spirulina, 198
as source of human food, 198
Stability of foods, *see* Foods, stability of
Stachyose
as causative factor in flatulence, 235, 237
in plant foodstuffs, 234
Staphylococci, growth of, effect of pH on, 179
Staphylococcus aureus, 180, 182
growth of, effect of moisture on, 184
Starch, in plant foods, improvement of digestibility of, 238
Starchy foods
consumption in different regions of world, 20–22
world consumption of
cassava, 22
plantains, 23
potatoes, 20–21
sweet potatoes and yams, 21
Starchy roots, *see also* Root crops
arable land used for production of, 37
production by region, 38–41
world area and production of, 36
Starvation, crop pests as factor in bringing about, 166
Steer, body composition of, during postnatal life, 217
Stem rust, resistance in Mexican wheat varieties to, 169
Storage, transportation and marketing, system for, and crop production, 106
Storage life
of foods
effect of anatomical features of commodities on, 185
effect of temperature on, 179
factors, determining, 178
Storage temperature and relative humidities of commodities susceptible to cold injury when improperly stored, 183
Strawberry, nutrient composition of, effect of nitrogen, phosphorus potassium, or magnesium on, 204
Streptococcus lactis, 179
Stress, as factor in evaluation of protein quality, 208
Sudan
calorie and protein intake in, 71
crop losses caused by locust in, 171
crop yields in, 114–115
food supplies of
animal protein in, 149
calories, total protein, and animal protein in, 148
milk, meat, eggs, and fish in, 150
total protein and proportions of animal and plant protein in, 149
PCM in, 8
Sugar
consumption in different regions of world, 31, 32
enrichment of, with vitamin A, 266, 267
fortification of, with vitamin A, 245
production by region, 38–41
world area and production of, 36
Sugar beets
area and production by region, 38–41
world area and production of, 36
Sugar cane, 205
area and production by region, 38–41
maximum photosynthetic efficiency of, 120
molasses derived from, use in livestock feeding, 140
ways of evaluation, its nutritional status, 205
world area and production of, 36
Sulfate, effect on selenium uptake by plants, 212
Sulfur
in soil availability of, effect of pH on, 96
requirement by plants, 93
Sulfur deficiency, of plants, symptoms of, 95, 97
Sulfur requirement, of plants, 95
Sunflower flour, use of, in nutritious food products, 257–258
Sunflower, world production of, 196
Sunlight, intensity of, effect on crop yields, 118
Superamine, ingredient composition of, 257
Surinam
calorie and protein intake in, 71
crop yields in, 116–117
food supplies of

animal protein in, 149
calories, total protein, and animal protein in, 148
milk, meat, eggs, and fish in, 150
total protein and proportions of animal and plant protein in, 149
Surpluses
of by-products, use in livestock industry, 140
of cereals, use in livestock industry, 139
Sus scrofa, 215
Swaziland
calorie and protein intake in, 71
crop yields in, 114–115
Sweden
crop yields in, 114–115
food supplies of
animal protein in, 149
calories, total protein, and animal protein in, 148
milk, meat, eggs, and fish in, 150
total protein and proportions of animal and plant protein in, 149
Sweet potatoes, *see also* Root crops
area and production by region, 38–41
consumption in different regions of world, 20–22
world area and production of, 36
yield increase compared to farmed area increase by region, 111
yields
and yield increases by country, 115, 117
and yield increases by region, 112
potential, 121
realized record, 122
Swine production, effect of religious belief on, 152
Switzerland
crop yields in, 114–115
food supplies of
animal protein in, 149
calories, total protein, and animal protein in, 148
milk, meat, eggs, and fish in, 150
total protein and proportions of animal and plant protein in, 149
Symbiotic bacteria, nitrogen fixation by, 93
Synthetic food, *see* Food, synthetic
Synthetic nutrients, use in formulation of new nutritious food products, 254
Syria
calorie and protein intake in, 71
crop yields in, 116–117
food supplies of
animal protein in, 149
calories, total protein, and animal protein in, 148
milk, meat, eggs, and fish in, 150
total protein and proportions of animal and plant protein in, 149

T

Taboos, effect on consumption of animal products, 135
Taiwan
calorie, total protein, and animal protein intake in, 71
crop yields in, 116–117
food supplies of
animal protein in, 149
calories, total protein, and animal protein in, 148
milk, meat, and eggs, and fish in, 150
total protein and proportions of animal and plant protein in, 149
salt iodization in, 246
Tamunuts, preparation from cottonseed, 268
Tanzania
calorie and protein intake in, 72
crop yields in, 114–115
food supplies of
animal protein in, 149
calories, total protein, and animal protein in, 148
milk, meat, eggs, and fish in, 150
total protein and proportions of animal and plant protein in, 149
kwashiorkor and marasmus in, prevalence of, 9
Taro, consumption of, 22
Tartaric acid, in foods, 186
Tea, fortification of, with vitamin A, 245
Technical inputs, at farm level, future use of, 174
Technical measures, to increase crop production, 91–107
Technological measures, for implementation of food and nutrition policies, 285
Technology
effect on farming, 84
effect on improvement of world food production, 53
Teff, use of, in nutritious food products, 257–258
Tempeh
effect of fermentation on nutritive value of, 236
tryptophan in, increase by fermentation, 237
vitamin E in, increased availability by fermentation, 237
Temperature
as factor in food spoilage, 178–179
effect on crop production, 99
effect on enzyme activity, 179
effect on microorganisms, 179
effect on milk production, 135
effect on plant growth, 118
effect on poultry production, 135
optimal, for growth and survival of microorganisms, 180
Temperature requirement, crop variation in, 100
Termite mounds, 206
Textured foods
soybean, protein quality of, 269
uses of, 190
vegetable protein, 268–269
Thailand
AID supported rice fortification studies in, 246
calorie and protein intake in, 71
crop yields in, 116–117
PCM in, 8
salt iodization in, 246
Thermophilic organisms, 179
Thiamine
destruction by thiaminase, 187
in rice, increased retention by parboiling process, 235
intake of, in developing countries, 252
Thiamine fortification, 246
of bread, 244

of food, 261
of white flour, 245
Thiaminase, in raw fish, 187
Threonine content, effect on protein quality of rice, 260
Tillage
effect on soil tilth, 99
objectives of, 99
practices, favoring higher rate of water absorption, 98
Time, as factor in food spoilage, 177–178
Tissue response, in livestock, to plane of nutrition, 221–224
Tobago
calorie and protein intake in, 72
crop yields, 116–117
Togo
calorie and protein intake in, 71
crop yields in, 114–115
Tomatoes
consumption of, 24, 25
provitamin A content of, effect of breeding on, 210
Toned milk, 267
Topography, effect on crop growth and yield, 206
Torolupsis utilis, 254
Tortilla flour, nutritive value of, effect of fortification with lysine, tryptophan, and vitamins on, 261, 262
Tortilla, nutrient restoration of, 264
Torula yeast
use of
as protein concentrate, 263
as protein supplement of lime-treated corn and rice, 260
in nutritious food products, 257–258
Tourne bacilli, wine deterioration by, 186
Town-and-country, development, 81
Trace elements
deficiency in soil, improvement of pastoral farming by correcting, 140
in plants, clinical evaluation of, 208
uptake by plants, effect of fertilizer on, 211
problems of, in U.S., 211
Trade
effect of purchasing power on, 154
restrictions in, effect on agricultural development, 53
Tradition, effect on animal production, 135–136
Translocation
of water, 98
losses of water through, 98
Transportation, dependence of agricultural productivity on, 106
Transportation system, effect on development of new agricultural land, 52
Trifolium alexandrinum, 139
Trifolium hirtum, 204
Trinidad
calorie and protein intake in, 72
crop yields in, 116–117
Triticum aestivum, 211
TRL, ingredient composition of, 258
Tropical rain forest, difficulties in developing potentially arable soil in, 87–88
Tropics
pastoral farming in, 141
potential and target crop yields in, 121
Trypanosome-tolerant cattle, 138
Trypanosomes
dry reistant, 138
transmitted by tsetse fly, 138
Trypanosomiasis
animal, 134
effect on livestock development in Africa, 160
in animals and man, control of, 137
Trypsin inhibitor
content of, effect of germination on, 237
of plant and animal origin, 187
in soy flour, destruction by alkali treatment of, 236
Tryptophan
effect on nutritive value of corn-bean diet in presence and absence of vitamins and minerals, 263
effect on protein quality of corn, 260
improvement of cereal protein quality by, 259
Tryptophan content
of pearl millet, effect of nitrogen fertilizer on, 211
of tempeh, increase by fermentation, 237
of wheat, effect of fertilizer on, 210
Tryptophan deficiency, of corn, 255
Tryptophan fortification
of corn with, 259
of corn-bean diet, 262, 263
of tortilla flour, 262
Tsetse fly
control of, 137
effect on cattle production, 151, 156, 160
effect on development of potentially arable land, 44
eradication of, 134
effect on animal production in Africa, 134
Glossina species, control of, 138
nagana transmitted by, 134
seasonal variations in incidence of, 135
Tunisia
AID supported lysine fortification study in, 247
calorie and protein intake in, 71
crop yields in, 114–115
food supplies of
animal protein in, 149
calories, total protein, and animal protein, 148
milk, meat, eggs, and fish in, 150
total protein and proportions of animal and plant protein, 149
Turkestan, effect of taboos on meat consumption in, 136
Turkey
calorie and protein intake in, 71
crop yields in, 116–117
foot-and-mouth disease in, 134
food supplies of
animal protein in, 149
calories, total protein and animal protein in, 148
milk, meat, eggs, and fish in, 150
total protein and proportions of animal and plant protein in, 149
Turkeys, protein content of, 218

U

Uganda
calorie and protein intake in, 72

consumption of plantains and bananas in, 22
crop yields in, 114–115
food supplies of
animal protein in, 149
calories, total protein, and animal protein in, 148
milk, meat, eggs, and fish in, 150
total protein and proportions of animal and plant proteins in, 149
kwashiorkor and marasmus in, prevalence of, 9
U.N., 57, 59, 60, 61, 63, 70
U.N. Demographic Yearbook, 64
U.N. Development Program, locust control project sponsored by, 172
Unconventional foods, *see also* Food, unconventional
need for, 191–192
sources of, production and use of, 189–202
use of, 190–191
UNCTAD, 202
Undernutrition
effect on carcass quality of livestock, 222
nutritional structure of diet in, 67
Unemployment, rural, in developing countries, 145
UNESCO, 81
UNICEF, 245, 246
United Arab Republic
food supplies of
animal protein in, 149
calories, total protein, and animal protein in, 148
milk, meat, eggs, and fish in, 150
total protein and porportions of animal and plant proteins in, 149
United Kingdom, *see also* Great Britain
crop yields in, 114–115
iron fortification in, 246
vitamin D fortification in, 245
Unsaturated fats, effect on adipose tissue composition of livestock, 225
Upper Volta
calorie and protein intake in, 71
crop yields in, 114–115
Urban population, *see* Population, urban
Urea
as source of nonprotein nitrogen
for ruminants, 140
use in pastoral farming, 140
Uruguay
calorie and protein intake in, 72
crop yields in, 116–117
food supplies of
animal protein in, 149
calories, total protein, and animal protein in, 148
milk, meat, eggs and fish in, 150
total protein and proportion of animal and plant protein in, 149
U.S.
agriculture in, reliance on fertilizers, 49
arable land and population of, 43
cereal grain product fortification in, 246
Colorado beetle in, 164
crop yields in, 116–117
donation programs in, 245
epidemic of Southern Corn Leaf Blight in, 165
food supplies of
animal protein in, 149
calories, total protein, and animal protein in, 148
milk, meat, eggs, and fish in, 150
total protein and proportions of animal and plant protein in, 149
hybrid maize development within, 105
iron deficiency anemia in, 7
iron fortification in, 246
land in, major uses of, 43
losses caused by pear decline disease in, 165
losses caused by plant parasitic nematodes, 165
losses caused by potato mosaic virus, 165
losses caused by weeds in, 100
malnutrition in, 190
minimum tillage systems used in, 99
number of farm animals vs. animal productivity in, 152
production of major food crops in, 38, 40
salt iodization in, 246
trace element problems in, 211
vitamin A fortification in, 245
yields of selected crops for 1930, 1950, and 1970 in, 104
U.S. Corn Belt, soil management practices in, 92
U.S. Department of Agriculture, 33, 46, 47, 54, 81, 83, 153, 178
soil surveys by, 81
U.S. Fish and Wildlife Service, 188
U.S. President's Science Advisory Committee, 65
U.S. Public Health Service, 190
U.S.S.R.
arable land and population of, 43
cereal consumption in, 18
collective agriculture in, 51
crop yields in, 114–115
crop yield increase, compared to farmed area increase in 1950 and 1970, 111
crop yields in 1950 and 1970, 112
crude birth rate, crude death rate, and gross reproduction rate for 1965
crude productivity of cattle and buffalo in, 130
crude productivity of pigs, 130
farm animal population in, 129
food supplies of
animal protein in, 149
calories, total protein, and animal protein in, 148
milk, meat, eggs, and fish in, 150
total protein and proportions of animal and plant protein in, 149
land in, major uses of, 43
productivity of farm livestock in, 128
population and expectation of life for 1960 and 2000, 57
production of major food crops in, 38, 40
selenium poisoning of cattle in, 133
urban and rural population of, 62
wheat consumption in, 18

V

Vaccination
of livestock
against bovine pleuropneumonia, 138

against foot-and-mouth disease, 137
against pasteurellosis, 138
against rinderpest, 137
Value income elasticity
computation of, 72–73
for selected commodities, 74
Vampire bat, rabies transmitted by, 133
Veal
production and consumption of
in Europe, 157
in North America, 158
in Oceania, 158
Vegetable farming, commercial, 50
Vegetable milk, 267
Vegetable oils, consumption of, 30
Vegetable protein foods, textured, 268–269
Vegetable protein sources, use of, in preparation of milk substitutes, 267
Vegetable sources, use in formulation of highly nutritious food products, 253
Vegetables
antinutritional factors in, 233–234
arable land used for production of, 37
as source of food protein, 193
as source of vitamins, 109
consumption in different regions of world, 24–26
inhibitory substances in, 186–187
popularization of, 193
Vegetarians, calorie and protein requirements of, 109
Venezuela
calorie and protein intake in, 71
crop yields in, 116–117
food supplies of
animal protein in, 149
calories, total protein, and animal protein in, 148
milk, meat, eggs, and fish in, 150
total protein and proportions of animal and plant protein in, 149
Vermin, wastage of food due to, 177
Vertical resistance, 175
nature of, 169
Veterinarians, number of, in developed vs. developing countries, 138–139
Vicia faba, 234
Vicia sativa, 233, 235
Victoria, pastoral sheep husbandry in, 140
Vietnam (North)
calorie and protein intake in, 71
crop yields in, 116–117
Vietnam (South)
calorie and protein intake in, 71
crop yields in, 116–117
Vigna, 195
Virus, responsible for paralytic rabies in cattle, 133–134
Vitalia, ingredient composition of, 258
Vitamin deficiency diseases, identification of, 1
Vitamin fortification
of corn-bean diet, 262
of food, 261
of tortilla flour, 262
Vitamin A
effect of lipoxidase on, 234
low intake in developing countries, 252
prevention of xerophthalmia by, 9
Vitamin A deficiency, 245
prevention of, 243, 245
Vitamin A enrichment
of margarine, 266
of sugar, 266, 267
Vitamin A fortification
of flour, 245
of food, 245, 261
of margarine, 244
prevention of vitamin deficiency by, 243, 245
of skim milk powder, 245
of sugar, 245
of tea, 245
of tortilla flour, 262
Vitamin B complex, fortification of foods, 244
Vitamin B_6, effect of antipyridoxine on, 233
Vitamin B_{12}, plant inhibitor of, 234
Vitamin B_{12}, deficiency, megaloblastic anemia due to, 8
Vitamin C deficiency, scurvy due to, 10
Vitamin C, destruction by ascorbic acid oxidase, 233
Vitamin C fortification, 246
Vitamin D
as preventive measure in rickets, 11
destruction by inhibitors in cereals and liver, 187
low intake in developing countries, 252
Vitamin D enrichment, of milk, 266
Vitamin D fortification, 245
of cereals, 245
of infant formulas, 245
of margarine, 245
of milk, 244, 245
prevention of rickets by, 243
Vitamin D requirement
effect of oxalic acid on, 233
effect of phytic acid on, 233
Vitamin D toxicity, 245
Vitamin E
destruction in fish oils, 187
in tempeh, increased availability by fermentation, 237
Vitamins
effect on protein quality of corn, 255, 263
fortification of foods with, 261
in foods, 185–186
sources of, 191
synthesis of, 200
use of, in nutritious food products, 257–258
Voandzeia, as source of protein, 193
VPM, ingredient composition of, 258
Vulnerable groups, requirement of foods by, 252

W

War, effect on population growth, 60
Wastes and by-products, inedible, as source of feed for ruminants and nonruminants, 197
Wastes, use of, in food fermentation, 199
Wasting disease, of livestock, 133
Water
absorbing and holding capacity, of soils, effect of

organic matter on, 96
absorption of, tillage practices favoring, 98
availability of, and fertilization of crops, 101
content of body, interrelationship between body fat and, 217
content of carcass, of Holstein steer, 217
content of foods, effect on storage life of foods, 178
content of pig, during prenatal and postnatal stages of life, 216, 217
content of sheep, breed differences in, 220
effect on crop yields, 118
quality of, effect on plants, 98
requirement by plants, 98
as provided by soil, 92
treatment, increase in nutritive value of foods by, 235
Water activity
as factor in food spoilage, 181–184
definition of, 181
values for various meats, 182
Water control
in soil management, 84
methods of, 84
Water deficiency, in plants, 98
Water holding capacity, of soil, 98
Water management, 98–99
Water penetration, effect of hard-pan on, 99
Weather
effect on animal production, 135
effect on parasites and disease vectors, 135
Weed control, 100
Weeds
damage caused by, history of, 163
economic losses in U.S., caused by, 100
Weevils
development of resistance in alfalfa to, 103
food deterioration due to, 187
West Africa coconut disease in, 167
West Europe,
crop yield increase compared to farmed area increase in 1950 and 1970, 111
crop yields in 1950 and 1970, 112
WFP, 284
Whale, as source of food, 197
Wheat, *see also* Cereals
area and production by region, 38–41
average yield in U.S., 104
calculated and obtained yields in Netherlands since 1965, 122
consumption in different regions of world, 17, 18–19
genetic improvement of, 210
high nitrogen varieties, 193
lysine in, increased availability by fermentation, 237
new varieties
loss of resistance to pathogens in, 169
use of, 169
prices of, effect of drought on, 275
protein content of
effect of breeding on, 209
effect of fertilizer on, 210
effect of nitrogen fertilizer on, 209
use of, in nutritious food products, 257–258
world area and production of, 36
yield increase compared to farmed area increase between 1950 and 1970, 111
yields
and yield increases, 112
and yield increases by country, 114, 116
and yield increases by region in 1950 and 1970, 116,
potential, 121
realized record, 122
targets for increases in, 124
Wheat bran, nutrients in, increased availability by treatment with cellulotyc enzymes, 237
Wheat cultivars, bread-making quality of, effect of environmental vs. genetic factors on, 210
Wheat flour
nutritive value of, effect of replacement with wheat protein concentrate on, 265
replacement with cassava flour, in bread making, 265
white, fortification of, 245
Wheat protein
nutritionally superior fraction of, 234
Wheat protein concentrate
effect of fractionation on quality of, 232
effect on nutritive value of wheat flour, 265
preparation of, 195
Wheat shorts, effect on nutritive value of corn flour, 264
Whey, use of, in food fermentation, 199
Wheat shorts, effect on nutritive value of corn flour, 264
Whey, use of, in food fermentation, 199
White muscle disease, of livestock, 133
WHO, 7, 9, 11, 202, 246, 247
Wild carnivores, rabies transmitted by, 134
Wild herbivores, as source of human food, 197
Wildlife
as source of meat in Africa, 161
its potential for increasing animal production, 155–156
production for meat, management of, 156
Wine, consumption of, 32
Work, effect on calorie requirements, 65
Working hours in rice fields, reduction in, from mechanization and herbicide use, 173
World Food Congress, 1963, 189

X

Xeromyces, 182

Xerophthalmia, 8–9, 245
prevalence of, 9

Y

Yams, *see also* Root crops
area and production by region, 28–41
as source of food protein, 195
consumption in different regions of world, 20–22
world area and production of, 36
yield increase compared to farmed area by region, 111
yields
and yield increases by region, 112
potential, 121
realized record of, 122
Yeast
growth of

effect of pH on, 179
effect of temperature on, 179
effect of water activity on, 183, 184
in bread, hydrolysis of phytic acid by, 237
temperature relations for growth and survival of, 180
Yeast protein, use in formulation of new nutritious food products, 254
Yemen, crop yields in, 116–117
Yield
of crops, increased relation between protein content of grain and, 204, 209
of rose clover, relation between magnesium content and, 204
Yield increases, of food crops, between 1950 and 1970 by region, 112
Yugoslavia
crop yields in, 114–115
food supplies of
animal protein in, 149
calories, total protein, and animal protein, 148
milk, meat, eggs, and fish in, 150
total protein and proportions of animal and fat protein in, 149

Z

Zaire
cretinism in, 10
crop yields in, 114–115
Zambia
calorie and protein intake in, 72
crop yields in, 114–115
Zea Mays L, 204, 211
Zebu, as source of human food, 156
Zebu cattle, 141, 142
as milk producers, 142
cross breeding studies with, 142
response to nutritional inputs by, 142
Zinc
absorption of, interference of phytic acid with, 233
application of, to soil, 211
in *Agrostis tenuis,* high levels of, 211
in soils effect of pH on availability of, 96
Zinc deficiency, in corn, 211
Zinc requirement
effect of metal-binding constituents on, 234
by plants, 93
Zoonoses, 133